Textbook of Surgery

Textbook of Surgery

Edited by
David A. Macfarlane BSc MCh FRCS
Senior Consultant Surgeon, St Stephen's Hospital, London; Member of the Court of Examiners of the Royal College of Physicians and Surgeons of Glasgow; Past Chairman and Member of the Court of Examiners, Royal College of Surgeons of England; Examiner in Surgery, University of London; Honorary Senior Lecturer, Charing Cross and Westminister Hospital Medical School; Teacher of Surgery, University of London; Formerly Surgical Tutor, Medical College of St Bartholomew's Hospital, London; Hunterian Professor, Royal College of Surgeons of England.

Lewis P. Thomas BSc MCh FRCS
Senior Consultant Surgeon, Royal Gwent Hospital, Newport; Formerly Senior Lecturer in Surgery, Welsh National School of Medicine, Cardiff.

Foreword by the late
Norman C. Tanner MD FRCS FACS(Hon) FRCSI(Hon)
Formerly Honorary Consulting Surgeon, Charing Cross and St James's Hospitals, London.

FIFTH EDITION

CHURCHILL LIVINGSTONE
EDINBURGH LONDON MELBOURNE AND NEW YORK 1984

CHURCHILL LIVINGSTONE
Medical Division of Longman Group Limited

Distributed in the United States of America by Churchill Livingstone Inc., 1560 Broadway, New York, N.Y. 10036, and by associated companies, branches and representatives throughout the world.

First edition 1964
Second edition 1968
Third edition 1972
Italian edition 1974
Fourth edition 1977
Fifth edition 1984

ISBN 0 443 02768 4

British Library Cataloguing in Publication Data
Textbook of surgery.—5th ed.
1. Surgery
I. Macfarlane, David A. II. Thomas, Lewis P.
617 RD31
ISBN 0-443-02768-4

Library of Congress Cataloging in Publication Data
Main entry under title:
Textbook of surgery.
Includes bibliographies and index.
1. Surgery. I. Macfarlane, David A. II. Thomas, Lewis P. [DNLM: 1. Surgery. WO 100 T355]
RD31. T47 1984 617 83-13196
ISBN 0-443-02768-4

Printed in Singapore by Selector Printing Co (Pte) Ltd

Foreword to the Third Edition

In such a live science and art as surgery, new ideas, technical innovations and the need to discard discredited concepts all demand a selective but voluminous output of medical literature. This in turn leads to a steady demand for the production of new editions of the standard textbooks or of new books. For the student's and particularly the undergraduate student's textbook, it is unnecessary to reflect every passing surgical fashion or to be in the vanguard of surgical thought. The student reader, with his ever more crowded curriculum, requires the help of writers who can provide a readable and sound basis of surgery, in a book which will also serve as a reference book. Such a book must be firmly pruned of outworn or discarded ideas and should not contain the minutiae of technique required only by the specialist.

The immediate and continuing success of this book demonstrates that students and their teachers have found that it amply fulfils these requirements. The editors and writers of this textbook are surgeons practised in undergraduate and postgraduate student teaching and perhaps no less important, mature operating surgeons. They have incorporated in it the physiological principles required in modern surgical treatment and aftercare.

In the foreword to the first edition the hope was expressed that the book would become the student's friend not only when confronted in the final clinical examinations, but also when he was at the bedside or in the out-patients' department. This objective has been attained.

By its skilful variation in emphasis it is hoped that it will long continue to reinforce the efforts of the clinical teachers to impart a balanced and sound surgical judgement to the student.

Norman C. Tanner

Preface to the Fifth Edition

In the preface to the first edition we stated that our aim was to provide surgical information in a concise and didactic form that would enable the student both to understand and retain the essentials in logical sequence, and thereby provide a sound basis for future surgical practice. Throughout subsequent editions every effort to present in a clear manner well accepted facts concerning surgical disease and management has been attempted and would appear justified. In this fifth edition we still consider this to be our principal endeavour.

In times of rising costs and in order to be easily handled, maintenance of size has been given consideration. Topographical anatomy has been largely discarded as standard texts may easily be consulted. It has nonetheless been retained as a separate entity where inclusion was deemed important, otherwise reference to salient aspects has been included in the text. The importance of physiology to the scientific basis of surgery is recognised and these sections have been up-dated.

Advances in endoscopic, radiological and scanning techniques have altered patterns of management in many conditions, and the chapters on gastro-enterology and liver disease and biliary tract have been revised to include these changes. Outmoded methods of management have been discarded in the chapter on chest and heart, where Mr Gareth Rees writing in his specialist field has entirely altered this section to include the latest progress.

Radical changes have also been made in the chapters on skin and pain where Mr Derek Sibson has taken over from the previous contributor. New technology and altering chemotherapy have accounted for a thorough re-appraisal of the chapter on malignant disease and changing antibiotic therapy has been updated. Present day nutritional aspects and metabolic changes together with appraisal of organ transplantation have been incorporated. The fluctuations in thought of the management of breast cancer have been summarised. New illustrations have been added where appropriate and some older ones withdrawn to maintain a correct balance between text and drawing.

It is a pleasure to record our thanks to Mr Gareth Rees and Mr Derek Sibson who have undertaken the new chapters and to Mr B. Ferris, FRCS, for compiling the index and careful proof reading. We appreciate the help received from our medical artist, Mr S. McAllister, and also from Mr Andrew Stevenson, Publishing Director of Churchill Livingstone, who has greatly assisted our discussions.

London, 1984

David A. Macfarlane
Lewis P. Thomas

Contributors

Martin Birnstingl MS FRCS
Consultant Surgeon, St Bartholomew's Hospital and Consultant in Peripheral Vascular Surgery, Royal National Orthopaedic Hospital, London. Chapters 18, 19 and 20

Thomas M. Bucknill FRCS
Consultant Orthopaedic Surgeon, St Bartholomew's Hospital, London. Chapters 27 and 28

Harold Ellis DM MCh FRCS
Professor of Surgery, University of London. Chapter 1

N. Alan Green MS FRCS
Consultant Surgeon, Norfolk and Norwich Hospital, Norwich. Chapters 7, 12, 22, 23, 24 and 25

David A. Macfarlane MCh FRCS
Senior Consultant Surgeon, St Stephen's Hospital and Honorary Senior Lecturer, Charing Cross and Westminster Hospital Medical School, London. Chapters 4, 5, 6, 8, 9, 13, 16, 17, 21 and 30

Gareth M. Rees MS FRCS MRCP
Consultant Surgeon, St Bartholomew's Hospital, London. Chapter 10

Robert Shields MD FRCS FRCSEd
Professor of Surgery, University of Liverpool, Liverpool. Chapter 2

Derek E. Sibson FRCS
Consultant Surgeon, Kettering and District General Hospital, Kettering, Northamptonshire. Chapters 3, 7 and 31

Lewis P. Thomas MCh FRCS
Senior Consultant Surgeon, Royal Gwent Hospital, Newport. Chapters 11, 14, 15, 26 and 29.

Contents

1

Surgical aspects of infection

INFLAMMATION

Inflammation is the response of living tissues to injury. Although usually bacterial in origin, similar tissue changes result from any form of trauma.

Bacterial infections

Fortunately only a few of the vast numbers of bacteria are noxious to man. Their effect is the result of the production of toxins, either from the breakdown of the bacteria (endotoxins) or from a secretion of toxin into the tissues or blood (exotoxins) of which the clostridia are typical examples. The clinical picture and the course of an infection depend on an interplay between the defence mechanisms of the host and the size and virulence of the bacterial invasion.

The defence mechanisms of the host include the intact epithelia of the skin and of the respiratory, alimentary and urinary tracts, as well as the local tissue reactions of acute inflammation, which constitute an important means of containing and destroying invading organisms. It also includes immunological defences, with the production of specific antibodies in response to foreign protein.

These natural defences can be reinforced artificially by immunisation and chemotherapy. **Active immunisation** makes use of killed organisms such as T.A.B. vaccine for typhoid, attenuated living organisms as in B.C.G. vaccine for tuberculosis, or inactivated toxins (toxoids), for example, formalin-inactivated tetanus toxoid. **Passive immunisation** employs the anti-serum produced by injecting the organisms or toxins into an animal, for example, tetanus and diphtheria anti-toxins. **Chemotherapeutic agents** act by either preventing the multiplication of invading organisms (Bacteriostatics) or by destroying the organisms (Bactericidals) (p. 11).

Chemotherapeutic agents are dependent upon an adequate blood supply to carry them to the affected tissues and are highly efficient in dealing with sensitive organisms free in the blood stream as in septicaemia, the tissues as in cellulitis or pneumonia, or the serous surfaces such as diffuse pleurisy or peritonitis. Where bacteria are walled off within slough or an abscess cavity, these agents can only penetrate by slow diffusion and in addition, the sulphonamides are inhibited by the action of pus. Thus the contained organisms are unlikely to be destroyed, the mass of dead and infected tissue persisting as an irritant to surrounding structures with the increasing formation of chronic inflammatory tissue, and the absorption of breakdown products will continue to cause toxaemia. In such cases surgical drainage will nearly always be required.

In addition to such specific mechanisms there are certain general factors which are important in the defence mechanism of the host. These are the age of the patient, his nutritional state, the presence of anaemia, protein deficiency or severe systemic disease of which the two most important are diabetes and renal failure. In any such associated conditions, as well as in the extremes of age, infection is more likely to be serious.

The bacterial invasiveness depends on the size of bacterial inoculation and the virulence of the bacteria. The latter consists of two components: (*a*) toxicity, the power of the organism to injure the host tissues, and (*b*) invasiveness, the ability to attack and spread in the body. Organisms may be highly lethal, although their invasiveness is low.

Thus *Clostridium tetani*, despite remaining localised at the site of inoculation, produces serious effects by the formation of a powerful exotoxin.

The environment in which the bacteria find themselves within the body is important. Organisms rarely become established in healthy tissues with an abundant blood supply, but favour haematomas, necrotic tissue and serous collections. Clostridia thrive only in anaerobic conditions.

ACUTE INFECTION

Cellulitis

Cellulitis is a spreading inflammation of connective tissues. The term usually refers to subcutaneous infection, but may also be applied to pelvic, retroperitoneal, perinephric, pharyngeal or intraorbital connective tissue infection. The common organism is the β-haemolytic streptococcus which usually gains entrance through a scratch or prick. The skin becomes dusky red around the site of inoculation and there is local oedema, heat and severe pain. Vesicles may appear in the involved area of skin, and in advanced cases there may even be cutaneous gangrene.

Cellulitis is frequently accompanied by *lymphangitis* and *lymphadenitis*, red streaks being seen along the lymph channels and the regional glands becoming enlarged and tender. Not uncommonly there is an associated *septicaemia* which originates either from a septic thrombophlebitis in the affected area or from spread of bacteria from the lymphatics to the blood stream by way of the thoracic duct (Fig. 1.1). The spreading invasiveness of *Streptococcus pyogenes* is due, at least in part, to its ability to produce hyaluronidase which dissolves the intercellular matrix, and a fibrinolysin called streptokinase which is able to destroy the fibrin inflammatory barrier to bacterial spread.

Treatment

Immobilisation of the affected part is essential and may necessitate bed rest. Antibiotics will often resolve a spreading infection. Local heat is frequently soothing and can best be achieved by shortwave diathermy which does not macerate the skin.

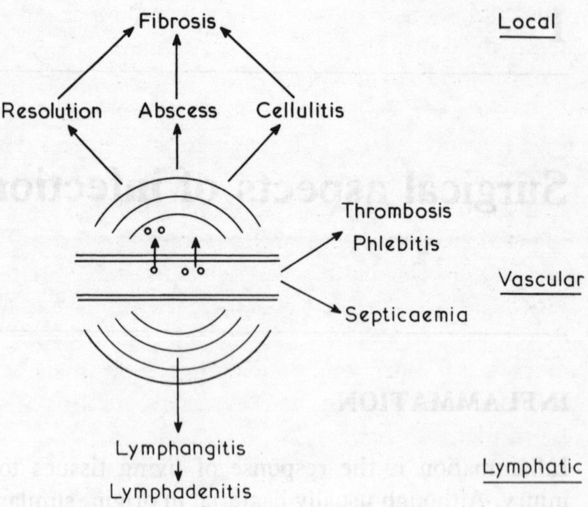

Fig. 1.1 The course and complications of acute infection

Incision is required to evacuate a localised collection of pus.

Abscess

An abscess is a localised collection of pus and is usually, but not always, the result of invasion by pyogenic organisms. Polymorphs ingest and kill these organisms, and in dying liberate enzymes which liquefy the resulting dead tissue. The pus becomes surrounded by a 'pyogenic membrane' of living polymorphs embedded in fibrin and granulation tissue, which in turn is contained by a zone of intensely hyperaemic tissue infiltrated with polymorphs. Septic thrombosis occurs in adjacent small blood-vessels, and the detachment of fragments of infected blood clot accounts for the septic emboli which may complicate a relatively insignificant abscess.

An abscess may result from a number of causes. There may be direct implantation of organisms, as occurs in the infection of a clean surgical incision, or that which results from inoculation of the subphrenic spaces with bacteria after perforation of a peptic ulcer. Lymphatic spread of infection may occur to regional nodes which can then undergo suppuration. Haematogenous spread may take place from even a small septic focus such as a boil. This is exemplified in osteomyelitis or in the production of a perinephric, cerebral or lung abscess.

Pus formation is not entirely dependent on bacterial invasion, and may occur wherever there is intense local tissue death; thus inadvertent injection of caustic fluids, thiopentone or other irritants into the soft tissues will result in an abscess, the contents of which are sterile. Clinically an abscess first manifests itself as a hard, red, painful swelling which later softens and becomes fluctuant. If not drained at this stage it may discharge spontaneously through the skin or internally into a viscus or serous cavity. There are the associated features of bacterial infection; a swinging fever, malaise, anorexia and sweating, and an accompanying polymorph leucocytosis.

Treatment

Drainage is required for all abscesses. The continued use of antibiotics without drainage is a dangerous practice. Chemotherapeutic agents cannot diffuse in sufficient quantity to sterilise an abscess completely; the pus collection continues to act as a source of toxaemia and becomes surrounded by a dense mass of fibrous tissue. Hard fixed swellings in the breast or pelvis are occasionally encountered following the attempted treatment of an abscess in these sites by prolonged chemotherapy. These have been referred to as 'antibiotic tumours.'

Boils

A boil or furuncle is a small abscess involving a hair follicle and its associated glands, it is usually due to *Staphylococcus aureus*. Boils do not therefore occur on the hairless palm and sole. They are encountered particularly in areas where the skin is injured by friction, such as the neck, or where the skin is dirty and macerated by sweat, such as the axilla, groin and perianal region. Staphylococcal septicaemia and embolic infection causing osteomyelitis or a perinephric abscess may occasionally occur. On the face and around the lip spread may take place via the facial veins to the cavernous sinus with development of the highly dangerous septic cavernous sinus thrombosis. Crops of boils, particularly on the neck and in the axilla, are a distressing and common complaint of adolescents and young adults, and may be due to a hormonal factor. They are more prone to occur when the general health is affected and this aspect of the condition is important.

Treatment

A boil should initially be left undisturbed, but when pus becomes visible it should be incised and evacuated. A course of ultra-violet light or short-wave diathermy to the affected area is also helpful. Carrier sites can be detected by taking nasal and perineal swabs. In positive cases daily treatment of these areas by neomycin ointment together with hexachlorophene baths should be carried out for two or three months. In some intractable instances a positive carrier will be found in the patient's immediate family and should be treated. In severe cases a long holiday, fresh air and a nourishing diet are to be recommended in preventing recurrence. Systemic chemotherapy should not be employed; it will not prevent either recurrence or spread.

Carbuncle

A carbuncle is an area of subcutaneous necrosis discharging on to the skin through multiple sinuses. It usually commences as a staphylococcal boil with spread of infection into the surrounding tissues, which later become honeycombed by small abscesses separated by trabeculae of fibrous tissue. Carbuncles are generally seen on the neck, shoulders and back of the hands. The affected area is swollen, brawny and painful; the overlying skin is dusky red and exhibits characteristic sinuses which discharge small amounts of yellow pus. General debility or diabetes are often associated with the condition; the urine should therefore be tested for sugar in all cases.

Treatment

Chemotherapy alone may cure the condition if commenced at an early stage. Short-wave diathermy is valuable and the affected area may be covered with a protective sterile dressing. Incision is rarely required but it may be necessary to excise the necrotic slough. When a large raw area remains, subsequent skin grafting may be necessary. Associated diabetes should be controlled.

SPECIFIC INFECTIONS

Gas gangrene

This serious infection of muscle and soft tissue is caused by a mixed group of Clostridia, such as *Cl. welchii*, *septique* and *oedematiens*, which are usually found in faeces and in the soil. They are anaerobic, spore-forming and gas-producing bacteria which secrete a powerful exotoxin. They also produce hyaluronidase which facilitates their spread in the tissues. Their anaerobic nature and usual habitat account for the danger of gas gangrene when deep wounds with a poor blood supply and with contained dead tissues are contaminated by soil or faecal material. War wounds are particularly liable to gas gangrene infection due to tissue destruction and unavoidable delay in treatment. In developed countries the majority of cases are autogenous infections in those who have had amputations or extensive orthopaedic procedures involving much tissue damage.

Clostridia include both saccharolytic and proteolytic groups. Gas formation is due partly to carbon dioxide and hydrogen liberated by fermentation of sugars and partly to ammonia produced by destruction of muscle protein. Bubbles of gas spread along tissue planes and throughout the length of affected muscles thus opening up pathways for bacterial diffusion. Profound toxaemia results due to the absorption of exotoxin and breakdown products from the destroyed muscle. Occasionally gas gangrene of the abdominal wall or peritoneal cavity follows appendicetomy or bowel resection, Clostridia reaching the damaged tissues from the intestinal tract of the patient. Gas gangrene of the uterus may occur after a septic abortion.

Clinical features

The incubation period is about 24 hours. There is profound toxaemia with rapid pulse, low blood-pressure, anorexia, vomiting, apathy and coma. Haemolytic anaemia may also accompany septicaemia. The temperature is at first elevated but becomes subnormal as the condition progresses. Severe pain in the injured area is an early and important symptom. The tissues around the wound become swollen and crepitant due to the infiltration of gas. The adjacent skin becomes discoloured and later gangrenous, and from the wound itself there is an unpleasant odoriferous watery brown discharge, heavily contaminated with Clostridia. On exploration of the wound the affected muscles are found to be dark red, swollen, soft and crepitant and are non-contractile when pinched with dissecting forceps; later they become completely gangrenous.

Treatment

(*a*) *Prophylactic*. Dead and soiled tissues should be excised from all wounds as soon as possible after injury to remove both the bacteria and the pabulum on which they thrive. War experience has shown the value of prophylactic penicillin; anti-gas gangrene serum is seldom employed. Pre-operative prophylaxis with penicillin is also indicated for mid-thigh amputations performed for senile gangrene and where necrotic bowel is resected since both of these procedures carry a high risk of gas gangrene.

(*b*) *Curative*. Large doses of penicillin, 300 to 600 mg intramuscularly six-hourly, should be coupled with blood transfusion and exploration of the wound. Any involved muscle must be completely excised, and if all groups of a limb are affected a guillotine amputation must be performed. When available, a hyperbaric oxygen chamber should be used, permitting a high concentration of oxygen in the affected tissues with often good clinical response. In some hospitals anti-gas gangrene serum is still used, but its efficacy has never been proved and there is a high risk of anaphylaxis. The prognosis of gas gangrene is serious but vigorous treatment is often effective in saving life if not limb.

Tetanus

Tetanus, or lock-jaw, is caused by *Cl. tetani*, an anaerobic spore-forming and exotoxin-secreting bacillus which is present in faeces and soil. The tetanus organisms require strictly anaerobic conditions, thrive in deeply penetrating wounds and may enter the body through minute puncture wounds.

The tetanus bacteria remain confined to the area of inoculation and exert a virulent effect by the production of a powerful exotoxin which becomes fixed in, and acts specifically upon, the cerebrospinal motor cells. The exact mode of spread of the exotoxin is still uncertain, but it is probably conveyed to the central nervous system directly along the peripheral nerves from the affected part rather than via lymphatic or vascular pathways.

Clinical features

Incubation varies from 24 hours to three weeks. Premonitory headaches, anxiety and sleeplessness are followed by local muscle spasms around the wound, which may not always be observed. Muscle spasm then spreads to the neck, spine and trunk, but rarely affects the limbs. The typical risus sardonicus due to painful trismus is a characteristic but late development. Dysphagia and difficulty in coughing are important and distressing features. Except in mild cases this stage is followed after one to three days by intense convulsions in which the patient remains completely conscious and between which muscle spasm persists. Death may occur from exhaustion, intercurrent infection such as pneumonia, or the aspiration of vomit and secretions. The prognosis where the incubation period is under one week or where convulsions follow in under 48 hours is grave; the outlook is also serious at the extremes of age.

Differential diagnosis must be made from tetany, which characteristically affects the limbs (carpopedal spasm) and not the head and trunk; strychnine poisoning, in which muscle flaccidity occurs between otherwise identical convulsions; meningitis, where neck stiffness and opisthotonos may be confused with tetanic spasm; other causes of trismus, including arthralgia of the temporomandibular joint due to the anaphylactic response to antitetanus serum; and, finally, hysteria.

Treatment

(*a*) *Prophylaxis*. Active protection against tetanus can be achieved by the intramuscular injection of alum precipitated toxoid and all should be encouraged to be immunised. In Great Britain tetanus toxoid is included with the antigens of diphtheria and pertussis in the triple vaccine recommended for all children in the first year of life. It is important that those in occupations carrying a high risk of injury should maintain a level of active immunity and booster doses of toxoid should be given at 5- to 10-year intervals and after an injury involving a contaminated wound. In the treatment of the wound itself, surgical toilet is of prime importance and is usually sufficient for tetanus prophylaxis in patients with wounds that are less than six hours old, clean, non-penetrating and with negligible tissue damage. In more serious injuries, penicillin is the antibiotic of choice and is an effective means of preventing growth of the tetanus organisms. If the patient has had a complete course of toxoid within the past five years, nothing more than this is required, but if outside this period a booster dose of toxoid should be given. If the patient has not previously recieved toxoid and the wound is considered serious, then human tetanus immunoglobulin should be given. The use of antitetanus serum has generally now been abandoned as it carries a high risk of reaction.

(*b*) *Curative*. Nursing should be carried out in an isolated, quiet and darkened room to reduce extraneous stimuli, which readily provoke convulsions. Swallowing may be difficult, and feeding is undertaken through a fine polythene nasogastric tube. An infected wound should be excised and drained under general anaesthesia, a bacteriological swab and excised tissue taken for culture, the area washed with hydrogen peroxide and the wound left open. A healed wound should not be disturbed.

Heavy doses of sedatives are given as anticonvulsants and chlorpromazine is preferable for this purpose. Penicillin in high dosage should be administered to destroy the organism and to prevent the production of toxin.

Tracheostomy, curarisation and mechanical ventilation are indicated in cases of poor prognosis, that is, where the incubation period is under seven days or where convulsions occur in less than 48 hours from the onset of symptoms, or where convulsions are not controlled by conventional treatment. Tracheostomy and the passage of a cuffed tube enable adequate bronchial suction toilet to be performed. Convulsions are completely controlled by repeated doses of muscle-relaxant drugs, and breathing is maintained by a mechanical ventilator. Curarisation may have to be continued for two to four weeks; it is terminated when spasms or rigidity do not present during a trial period without relaxants. This treatment is preferably carried out in a special unit and has considerably improved the prognosis in severe cases.

Anthrax

Anthrax is caused by the spore-forming bacillus *B. anthracis*. It principally affects cattle and sheep; human cases are seen amongst leather workers, butchers and wool-workers. Infection occurs either through a skin graze on exposed areas, such as the face, hands and forearms, or by inhalation; both may be followed by septicaemia.

The skin inoculation results, after one or two days incubation, in the formation of a 'malignant pustule' which, when fully developed, comprises a central black slough surrounded by vesicles and a zone of intense oedema. Inhalation of the organism results in a virulent pneumonia ('wool-sorter's disease'). The diagnosis is confirmed by bacteriological examination either of a swab of the pustule or of the sputum.

Treatment involves isolation and antibiotic therapy.

Candida albicans

This fungus is a normal mouth commensal but may produce an infection of the mouth and throat known as *thrush*, or spread to involve the lungs or alimentary tract. It occurs frequently in the vagina. The infection, with its characteristic plaques of white material on the mucosae of mouth and pharynx, is seen particularly during the administration of broad spectrum antibiotics; the oral bacteria are destroyed, leaving the fungus to grow in uncompetitive surroundings.

Treatment

Nystatin lozenges are specific for the oral form of this infection and relief is obtained within 24 hours. Amphotericin B is the drug of choice in treating severe systemic fungal infections. It is poorly absorbed from the gut and must be given intravenously. It is a highly toxic substance with many side effects.

CHRONIC INFECTION

An acute inflammatory process may fail to subside completely and pass into a chronic phase. Examples of this are encountered when an abscess is inadequately drained, when there is dead tissue or inert material present, such as a sequestrum, or when the local defences are impaired by a poor blood supply. Another group of chronic infections is due to the particular nature of the responsible organism, the most important being tuberculosis, syphilis and actinomycosis.

Characteristic of all these chronic infections is the presence of lymphocytes, plasma cells, macrophages, giant cells and fibroblasts; the polymorphonuclear leucocytes and intense vascular response seen in acute inflammation are not in evidence. The lymphocytes and plasma cells are both probably concerned with antibody production. The phagocytic macrophages are derived partly from histiocytes in the surrounding tissues and partly from monocytes in the blood; giant cells are formed by fusion of a number of these macrophages. Fibroblasts are usually present in large numbers around the margins of the chronic inflammatory focus, and fibrous tissue formation is generally a marked feature of the condition.

Tuberculosis

Tuberculosis is caused by infection with *Mycobacterium tuberculosis*, a slender rod-shaped organism which is acid and alcohol fast when stained by the Ziehl-Neelsen method. Two varieties of the organism are pathogenic to man; the *human* type is spread by sputum and dust and may be inhaled or ingested; the *bovine* type is ingested with milk contaminated from the tuberculous udder of the cow. The two varieties can be distinguished by their cultural characteristics. In addition, the human type is less toxic to rabbits than the bovine variety.

The effects of an inoculation of the tubercle bacillus depend on its size and virulence and on the resistance of the host. This in turn depends on the general health of the subject and on the presence of immunity acquired either naturally from previous infection, or artificially as a result of inoculation with B.C.G., which is an attenuated strain of the organism.

The tissue reaction to invasion by *Myco. tuberculosis* results in the formation of the characteristic tubercle. The bacilli are first ingested by polymorphs, which usually do not succeed in destroying them. Within a day or two the polymorphs are replaced by macrophages which become converted into epithelioid cells, oval or spindle-shaped, with large amounts of clear cytoplasm. Some of these cells fuse together into giant cells, which contain numerous small round nuclei lying peripherally within the cell. Around this focus collects a cuff of lymphocytes. Within a few weeks the centre of the tubercle undergoes necrosis as a result of the destruction of cells by the bacterial toxins; this necrosis produces the typical cheesy or caseous tuberculous material which may later liquefy into pus.

A tubercle may heal completely, leaving only a fibrous scar. It may become surrounded by dense fibrous tissue which subsequently may calcify, or it may spread. Dissemination of tuberculous disease can be along anatomical pathways, such as the bronchial tree, by lymphatic spread to the regional lymph nodes or by the blood stream. The last method may result in the production of a few scattered lesions, or there may be generalised and fulminating dissemination known as miliary spread.

Tuberculosis carried, until recent years, a high mortality particularly in children and young adults. The present fall in incidence is due to the discovery of specific chemotherapy (streptomycin, para-aminosalicylic acid, isoniazid, rifampicin and ethambutol (p. 13)), B.C.G. inoculation, improved general health and hygiene, the elimination of tuberculous cattle together with pasteurisation of milk, and earlier diagnosis by extensive mass radiography campaigns.

Syphilis

The causative organism is the *Treponema pallidum*. Infection is venereal in 95 per cent of cases although it may occasionally be acquired on the lips by kissing or on the fingers by contact with the lesion.

The **primary lesion**, or chancre, appears from two to six weeks after infection, and is usually found on the glans or on the inner aspect of the vulva. Initially there is an indurated papule which ulcerates into a painless ulcer, and even if untreated heals within a few weeks. Painless enlargement of the regional nodes is also present. The treponema can be found both in the serous discharge from the chancre and in the fluid aspirated from the affected nodes.

The **secondary stage** appears two to four months later and is characterised by malaise, fever and headache, a widespread dull-red skin rash and generalised lymphadenopathy. Shallow serpiginous greyish ulcers may be seen in the throat ('snail-track ulcers') and there may be condylomata around the anus and vulva.

Tertiary syphilis may develop at any time from one to thirty years after the initial infection. The *localised* form of the disease is characterised by the development of a *gumma*—a mass of necrotic rubbery material surrounded by chronic inflammatory cells and fibroblasts. When superficial, a gumma may ulcerate to form a typical lesion with a circular or serpiginous margin, punched-out sides and a 'wash-leather' slough on its floor. Usual sites include the skin, particularly on the leg just below the knee, the scalp, the face, the hard palate or the tongue. Gummata may also involve the liver, testis, bones and brain. The *generalised* variety of late syphilis affects the cardiovascular and central nervous systems. There may be aneurysmal dilatation, particular of the ascending aorta, and fibrosis and incompetence of the damaged aortic valves. Involvement of the posterior columns of the spinal cord produces tabes dorsalis, or diffuse degenerative changes in the brain cause general paralysis of the insane.

Congenital syphilis is the result of transplacental infection of the foetus from the affected mother. It is now rare as a result of efficient treatment of infected women during early pregnancy.

Diagnosis is confirmed in the early weeks by identification of the spirochaetes in dark-ground illumination microscopy of fluid expressed from the chancre. From six to eight weeks after infection and in congenital cases confirmation depends on the positive Wassermann reaction and the positive complement fixation test of Kahn. More specific tests such as the treponema immobilisation test or the fluorescent antibody test may be used to confirm the diagnosis or to eliminate the occasional case which gives a positive test with the less specific standard ones, such as malaria and virus diseases.

Treatment

Penicillin is employed in all three stages. Occasionally it may be accompanied by the Herxheimer reaction, which is an acute exacerbation of the local manifestations of the disease with pyrexia.

Actinomycosis

Actinomycosis is an infection produced by the *Actinomyces israelii*, a micro-aerophilic fungus found as a saprophyte in the mouth and alimentary canal. Although other varieties of actinomyces grow on grasses, they are not pathogenic to man and infection by chewing a contaminated straw is a myth. The organisms invade through a breach in the mucosa which may follow dental extraction or the perforation of a gangrenous appendix. The infection results in a dense fibrous tissue reaction within which pockets of pus may form. The latter contains the characteristic 'sulphur granules,' yellow specks which consist of large clumps of the mycelium. Spread occurs along fascial planes, and occasionally by the bloodstream, but not via the lymphatics, probably because the mycelia are too large to disseminate along these channels.

The common sites of the disease are cervico-facial, abdominal and pulmonary.

Cervico-facial actinomycosis occurs after teeth extraction, tonsillitis, or in gross dental caries. A swelling arises in the region of the angle of the jaw, is accompanied by trismus and at times by pain. The tissues over the jaw and neck become greatly indurated and assume a bluish discoloration. One or more sinuses develop, exuding thin yellow pus from which the actinomyces can be recovered. Spread is by direct infiltration; the mediastinum and vertebral column may be involved or, if the upper jaw is the site of origin, the orbit, base of skull, meninges and even the brain may be invaded.

Abdominal actinomycosis follows appendicitis, the abrasion of the alimentary mucosa by a foreign body or perforation of a peptic ulcer. A hard fibrous mass forms, becomes honeycombed with abscess cavities, and may spread to the abdominal wall. Actinomycosis is an uncommon cause of a persistent discharging wound sinus after appendicectomy. In advanced cases spread may occur by the portal vein to the liver, which becomes extensively involved with multiple abscesses.

Pulmonary actinomycosis may follow inhalation of the actinomyces from the mouth. Spread then occurs from the affected lung to the pleura and chest wall. Rarely pulmonary involvement is secondary to abdominal disease as a result of extension through the diaphragm.

Treatment consists of a three-month course of penicillin, 300 mg daily, supplemented by Lugol's iodine by mouth. Any obvious collection of pus should be drained. Early cases respond satisfactorily to this regime, although the prognosis in advanced disease is not favourable.

HOSPITAL INFECTION

The introduction of antibiotics appeared at first to herald an end to the infection of clean surgical wounds, infection of the urinary tract after prolonged catheterisation and the many other manifestations of cross-infection which occur in hospital practice. The problem has again recurred in recent years and this may be related to the following facts: (1) extensive and prolonged operations are now performed, exposing large raw surfaces to possible infection for many hours; (2) the emergence of strains of bacteria, particularly *Pseudomonas aeruginosa* (*pyocyanea*) and *Staph. aureus*, which are frequently resistant to antibiotics and appear to be of enhanced virulence; (3) a lowering of the standards of aseptic technique, initially produced by a false sense of security which accompanied the discovery of antibiotics; (4) an increasing number of seriously ill hospital patients being kept alive on marrow depressant drugs and on therapy which reduces the body defences, such as steroids.

Causes of hospital infection

When sepsis occurs in hospital practice, it is important to attempt to trace the source of the bacterial infection (Fig. 1.2). This may be associated with the **patient**, for example, a compound fracture may be contaminated by dirt, and infection might already be established by the time of arrival in hospital; similarly the incision in cases of general peritonitis becomes flooded with organisms and the chances of subsequent wound sepsis are high. The patient subjected to a 'clean' operation may be a nasal or skin carrier of pyogenic organisms or may have a cutaneous infected lesion; there is sound evidence that in such individuals there is a higher incidence of post-operative wound infection than in non-carriers.

The source of infection may arise in the **operating theatre**. Direct inoculation of organisms into the wound from the hands of the surgeon or assistant or from inadequately sterilised instruments or dressings may occur. Aerial contamination may take place from the noses and mouths of the theatre staff or from clothes and blankets. Suction fans or unsatisfactory ventilation are a source of particular danger in extracting organisms from the adjacent corridor or ward and blowing them into the wound.

Post-operative cross-infection may occur in the **ward**, either directly from the hands of the attending staff and from contaminated instruments or dressings, or indirectly from nearby infected wounds or dust particles produced during bed-making and other ward activities.

Staph. aureus is the most important organism responsible for hospital infections; it has replaced the β-haemolytic streptococcus in this role principally because the latter has remained sensitive to the sulphonamides and to penicillin. Strains of antibiotic-resistant staphlococci are now responsible for the majority of wound infections which follow 'clean' surgical procedures. The staphylococcus is also concerned in outbreaks of cutaneous infection in neonatal units, breast abscesses in nursing mothers delivered in hospital, skin infection among medical and nursing staff and outbreaks of staphylococcal pneumonia. The exact epidemiology of many outbreaks is not fully understood. The presence of cutaneous infection in hospital personnel will result in epidemics of wound infection, but the part played by droplet infection from nasopharyngeal carriers or from contaminated dust particles in the wards and operating theatre remains to be accurately assessed. Bacterial counts of wounds and air are not necessarily correlated with the amount of wound infection. The pathway of spread may be indirect, for example, the nasal carrier may cause

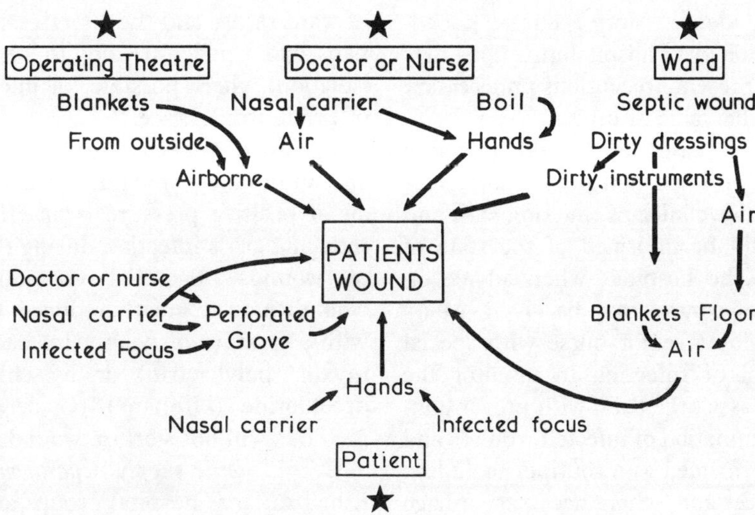

Fig. 1.2 The sources of hospital wound infection

infection not by a droplet route but by initial inoculation of the hands, whilst occasionally the perineum serves as an intermediate depot.

Gram-negative sepsis due to the coliform organisms, proteus and pseudomonas as well as anaerobic infection due to *Bacteroides* sp. is becoming increasingly important. These pathogens have their normal habitat in the large bowel and are often resistant to many of the antibiotics; in addition, resistance to antibiotics may develop during treatment. Infections with Gram-negative bacilli are important in surgical wounds, burns, the urinary and biliary tracts and in infant and premature baby units. Infection of the eye with *Pseudomonas aeruginosa (pyocyanea)* is especially serious. In respiratory units these organisms are commonly responsible for infection of the tracheoestomy wound. The pseudomonas in particular can remain alive for long periods on damp surfaces and is a persistent hazard in ward infections. An important complication of Gram-negative infection is profound shock. This may accompany the septicaemia which can complicate infection with these organisms (p. 23).

Control of hospital infection

No single measure will control hospital cross-infection; recent careful studies have shown that only a wide range of precautions will lead to a significant lessening of the incidence. More accurate knowledge of the epidemiology of hospital infections may render some of the present precautions unnecessary whilst reinforcing the value of others.

Notification of all cases of wound infection within a hospital is an important preliminary step. A committee of senior clinicians, nursing staff and bacteriologist should be informed of the state of affairs throughout the hospital, when advice on uniform methods of control may be given. Many hospitals now employ a senior nurse with special training in Control of Infection to monitor the infection rates and assist the team with prevention. Bacteriological examination of infected wounds and urine should be performed as a routine, including antibiotic sensitivities and, where necessary, phage typing. The spread of infection due to a specific causal organism may thus be traced to a source of infection in the ward. This may be a discharging wound, an infected bladder or a septic lesion on nurse or doctor. It is important that all medical or nursing personnel with any infection should be excluded from the ward or operating theatre. It is of value to keep a Wound Book in each ward, in which details of the operation, including the names of the surgical team, the use of antibiotics and the post-operative course are recorded. It is not possible to determine the immediate implications of an outbreak of infection without such a record.

Scrupulous aseptic technique in the operating theatre is essential and ideally includes the positive pressure ('plenum') air conditioning which provides a current of filtered air over the operation field. The methods of instrument and dressing sterilisation in both theatre and ward should be kept under close supervision and bacteriological review. Droplet contamination is reduced by the universal use of adequate face masks. Contamination of the skin of staff and patients with organisms can be adequately controlled by the use of soap containing hexachlorophene. A cream to which the organism is sensitive applied to the anterior nares is effective against nasal staphylococci and should be used to eliminate resistant infection.

Simple hygienic methods such as adequate spacing between beds in the ward, the provision of sufficient ventilation and sunlight, the avoidance of dressings during bed-making or toilet rounds when air contamination is maximal, the efficient disposal of ward refuse and the effective sterilisation of bed pans and urinals are not to be overlooked. The isolation, where possible, of infected cases is also of prime importance.

The use of a special dressing-room provided with air-conditioning apparatus which supplies filtered air at positive pressure is an effective method of reducing cross-infection during the actual dressing of wounds. Bacterial contamination of open wounds may be greatly reduced it they are sprayed with a mixture of neomycin, bacitracin and polymyxin (polybactrin) or by chlorhexidine dihydrochloride (Hibitane) powder, although these methods will not sterilise wounds already infected.

Central sterile supply departments are now established in large hospital groups and provide sterile dressings, instruments and surgical sundries such as syringes, needles and catheters. An increasing amount of disposable items is now available for use on one occasion only but more expensive instruments are re-sterilised in autoclaves or hot-air ovens. The adequate sterilisation of mattresses, blankets and curtains is a problem since these expensive items deteriorate rapidly on repeated cleaning. The use of cotton instead of woollen blankets enables sterilisation to be carried out frequently without affecting quality and disposable plastic bags can be used to enclose mattresses and render their sterilisation unnecessary.

Established infection is managed as previously indicated (p. 2). Indiscriminate use of cloxacillin to which the staphylococci are still mainly sensitive is to be avoided, since there is the likelihood of the development within the hospital of strains resistant to this drug. They should be reserved solely for use in cases of serious infection.

Antibiotic associated enterocolitis

Although sporadic cases of enterocolitis were recorded in the pre-antibiotic era, enterocolitis is seen particularly in patients who have received broad spectrum antibiotic therapy and seems especially likely to occur in patients who have also recently undergone surgery. The probable mechanism is the destruction of the normal bowel flora with overgrowth of resistant bacteria. In early epidemics the *Staph. aureus* was implicated, but more recently there is strong evidence to support the role of toxin-producing strains of *Cl. difficile* which can be recovered from patients with this condition.

The entire bowel shows intensive mucosal inflammation with pseudo-membrane formation. The intestine becomes dilated and may hold many litres of green watery fluid.

Clinical features

The condition usually occurs in the first week after a major surgical procedure in a patient who has received antibiotic therapy; there is a strong association with preceding administration of lincomycin or clindamycin. Mild cases present with watery diarrhoea. Severe cases have a cholera-like picture. The abdomen is distended, the patient feverish, weak and lethargic and there may be all the features of shock. There is copious diarrhoea with the passage of green watery stools which contain mucus and shreds of pseudomembrane. Sigmoidoscopy demonstrates a friable, reddened mucosa with whitish-yellow plaques which may run together to form a continuous pseudomembrane.

Treatment comprises urgent replacement of fluid and electrolytes; blood, plasma or dextran together with hydrocortisone are given if shock is severe. Other antibiotics are immediately discontinued and oral vancomycin is prescribed; this rapidly eliminates *Cl. difficile.*

CHEMOTHERAPY

Chemotherapeutic agents may be employed to overcome bacterial invasion. They can act in a bacteriostatic manner by preventing the reproduction of the organisms; sulphonamides, chloramphenicol and the tetracyclines being examples of this: or they can be bactericidal and destroy the organisms; penicillin, streptomycin, erythromycin and neomycin being in this category. Originally antibacterial substances were divided into chemotherapeutic agents, produced by chemical synthesis and antibiotics, extracted from moulds and bacteria, but the synthesis of antibiotics has rendered this classification only of historical interest.

The probable mode of action of these substances is their interference with an essential metabolic process in the bacterial cell. Streptomycin appears to disturb the Krebs cycle of carbohydrate metabolism; the tetracyclines interfere with phosphorylation and the sulphonamides prevent the utilisation of para-aminobenzoic acid, essential for bacterial reproduction, by the substitution of para-aminobenzene sulphonamide.

General considerations in the use of chemotherapeutic agents

The causative organism should be identified whenever feasible and its sensitivities determined in order that the appropriate antibiotic can be prescribed. If the condition is too urgent to warrant such delay, clinical judgment should be used to select the agent which is most likely to be effective in the paticular case. A specimen of pus, infected urine or blood for culture should first be obtained so that subsequently the bacterial sensitivity can be checked and the chemotherapeutic agent changed if necessary. Although chemotherapy is ineffective in the treatment of an established abscess and cannot be a substitute for surgical drainage, in acute spreading infections it should prove efficacious in 24 to 48 hours. If clinical improvement is not then evident the problem must be reviewed and consideration given to changing the antibiotic or to the likelihood of a localised collection of pus requiring evacuation. Combined therapy employing two bactericidal or two bacteriostatic antibiotics has the advantage of preventing the emergence of resistant bacteria.

The sulphonamides

The sulphonamides are readily absorbed from the small intestine and distributed throughout the body, including the cerebrospinal fluid. They are excreted in the urine partly unchanged and partly in the conjugated, inactive form after acetylation in the liver. In modern surgical practice sulphonamides are employed in coliform urinary infections and in the pre-operative preparation of the large bowel for resection, in which one of the relatively non-absorbable sulphonamides is used. Toxic effects include nausea, vomiting, skin rashes and occasionally neutropenia or agranulocytosis. Anuria may follow renal deposition of sulphonamide crystals, but this is rare with the modern highly soluble preparations.

Sulphadiazine and sulphadimidine are two of the sulphonamide compounds which are of general application; they are relatively non-toxic, are slowly excreted and are highly soluble, therefore carrying little risk of deposition in the urine. Sulphamethizole (Urolucosil) is a highly soluble sulphonamide and is useful as a urinary bacteriostatic in a dosage of 200 mg eight-hourly. Phthalylsulphathiazole (Sulphathalidine) is relatively (95 per cent) unabsorbed from the alimentary tract and is used in the pre-operative sterilisation of the colon. It is given in divided doses of a total of 10 g a day for five days.

Co-trimoxazole (Septrin) is a mixture of trimethoprim and sulphamethoxazole. These two anti-metabolites act on the same metabolic pathway affecting sequentially two enzymes in the biosynthesis of folinic acid. Their action is synergistic and Septrin is bacteriostatic. It is effective against all common pathogens except *Myco. tuberculosis, Tr. pallidum* and *Ps. aeruginosa* (*pyocyanea*) and is particularly useful in respiratory and urinary tract infections. The dosage is two tablets two or three times daily, or for long-term therapy, one tablet twice daily, each tablet containing 80 mg trimethoprim and 400 mg sulphamethoxazole.

Penicillin

Penicillin was originally obtained from the mould *Penicillium notatum* but is now produced as white crystalline *benzyl penicillin.* It is destroyed by the acid in the stomach and except in infants, who have low gastric acidity, it is ineffective when given by mouth and the intramuscular route is therefore used. Phenoxymethyl penicillin ('Penicillin V') is acid-stable and may be employed orally, but due to variable absorption intramuscular penicillin is preferable in most surgical conditions.

Penicillin does not enter the cerebrospinal fluid when given systemically and therefore must be introduced intrathecally when employed for meningeal infections. It is effective against the haemolytic streptococcus, pneumococcus, gonococcus, the clostridia and the *Tr. pallidum.* The original highly effective bacterial action against the *Staph. aureus* has now to a great extent been lost with the emergence of resistant strains of this organism which produce a penicillin-destroying enzyme (penicillinase). At present up to one-third of all staphylococcal infections acquired outside of hospital are resistant to penicillin and the staphylococci endemic within hospitals are mainly resistant strains.

Cloxacillin (Orbenin) is not inactivated by penicillinase and is used in the treatment of resistant staphylococcal infections. It is acid-resistant and can therefore be administered orally.

Ampicillin (Penbritin) is of value in urinary infections due to coliform organisms or *Proteus* as well as in the treatment of respiratory tract infections. It has a broader spectrum of antibacterial activity than the other penicillins and is useful in infection due to Gram-negative bacilli and *Strept. faecalis,* being frequently employed in peritonitis. It is however inactivated by penicillinase and is therefore of no value in the treatment of penicillin-resistant staphylococcal infections. Dosage is 250 to 500 mg six-hourly by mouth or by intramuscular injection.

Flucloxacillin (Floxapen) and *amoxycillin* (Amoxil) have similar spectra of antibacterial activity to cloxacillin and ampicillin respectively, but, being better absorbed, require lower dosage. Flucloxacillin will probably replace cloxacillin as the drug of choice in the treatment of resistant staphylococcal infection. Higher blood levels of ampicillin may also be obtained with the ampicillin esters such as *talampicillin* (Talpen).

Carbenicillin (Pyopen) is a semi-synthetic penicillin with a wide spectrum of antibacterial activity which includes the Gram-negative bacteria including pseudomonas. It is not absorbed orally and must be given by intramuscular or intravenous injection in divided doses to a total of 8 to 30 g per day. *Ticarcillin* (Ticar) and *azlocillin* (Securopen) have greater activity against *Ps. aeruginosa* than carbenicillin, but still require parenteral administration. *Carfecillin* (Uticillin) can be given by mouth in pseudomonas urinary infections.

Penicillin remains the antibiotic of choice in streptococcal infections, gas gangrene and tetanus; it is still of value in staphylococcal sepsis acquired outside hospital practice. Toxic effects are remarkably uncommon, rare instances of anaphylaxis having been noted, but the danger of monilial infection or of enterocolitis does exist. The usual dosage is 300 to 600 mg every six hours by intramuscular injection. In fulminating infections, such as acute osteomyelitis, this dose may be doubled.

Streptomycin

Streptomycin is obtained from the mould *Streptomyces griseus*. It is of particular importance in the treatment of tuberculosis. Toxic effects include vertigo, tinnitus and eighth nerve deafness, which may be permanent and occur particularly during prolonged treatment. In the treatment of tuberculosis streptomycin is not used alone because of the emergence of resistant strains during the course of therapy but, in a dosage of 1 g by intramuscular injection daily, it is combined with isonicotinic acid hydrazide (isoniazid or INAH), 300 mg daily, and para-aminosalicylic acid (PAS), 12 g daily, given by mouth in divided doses in a combined cachet (Pasinah). Pyridoxine, 50 mg twice daily is essential with isoniazid to prevent peripheral and optic neuritis. Streptomycin is given for a minimum period of three months and the other drugs continued for at least a further year. Rifampicin, 600 mg daily by mouth, in combination with isoniazid, is being increasingly used and is at least as effective as streptomycin with isoniazid, without such serious toxic effects.

The tetracyclines

This group of antibiotics comprises chlortetracycline (Aureomycin), oxytetracycline (Terramycin) and tetracycline (Achromycin). All possess a similar range of activity and sensitivity. The tetracyclines are rapidly absorbed when given orally, but do not achieve a high concentration in the cerebrospinal fluid. They exert a 'broad spectrum' of activity to bacteria, rickettsiae and certain viruses, the important exceptions being Proteus and some strains of *Ps. aeruginosa* (*pyocyanea*). The tubercle bacillus is slightly sensitive to oxytetracycline. Resistant strains, particularly of the *Staph. aureus*, are becoming increasingly common.

The tetracyclines are of value in the treatment of severe peritonitis. They may also be used in sulphonamide-resistant urinary infections and staphylococcal sepsis, when bacteriological studies confirm the sensitivity of the infecting organism to these drugs. Toxic effects include nausea, vomiting, anorexia, heartburn and diarrhoea; these are more common with the chlor- and oxy-derivatives than with tetracycline. In addition, there are risks of superinfection of the alimentary tract by resistant bacteria with effects which vary from mild diarrhoea to severe enterocolitis (p. 11). Monilial infection of the mouth is not uncommon and the fungicide nystatin is often simultaneously prescribed. The tetracyclines are stored in bones and teeth and can stunt the growth and stain the teeth of children.

The usual route of administration is by mouth, 1 g daily being given in divided doses for five to ten days. Intravenous preparations are available as well as intramuscular preparations of oxytetracycline and tetracycline; these are used in fulminating infections or where the oral route cannot be employed.

Table 1 Chemotherapeutic agents in common usage

Approved name	Proprietary name	Principal application
Sulphadiazine		General Meningeal
Sulphadimidine		General
Phthalylsulphathiazole	Sulphathalidine	Bowel sterilisation
Sulphamethizole	Urolucosil	Urinary tract
Co-trimoxazole	Septrin	Respiratory and urinary tract
Benzyl penicillin	Crystapen	General
Phenoxy-methyl penicillin	Distaquaine V	General
Ampicillin	Penbritin	Gram-positive and Gram-negative
Cloxacillin	Orbenin	Resistant staphylococci
Flucloxacillin	Floxapen	Resistant staphylococci
Carbenicillin	Pyopen	*Ps. aeruginosa* (*pyocyanea*)
Streptomycin		Coliform organisms Tuberculosis
Isonicotinic acid hydrazide	Isoniazid	Tuberculosis
Rifampicin	Rifadin	Tuberculosis
Oxytetracycline Tetracycline Chlortetracycline	Terramycin Achromycin Aureomycin	Broad range
Chloramphenicol	Chloromycetin	Broad range
Erythromycin	Erythrocin	Gram-positive
Neomycin		Bowel sterilisation
Kanamycin	Kannasyn	*B. proteus* and *Ps. aeruginosa* (*pyocyanea*)
Gentamicin	Cidomycin	Gram-negative septicaemia and *Ps. aeruginosa* (*pyocyanea*)
Colistin	Colomycin	*Ps. aeruginosa* (*pyocyanea*)
Clindamycin	Dalacin C.	*Bacteroides* sp., and anaerobic Gram-negative septicaemia
Nitrofurantoin	Furadantin	Urinary tract
Sodium fusidate	Fucidin	Resistant staphylococci
Cephaloridine	Ceporin	Resistant staphylococci and broad range
Nalidixic acid	Negram	Urinary tract
Metronidazole	Flagyl	Bowel sterilisation Peritonitis Certain protozoal infections

Chloramphenicol

This antibiotic also has a wide spectrum of antibacterial activity, which includes the typhoid and paratyphoid bacilli. Rarely aplastic anaemia may follow administration, although generally it only occurs after long or repeated courses. It should only be employed when there is a specific indication, such as typhoid fever, or in resistant staphylococcal or other bacterial infections. Dosage is 2 g daily in divided amounts by mouth, and this should not be continued for more than 10 days and the course not repeated. A total dosage of 24 g should never be exceeded.

Route	Dosage (Average)	Duration
Oral	2 g statim then 1 g every four hours	5 to 10 days
Oral and intramuscular	2 g statim then 1 g every four hours	5 to 10 days
Oral	2.5 g every six hours	5 days
Oral	200 mg every eight hours	5 to 10 days or prolonged
Oral	Tabs. 2 every eight hours	10 to 14 days
Intramuscular	300 to 600 mg every six hours	5 to 10 days
Oral	250 mg every four hours	5 to 10 days
Oral, intramuscular and intravenous	500 mg every six hours	5 to 10 days
Oral, intramuscular and intravenous	500 mg every six hours	5 to 10 days
Oral, intramuscular and intravenous	250 to 500 mg every six hours	5 to 10 days
Intramuscular and intravenous	8 to 30 g daily in divided doses	10 to 14 days
Intramuscular	1 g twice daily	5 days maximum
Intramuscular	1 g daily	3 to 6 months
Oral	300 mg daily in divided doses	1 year
Oral	450 to 600 mg daily	1 year
Oral, intramuscular and intravenous	250 mg every six hours 100 mg every six hours 1 to 2 g daily in divided doses	5 to 10 days
Oral, intramuscular and intravenous	500 mg every six hours	10 days maximum
Oral, intramuscular and intravenous	500 mg every six hours	5 to 10 days
Oral	1 g hourly for four hours then four hourly for 24 hours	28 hours
Intramuscular	500 mg twice daily	10 days maximum
Intramuscular and intravenous	Weight-related with laboratory control	7 to 10 days
Oral and intramuscular	3 million units eight-hourly 1 to 5 million units eight-hourly	7 to 10 days
Oral	150 to 450 mg every six hours	5 to 10 days
Oral	100 mg every eight hours	7 to 10 days
Oral	500 mg every eight hours	7 to 10 days
Intramuscular and intravenous	500 mg every eight hours	7 to 10 days
Oral	1 g every six hours	7 to 10 days
Oral Intravenous Rectal	400 mg every eight hours 500 mg every eight hours 1 g every eight hours	5 to 7 days

Erythromycin

Erythromycin resembles penicillin in its spectrum of activity. The principal use is in the treatment of penicillin-resistant staphylococcal infections, when it should be given in doses of 500 mg six-hourly by mouth or by intramuscular or intravenous injection. It is also of use where penicillin allergy exists and when penicillin would be the drug of choice. Novobiocin, vancomycin and lincomycin are other examples of antibiotics which are of value in certain resistant and severe staphylococcal infections especially in patients with penicillin sensitivity.

Neomycin

Neomycin is too toxic for routine systemic administration; deafness and renal damage are not uncommon following such use. It is of value when given orally in producing rapid sterilisation of the alimentary canal but is not without some dangers. Antibiotic associated enterocolitis may be encouraged by its use and a neomycin-resistant strain of staphylococci in the nose or throat may adversely affect the patient with subsequent spread throughout the ward and hospital. It is often employed as a pre-operative measure before surgical procedures involving the large intestine; 1 g hourly for four hours followed by 1 g four-hourly for 24 hours is considered effective, providing the colon is not loaded with faeces. In the management or prevention of hepatic coma in severe liver disease it is used to destroy the intestinal flora which produce ammonia, the absorption of which contributes to the toxaemia of hepatic failure. Neomycin is also of value for surface application to infected wounds or ulcers. It seldom produces skin sensitisation which is a serious hazard of the use of penicillin, streptomycin or chloramphenicol. It is combined with hydrocortisone for topical application to surface lesions associated with infection.

Kanamycin

Kanamycin, isolated from *Streptomyces kanamyceticus*, is of value in the treatment of infections resistant to other antibiotics, particularly the staphylococci, proteus and pseudomonas. In addition it is useful in treating resistant cases of tuberculosis. It is given in doses of 1 g daily by intramuscular injection; absorption does not occur from the alimentary canal. It is more toxic than streptomycin, affecting principally the kidney and eighth cranial nerve. It should not be used if there is any impairment of renal function.

Gentamicin

This drug is produced from *Micromonospora purpurea* and is related to kanamycin. It has a similar range of antibacterial activity to both Gram-positive and Gram-negative organisms but a notable feature is a high degree of activity against *Ps. aeruginosa*. It is excreted by the kidneys and is valuable in the treatment of pseudomonas infection of the urinary tract. It may be used as a local application for burns infected with this organism. It is most important in combating Gram-negative septicaemia. Gentamicin resembles streptomycin in producing ototoxicity but disturbs vestibular rather than auditory function. The dosage should thus be limited to 80 mg three times a day by intramuscular injection, but it is preferably controlled by laboratory estimations. Other aminoglycosides for use in gentamicin-resistant infections include amikacin, netilmicin and tobramycin.

Colomycin

Colomycin is obtained from the micro-organism *Bacillus colinistinus*. It possesses selective activity against pathogenic Gram-negative bacilli, and is of value in dealing with *Pseudomonas* infections of the urinary tract. It may be given orally (three million units three times a day) or intramuscularly (four million units daily in divided doses).

Clindamycin

Clindamycin (Dalacin C) is a synthetic modification of lincomycin. It is active against staphylococci, pneumococci, *Bacteroides* sp., for which last organism it is the drug of choice. It is given orally in a dosage of 300 to 450 mg six-hourly for serious infection, and has proved of great value in anaerobic Gram-negative septicaemia. Enterocolitis may complicate its use, probably as a response to the profound change in intestinal flora. This complication can be avoided with metronidazole (Flagyl) which is now being preferred for anaerobic infection.

Fucidin

Fucidin is the sodium salt of fusidic acid obtained from *Fusidium*. It is effective against most varieties of *Staph. aureus*, is well tolerated by mouth and is given in doses of 500 mg eight-hourly. It is of particular value in treating staphylococcal infections which cannot be treated by the penicillins because of sensitivity or drug resistance. Due to the possibility of the staphylococcus rapidly developing resistance to sodium fusidate, it can be given with another antibiotic to which the organism is sensitive, such as erythromycin. The ability of the drug to penetrate into bone makes it of value in the treatment of staphylococcal osteomyelitis. Local application is useful in the management of staphylococcal skin sepsis.

Cephaloridine

This semi-synthetic antibiotic is effective against both Gram-positive and Gram-negative organisms, as well as being useful in staphylococcal infections resistant to other antibiotics. It is inactivated by Staph. penicillinase although not as rapidly as benzyl penicillin. Its main value is in those patients who are allergic to penicillin and for whom this drug would be the choice. Side-effects are rare but skin sensitivity may occur and renal dysfunction if already present may be aggravated. The dosage is 500 mg eight-hourly by intramuscular injection. Other cephalosporins include cephalothin for parenteral administration, cephalexin for oral administration and cephradine for both parenteral and oral administration but a large range of them is now available.

Nalidixic acid

Nalidixic acid is effective against Gram-negative organisms, particularly in the urinary tract, with the exception of pseudomonas which is resistant to it. Further resistant organisms do emerge during treatment particularly if the dosage is inadequate. Side-effects are uncommon but include nausea, vomiting, diarrhoea, skin rashes, headache, dizziness and rarely photosensitivity. The drug is administered orally in a dosage of 1 g six-hourly for seven to ten days in acute infections but for periods of two to three months in chronic infections.

The nitrofurans

A group of chemicals synthesised from 5-nitrofuran have a broad bacteriostatic activity. Nitrofurantoin (Furadantin) is the most widely used and is active against strains of *Escherichia coli*, *Proteus*, *Pseudomonas*, *Strept. faecalis* and *Staph. aureus*. When adminstered orally about 40 per cent is excreted in the urine and this, together with its range of bacterial sensitivity, renders nitrofurantoin useful in urinary tract infections.

Nausea, vomiting, heartburn and skin rashes may occur, although alimentary symptoms can be reduced by giving the drug with milk or at mealtimes. A more serious side-effect is peripheral neuropathy, especially in the presence of impaired renal function. Dosage is 100 mg eight-hourly in a seven to ten day course.

Metronidazole

Metronidazole (Flagyl) is an imidazole compound which is effective against a number of protozoa, particularly trichomonas, *Entamoeba histolytica* and intestinal infestation with *Giardia lamblia*. It is of particular importance to the surgeon because most strains of *Bacteroides*, as well as anaerobic cocci and *Clostridia*, are very sensitive to this drug. It is now widely used in the preparation of the bowel before colon surgery and also in the prophylaxis and treatment of peritonitis due to bowel organisms, for example, gangrenous appendicitis. In severe peritoneal infections it is usually combined with gentamicin or one of the new generation of cephalosporins. Although nausea and skin rashes may occur, tolerance to the drug is high and it may be given either orally, by suppository or intravenously.

FURTHER READING

Keighley, M. R. B. & Burdon, D. W. (1979). *Antimicrobial Prophylaxis in Surgery*. Tunbridge Wells: Pitman Medical.

Lowbury, E. J. L., Ayliffe, G. A. J., Geddes, A. M. & Williams, J. D. (1975). *Control of Hospital Infection. A Practical Handbook*. London: Chapman and Hall.

Watts J. M., McDonald, P. J., O'Brien, P. E., Marshall, V. R. & Finlay-Jones, J. J. (1981). *Infection in Surgery. Basic and Clinical Aspects*. Edinburgh: Churchill Livingstone.

2

Surgical aspects of injury and repair

On receipt of an injury, whether accidental or planned, as in a surgical operation, there occurs a series of events designed to restore the injured person to health and to return body function to normal. The responses of an individual to injury may be classified as local and general.

LOCAL RESPONSE

The local result of an injury is a wound, whose healing will depend upon its severity and extent. A clean-cut incision will heal with minimal scarring (i.e. by first intention) provided that

(i) there is minimal damage to adjacent tissue.
(ii) loss of tissue is minimal.
(iii) the wound is not contaminated by foreign material.
(iv) bleeding is controlled.
(v) infection is prevented.
(vi) the edges of the wound are brought together without tension by carefully inserted sutures.

If the wound is allowed to heal without approximation or suture of its edges, the defect becomes filled with granulation tissue. This is ultimately covered by epithelial cells which have migrated from the edges of the wound (healing by *second intention*).

Primary healing

The process of primary healing of a wound may be regarded as occurring in three phases which overlap considerably. Each phase has distinctive microscopic and biochemical features.

Phase I (preparative or exudate phase)

The space between the edges of the wound quickly fills with blood clot and the wound is sealed with fibrin. Within a few hours, adjacent capillaries become dilated and fluid is poured into the interstitial space. This protein-rich fluid quickly forms an impermeable coagulum which has valuable antibacterial properties. This stage closely resembles the early response to bacterial invasion. Leucocytes and macrophages invade the wound to destroy, ingest and remove dead and damaged tissue. Fibrin, endotoxins, foreign body and bacteria 'activate' the macrophages to release factors which stimulate the growth of fibroblasts and blood vessels.

At the same time in the wound there is a rapid increase in a number of chemical substances, later required for the process of healing. The major substances in this phase are the mucopolysaccharides of the ground substance, of which the best known is chondroitin sulphate.

This phase, often called the *lag* or *substrate* phase, lasts from four to six days during which the wound has no tensile strength. The wound edges would fall apart if the sutures were removed. This phase may be prolonged by the development of wound infection.

Phase II (reparative or proliferative phase)

The congestion within the wound subsides and the formation of collagen begins. New capillaries sprout from the side of existing ones, and fibroblasts appear and align themselves to the capillaries. The granulation tissue becomes vascular, bleeds easily but affords some protection against bacterial invasion. Fine fibrils appear in the intercellular space and aggregate to form collagen fibres.

At the same time, epithelium from the cut edges migrates inwards over the connective tissue of the skin, comes into contact with the deeper structures and undergoes hyperplasia and thickening. Tongues of epithelial tissue also pass down between the cells of this newly forming connective tissue. Epithelial elements in hair follicles, sebaceous glands and sweat glands, lying in the epidermis, form an invaluable source of epithelium for the repair of wounds in which most of the epidermis is lost, such as in abrasions and burns.

The important biochemical substance is collagen whose concentration rapidly increases while that of mucopolysaccharides correspondingly decreases. Collagen which is of mesodermal origin is a fibrous protein, one of whose unique features is a high content of hydroxyproline. Strong collagen fibres are formed through polymerisation of sub-microscopic particles and in this way the wound is bridged. Intra-molecular cross-linking is the source of the tensile strength. Coincident with this deposition of collagen is simultaneous collagen lysis; by successive deposition and removal, the wound collagen is slowly modelled into mechanically more useful patterns. Consequently wound strength no longer parallels collagen content but continues to increase long after total collagen is stable and even diminishing.

This phase of wound healing, the *proliferative* phase, lasts four to fifteen days and begins to subside thereafter. During this phase there is a rapid increase in the tensile strength of the wound.

Phase III (*contraction or maturative phase*)

The hyperplastic wound tissue, composed of fibroblasts, capillaries and young collagen begins to be reabsorbed. Collagen fibres become larger, longer and intertwined. The wound then begins to contract. This *contraction* is a normal physiological process with minimal scarring, and is probably caused by active movement of fibroblasts, within the granulation tissue, to pull the wound edges together by cell contraction. The skin around the contracting defect appears to play a part in the process, possibly by forming a rim which protrudes into the centre of the defect. In this way an open soft-tissue wound spontaneously closes by the centripetal migration of normal tissue. The process must be distinguished from contracture, the end result of poor or delayed healing, which in the region of a joint may restrict its movement.

As a result of contraction, the red scar of the wound becomes replaced by a silver, flat hairline one. Tensile strength continues to increase until normal strength is gained after about three months.

Delayed healing

When the healing of a wound is delayed, epithelialisation is retarded. The gap between the wound edges becomes bridged by granulation tissue consisting of capillary buds, fibroblasts, macrophages and leucocytes, the epithelium gradually covering the wound from its edge. A defect may thus remain partly or wholly covered with fragile epithelium. Excessive fibrous tissue formation may produce a contracture and deformity. The effects of second intention healing may be minimised by suture of the wound or by the application of skin grafts which will ensure reduction of fluid and blood loss from the wound, and protect the underlying tissues against bacterial invasion. Pain is diminished and deformity minimised.

Factors implicated in wound healing

A wound may not heal as rapidly or effectively as has been described, because certain factors required for prompt and complete healing are absent or other factors are present which interfere with the process of repair.

Local factors

1. Inaccurate skin apposition or a large tissue defect causes a delay in healing until the gap has been bridged.
2. The presence of dead or damaged tissue, foreign bodies and blood clot also delays healing and their removal facilitates the early phase of wound repair.
3. An impaired blood supply will slow healing, inhibit fibroblasts and weaken the defences against

infection. The blood supply to the part may be impaired by associated damage to an artery or suture of the wound under excessive tension. Venous and lymphatic stasis may cause oedema and so lead to deficient perfusion of the tissue. Regional differences in wound healing, e.g. rapid healing of facial wounds, are largely related to differences in local blood supply.

4. The most common cause of delay in wound healing is local infection. The constant aim should be to prevent bacteria reaching the wound, rather than subsequent treatment, because antibiotics and antiseptics may interfere with subsequent healing.

5. Complete immobilisation of the wounded area may enhance repair by avoiding damage to the delicate capillaries and regenerating cells. The value of immobilisation is apparent in dealing with fractures, but, though beneficial, may not be quite so necessary in soft tissue injuries and occasionally, as in wounds of the heart, lungs and arteries, is impossible to achieve. Increased mechanical stress on a wound delays healing. Thus rupture of an abdominal wound after operation is frequently preceded by repetitive coughing, vomiting or intestinal distension, and is commoner in the obese patient.

The nature of the suture material and method of suturing play a lesser part in wound healing. Breaking of sutures and slipping of knots can be avoided by careful selection of materials and good technique. In general, non-absorbed suture materials, such as stainless steel, are less frequently associated with wound disruption than catgut.

General factors

1. *Protein deficiency* may lead to delayed repair due to lack of collagen in the wound and dehiscence is common in the malnourished. The essential amino-acids, cysteine, lysine and methionine, are particularly important.

2. Lack of *vitamin C* leads to defective formation and maintenance of collagen. In scurvy there is no evidence of healing but this disease is rare in Western countries; less severe forms of vitamin C deficiency are probably not uncommon in those with inadequate diets, as in the elderly, the poor or ill-educated. Wounds in the scorbutic are fragile and tear apart easily.

3. *Anaemia*. There is little evidence that anaemia alone interferes with wound healing and when delay occurs in an anaemic patient it is usually caused by associated hypoproteinaemia.

4. *Hormones*. It has not been conclusively proved in man that cortisone, or other adrenal corticosteroids, will impair wound healing except in high doses, above those usually given therapeutically. In any case steroids do not inhibit primary repair when given after the development of the acute inflammatory phase, i.e. after the fourth day.

5. *Age*. The young heal better than the elderly but the factors involved are not obvious.

6. *Other diseases*. Healing is probably deficient in a number of systemic disease such as diabetes, uraemia, jaundice, Cushing's disease and in disseminated neoplasia but evidence is lacking that there is any specific factor involved other than hypoproteinaemia and vitamin C deficiency.

Complications of wounds

1. Haemorrhage may occur immediately due to severance of a blood-vessel (*primary haemorrhage*) or it may be delayed. Delayed haemorrhage may occur within a few hours of the infliction of an injury when the blood-pressure of the patient is restored to normal (*reactionary haemorrhage*). Occasionally severe bleeding may result several days after injury and is usually due to wound infection with erosion of the blood-vessel wall (*secondary haemorrhage*).

2. Infection in a wound may allow organisms to enter the circulation (Bacteraemia, p. 2).

3. The scar may (*a*) be delicate, poorly nourished and break down easily; (*b*) adhere to underlying tendon or bone, delaying healing and interfering with function; (*c*) develop a contracture with subsequent deformity and limitation of joint use; (*d*) fail to regress, becoming raised and extending into adjacent tissues (*keloid*). The last is more liable to occur in the young, in Negro races or if healing has been delayed.

Treatment of wounds

The injured part should be handled gently to avoid further injury. Bleeding should be controlled, pain relieved and shock prevented or treated (p. 25).

Prophylactic measures against tetanus and gas gangrene may have to be instituted.

Local management

A sterile protective dressing should be immediately applied. The surrounding skin should be cleaned and shaved. Under local or general anaesthesia the wound should be cleaned, irrigated with sterile saline, and all foreign bodies removed. The edges should be excised up to 3 mm except in facial and hand injuries. Damaged fat, fascia and muscle should be removed but essential structures such as blood-vessels and nerves should be carefully preserved. Small detached fragments of bone may be excised but if excessive comminution exists the fragments may require to be used in reconstructing the bone. If a wound has only been lightly contaminated and has been well cleansed the wound edges should be brought together (primary suture) by meticulous insertion of fine sutures. A drain is inserted only if infection or haemorrhage are likely to follow or discharge occur from a hollow organ such as the intestine. If the wound is heavily contaminated or infection is already present or if there is a considerable amount of tissue necrosis, suturing may be delayed for five or six days (delayed primary suture). The employment of skin grafts, relieving incisions or advancement flaps may be necessary to ensure primary closure at certain sites when skin approximation is difficult and yet primary healing is a necessity to protect underlying structures such as an exposed joint or bone. Sutures should be removed when adequate tensile strength has developed. To set a finite period for the removal of stitches implies a standard rate of wound healing. Rather the wound is inspected and one or two sutures can be removed to see if the skin edges are sufficiently adherent to permit removal of all of the sutures. In general, stitches may be removed from facial wounds within 24 hours, whereas a long abdominal wound may need the sutures retained for up to 10 to 14 days.

GENERAL RESPONSE

In addition to the local response to an injury there is a sequence of clinical, metabolic and hormonal events of a general nature which we call recovery or convalescence which are designed for an ultimate return to full health.

Clinical events

Four phases can be recognised:

Initial. The patient lies quietly in bed and may sleep for many hours, resenting movement and disturbance and usually refusing food. Urine output is scanty and there may be tachycardia and pyrexia. The intensity and duration is dependent on the severity of the injury and freedom from complication. It usually lasts for two to three days after a major operation, but may extend to a week or more if the injury is serious or becomes complicated.

'Turning point'. A sense of well-being is experienced, the appetite returns and ambulation is requested, but weakness is still marked.

Weight gain. The chief feature of this phase is restoration of body protein with the build-up of skeletal muscle. It may last three to ten weeks and is accompanied by increased appetite and muscular strength. There is little gain in body fat.

Fat gain. This stage may last for weeks or months depending on the losses incurred after injury. The body-weight and appearance are restored with the resumption of storage of body fat. Obesity may follow unless care is exercised.

Metabolic events

After injury or operation three major metabolic changes can be observed:

(*a*) The most obvious feature is weight loss. Between 5 and 10 per cent of bodyweight may be lost after a major abdominal operation, largely the result of breakdown of cellular protoplasm, with the release of amino-acids and intracellular electrolytes. Cellular protein from skeletal muscle and organs is hydrolysed, the nitrogen being excreted in the urine mainly as urea. Potassium is released from the cells and floods the extracellular fluid—as much as 100 to 300 mmol per day.

(*b*) The volume of urine is scanty and the urinary losses of sodium chloride and bicarbonate are reduced, due to selective changes in the renal handling of water, salt and acid. In contrast, the urinary excretion of potassium is normal or often increased. A mild metabolic alkalosis may develop. These changes in renal function are more marked if the circulatory blood volume has been reduced. The result will be to restore the volume of extracellular fluid.

(*c*) A patient may not eat after an operation, but if he is healthy and well-nourished, starvation for a few days will make little difference to him. He will exist on his own stores of fat and protein. There are three endogenous sources of energy: first, after injury glycogenolysis and gluconeogenesis are increased with accompanying reduction in glucose tolerance; but these mechanisms provide only a small source of calories (about 1600 calories) which is rapidly exhausted; second, the breakdown of protein in muscle is of some help but is an expensive source of calories and is relatively inefficient; third, oxidation of stored body fat meets most of the caloric needs of the body after injury. This process involves the mobilisation of free fatty acids from storage triglycerides with their subsequent hydrolysis and metabolism in the Krebs cycle. The factors influencing this post-traumatic mobilisation are not clear. If there are no complications, energy requirements are normal. Additional energy may have to be supplied if there is excessive tissue destruction, complicating sepsis, increased mechanical work as in dyspnoea, or increased thermal work as after a burn, or in a fever, or if the patient has been depleted beforehand, such as in malignant disease. After such complicated injury, 300 to 500 g of fat are oxidised daily with the production of 2700 to 4500 calories; at the same time there is release of a considerable amount of water (1 litre for each kg of fat).

Endocrine events

Certain changes in function of the endocrine organs accompany the metabolic events.

Adrenal cortex. Due to increased secretion of adrenocorticotrophic hormone from the pituitary gland, *cortisol* production is also increased, being one of the earliest changes noted after injury. There is a consequent rise in the level of cortisol metabolites in the urine for several days. The factors responsible for the increased secretion of the adrenocorticotrophic hormone are not clear but are probably the result of nervous and humoral stimuli arising in the injured area. A raised aldosterone output, stimulated by acute reduction in blood volume, is brought about by increased secretion of adrenocorticotrophic hormone by the pituitary, of glomerulotrophic hormone in midbrain and of renin which is converted to angiotensin, thereby stimulating the adrenal cortex directly to produce aldosterone. The result is a reduced excretion of sodium bicarbonate in the urine with an increased loss of potassium. The metabolic response to surgery cannot be entirely explained in terms of increased adrenocortical activity, and it is most likely that the adrenal steroids play a permissive role in the metabolic and endocrine responses.

Adrenal medulla. A reduced blood volume and associated hypoxia stimulate the secretion of adrenaline and noradrenaline. In addition to their action on peripheral blood-vessels these substances also promote hepatic glycogenolysis.

Antidiuretic hormone. The secretion of antidiuretic hormone from the posterior pituitary gland is increased after injury as a result of a reduction in blood volume. Urinary output is diminished. This effect may be prolonged if an injury is severe or complicated. Excessive intake of water as by injudicious intravenous fluid therapy may cause severe dilution of the constituents of the serum.

Gonads. Amenorrhoea in the female and loss of libido in the male are usual after an injury. These gonadal functions usually return when the patient enters into the phase of nitrogen anabolism.

Factors affecting the metabolic response

Several factors can influence the extent and duration of the metabolic response to injury.

1. *Nutrition of the patient*. Patients who are underweight, or, more properly, have a reduced lean body mass, will excrete less nitrogen after injury and as a result they can be kept in positive balance by a modest intake. Consequently the breakdown of protein is much less in women and the greatest loss is found in muscular men.

2. *Nutrition intake*. The transient reduction in intake of food after an operation is not particularly harmful to well-nourished patients, despite increased protein catabolism. Greater reduction in body stores of nitrogen may occur in those with more severe injury, but a modest increase in intake

is capable of overcoming the net losses. In patients unable to eat, intravenous nutrition may combat the losses in the post-operative period but there is little evidence that the continuous intravenous infusion of calories and amino-acids will benefit the vast majority of patients undergoing elective surgery. The maintenance of an adequate nutritional intake is of some importance in those already under-nourished and who have undergone a major operation, after which normal oral feeding would be impossible for a week or more. Prolonged loss of nitrogen, uncompensated by adequate intake, will delay wound healing, increase susceptibility to infection and lead to excessive weight loss, often associated with an increase in mortality.

3. *Severity of injury*. The amount of protein catabolised and therefore the amount of weight loss after an injury are related to its severity. Post-operative complications such as wound infection or venous thrombosis prolong the catabolic phase.

4. *Hypovolaemia*. If hypovolaemia (reduction of blood volume) is prevented or treated effectively, the breakdown of protein is greatly reduced.

Significance of metabolic response

The endocrine and metabolic changes, in response to injury, seem to be directed towards water and salt conservation, maintenance of blood pressure, general mobilisation of carbohydrates and fat, elaboration of hormones essential for cell life, and the production of energy for muscles, heart and brain. Most of the components of the response are quantitatively related to the severity of the injury so that the first step in a smooth short convalescence after injury is the skilful and gentle operative technique. The metabolic changes observed after injury are normal and attempts to overcome them are not beneficial.

SHOCK

Shock is a clinical syndrome resulting from inadequate perfusion of the tissues with blood. There is restlessness, anxiety and agitation. The skin is cold and clammy, quickly becomes mottled and ultimately cyanosed although initially in septic shock it may be warm, dry and pink. The pulse is rapid, weak and thready, the blood-pressure low and the nail beds are cyanosed with poor capillary refill after compression. The respirations may become stertorous and the urine output scanty.

Aetiology

So many factors are involved in the production of shock that the use of a single term to cover the many causes and the various clinical manifestations has to be deprecated. In the production of the clinical syndrome three factors must be considered—the heart as a pump, the blood volume and the peripheral circulation. Each may be abnormal for more than one reason, to varying degree and at various times during the course of the syndrome. In any one particular type of shock one form of abnormality usually predominates.

Types of shock

The major types of shock are:

1. **Oligaemic shock**—the blood volume is reduced due to loss of blood, plasma or fluid from the circulating blood volume. Such loss may be obvious as in bleeding from a severed artery (haemorrhagic shock), exudation of plasma from burned skin or excessive vomiting. The loss may be occult and the cause of the shock not immediately evident, as in the considerable loss of blood into the body cavities and tissues after severe injury (traumatic shock), the exudation of plasma into the peritoneal cavity in peritonitis or the sequestration of water and salt in dilated coils of obstructed intestine.
2. **Cardiogenic shock** occurs in myocardial infarction, cardiac tamponade and pulmonary embolism and is brought about by the failure of the heart as a pump.
3. **Arteriolar and capillary vasodilatation** as observed in the following:
   (a) *Septic shock* (endotoxic shock) can be caused by either Gram-negative or Gram-positive organisms. The Gram-negative organisms frequently encountered are *Esch. coli* and *Proteus*. Shock is probably produced by the action of endotoxins released by bacteria; lipopolysaccharides produce an initial intense vasoconstriction, partly by direct

action on the blood-vessels and partly by the release of endogenous catecholamines. Vasoconstriction is quickly replaced by vasodilatation due to exhaustion of the adrenal cortex and the release of histamine. Blood begins to pool and sludge in capillaries and veins and clotting may occur. Gram-negative septicaemia is particularly liable to occur after colonic and biliary operations and urological procedures.

(b) *Anaphylaxis* which results from an antigen-antibody reaction, previous sensitisation by an antigen having occurred. The latter reacts with the antibody bound to the surface of the mast cell releasing a number of chemical substances, chiefly histamine. These substances cause intense constriction of the bronchioles, congestion of the small veins and increased permeability of capillaries.

(c) *Acute adrenal failure*. The normal response to shock or injury is accompanied by increased secretion of glucocorticoids from the adrenal glands whose main effect in this context is to sensitise the arterioles to the action of catecholamines. Lack of glucocorticoids, due to destruction or absence of the adrenals, can lead to a clinical state similar to shock.

4. **Neurogenic shock** (vasovagal shock). This is a simple faint, often precipitated by pain or fear. The heart action slows due to reflex vagal action. There is rarely any confusion with other forms of shock because of its transient nature and the accompanying bradycardia.

Pathophysiology of shock

The pathophysiology of shock can best be understood by describing the type of shock about which most is known—haemorrhagic shock. In the early stages after a small haemorrhage, reduction in blood volume leads to a diminished venous return to the heart. Cardiac output falls with consequent reduction in the arterial blood-pressure. Various compensatory reflexes, originating in receptors in the aortic arch, carotid sinus and other great vessels are stimulated, and counteract a threatened reduction in cerebral circulation. As a result medullary sympathetic neurones are stimulated to produce constriction of small vessels, increased return of blood to the heart and more forceful cardiac contractions. Catecholamine secretion causes increased vasoconstriction which is most marked in the skin, kidney and intestinal mucosa. Reciprocal inhibition of vagal efferents leads to a tachycardia; the cardiac output is increased. There is complete compensation for a moderate haemorrhage, at the expense of hypoxia in the vasoconstricted area.

If bleeding persists the reflex compensatory mechanisms no longer suffice, cardiac output may be reduced and the blood flow to vital organs will be decreased. Some degree of protection is accorded by a redistribution of blood flow away from less vital areas to the heart and brain. Thus ischaemia of the skin will produce its characteristic cold clammy feeling and reduction of renal blood flow will lead to a diminished excretion of urine. Impairment of cerebral circulation will cause the characteristic restlessness, confusion and agitation. Such redistribution of blood may initially maintain a supply to the critical organs but ultimately this flow will also be impaired. The intestine suffers partly due to the general reduction in cardiac output and partly as a result of intense vasoconstriction in the mucosa, so that the normal barrier to the absorption of bacteria and other noxious agents within the intestinal lumen may be overcome. Such absorption and a reduced ability of the reticulo-endothelial system to detoxify may be the cause of eventual deterioration.

Vasoconstriction, the principal factor in the body's response to blood loss, eventually becomes a destructive force. The reduced renal blood flow leads to a fall in the glomerular filtration rate with consequent impairment of the renal regulation of acid-base status and fluid and electrolyte balance. Renal tubules are particularly vulnerable to ischaemia and acute tubular necrosis may follow. In prolonged shock, acidosis becomes extreme not only due to renal failure but also as a result of tissue hypoxia which shifts cellular metabolism towards anaerobic glycolysis. Acidosis impairs the heart action. Almost all patients who suffer major injury show an abnormal pattern of ventilation with increased rate of breathing, decreased tidal volume and increased arterio-venous pulmonary shunting. These features are the result of an increase in 'lung stiffness', due to an increased interstitial accumulation of sodium and water. In the terminal stages blood pools and sludges in the under-perfused capillaries and intravascular clotting leads to further ischaemia. Perfusion of the tissues becomes almost non-existent and the heart begins to fail. Fluids and proteins leak into the extravascular space and ventricular fibrillation may occur at any time resulting in death.

An important homeostatic mechanism after severe haemorrhage is compensatory haemodilution. Fluid is mobilised into the intravascular compartment, sometimes at rates of up to 1 litre per hour. As a result oligaemia can be quickly corrected with, of course, the production of a secondary anaemia. Within a few days, provided hepatic function is unimpaired, plasma proteins will be mobilised from the body protein pool. Ultimately, the marrow will produce new blood cells.

The underlying mechanisms in other types of shock are less clear.

(a) *Septic shock.* In some forms of septic shock the myocardium is chiefly affected; as a result congestive cardiac failure may be a prominent feature and in contrast to the patient with oligaemic shock, the central and neck veins are congested. In these patients therapeutic efforts are directed to improving cardiac action using digitalis and infusions of isoprenaline. In other types of septic shock the precipitating cause of the shock is generalised vasodilatation with pooling of blood in the tissues and loss of fluid through capillary walls which have become increasingly permeable. White cells and platelets are affected by the damage to capillary endothelium, producing widespread arteriolar and capillary thrombosis (disseminated intravascular coagulation). Platelets are consumed in excess and, as a result, there is an increased predisposition to bleeding, especially from the gastrointestinal tract. In the early stages of this type of shock, the skin is warm and flushed compared with the pallor and clamminess of oligaemic shock. There is some evidence that the severe effects of bacteraemic shock are largely the direct result of endotoxic damage to organs, particularly the liver and heart.

(b) In *cardiogenic shock*, as after a myocardial infarction, the primary defect is the failure of the heart as a pump, but autonomic dysfunction with generalised vasoconstriction may also contribute to the deterioration. Of particular importance is the fall in diastolic blood-pressure.

Treatment

The principal aims in treatment are to restore perfusion of all critical tissues, to ensure an adequate supply of oxygen and nutrients and to remove metabolites. The details depend on the type and cause of the shock. A vaso-vagal attack responds rapidly to relief of pain, warmth, reassurance and the head-down position.

Oligaemic shock. The immediate treatment is to arrest haemorrhage by elevation of the bleeding area, compression of the affected part and, if necessary, clamping of the bleeding vessel with a haemostat and subsequent ligature. Tourniquets should be avoided because of the considerable damage to muscles and nerves that may result. The blood volume should then be restored by infusion of the type of fluid lost. Thus blood should be given to the patient with haemorrhagic or traumatic shock, plasma to the burned patient and electrolyte solutions in severe vomiting and diarrhoea, although in the last instance rapid restoration of the blood volume may occasionally be required to save life and this is better achieved by the administration of a plasma expander (p. 29), or of balanced salt solution containing potassium and lactate as well as sodium and chloride.

Except where blood loss is directly measured as during an operation, the amount has to be estimated by clinical examination, special investigations and the response to treatment. Although the general appearance and altered blood-pressure and pulse-rate do not provide an accurate estimate of the volume lost, their return to normal is a good guide to adequacy of replacement. The amount of blood loss into soft tissues after their injury can often be estimated by the approximate relationship between volume loss and the extent of injury (Table 2).

A reliable guide to transfusion is the measurement of the pressure within the great veins and the right atrium of the heart, or Central Venous Pressure (C.V.P.), by means of a catheter inserted into an elbow or neck vein and passed into the great veins or right atrium. A single measurement is usually of little value but observation of changes in

Table 2 Relationship between blood loss and tissue injury

Volume of soft tissue injury*	Fracture	Approximate volume of blood lost (litres)
Less than 1 'hand'	Ankle	Less than 0·5
1 to 3 hands	Both bones of leg	0.5 to 1.5
3 to 5 hands	Femur	1.0 to 2.0
Greater than 5 hands	Pelvis	More than 2

*Given as volume of clenched fist.

pressure levels following blood volume replacement is helpful. If the central venous pressure is normal or below normal and there is arterial hypotension, a test infusion of a plasma expander should be given. A rise in central venous pressure may warn against further transfusions. Interpretation requires considerable skill particularly if the patient is on certain drugs, is receiving artificial ventilation, or in the terminal stages of shock where the heart is beginning to fail because of poor coronary perfusion. There is some experimental evidence that measurement of the pulmonary artery pressure or pulmonary wedge pressure may be a better guide to treatment but such intensive monitoring is usually confined to the intensive care unit and has not found widespread application in clinical practice.

Septic shock. There is no drug with specific effect on the tissue damage produced by endotoxin, but drugs are used to restore cardiac output and to improve tissue perfusion, whilst antibiotics are given to counteract organisms in the blood stream. The choice of antibiotics will be dictated by the sensitivity of the organism isolated from the blood on culture. In most cases the organism is sensitive to gentamicin, lincomycin or metronidazole which are the antibiotics of choice until the results of culture and antibiotic sensitivity results are available. The dose of the drug is related to the blood levels produced. Oxygen is given, usually by intermittent positive pressure ventilation. Digitalisation of the heart is beneficial to avoid atrial fibrillation. Failure to respond to this treatment suggests a continuing surgical catastrophe such as collections of pus or segments of gangrenous bowel which should be diagnosed and treated as quickly as possible.

To improve myocardial contractility, positive inotropic drugs are administered, especially in septic shock. Catecholamines are widely used and given by continuous intravenous infusion. Isoprenaline (0.02–0.18μg/kg/min) which acts on beta-adrenergic receptors, increases cardiac output but reduces arterial pressure and therefore may reduce renal vascular perfusion. Noradrenaline (0.01–0.07 μg/kg/min) has a predominantly pressor action so that at high dose cardiac output is reduced and renal blood flow may fall. Dopamine (1–30 μg/kg/min) shows the haemodynamic effects of the two previous drugs but in addition will produce vasodilatation of the renal and mesenteric vessels, through its action on specific dopamine receptors. Dopamine therefore seems to combine the advantageous action of the catecholamines.

The following agents are also of value in the management of shock.

Oxygen. Tissue hypoxia in shock is the result of the reduction in cardiac output and consequent poor peripheral perfusion. There is also evidence of intrapulmonary shunting of blood from the venous to arterial side of the circulation with reduced contact of blood with alveolar air. Oxygen therefore is administered in an attempt to correct tissue hypoxia.

Vasoconstrictor and vasodilator drugs. Vasoconstrictor drugs, such as the catecholamines, increase the blood-pressure by constricting the renal, skin and splanchnic vessels, but may cause irreversible ischaemic changes. Drugs which block the effect of adrenaline on alpha receptors, such as phenoxybenzamine, are used. Their vasodilator effects produce a fall in blood-pressure and during their administration adequate replacement of blood to maintain the circulating blood volume is necessary. Overloading is also to be avoided and the central venous pressure should be frequently measured to control the rate of fluid replacement. In this type of treatment the blood-pressure may remain low but perfusion of tissues improves, extremities become warm and flushed and the urine output increases.

Steroids. In shock due to acute adrenal failure administration of hydrocortisone is mandatory. The use of adrenal cortical steroids in other types of shock is less well-founded, although they may have a direct pharmacological action on blood vessels to reduce arterial vasoconstriction, which may make their use valuable in septic shock.

Digitalis. This is often required in cardiogenic shock. In severe septic and haemorrhagic shock digitalis may be occasionally indicated as poor filling of the coronary vessels may impair cardiac function.

Analgesics. Morphine should only be given when pain is severe as sedatives may suffice to relieve anxiety. The intravenous route is preferable to ensure rapid and controlled absorption.

BLOOD TRANSFUSION

Blood is most frequently transfused to restore a depleted blood volume and so permit adequate perfusion of the tissues. It may also be given to overcome a specific defect in the blood components as in restoring red cells in anaemia before an urgent operation or occasionally to supply platelets in thrombocytopenia. Blood transfusion carries some risk and alternative methods should be chosen whenever possible. Anaemia is often better corrected before operation by prescribing oral or parenteral iron. Blood is also used extensively in the preparation of various forms of apparatus, such as an extra-corporeal circulation in cardiac surgery or an artificial kidney for dialysis.

Compatibility

Before transfusion, the serum of the recipient should, whenever possible, be matched with the cells of the donor. Although as many as fifteen, genetically independent, major systems of red cell blood groups have been described, in practice it is necessary to have blood homologous in respect of ABO and Rh antigen D for a transfusion to be successful. In the ABO blood-group system, antigens (agglutinogens) of two types exist in red blood corpuscles. They are denoted A and B; they may occur in the combination A, B and AB or they may be absent. The four blood groups which thus result are given the symbols A, B, AB and O respectively to denote which, if any, of these antigens is present in the cells.

Agglutination of the corpuscles is caused by reaction with antibodies (agglutinins) present in the serum; these are termed anti-A, which reacts with any corpuscles containing antigen A, and anti-B, which reacts similarly with cells containing antigen B. The grouping of the blood of a patient depends on the reaction of the red cells to stock specimens of anti-A and anti-B sera. This should be cross-checked by typing the patient's serum against known A and B red cells. Numerous other blood-antigens exist, of which the most important is the *Rhesus (Rh) Factor*. An Rh-positive person (83 per cent of the British population) possesses the Rh antigen D, which an Rh-negative person lacks. The clinical importance of the Rh system depends primarily on the ability of the D antigen to induce antibody formation when it is introduced into a circulation which lacks it. Rh-negative subjects may be sensitised with Rh-positve blood; an Rh-negative mother may be sensitised when she bears an Rh-positive child. Later transfusions of Rh-positive blood in a thus sensitised Rh-negative patient will then give rise to agglutination and haemolysis of the transfused blood.

Accurate cross-matching of blood is a complex procedure, details of which may be sought in appropriate textbooks. Routine cross-matching can normally be done in two hours, but emergency techniques are available whereby accurate cross-matching can be speeded up and reported in half an hour. If the emergency is greater than this it is preferable to give uncross-matched Group O blood (containing no A or B antigens) which is Rh negative, but it must be accepted that there is an element of risk in using any form of uncross-matched blood.

Complications and hazards of blood transfusion

Blood transfusion is a serious procedure carrying the risk of complications which may be classified into:

1. The dangers associated with transfusion of any fluid; thrombophlebitis, fever, allergic skin rashes and painful joints due to contaminating foreign proteins (less common with plastic disposable transfusion sets), right heart failure from overloading the circulation and air embolism. Over-transfusion causes a rise in the venous pressure and later pulmonary oedema, particularly in the elderly or debilitated or in

those with pre-existing cardio-pulmonary disease. It may be prevented by accurate monitoring of the venous pressure, and where indicated by the use of packed red cells rather than whole blood. Over-transfusion can be treated by the rapid removal of blood by venesection, the use of limb tourniquets inflated to above diastolic pressure and by the administration of diuretics.

2. The especial dangers of using blood.
   (a) *Infection*. Accidental bacterial contamination of the blood at the time of collection is rare, and the storage of blood at an acid pH between 2 and 6 °C prevents bacterial proliferation and survival. Occasionally bacterial endotoxins may be present in transfused blood and on transfusion lead to a severe pyrexial reaction with cardiovascular collapse. The main source of bacterial contamination is the drip insertion site. While syphilis, malaria and brucellosis may also be transmitted, the most serious problem is serum hepatitis due to the transmission of a virus (p. 235).
   (b) *Hyperkalaemia*. Prolonged storage of blood causes a rise in the plasma potassium concentrations to 20 to 30 mmol per litre but there is little danger of producing hyperkalaemia because the stored cells when transfused act as a sponge. Hypokalaemia may be a problem.
   (c) *Hypocalcaemia*. Citrate is added to stored blood as an anticoagulant and acts by removing all ionised calcium. An excess of citrate in stored blood may also remove calcium ions from the recipient's blood and so potentiate the action of potassium on the heart leading to impairment in myocardial contraction. There are muscle tremors and circulatory depression. With massive transfusions of blood the patient should therefore be protected by giving calcium gluconate, 1 g for every 1000 ml of blood transfused. The risk of citrate intoxication is particularly important in children or in the presence of liver disease. The injection of ionised calcium solutions may only be partially helpful and where rapid and massive transfusions are required citrated blood is better avoided.
   (d) *Hypothermia*. The rapid transfusion of large quantities of cold blood may lead to a general reduction in the body temperature. Cooling of the heart may predispose to cardiac arrest and blood should be warmed during infusion.
   (e) *Haemostasis*. The storage of blood results in a reduction in the number of platelets and the loss of factors essential for coagulation. Where large transfusions are being given rapidly, the recipient's own coagulation factors are diluted so that oozing of blood may become general.

Serological incompatibility

The clinical picture of a patient who receives a transfusion of incompatible blood is that of headache, fever, rigors, paraesthesiae, dyspnoea, severe loin pain, jaundice which commences about 12 hours after transfusion, haemoglobinuria, occasionally oliguria and even anuria due to renal tubular damage. Severe collapse with low blood-pressure may occur. Diagnosis may be difficult since fever and rigors may result from pyrogens present in the transfusion apparatus or infected blood. Loin pain although characteristic may not occur, or the patient may be anaesthetised during the transfusion so that this symptom will not be manifest. When untoward reaction occurs the transfusion must be stopped, the blood carefully rechecked, and the pathologist informed and supplied with a specimen of blood and urine from the patient. The donor's blood should also be rechecked. Collapse may require the use of intramuscular methedrine and occasionally intravenous noradrenaline. Loin pain may be severe enough to require morphine for its relief. A careful record is kept of the urinary output and a catheter should be inserted into the urinary bladder. Damage to the kidney is related to the rate of urine production and its *p*H; alkalinisation of the urine prevents the precipitation of haemoglobin within the tubules and therefore attempts are made to initiate a diuresis and alkalinise the urine, by giving 20 per cent mannitol and sodium bicarbonate. Should there be oliguria or anuria, the prognosis is reasonably good providing the general condition can be maintained during the critical period of three weeks before tubular recovery and diuresis occur. Detailed management of such patients is considered on p. 273.

An incompatible blood transfusion is preventable by meticulous care in the checking of blood before its administration, both in the pathological laboratory and again in the ward or operating theatre.

Blood substitutes

The potential dangers of blood transfusion and the high cost and occasional scarcity of blood have led to the search for some form of substitute. For the treatment of shock, the essential characteristic of a substitute solution is that it should restore and maintain the volume of fluid circulating in the vascular system of the shocked patient.

Plasma. At one time plasma was available in a dried form which, by the addition of sterile water, could be stored for many years without refrigeration. Dried plasma is now being replaced by plasma protein fraction, which is a 4.5 g per 100 ml protein solution with the same colloid osmotic pressure as reconstituted dried plasma. Plasma protein fraction, mainly albumin, is superior to dried plasma because it is ready for infusion (not requiring the delay of reconstitution) and does not carry the risk of homologous serum hepatitis.

Plasma is rarely indicated for the treatment of the shocked patient. In emergency circumstances Ringer's lactate or other buffered saline solution is as effective with fewer complications. Rapid expansion of blood volume can be brought about by the administration of dextran (q.v.).

Fresh frozen plasma obtained from one individual and so carrying little risk of hepatitis, contains most of the factors responsible for blood clotting, particularly factors V and VIII which are destroyed in stored blood.

Dextran. Dextran is a glucose polymer of high molecular weight produced by the fermentation of sucrose by *Leuconostoc mesenteroides*. Various molecular ranges have been produced, but for the emergency treatment of haemorrhage the most useful are dextran 110 and dextran 70. Low molecular weight dextran of 30 000 to 40 000 is said to reduce in shock the clumping of red blood cells in the microcirculation, but its role has not been fully substantiated and in the treatment of shock dextrans 110 and 70 are preferred. They have a colloidal osmotic pressure comparable with plasma and can be given to patients of any blood group. They are easily stored and there is no risk of hepatitis.

Blood component replacement

With modern techniques it is now possible to prepare and administer with safety products, fractions and concentrations of whole blood.

Of the cellular components, red cells are easily separated and are useful for the treatment of anaemia in patients in whom circulatory over-loading may be a hazard. To minimise damage to red cells and encourage their rapid recovery after thawing, red cells freed from donor plasma, leucocytes and platelets, can be frozen. Although frozen blood cells are being increasingly used, especially in the United States, red cells freed from plasma and other cellular elements can also be preserved by the addition of adenine to the conventional citrate phosphate dextrose to enhance red cell viability. Platelets can also be separated and presented as either a platelet-rich plasma or as a platelet concentrate. Although the function of platelets is partially impaired in the preparation of these products, they can be effective in arresting bleeding due to severe thrombocytopenia. It is not yet possible to transfuse white cells satisfactorily because they carry histocompatibility antigens.

The other products which are available include antihaemophiliac globulin (A.H.G.) concentrate and factor IX concentrate, the former as a plasma cryoprecipitate. Desiccated human fibrinogen is commercially available and albumin has also been concentrated and has the advantage that it is a hepatitis-free product. Salt-poor albumin is available for use in patients with sodium retention.

WATER AND ELECTROLYTE BALANCE IN SURGICAL PATIENTS

In health the volume and composition of the body fluids remain relatively constant, but in disease and after injury the regulatory mechanisms which maintain this constancy may be impaired to an extent that the surgeon may have to intervene and impose external control upon the fluid balance. In surgical practice derangements in fluid and electrolyte balance originate, for the most part, in the gastro-intestinal tract, either because of defective intake such as malignant obstruction of the oesophagus, or because of excessive loss, as in the persistent vomiting of intestinal obstruction.

To recognise and treat disorders of water and electrolyte balance, it is necessary to know: (*a*) what is normal—namely, the distribution of water and electrolytes throughout the body and the regulating mechanisms involved and (*b*) what abnormalities may arise and recognise and treat the appropriate disorder.

Body water

The total amount of water in the body varies with age, sex and adiposity. The amount of water in the body is proportional to the lean body mass, so that there is proportionately less water in fat people than in thin. For example, females having a smaller lean body mass have proportionately less body water. In a 70 kg adult male, body water represents 60 per cent of the body-weight, more in children, and tends to decrease with age and obesity. Body water is divided into two major compartments:

Intracellular water (40 per cent of body-weight) and

Extracellular water (20 per cent of body-weight) which is subdivided into:

(a) an *intravascular compartment* (3.5 to 5 per cent body-weight) which carries the cellular elements of the blood, has a protein content higher than the extravascular (interstitial) fluid and

(b) an *extravascular compartment* which can be further divided into *interstitial fluid*, which is in contact with the cells (separated from them only by cell membranes) and with the plasma (separated by the capillary membranes which permit the flow of all except the cellular elements and large protein molecules), and *transcellular fluid*, which is produced by cells and has an electrolyte composition different from plasma and the interstitial fluid, *e.g.* cerebrospinal fluid, secretions of the gastro-intestinal tract and fluid in serous spaces.

Electrolytes

The major cation of the *extracellular fluid* is sodium (approximately 140 mmol per litre) and the major anions are chloride, bicarbonate and protein; the concentration of potassium in the extracellular fluid is only 4 mmol per litre. In the *intracellular fluid* compartment the major cation is potassium and the major anions are protein and organic phosphate; the concentration of sodium is low. The maintenance of the difference between the extracellular and intracellular concentrations of cations depends largely upon the active extrusion of sodium ions from the cell by sodium pump. Damage to the cells as in hypoxia can interfere with the pump, so that sodium will enter easily and potassium will leak out of the cells. Because of the predominant presence of sodium in the extracellular fluid, the estimation of plasma sodium will give a rough approximation of total body content of sodium, whereas the potassium level in plasma gives little index of the total body content of potassium.

Osmotic pressure

The concentration of osmotically active particles remains remarkably constant among the body compartments because of the free mobility of water across cellular and capillary membranes. As the principal osmotic particles in the compartments are the major cations, the osmolarity of the extracellular compartment is related to its concentration of sodium and that of the intracellular compartment to that of potassium. The osmotic pressure of serum and urine is measured usually by the depression of the freezing point of the fluid, and expressed as the *osmolality* (mosmol/kg) rather than the osmolarity (mosmol/l). The normal serum osmolality is 270 to 300 mosmol per kg. The normal urinary osmolality varies widely from 50 to 1200 mosmol per kg and in the most concentrated urines may attain a value approximately four times that of the plasma from which it is derived. If the solute content of one compartment is changed, the volume of that compartment will be altered to maintain isotonicity with the other compartments. Thus the addition or removal of sodium ions will cause expansion or contraction of the extracellular space.

Regulatory mechanisms and baseline requirements

In spite of large variations in intake, the composition of the body remains constant as the result of regulatory mechanisms which precisely balance the intake and output of water and electrolytes.

Water intake has to provide for (*a*) an adequate *output of urine*: if all products of metabolism are to be excreted, this may be as little as 600 ml in 24 hours in a young healthy adult but may amount to more than 1.0 to 1.5 litres in a sick patient after an operation and with some impairment of renal function; and (*b*) *insensible loss* which is incurred by the evaporation of water from the respiratory tract and from skin surfaces. The volume of fluid lost by evaporation is approximately 500 to 800 ml as electrolyte-free water.

The requirement for water is largely met from the intake but is supplemented from endogenous sources, from cellular breakdown and the oxidation of fat. The basal requirement to maintain balance is approximately 1.0 to 2.0 litres per 24 hours. Water balance is controlled through the thirst-neurohypophysis-renal axis, adjusted to maintain a plasma osmolality of approximately 300 mosmol per kg. In health, thirst controls the intake of water and the neurohypophysis regulates the release of antidiuretic hormone which controls the selective excretion of water by the kidney.

Sodium balance is largely maintained by precise regulation of its excretion. The average intake of sodium is about 100 mmol per day but about 75 mmol of sodium only are required to meet basal requirements. Sodium is largely lost through the kidneys. Most of the sodium in the glomerular filtrate is removed by active reabsorption in the proximal tubules, where the regulatory mechanisms are incompletely understood. Further adjustment of sodium balance is made in the distal tubules, under the control of adrenocortical hormones, in particular aldosterone, whose own secretion is controlled by several mechanisms, activated largely by variations in blood volume. Only small amounts of sodium are lost in the stool or in the sweat. When the sodium intake is low, sodium may therefore disappear from the urine completely, so efficient is the mechanism for its conservation.

Potassium intake varies but the basal requirements are usually met by a daily intake of 40 mmol. In health, losses of potassium from the body are mainly in the urine and potassium balance is primarily regulated by its renal excretion. This is largely dependent on the tubular secretion of potassium in exchange for sodium. Thus the control of the external balance of potassium is much less effective than that of sodium and frequently the body ensures sodium balance at the expense of that of potassium.

The baseline requirements for water and electrolytes, as detailed above, vary greatly. These baseline requirements will be increased in fever, excessive sweating, in the young and in the large (but not in obesity) and in hyperthyroidism. Baseline requirements will be correspondingly reduced in the old, the small, the obese and in those who have hypothyroidism.

Disorders of fluid and electrolyte balance

In surgical patients deficiency of water and electrolytes is more common than excess, the latter being usually the result of unwise treatment. Pure water and pure sodium deficiencies are uncommon; the more usual presentation is that of a mixed deficiency. To give a clear picture of the method of production and results of the deficiency, however, the 'pure' abnormalities will be described.

Water depletion

This deficiency largely results because the patient cannot or will not drink. It is therefore seen in the untreated unconscious patient, in the apathetic and the old, or in malignant obstruction of the oesophagus. Increased loss of water may occur from the skin when the body temperature is raised, from the lungs when there is an increased respiratory rate due to the rise in body temperature or hyperventilation, or from the urine, as in diabetes insipidus caused by the absence of vasopressin. In the presence of reduced intake and continuing insensible losses, the total amount of water in the body is decreased and, because water moves freely from one compartment to the other, this loss is distributed throughout all body compartments. Initially, to maintain isotonicity of the extracellular compartment, water flows out of the cells to produce cellular dehydration. At first there is only a small decrease in blood volume and oligaemic shock is a late feature. The patient becomes thirsty and has a dry mouth and skin, and the eyes are sunken. Urine with a high specific gravity is passed in greatly reduced amounts. Treatment is by the administration of water either by mouth or by means of a nasogastric tube, or by intravenous infusion of 5 per cent dextrose solution.

Sodium depletion

In surgical practice this is usually due to extrarenal loss of body fluid containing isotonic concentrations of the extracellular electrolytes. The common cause is loss from the gastro-intestinal tract by vomiting, nasogastric suction, diarrhoea or intestinal fistulae. Large volumes of fluid may also be lost from the extracellular compartment into physiologically inert sites, for example into the distended bowel in intestinal obstruction or into the peritoneal cavity in peritonitis. The fluid lost from the body derives initially from the plasma compartment which in turn is replenished from the tissue fluid compartment under the influence, partly, of a rising plasma protein concentration. Since the osmotic pressure of the tissue fluid tends to continue to fall, or at least not to rise, as sodium is lost, there will be no compensatory osmotic movement of water from the cells into the tissue fluids, as occurs in water deficiency. Hence the dehydration of sodium deficiency is mainly extracellular and results in a more rapid fall of plasma volume and of blood-pressure than in water deficiency. Oligaemia is encountered early and in acute sodium depletion the clinical features of shock rapidly develop. In the chronic situation, when water is retained by the kidneys to maintain plasma volume, there may be apathy and disorientation with anorexia, muscle cramp and weakness. There are usually no specific symptoms such as thirst.

In acute sodium depletion the urgent need is rapid replenishment of the blood volume, which can be achieved by administering colloidal solutions such as plasma or dextran or by infusion of isotonic electrolyte solutions. In more chronic loss the type of solution infused largely depends on the cause of the fluid loss; if this results from vomiting, sodium chloride solution (0.9 per cent) should be given. If the loss has been the result of diarrhoea or intestinal fistula, replacement should be with a balanced electrolyte solution which is isotonic with plasma and contains electrolytes in approximately the same concentration as the fluid being lost, for example Ringer-lactate solution. Potassium chloride should be given only when the renal output increases to normal volume.

In the most severe cases of loss of salt, the extracellular volume is much less reduced and therefore the requirement for water is restricted and hypertonic salt solution (3 per cent NaCl) may be required.

Water excess (water intoxication)

The usual cause is ill-advised and excessive intravenous infusion of glucose and water, particularly to those unable to excrete water due to antidiuresis, as in chronic illnesses, malignant disease and after operation. In normal circumstances the excess of water would be excreted but the post-operative secretion of antidiuretic hormone may prevent such excretion and result in water overloading. The water accumulates in the lungs and skin where intercellular space can be relatively easily expanded. Excess water in brain and muscle gives rise to oedema, headache and convulsions, nausea and vomiting. There is marked reduction of the concentration of electrolytes in the plasma. Early recognition of the abnormality and restriction of water intake provides adequate treatment.

Sodium excess

The cause is usually the excessive administration of solutes, both salt and protein (*e.g.* tube feeding), in the absence of sufficient water to permit renal excretion of the solute load. There are usually contributory mechanisms such as the relative impairment of renal function in the early stages after injury or in renal disease. Since the excessive quantities of sodium are slowly excreted in the urine the extracellular compartment is greatly expanded and the blood volume is increased, with subsequent development of congestive cardiac failure, pulmonary oedema and anasarca. The cardinal feature is an increase in the serum sodium concentration. Treatment consists of restricting the intake of sodium chloride and of providing sufficient water to permit urinary excretion of the large solute load. Water may be given orally, or intravenously as 5 per cent dextrose solution. Diuretics may be needed in some instances.

Potassium

Following injury or operation, potassium is lost from the cells and appears in the urine. In these circumstances there may be a transient rise in the plasma potassium concentration particularly in debilitated patients, but the concentration of potassium in the plasma is not a reliable index of the total body potassium or of the need for potassium administration. Thus in potassium deficiency, with a reduction in the body content of potassium, the plasma potassium concentration may be low, normal or even elevated.

(*a*) Potassium deficiency. This is usually the result of inadequate replacement of an abnormal *extrarenal* loss, which may result from vomiting or diarrhoea. Potassium deficiency may also be caused by abnormal *renal* loss, which may occur either after operation or during the administration of cortisone or diuretics or in chronic renal disease or hyperaldosteronism.

Reduction in plasma potassium concentration (*hypokalaemia*) may produce disorders in muscle function; thus paralytic ileus may be aggravated, muscle reflexes become depressed (occasionally proceeding to skeletal muscle paralysis) and cardiac arrhythmias may occur along with sensitivity of the heart to the action of digitalis. Weakness and extreme lethargy are common features of this disorder. There is often an associated alkalosis. The treatment of potassium deficiency consists of the administration of potassium chloride, preferably by mouth. Occasionally intravenous infusions have to be set up but precautions must be taken to avoid the considerable risk of potassium overdosage. Potassium should not be given intravenously to patients with a low urine output or in whom the concentration of plasma potassium is high. For these reasons it is not usually given in the early post-operative phase. Potassium should be given slowly, the rate not exceeding 30 mmol per hour and the total daily dose should be restricted below 100 mmol. It must never be given directly into a central venous pressure infusion.

(*b*) Potassium excess. This is often manifested as hyperkalaemia in which the plasma potassium concentration is above 6 mmol per litre. It is a potentially dangerous condition and death can occur due to cardiac arrest. It is a common accompaniment of renal failure, the rapid infusion of potassium solution or the transfusion of stored blood. When intracellular protein breakdown is excessive, as after injury, the extracellular potassium concentration may increase, particularly if at the same time there is diminished renal excretion. The aim of treatment is rapid reduction of the plasma concentration of potassium by the administration of glucose with insulin, and the prevention of the cardiac effects of potassium by infusion of calcium gluconate. In renal failure peritoneal dialysis or haemodialysis may be required.

Acid-base disorders of body fluids

Closely related to disturbance in water and electrolyte balance are alterations in the acid-base status of the body. Acid-base disturbances alone rarely cause death but combined with other disorders such as respiratory disease or electrolyte abnormalities they may threaten life. Acid-base abnormalities cannot be identified solely by clinical observation and precise biochemical techniques are required for diagnosis and treatment.

Management of these disorders has previously been difficult because of insufficient understanding of the modern acid-base theories of physical chemistry and by the lack of easy, reliable methods of measuring the *p*H of body fluids. In the now widely accepted Brønsted-Lowry system, attention is focused on the hydrogen ion (proton). An acid is defined as a proton (or hydrogen ion) donor and base as a proton acceptor. Strong acids are those which dissociate completely, or nearly so, to release protons; strong bases associate strongly with protons. With modern *p*H electrodes, the reaction of the blood can be determined rapidly from small volumes. The blood *p*H may be normal (7.35 to 7.45), low indicating acidosis, or high indicating alkalosis.

The reaction of the blood and other body fluids is maintained relatively constant by a variety of mechanisms; some of these are physiological, involving the function of the kidneys and the lungs, but more rapid alterations utilise buffer systems.

Buffers are substances which maintain a solution at a relatively constant *p*H, when strong acids or bases are added. A buffer system consists of two parts, a weak acid and a salt of that acid. The principal buffers in the extracellular fluid are carbonic acid and bicarbonate and in the intracellular fluid protein (haemoglobin in red cells) and proteinic anion.

The functions of the buffer system are expressed in the Henderson-Hasselbalch equation, which defines the *p*H in terms of the ratio of the salt and acid. The *p*H of extracellular fluid is defined primarily by the ratio of the amount of base bicarbonate (majority as sodium bicarbonate) to the amount of carbonic acid (related to CO_2 content of alveolar air) present in the blood:

$$pH = pK + \log\frac{BHCO_3}{H_2CO_3} = pK + \log\frac{27\,\text{mmol/l}}{1.33\,\text{mmol/l}}$$

$$= pK + \log\frac{20}{1} = 7.4$$

pK represents the dissociation constant of carbonic acid in the presence of base bicarbonate and by measurement is 6.1.

A corollary of the Henderson-Hasselbalch equation is that the *p*H of the blood sets the ratio [base]/[acid] for all buffer systems and indicates the status of the acid-base equilibrium. To determine the acid-base status we need to know the concentrations of one buffer pair. In clinical practice the usual ratio determined is [bicarbonate]/[carbonic acid]. The concentration of carbonic acid in the blood is related to the partial pressure of carbon dioxide (PCO_2) which can be easily measured. The PCO_2 is determined by alveolar ventilation.

Thus in alveolar hypoventilation, PCO_2 will rise above its normal mean pressure of 40 mmHg—a condition known as **respiratory acidosis** (the blood *p*H may be normal or low). This condition is seen in respiratory disorders such as an obstructed airway or depressed respiratory centre due to anaesthetic agents. The patient becomes restless and flushed, with a rise in blood-pressure and pulse-rate. The condition can be treated by clearing the airway and assisting ventilation by artificial means.

Conversely, the PCO_2 of the blood may be low, *i.e.* below 35 mmHg—a condition known as **respiratory alkalosis** (in which the blood *p*H may be normal or high). This condition is usually brought about by hyperventilation because of excessive stimulation of the respiratory centre caused by fear, or because of excessive artificial ventilation. Mild degrees of this condition are usual after operation and do not require treatment. Severe grades, which may lead to tetany and twitching of muscles, may be treated by depressing the ventilatory rate with narcotics. If hypoxia is the cause of excessive respiratory drive, oxygen should be administered.

There are several **non-respiratory** (formerly called metabolic) causes for disorders of acid-base status.

(1) A *non-respiratory* (*metabolic*) *acidosis* is brought about by the addition of strong acid. This may be due to the production of ketoacids in diabetes or of lactic acid in hypoxia, occurring after cardiac arrest, or retention of acids in renal failure. The removal of strong bases also leads to acidosis and may follow the loss of pancreatic juice or intestinal secretions in diarrhoea. Severe acidosis affects the actions of the heart leading to reduction in cardiac output and contributing to the severity of shock. The harmful effects of acidosis may be aggravated by associated abnormalities such as hypoxia and other electrolyte disorders. A non-respiratory acidosis may be corrected by administering sodium bicarbonate. To assess the severity of the acidosis and thus determine how much sodium bicarbonate should be given, it is necessary to calculate the non-respiratory (metabolic) component of the acid-base disorder. This calculation can be made by determining the buffer bases of the blood. The important *buffer bases* are bicarbonate, haemoglobinic anion and organic phosphate anion—amounting, in normal blood, to 42 mmol per litre. This amount of buffer base is unaffected by changes in the *p*H of the blood due to the respiratory component, that is carbonic acid or PCO_2. On the other hand the concentration of buffer base in the blood is significantly altered by metabolic processes which add strong acids or bases to, or subtract them from, the body fluids. Since the *p*H, PCO_2, total CO_2 in the blood or plasma and buffer base are related, it is feasible to derive the values of all if any two are known. This is usually done with the help of a nomogram. The appropriate quantity of sodium bicarbonate which should be given can then be calculated by a simple formula.

(2) *Non-respiratory* (*metabolic*) *alkalosis* results either from the addition of base or the loss of acid. The former may result from the excessive administration of alkalis in the treatment of peptic ulcer and the latter from vomiting of the acidic gastric juice in pyloric stenosis. The treatment of this condition mainly involves the correction of the cause.

To separate the respiratory and metabolic components of acid-base disorders, the most popular approach is the used of *standard bicarbonate* and base excess values.

The determination of *p*H and PCO_2 is preferably made by micro-methods. The non-respiratory (metabolic) component is measured as buffer base or 'base excess'. The latter value is calculated from the determination of plasma bicarbonate after standardisation of the blood with a standard partial pressure of CO_2 of 40 mm of mercury. The arbitrary normal for base *excess* is zero; any values above the upper limit of normal (+12) indicate a non-respiratory alkalosis; values below the lower limit of normal (−12) indicate non-respiratory acidosis.

Maintenance of fluid balance in surgical patients

In the majority of instances a well-hydrated individual on a normal intake until a few hours prior to surgery, during which there is not excessive fluid loss, presents no problem in regard to fluid and electrolyte balance. During the 24 hours of post-operative water retention, sips of fluid by mouth are sufficient. A simple fluid intake and output chart should be maintained, and provided that more than 1 litre of urine is passed during the 24 hours after operation and that there are no abnormal losses, no problem arises. Normal intake may then gradually be resumed.

The routine use of gastric aspiration and intravenous replacement is to be deprecated as unnecessary and potentially dangerous. Over-infusion of water from solutions such as glucose in the first 48 hours post-operatively may result in water intoxication (p. 32). Over-transfusion of saline during the same period may lead to salt retention (p. 32).

Certain major procedures, such as gastric or intestinal resection or development of paralytic ileus may necessitate gastric aspiration and intravenous fluid replacement. A careful record of the daily intake and output must be charted. In the early post-operative phase (48 hours) the basic requirements for fluid balance can be maintained by giving 1.5 to 2.0 litres of 5 per cent dextrose. After this the amount of fluid should be increased to 2.5 to 3.0 litres, made up of 1.0 litre Ringer lactate solution (supplying 150 mmol of sodium) and the remainder as 5 per cent dextrose solution. In addition to the basic requirements any abnormal loss from gastric aspiration, excessive sweating, fistula or diarrhoea must be replaced, and this should be done volume for volume by 0.9 per cent sodium choride solution or Ringer lactate. Potassium is added provided the urinary output is adequate, the normal daily requirement of 40 mmol being provided in 3 g of potassium chloride. The clinical condition, urinary output and estimation of haemoglobin, haematocrit, blood urea, serum electrolytes, urine specific gravity and the patient's weight, especially in children, should all be considered to ensure that the regime progresses satisfactorily.

Where dehydration and electrolyte imbalance have been present for some time before operation, measurement of the losses due to vomiting, naso-gastric aspiration or fistulous discharges and urinary output should be made and their electrolyte composition estimated. The previous losses may not be known if the patient has recently been admitted to hospital and the amount present in distended coils of intestine or as peritoneal exudate also cannot be measured. Assessment of the degree of deficiency can usually be made by a careful history and examination for laxity of subcutaneous tissues, the degree of dryness of skin and tongue, pulse volume, blood-pressure, type of respiration and mental state. Repeated vomiting accompanied by lassitude and giddiness on standing indicate a loss of 3 litres of extracellular fluid whilst up to 6 litres may have been lost where there is fainting, nausea and mental confusion with a reduction in blood-pressure. The estimation of haematocrit, serum electrolytes and blood urea are essential in providing a baseline for therapy but too much reliance should not be placed on them as they may be normal even in gross fluid and electrolyte depletion.

Initially the oligaemia should be treated by giving colloids such as plasma or dextran followed by electrolyte solutions. In severe deficiency it is inadvisable to attempt the restoration to normality at a rapid rate and replacement may be spread over two to three days. It is important to attempt restoration to as near a correct balance as possible before surgery in order to avoid any post-operative difficulty due to the further biochemical disturbance which is the normal sequel to operative trauma.

Frequent clinical observations must be made to evaluate rehydration, aided by daily estimations of haemoglobin, blood urea and serum electrolytes. It is important to look for signs of over-infusion.

Intravenous nutrition

Most patients undergo elective surgical operations without special nutritional problems but in some instances it is evident before operation that, because of weight-loss and depleted energy reserves, the patient will, during and after operation require nutritional support. In others, recovery from operation is delayed because of an inability to eat or absorb nutrients from the gastro-intestinal tract and for the maintenance of energy and the restoration of losses the intravenous route has to be used.

The ordinary Western male requires daily about 40 to 60 kcal per kg, of which 40 per cent is carbohydrate and 40 per cent fat. These requirements are increased by about 10 per cent in a patient undergoing elective surgery and are further increased by major injury or burns and by complications such as peritonitis. The caloric requirements of a 70 kg male after a complicated operation may be as high as 6000 kcal. The protein requirements are usually between 1 and 2 g per kg per 24 hours.

Although the body reserves of energy are considerable, only a fraction can be obtained from readily accessible stores. Carbohydrate as a source of calories is readily obtained from glycogen stored in the liver, but supplies only 1600 kcal and so provides the energy requirements for less than 12 hours. Energy can be obtained from protein, mainly in muscles. Although theoretically up to 25 000 kcal could be supplied from the muscle bulk of the body, there would be cellular breakdown to a level incompatible with life. Energy is stored in a relatively accessible form as fat in adipose tissue, which can supply up to 140 000 kcal, lasting for up to 25 days.

It is generally regarded that the consumption of these body stores for the supply of energy and protein (to any great extent) is on the whole deleterious and management is directed to prevention of catabolism, to rapid restoration of any losses which have been incurred and to promotion of anabolic repair.

Energy may be supplied to the body in several forms. Carbohydrate can be given as glucose which supplies 4 kcal per g. Glucose should be used as the source of carbohydrates because it is a normal constituent of blood and because it stimulates insulin release which may encourage the retention of nitrogen in muscle. An isotonic solution (200 kcal per l) would not meet energy requirements to any great extent. Hypertonic carbohydrate solutions are used but after operation there may be impaired tolerance to glucose, much of which may be lost in the urine; hypertonic solutions are also highly irritating to the vein endothelium. Fructose has been advocated, principally because its metabolism is independent of insulin and it undergoes more rapid metabolism in the liver, but fructose is also excreted in the urine and can induce lactic acidosis. Other carbohydrate solutions, such as sorbitol and xylitol, as well as ethanol have their disadvantages. Fat as an energy source has many advantages. It is a concentrated source of calories, it can be prepared in isotonic forms and the risk of thrombophlebitis is rare. A litre of 20 per cent fat emulsion will provide the same quantity of calories as a litre of 50 per cent glucose. Moreover it can supply essential fatty acids. Fat is prepared in an emulsion which is handled by the body in the same way as chylomicrons. Hyperlipaemia can occur with a fall in the number of platelets.

Protein is given to reduce, if not prevent, protein catabolism. A 5 per cent aminoacid solution can provide 50 g of protein. Protein requirements of an ordinary individual lie between 1 and 2 g per kg per day, but this requirement may be doubled or trebled after a major operation, particularly if it is complicated. Intravenous infusion of amino-acid solution must be accompanied by sufficient calories from sources other than protein so that the amino-acids are used for protein anabolism rather than for energy.

Intravenous nutrition in the adult may be required if there is prolonged paralysis of the intestine following major operation. Intravenous feeding is also indicated in patients whose oral intake is poor, but who have excessive metabolic requirements as a result of major injury, such as full thickness burns or major fractures. Patients who have intestinal fistulae or diseases of the intestine impairing the absorption of nutrients may require prolonged intravenous nutrition before operation can be carried out with safety. An intravenous regime should attempt to supply 2800 kcal, 3.5 to 4.0 litres water and 70 g protein. Greater quantities of fluid and nutrients may have to be given to patients with severe injuries but there is a risk of overloading the circulation especially if there is poor cardio-renal function.

Intra-gastric or intra-jejunal feeding. Feeding by means of a tube may have to be instituted in the unconscious or apathetic patient and is particularly valuable in patients with a high intestinal fistula. Liquid feeds are given in an attempt to provide balanced amounts of protein, fat and carbohydrate, but the feed must not contain an excessive amount of protein giving rise to azotaemia, or be osmotically irritating because diarrhoea may result with loss of fluid and electrolytes from the gut. Recently elemental diets have been introduced to provide nutrition in a form in which it may be easily absorbed from the proximal part of the small intestine with minimal residue. They have a restricted use in the treatment of fistula of the small intestine and in Crohn's disease, but their use is limited by the inability of patients to tolerate the taste and smell, and by certain side-effects, including diarrhoea.

PRE-OPERATIVE AND POST-OPERATIVE MANAGEMENT

Surgical care embraces both pre-operative and post-operative management which are of fundamental importance to the success of an operation. Technically brilliant achievements may be rendered unsatisfactory by failure to appreciate these aspects of surgical treatment.

Pre-operative preparation

The first essential is to establish the correct diagnosis and the initial step is a careful and accurate history. Sympathetic questioning obtains the confidence of the patient and may determine the presence of co-existing lesions. It should be followed by full clinical examination, accessory investigation and assessment, of which the following are important aspects.

General build

Obesity increases both the technical difficulties of operation and the liability to post-operative chest complications and venous thrombosis. Unless an emergency procedure is necessary, the obese subject should be treated by a rigorous low-calorie diet before admission to hospital. In others undernourishment and dehydration may be evident. Cachexia produced by advanced pyloric stenosis or oesophageal cancer should be improved by an initial period of intravenous or oral therapy.

Anaemia

Chronic bleeding from haemorrhoids, menorrhagia or gastrointestinal ulceration may produce marked anaemia. In some instances an incipient loss may not be observed by the patient or practitioner and clinical judgment can be unreliable. The haemoglobin level should be determined pre-operatively in all cases undergoing major surgery. A deficiency should be corrected by iron in minor and non-urgent cases, or by blood transfusion when major or if immediate surgery is required.

Cardiovascular system

The patient's cardiovascular system must have an adequate reserve of function so that cardiac output can be increased under the stress of operation. This is generally denoted by a good exercise tolerance. Breathlessness on mild exertion, paroxysmal dyspnoea at night or orthopnoea suggest serious disease, and operation should be undertaken only if urgent. A history of myocardial infarction is particularly significant as the risk of a second infarction is considerable if the operation is performed within 12 months of a previous episode. If angina occurs on mild effort, the cardiac reserve is limited and the risk of operation is great. All patients over the age of 40 should have an electrocardiogram performed, to determine the presence or extent of myocardial ischaemia. The presence of severe aortic stenosis or incompetence predisposes to ventricular fibrillation and surgery should be performed only when urgently indicated. Chest radiography should be performed before surgery.

Respiratory system

Respiratory complications are common after surgery, particularly abdominal operations and the respiratory function should be improved when feasible. Postponement of operation until the summer months in chronic bronchitis patients may be advisable. Intensive medical treatment, including an appropriate antibiotic, breathing exercises and postural drainage of the lungs is helpful. Smoking should be avoided for at least two or three weeks before operation.

Prolonged expiratory wheezing indicates a diminished ability to hyperventilate. Where impaired respiratory function exists pulmonary function tests should be carried out. The three main tests of ventilatory capacity are: (i) Forced vital capacity (F.V.C.)—the volume expired as rapidly and completely as possible after maximum inspiration. (ii) Forced expiratory volume (F.E.V.)—gas volume expired over a period of time. Thus $F.E.V._{1.0}$ = volume expired over one second during a forced expiration. (iii) Percentage of measured F.V.C. expired in t seconds ($F.E.V._{t\%}$)—usually $F.E.V._{1.0}/F.V.C. \times 100$—lower limit of normal being 70 per cent. Reduced value for F.E.V. % indicates obstructive disease in which the resistance of the airways is increased as in asthma and chronic bronchitis. Improvement in these indices follows intensive medical treatment. The measurement of blood gases and *p*H is also of considerable help in the evaluation of a patient. Hypoxia may be due to several causes such as hypoventilation, shunting of the blood past the gas exchanging tissues and impairment of diffusion due to thickened alveolar capillary membranes. In the presence of a head cold, tonsillitis or acute bronchitis operation should be postponed.

Genito-urinary system

In the young healthy adult with no history of renal disorder, it is usually sufficient to examine the urine microscopically and to ascertain the presence or absence of sugar and protein. In those over 50 years, the concentration of urea in the blood should be determined. If the blood urea concentration is greater than 12 mmol per litre blood, operation should be postponed and the cause of the azotaemia ascertained. If obstruction of the ureter, bladder or urethra is suspected, radiological examination of the urinary system may be required. Chronic renal disease may present as anaemia. The other major cause of a high blood urea is dehydration and consequent poor renal perfusion; correction of the dehydration or other electrolyte disorder should reduce the azotaemia.

In a patient with latent prostatic obstruction, acute retention may be precipitated by enforced bed rest or operation for even minor unrelated conditions. Evidence of mild symptoms is important.

Diabetes

Routine examination of the urine for sugar and ketones should be undertaken in all cases prior to surgery. Recognition is important because postoperative coma may develop in the unsuspected case, the disease being temporarily aggravated by surgical trauma and infection. Diabetics requiring non-urgent surgical treatment should be admitted to hospital at least two or three days before operation, and each individual assessed separately with regard to his diabetic state.

Preparation for surgery is dependent on the severity of the diabetes and the duration and magnitude of the operation. When the disease is controlled by diet alone or by oral hypoglycaemic agents, no special treatment for the diabetes is required on the day of surgery, except cessation of the tablets on the morning of operation and their recommencement when oral feeding is resumed. Local, spinal or regional block anaesthesia produce less metabolic disturbance.

When insulin is normally required to control the disease, approximately one-third of the usual daily dose should be given in the morning one hour before operation with 25 to 50 g of glucose in a 50 per cent solution intravenously. After only minor operation, insulin and food may be given on return to consciousness, if there is no contraindication to oral feeding.

After major operation glucose is administered by mouth as soon as possible; if oral feeding is contraindicated, the intravenous route is used and at least 100 to 150 g given daily. Insulin requirements are determined by a sliding scale based on four-hourly urine testing and checked by the absence of ketonuria and by daily blood-sugar estimations.

Gradual return to a normal regime is then permitted.

In emergency surgery, in the absence of ketonuria or heavy glycosuria, the immediate pre-operative regime already described should be instituted. In a precoma state 50 to 100 units or more of insulin, depending on the blood-sugar level and degree of ketonuria, should be given in intravenous saline combined with lactate solution. Whenever feasible, diabetes should be controlled before surgery is undertaken. Post-operatively, insulin requirements are assessed by frequent blood-sugar estimations, particularly within the first 12 to 24 hours.

Drugs

An accurate history of intake of drugs is essential to the pre-operative evaluation. Some may be the cause of the present disease, for example, aspirin predisposes to gastro-intestinal bleeding. Others, such as monoamine oxidase inhibitors may result in periods of low blood-pressure under anaesthesia. When steroid therapy is already required increased dosage is necessary before, during and after surgery. It is also advisable to administer steroids when there is a past history of such treatment although an interval of up to 12 months may have elapsed between cessation of the drug and operation.

Sepsis

Any site of inflammation increases the risk of wound infection and if possible should be treated before operation.

Psychological factors

The prospect of surgery is frequently viewed with apprehension. Kind and simple explanation of the intended procedure is reassuring to the patient. The proposal of an ileostomy, colostomy, amputation or mastectomy requires special tact, and it is often of help to effect an introduction to a completely rehabilitated patient prior to surgery. The disability can then be discussed in a practical manner with considerable benefit.

Post-operative management

The management of the patient after an operation consists of care directed towards his recovery and the prevention, early recognition and treatment of complications. In this section, only routine care and general complications after operation will be described. Complications related to particular operations will be discussed in the appropriate chapters.

Immediate post-operative period

Problems of the immediate post-operative period arise usually from the surgical procedure or the administration of the anaesthetic agent. Where possible, a patient should be transferred from the operating theatre to an adjacent recovery room where he will be closely supervised by trained staff and where all facilities necessary for urgent resuscitation will be available. The patient can be transferred back to his own room when the respiratory and circulatory state is stable, usually four to six hours from the end of the operation. The major considerations of this immediate post-operative period are largely concerned with respiratory problems, arterial hypotension, the relief of pain and the output of urine.

Respiratory problems. The most urgent problem of the immediate post-operative period is that of inadequate gas exchange in the lungs, often due to the residual effects of the anaesthetic agent or relaxant drug or to obstruction of the airway, either by the tongue falling back or from inhalation of vomit. Care has to be taken with the administration of opiates for the relief of pain because of their depressing action on the respiratory centre. An adequate airway can be ensured by careful timing of the removal of the endotracheal tube and of the mouth tube. The post-operative accumulation of secretions in the respiratory tract prevents effective ventilation of segments of the lung and can be a frequent cause of serious hypoxia. As soon as possible after recovery from the anaesthetic the patient should be encouraged to breathe deeply and cough up secretions in the trachea and bronchi. Occasionally the bronchial passages must be cleared by aspiration of mucus through a sterile suction catheter and by encouragement to cough. In the elderly and enfeebled, bronchoscopy may be required to remove such secretions. Severe respiratory distress suggests a major intra-thoracic complication such as massive collapse of a lung or tension pneumothorax.

Arterial hypotension. The commonest cause of severe arterial hypotension in this period is a reduction in blood volume because of haemorrhage. The management of oligaemic shock has already been discussed (p. 25). If post-operative hypotension cannot be explained by blood-loss, attention must be turned to other possible causes, such as hypoxia secondary to hypoventilation due to airway obstruction, myocardial infarction, narcotic overdose or acute gastric dilatation.

Relief of pain. The intensity and duration of pain which is experienced after an operation is partly related to the severity and extent of the procedure performed although there is marked individual variation. Simple measures such as loosening a tight bandage or emptying an overfull bladder may be helpful. Pain relief after an upper abdominal incision will also enable the patient to breathe more easily and therefore prevent diffuse pulmonary collapse. Morphine and its analogues are useful analgesics but their over-use should be avoided because of the respiratory depression which may ensue. It is better to avoid pain being experienced by the planned administration of analgesics in adequate dosage, rather than to delay administration until the patient is experiencing severe pain.

Output of urine. After a major operation, especially in the lower abdomen, pelvis or perineum, the patient may be unable to pass urine. This may result from difficulty in micturition (retention of urine) or reduced formation of urine by the kidneys (oliguria). The unaccustomed position of micturating whilst lying in bed may be a factor and simple measures such as early ambulation and the sound of a running tap may suffice. Over-distension of the bladder is to be avoided or atony and later infection follow. A catheter may need to be passed into the bladder and the urine drained. If prolonged retention is anticipated, continuous drainage for some days may be necessary until function has returned.

Less commonly, failure to pass urine is the result of impaired production of urine. Usually such post-operative oliguria is secondary to a decrease in cardiac output or deficit in blood volume, leading to a sudden reduction in renal blood flow. In these circumstances total anuria is rare and usually the daily output in such pre-renal failure lies between 70 and 300 ml of urine. After a major operation it is wise to insert a catheter into the bladder and measure the hourly output of urine. If the figure is between 25 and 50 ml per hour renal function is probably unimpaired but if the output is low, several causes may be responsible. Usually there is poor perfusion of the kidneys because of inadequate replacement of fluids, such as blood or plasma but the ureters may have been inadvertently injured during the operation. The procedures undertaken to avoid, diagnose and treat these complications are considered in Chapter 22.

Routine post-operative care

Nutrition. Gastric emptying is usually delayed after an operation, particularly those in the abdomen, and the intake of food should be curtailed and fluid restricted for 24 hours. After most intra-abdominal procedures the stomach should be kept empty by a nasogastric tube. On the day following the operation, small volumes (15 to 30 ml) of fluid may be given orally and if their onward passage is apparent as determined by judicious timed aspiration of gastric contents, the tube can be removed and the oral intake of fluids increased. Other favourable signs of a return of gastro-intestinal function are normal, propulsive bowel sounds, the passage of flatus and the absence of abdominal distension.

The reduction in oral intake combined with the aspiration of gastric contents will lead to an upset in fluid balance unless fluids are given parenterally. If the return of normal gastro-intestinal function is delayed because of prolonged ileus, leakage at an intestinal anastomosis or the development of a fistula, intravenous fluids may be required for some time and careful supervision of fluid balance will be necessary (p. 35). After about five to seven days if gastro-intestinal function has not been resumed, calories, vitamins and minerals may have to be given parenterally, particularly if the patient is malnourished or if it is evident that oral feeding will be further delayed. Usually after a major operation, particularly if complicated by infection, the appetite will be poor and considerable dietetic and nursing skills are required to prepare an attractive meal and to encourage the patient to eat.

The wound. The wound need not be disturbed until the skin sutures have to be removed. Occasionally a drain may be inserted into a wound, abscess, pleural or peritoneal cavity to drain blood, pus or bile which would otherwise accumulate and impair healing. The discharge from such drains is usually led into a plastic bag or, from the pleura, into a water-seal drainage bottle. Gradual removal is usually satisfactory, but in deep-seated regions such as a subphrenic abscess, radio-opaque material may be injected through the tube to check that the cavity is shrinking before the tube is finally withdrawn.

Post-operative complications

An operation cannot be entirely without risk related either to surgery or to anaesthesia. Intelligent anticipation can minimise and often avoid the risks or mitigate the effects. General complications include fever, pulmonary complications, gastric dilatation (p. 157), complications of the wound and deep venous thrombosis (p. 42). Local problems related to particular operations will be discussed in the appropriate chapters, but examples of these are as follows:

(a) *Intestinal obstruction*, caused by prolonged paralytic ileus secondary to an intraabdominal infection or leakage at an anastomosis, or mechanical obstruction due to oedema of an anastomosis or to adhesions.
(b) *Fistula*, which is the development of an abnormal communication between a hollow viscus and the skin after abdominal, urological or thoracic surgery.
(c) *Retention of urine* due to blood clot after genito-urinary surgery.
(d) *Formation of an abscess* in a body cavity, especially under the diaphragm, in the pelvis or in a paracolic space, particularly after emergency surgery for rupture of a hollow viscus.
(e) *Pulmonary collapse and infection* after thoracic and upper abdominal operations.
(f) *Occlusion of blood-vessels* after cardio-thoracic surgery.

Post-operative pyrexia

A slight increase in body temperature to 38° to 39°C in the first 48 hours after an operation is usual and is part of the metabolic response to surgery. This should be recognised as such and no treatment administered. If the temperature becomes more elevated a cause should be sought. A high temperature developing in the first day or so after operation usually means segmental collapse of the lung. A pyrexia developing within a week of an operation often indicates an infection in the wound and, if a high intermittent fever develops, a deep-seated abscess is usually present.

Post-operative pulmonary complications

The respiratory system has developed a number of defence mechanisms to prevent the invasion of the lower respiratory tract with organisms and so reduce the changes of infection, namely the cough reflex, the action of cilia, adequate ventilation of the lungs, warming and humidification of the inspired air. These defence mechanisms may be impaired after operation: the cough reflex is depressed, the cilia may be paralysed by anaesthetic agents and the respiratory passages irritated by dry anaesthetic gases. Ventilation of the lungs may be greatly reduced after operation and further embarrassed by tight bandaging especially after upper abdominal operations when inspiration can be particularly painful. The conditions for pathogenic organisms entering and proliferating in the lungs may be favoured by (*a*) pre-existing disease of the lungs such as chronic bronchitis and pneumoconiosis, (*b*) collapse of the lung due to the inhalation of viscid sputum.

The risk of a pulmonary complication is greatly reduced by the avoidance of smoking for at least two weeks before operation, by breathing exercises which encourage thoracic rather than abdominal muscles and by the vigorous treatment of any pre-operative infection. In the early stages, these complications may be prevented and treated by the inhalation of warm, humidified air, the use of drugs to lower the viscosity of sputum or to diminish painful respiration, postural drainage of the lungs and encouragement to cough. The commonest major post-operative pulmonary complication is that of diffuse collapse and atelectasis. The physical findings are diagnostic and appear many hours before a characteristic picture is visible on chest radiography: there is usually a rapid pulse and respiration; localised moist sounds and diminished breath sounds with bronchial breathing are detected, especially posteriorly towards the lung bases. This should be vigorously treated before infection becomes established; in the early stages, antibiotics are not required.

Complications in the wound

Haemorrhage may be an immediate complication of a wound. Such bleeding may be external evidence of a large serious haemorrhage from a major vessel in the depths of the wound or in a body cavity, but more often it is caused by bleeding from vessels in the skin. Occasionally the loss can be so severe as to lead to marked reduction in the blood volume. More frequently the bleeding ceases but a large clot of blood remains within the susbtance of the wound to delay its healing. Such a haematoma should be evacuated.

Rupture of the wound may occur from three to six days after operation. The presentation may be dramatic by the sudden dehiscence of an abdominal wound and prolapse of intestine on the skin surface. Frequently only the deep layers of the wound give way and the skin is seemingly intact. This type of deep rupture is often manifested by a considerable serosanguinous discharge from the wound and prolonged paralytic ileus. In all cases the layers of the wound should be carefully sutured, or a permanent weakness will persist and lead to the development of an incisional hernia.

Infection of a wound usually declares itself within four to seven days after operation by increasing pain and discomfort in the wound which may show the classical signs of inflammation. Ultimately pus may discharge. The infecting organisms may come from a variety of sources and the risk is best reduced by careful aseptic surgical technique. It is unwise to rely on antibiotics to prevent the development of wound infection, but when established, appropriate antibiotic treatment can be employed. If an abscess exists drainage is required.

Deep vein thrombosis

A major cause of hospital deaths in elderly and ill patients is pulmonary embolism, in which large clots of blood which have formed in the pelvic and lower limb veins become detached and lodge in the pulmonary arteries. During and after operation several factors predispose to venous thrombosis. The blood coagulates more readily due to a greater number of platelets and an increase in their adhesiveness. There is also, after an operation, an increase in the concentration of fibrinogen in the blood and a fall in its fibrinolytic activity. The tendency to coagulate is marked in polycythaemia, dehydration and in shock. There is also an increased risk of thrombosis in females on the oral contraceptive. Clotting may also occur because of pre-existing disease of the veins, such as varicosities or because of more recent damage to the vascular endothelium as in pelvic infection. The flow of blood may be greatly slowed during and after operation as a result of pressure on the lower limbs during surgery and subsequent inactivity. The condition is also more common in patients with malignant disease and cardio-respiratory disorders and those undergoing operations for prostatic disease or fractured neck of femur are particularly prone to this complication.

Thrombosis may occur in the superficial veins of the lower limbs and be accompanied by marked inflammation; such superficial thrombophlebitis is uncomfortable but rarely of serious importance. Clotting occurring in the deep veins and in the venous sinuses of the leg is of greater significance. These clots may become detached, but embolism is more likely when clotting occurs in the main deep veins of thigh and pelvis. Such deep vein thrombosis may be clinically manifest by swelling of the legs, low-grade fever and tenderness along the course of the vein, but thrombosis may occur without symptoms and the first sign may be pulmonary embolism. If clotting of the deep veins is suspected venography should be performed. Methods measuring venous flow and turbulence using ultrasonic techniques and the employment of external scanning after injecting radioactive fibrinogen are also being used to detect deep vein thrombosis.

The prevention of venous stasis in the legs by pneumatic compression of the calf, galvanic stimulation of the calf muscles during operation and exercise of the calf muscles immediately after operation is important in diminishing the frequency of deep-vein thrombosis. Small amounts of heparin, 5000 units subcutaneously, pre-operatively and two to three times daily post-operatively for five to seven days, may also lower the incidence of deep vein thrombosis and reduce the risk of pulmonary embolism. Post-operative bleeding and haematoma formation do not appear to be increased, and it may be advisable routinely where a special risk exists; that is, patients above the age of forty who are undergoing major abdominal or pelvic operations, who are obese, who have had a previous history of venous thrombosis, who have malignant disease or who are on an oral contraceptive. Although the regime of low-dose heparin is now widely used, its value is still in doubt.

The majority of cases improve spontaneously. The patient should be confined to bed with the foot elevated and firm stockings or elastic bandages applied. Anticoagulant therapy, which lowers the risk of embolism and limits the development of post-phlebitic swelling and ulceration of the leg, is commenced by giving intravenous heparin (15 000 units) together with an oral anticoagulant such as warfarin. Heparin is stopped after two to three days when the latter has become efficacious. Oral anticoagulant dosage is subsequently controlled by daily or ultimately twice weekly prothrombin estimations. The prothrombin time should be maintained at between two and two and a half times the control value. Haemorrhage due to over-dosage can occur and careful control of treatment is essential. Operative removal of the thrombus and the administration of drugs such as streptokinase, which were widely used at one time, are falling into disfavour. An exercise programme including walking, swimming and a hot bath are probably more important than other measures in deep venous thrombosis, because muscular exercise and heat both stimulate fibrinolysis and exercise increases blood flow.

Pulmonary embolism

A loose clot may be detached from a deep vein of the lower limb or pelvis, be carried in the blood stream and lodge in the pulmonary arterial tree as a pulmonary embolus. The condition is not necessarily confined to the post-operative patient. The severity of symptoms is related to the degree of occlusion. There may be rapid collapse and death due to obstruction of a major pulmonary artery, or collapse, dyspnoea and cyanosis can occur with a rapidly developing acute right ventricular failure which proves fatal in a few hours. In some instances there may be severe pain in the chest, aggravated by deep breathing, haemoptysis and the clinical signs of consolidation of the lung and a pleural friction rub; later a pleural effusion may develop. The diagnosis at this stage may be confirmed by radiography of the chest and an electrocardiogram which may show right ventricular strain. Occasionally a sudden fall in blood-pressure without any localising sign may be noted. Lastly repeated pulmonary emboli may gradually obstruct the pulmonary arterial system and pulmonary hypertension develops subsequently. When the clots are small there may be some difficulty in establishing the diagnosis of pulmonary embolus. A simple measure is a pulmonary scan following injection of radio-iodinated macro-aggregated human albumin and this may differentiate a major pulmonary embolus from acute myocardial infarction, although it is not as accurate in the diagnosis of pulmonary embolus as angiography. Dye is injected through a catheter placed in the right ventricle and a pulmonary embolus can show itself by an intraluminal filling defect or by an abrupt cut off of the vessel, or loss of its side branches.

Active treatment is of little avail when there is sudden acute respiratory distress and death within a few moments. In less severe conditions some time is usually available and the aim of treatment is to convert a shocked moribund patient into one whose condition is relatively stable and in whom definitive treatment can be carried out. External cardiac massage must be employed if indicated, and oxygen, anticoagulants and intravenous bicarbonate should be administered. Occasionally survival may be prolonged to permit removal of the pulmonary embolus, the patient being maintained with a cardio-pulmonary by-pass. The site of the embolus is determined by angiography and pulmonary embolectomy performed. Repeated small emboli require anticoagulant therapy with heparin and warfarin for several months. Recurrent pulmonary embolism may also require interruption of major veins between the site of origin of the embolus, usually in the pelvic vein, and the lung. Where the source of the embolus is in the lower extremity, the femoral vein can be ligated; but more usually the pelvic veins are the source of emboli and under these circumstances plication of the inferior vena cava is preferable.

BURNS

Each year 10 000 patients with burns are admitted to hospitals in the United Kingdom and between 900 and 1000 die. Burns are therefore common injuries, varying in severity from the trivial to the lethal and often resulting in permanent scarring, which may cause serious disfigurement or disability. The majority of burns and scalds are the result of accidents in the home. A burn is an injury caused by thermal, chemical or physical agents, such as heat, corrosive substances or irradiation. Local and general effects are produced and their understanding is of importance in subsequent clinical management.

Local effects

The local effect of a burn depends on the heat given out by the burning agent and is thus related to its temperature and the duration of contact with the skin. The severity of the local response can vary from simple reddening to destruction and charring of tissues. As far as the depth of a burn is concerned, the most important feature is the amount of living tissue remaining: with a superficial burn, only the surface layers of dermis are damaged and the *stratum germinativum* survives. In deeper burns this layer is destroyed but skin can be generated from the epithelial lining of sweat glands and hair follicles (Fig. 2.1). Such **partial skin loss** will usually heal spontaneously without scarring and skin grafting is not required. Where all the epithelial elements are destroyed, there is no prospect of spontaneous healing; a **whole thickness burn** has been produced. The distinction between the two major classes of skin loss is difficult because both types often co-exist in the same burned area, the area of partial skin loss being peripheral and that of whole thickness loss being central. The appearance of a burn is informative only of the surface and not of the more important deeper part and to determine the depth of a burn requires great experience. Skin sensitivity to pin-prick may be helpful, a sharp sensation indicating partial skin loss. Insensitivity may be due to whole or partial skin loss and the test is of no practical value in burns of the face, skull, palms and soles.

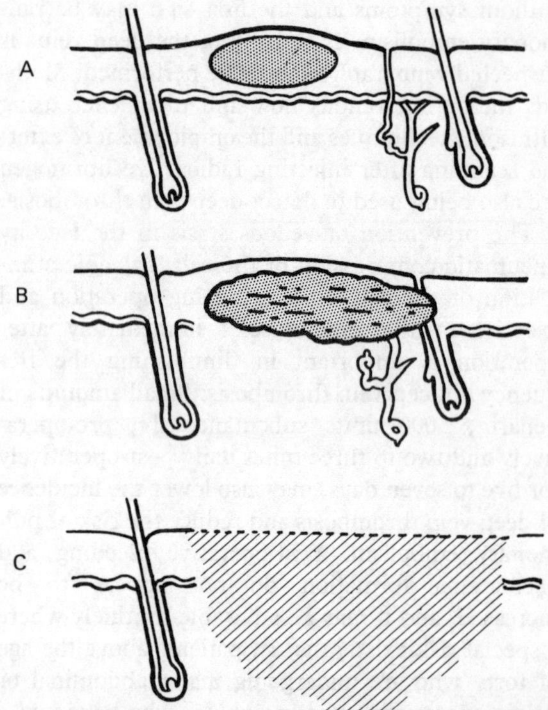

Fig. 2.1 The depth of burns. **A.** Superficial. **B.** Partial thickness. **C.** Whole thickness.

In addition to the epidermal injury there is also damage to the dermal capillaries which dilate and become more permeable. Fluid collects locally in the form of blisters and more generally as local oedema. It contains plasma protein with a predominance of smaller molecules such as albumin. The volume accumulating in the tissues reaches a maximum usually 48 hours after the burn and reabsorption then begins. The extent to which the oedema fluid collects is dependent on the increase in permeability of the capillaries and the number that have been damaged and it is limited by the pressure of the tissue fluid and overlying skin. The local loss of fluid in a large burn is sufficient to cause marked reduction in circulatory volume and is the cause of most of the systemic effects that ensue.

Although a burn is initially sterilised by the heat of injury, the normal barrier of the skin to infection is destroyed and replaced by dead tissue in which bacteria can proliferate. Infection remains the major problem in the treatment of burns and the biggest single cause of death.

Excessive colonisation of the burn by pathogenic organisms may increase the amount of tissue destruction, delay healing or interfere with the 'take' of skin grafts. It may also affect the general condition by absorption of toxins and, by invasion, lead to septicaemia and death. Organisms reach the burned surface by cross-infection and the pathogens commonly encountered are staphylococci, β-haemolytic streptococci, *Pseudomonas aeruginosa*, *Proteus vulgaris* and *Escherichia coli*. Haemolytic streptococci, although less of a problem than formerly, can rapidly destroy skin grafts and cause breakdown of recently healed surfaces. *Ps. aeruginosa* is particularly serious, since it not only causes local damage but may lead to septicaemia. Destruction of the skin also means that the normal barrier to the loss of water and electrolytes from the body is absent and up to 7 to 8 litres may be lost each day through extensive burns.

General effects

Plasma loss into the burned tissues leads to a marked reduction in blood volume. The blood becomes more viscous as the loss of plasma through the capillaries is much greater than that of the red blood cells. The volume of plasma loss is roughly proportional to the extent of the body surface burned. A burn of more than 10 per cent of the body surface in a child, or more than 15 per cent in an adult, will cause oligaemic shock within a few hours. In the untreated burn there is a period of apparent normality when compensatory reactions to the loss of plasma take place and the only sign of developing shock is haemoconcentration with a rise in haematocrit. Shock develops later with a fall in blood-pressure and an increase in pulse-rate. Red blood cells may be damaged in the burn and a greater number often show increased fragility and they are destroyed over the next few days.

Severe oligaemia can damage other organs, particularly the kidney. The glomerulus is mainly affected due to severe renal vasoconstriction; even in a minor burn the glomerular filtration rate is reduced. In a severe burn there is usually marked and progressive azotaemia with associated damage to the renal tubules. Occasionally, severe azotaemia develops without marked reduction in the urine volume, the urea concentration in the blood rising steadily whilst a relatively normal output of urine is maintained. Diagnosis of impending renal damage rests with monitoring not only the volume but also the composition of urine. An hourly urine output of less than 0.5 ml per kg per hour suggests acute renal failure. Insufficient perfusion, if prolonged, may lead to established renal failure. In a fatal burn, vascular engorgement and petechial haemorrhage in the alimentary wall are frequent and occasionally an acute duodenal ulcer may develop.

Severe loss of body protein often occurs, leading to serious weight loss, pressure sores, lowered resistance to infection, delayed healing and skin graft failure. Some protein is lost in the exudate from the damaged surface, but the main cause is the metabolic response to injury with excessive protein catabolism, resulting in urinary nitrogen secretion of up to 30 to 40 g per day. This protein catabolic phase continues until healing is well advanced.

Several days after a burn, the patient may become grey, cyanosed, pyrexial and vomit blood. Gradual drowsiness followed by coma may occur with hypotension and tachycardia. The toxaemia represents a combination of gross biochemical disturbances, loss of plasma and extensive infection of the burned area.

Treatment

The management of burns may be considered under four headings: first aid, general treatment, local treatment, and the treatment of special sites.

First aid

Those burns which involve more than 5 per cent of the body surface, facial burns, circumferential burns of the limbs and any deep burn should be regarded as urgent and the patient transferred to hospital. Attempts should not be made to remove clothes or to dress the burn, particularly avoiding the application of dressings of ointment. Blisters should not be pricked at this stage. In lesser burns the patient should be put to bed and the burned area covered with clean, dry material. Pain relief may be urgent and the intravenous route is preferable for analgesics in severe cases.

General treatment

Intravenous therapy is required to correct oligaemia when the burn is more than 15 per cent of the body surface of the adult or 10 per cent in a child. The choice of fluid varies from centre to centre—plasma is of known value in treating patients with extensive burns, or one of the synthetic plasma expanders, such as dextran, may be used. Alternating with these colloids a balanced salt solution, e.g. Ringer lactate, can be employed. In deep burns, or in superficial ones involving more than 20 per cent of the body surface, whole blood should also be given. Various formulae have been devised as a guide to fluid replacement such as the 'rule of nine' (Table 3) but these do not allow for the wide fluctuations in the requirements of badly burned patients. Correction of the formula is also necessary in children where the head forms a larger proportion of the body surface and the legs correspondingly less. Another measure that may be used is that of the outstretched palm and fingers which comprise 1 per cent of body surface. Most of the total volume of fluid replacement should be given in the first 12 hours—at least one-third in the first eight hours—and after 48 hours intravenous infusions should be curtailed as plasma losses will be diminishing. A formula is only used as an initial

Table 3

Site	Area (%)	Total area (%)
Head and neck	9	9
Each upper limb	9	18
Each lower limb	9 × 2	36
Front of trunk	9 × 2	18
Back of trunk	9 × 2	18
Perineum	1	1
		100

assessment of the probable fluid requirements and the quantity and rate of administration must be varied according to the patient's response.

Careful clinical observation is essential but the skilled use of clinical indices of adequate tissue perfusion is of great value in assessing the required amount of fluid.

(i) *Haematocrit*. On admission, the haematocrit commonly shows some degree of haemoconcentration corresponding to the loss of plasma. Plasma should be given to correct this and the degree of success can be checked by hourly repetition of the haematocrit determination. The appreciable loss of red blood cells in severe burns may make the use of the haematocrit, as an indicator of blood volume, less reliable. (ii) *Urine volume*—if a burn covers more than 20 per cent of the body surface a catheter should be inserted to obtain urine hourly. An output of 35 to 60 ml per hour in an adult may be regarded as satisfactory. (iii) *Physical signs*—pallor, coldness, restlessness and collapsed peripheral veins indicate oligaemia and further colloid is required. (iv) *Serum electrolyte estimations* of sodium and potassium concentrations and of osmolality and acid base balance may all assist in monitoring treatment at this stage.

After three to eight days from the receipt of the burn there is increased breakdown of cellular protein and a high protein intake then becomes essential. Prolonged discomfort, repeated operations and the fear of permanent disfigurement require emotional and psychological support.

Local treatment

The objects of local treatment are to minimise infection, to prevent further tissue loss and to provide the best conditions to encourage healing in a superficial burn and to facilitate surgical resurfacing of a deep burn. Initially the area should be cleaned with a mild antiseptic such as chlorhexidine. Removal of blisters is advisable since the contained fluid is a good culture-medium but in areas of thick skin such as the palm of the hand they should be left. Sepsis can be controlled by applying antibiotic creams, covered with gauze and a generous dressing which extends several inches beyond the edge of the burn. Bacterial contamination can also be reduced by moist compresses of 0.5 per cent solution of silver nitrate. Closed dressings prevent access of organisms and reduce the loss of water but they tend to be unsatisfactory if the burn involves the face and perineum and these areas should be exposed and kept dry. Careful bacteriological control and the judicious use of antibiotics is necessary to control infection.

Partial thickness burns usually heal in two or three weeks. In deep whole thickness burns, primary excision is not attempted except if the burn is small. Excision of areas of full thickness burn should begin as soon as possible because such tissue remains a hazard for infection, but with wide areas of full-thickness burns removal of all burned tissue cannot be done in one stage. Usually the programme of wound excision begins after the fifth post-burn day and is carried out in several stages until all totally destroyed skin has been removed. Grafting is undertaken immediately. The skin for such grafting is usually obtained from an unburned part of the body. Occasionally, in an extensive burn, skin, obtained in the fresh state from suitable donors, can provide temporary cover for up to two weeks before rejection. Cadaver homograft skin may be used to seal off large areas when donor sites are extremely limited. The value of these homografts lies in the reduction in bacterial infection and protein loss despite their transient survival. Penicillin is given for the first five days to all patients with burns exceeding 10 per cent of the body surface area. Broad-spectrum antibiotics are avoided initially and should be withheld until skin grafting is commenced or until there are definite clinical indications. Nutrition remains a major problem because despite increased requirements for protein and calories the intake is usually greatly impaired by poor appetite as a result of pain, infection and multiple operations. A vigorous feeding regime is required and if oral intake is inadequate, recourse must be taken to intravenous nutrition.

Special cases

Electrical burns. With electrocution, the current spreads through the body, the major local changes occurring at the sites of entrance and exit of the current. Initially tissue damage may appear small but extensive tissue necrosis usually ensues.

Inhalation burns. The inhalation of dry hot air can lead to extensive burning of trachea and larynx, occasionally necessitating a tracheostomy. With the inhalation of wet air, such as steam, the bronchial tree may be burned and the patient develop pulmonary oedema. If stridor develops immediate endotracheal intubation will be required for pulmonary oedema, suggested by chest radiography. Monitoring of blood gases and oxygen therapy, antibiotics and intubation with assisted respiration are required.

Face. In facial burns, chlorhexidine cream is lightly applied to the lips and nostrils, and moisture from the eyes, nose and mouth should be frequently wiped away with gauze swabs. Scalp hair should be shaved and subsequently kept short near the burn. Burns to the eyelids require close attention and may have to be softened with liquid paraffin if they become stiff and immobile with coagulum. Chloramphenicol ointment should be instilled between the lids twice daily. In deeper burns of the eyelids early skin grafting may be necessary to forestall lid retraction and corneal exposure. Chemical burns to the eyes require copious irrigation of the conjunctival sacs.

Hands. The hands should always be dressed in the position of function and elevated. Early movement is essential to avoid stiffness.

ORGAN TRANSPLANTATION

When an organ or tissue ceases to function due to disease, it can occasionally be replaced by artificial materials or by an organ taken from another individual. No material combines ideal mechanical characteristics with complete lack of toxicity and perfect compatibility with human tissues. Nevertheless many artificial devices, or prostheses, enjoy considerable success, as hip-joint prostheses in osteoarthritis of hip and artificial heart valves.

The replacement of a diseased organ by one removed from another individual is now in some instances, such as the kidney, a clinical reality. The major obstacle to wider application of transplantation is the process of **rejection** by which the body destroys the grafted organ. The process is essentially an immunological one. When skin of rabbit A is grafted on to rabbit B, the grafted tissue is accepted initially but after 10 days clotting occurs in the blood-vessels which have grown into the grafted tissue and the skin dies. Rejection has occurred. If a second piece of skin from rabbit A is grafted on to rabbit B, rejection is more rapid, occurring in three to five days. However, when skin from another rabbit, rabbit C, is grafted on to rabbit B, rejection will not be found until after 10 or more days. Thus the first experience of receiving a graft from rabbit A has produced a special relationship between A and B so that B rejects very rapidly a second set of skin grafts.

Tissue or organ grafts between individuals of the same species (allografts or homografts) are rejected with a vigour proportional to the degree of the genetic disparity between them. Grafts between individuals of different species (xenografts or heterografts) are rejected even more rapidly. Grafts between identical twins (isografts or syngenic grafts), or from an individual to himself (autografts) survive indefinitely once the vascular supply has been re-established to the host.

The reaction is immunologically specific for the antigens involved and the second set rejection occurs only when the recipient has previously encountered the antigens of the first graft. Tissue transplanted from one individual to another will be rejected if the new host can recognise that tissue as foreign. Foreignness is equated with the presence of antigens in the donor cells which the host does not possess. Foreign antigens on a tissue organ graft are considered histocompatibility antigens if they can be related to graft rejection. These antigens are known to be protein molecules situated on cell membranes. While they are distributed throughout various tissues, some tissues, like those of the lymphoid system, are particularly well endowed and for that reason lymphocytes are generally used for 'tissue typing'.

The transplantation antigens are genetically controlled according to Mendelian law. Several genetic loci can be identified which control antigen systems. Some are only of minor importance but one locus, or perhaps a combination of two closely placed loci (HL-A in man) overshadow all others in importance, strength and intensity of expression. Each individual carries four of some 30-odd antigens controlled by the HL-A system. Due to the method of inheritance it is therefore easy to appreciate why sibling or parent-donated kidneys have fared better than cadaver-donated transplants. Given the large number of HL-A controlled antigens, several thousand combinations are possible but fortunately some antigen combinations have been found to be more frequent than others with the result that some 5 per cent of the general population appears to have a close match in the specific HL-A antigenic arrangements. It is therefore possible to find well-matched cadaver kidneys for most recipients through organ-sharing programmes covering institutions in a large geographical area. Some dispute exists over the value of typing and matching procedures in forecasting the chances of acceptance or rejection of a donor organ, but it is preferable to match donor and recipient HL-A patterns as closely as possible.

There are two immunological systems controlled by two lymphoid systems. One seems mainly to be concerned with defence against micro-organisms by the manufacturing of antibodies. The second is responsible for graft rejection. The stem lymphoid cells, as created in the bone marrow, are not immunologically competent until they have passed through one of two organs, after which they begin to function. Transplantation is concerned with the cells that pass through and are acted upon by the thymus, the *T* cells. From the thymus small lymphocytes emerge which do not secrete antibodies. After contact with antigen, lymphocytes pass through a lymph node and emerge as the large 'blast' cells, which divide to form memory cells storing the memory of the contact, and other cells affector cells, which destroy the foreign graft. This is why a graft undergoing rejection is full of lymphocytes. The other type of immunologically competent lymphocyte probably also plays a part in graft rejection, but its role is less well defined; it is known as the *B* lymphocyte and produces antibody. The *B* cells are responsible for the manufacture of circulating immunoglobulins and thus are used in humoral immunity. The *T* cells represent the immuno-competent cell population responsible for the development of cell immunity. These reactions include delayed hypersensitivity reactions as well as many of the early reactions responsible for graft rejection. In immune responses *T* and *B* cells interact and the whole process is of considerable complexity.

The process of rejection may be modified in a number of ways.

1. *Tissue matching*. In general terms the aggressiveness of the immune reaction depends on the number and strength of the relevant incompatible antigens and on the immune capabilities of the recipient. For a given state of immune potential, the chances of a graft remaining unrejected are inversely related to the number and strength of incompatible antigens. Attempts have been made to determine compatibility between antigens of the donor and recipient. Several techniques are available for tissue-matching but at times some grossly mismatched kidney transplants do well, whilst some well-matched ones do poorly. Some clinicians give HL-A matching low priority, in comparison with factors such as the quality of the transplant and the availability of the recipient. Excellent results are achieved if all four HL-A antigens are compatible in donor and recipient. This situation occurs in identical twins but non-identical siblings have a 1 : 4 chance of inheriting the same HL-A antigens. A difference of one or more HL-A antigens gives uniformly poorer results. A direct cross-match of the ABO blood group is always done because if the patient's serum contains antibodies which react with the leucocytes of the prospective donor, there is a high probability that a transplanted organ will undergo acute rejection.

2. The process of rejection may be modified by the use of *immunosuppressive* techniques which depress the reactivity of the immune reacting centres of the recipient. The most successful have been drugs such as azathioprine and prednisolone but they tend to have undesirable depressing actions on other tissues, such as the bone marrow and the gastro-intestinal mucosa. The immunosuppressive drug, cyclosporin-A, is more promising. Other methods, such as total body radiation, thoracic duct drainage, splenectomy, thymectomy, have been tried but have not become established in practice. Antilymphocytic globulin, high levels of which can be raised in the horse, will, when injected into a recipient, reduce the number of circulating lymphocytes and may modify the process of rejection. The place of antilymphocytic globulin has not been fully defined and it carries some disadvantages, such as allergic reactions and variability in its immunosuppressive potency.

Transplant function

The transplanted organ must be capable of performing the function required of it immediately on being grafted or, alternatively, this need must be met temporarily in another way. Thus development of satisfactory methods of treating severe renal insufficiency by dialysis has solved the problem as far as kidney transplants are concerned, but the lack of comparable methods of support for recipients of liver and heart transplants has proved a major obstacle to progress.

The need for temporary support partly depends on the state of the organ when it was removed from the donor and the extent to which it has deteriorated subsequently during storage. This problem does not arise with organs removed from healthy volunteers and transplanted immediately, but the use of such donors raises important ethical questions and is not possible in respect of organs such as the heart or liver. The possibility of obtaining satisfactory organs from cadavers depends mainly on how quickly the organ can be removed and transplanted. This in turn depends on what is regarded as proper and ethical by both lay public and members of the medical and allied professions. Whatever criteria are used to diagnose death, all agree that organs for transplantation should not be removed until the donor has been pronounced dead by doctors independent of the transplant team.

Due to the inevitable delay in preparing the recipient for operation and in transporting the donor organ to a recipient with an appropriate tissue match, much effort is also being spent in developing methods of storing organs. It is now possible to store kidneys for some hours at a temperature of little above freezing point after flushing with a cold solution and storing in an iced vacuum flask.

Clinical applications

Transplantation of the kidney is now clinically acceptable and many centres exist where irreversible renal disease can be treated either by repeated dialysis or renal transplantation. Using live-related donors the two-year transplant survival rate is approximately 75 per cent, whilst with unrelated cadaver donors the figure is 50 per cent, but as important is the quality of life enjoyed by those patients with functioning transplants: many patients return to full-time work and can engage in outdoor activities. The donor kidney is transplanted usually into the right iliac fossa, the renal artery being anastomosed with the internal iliac artery and the renal vein end-to-side with the common iliac vein; the ureter is either joined to the recipient ureter or implanted into the recipient bladder.

The patient who has received a transplanted kidney is vulnerable not only to the complications of the transplantation itself, but to the complications of immunosuppression. The kidney may undergo acute tubular necrosis if the duration of its ischaemia between removal from the donor and insertion into the recipient was unduly prolonged. Acute rejection, in which the transplanted kidney swells and the patient shows a fever and oliguria, requires prompt addition to the immunosuppressive regime. Chronic rejection can be detected by renal biopsy and shows itself ultimately by albuminuria and the development of renal failure. Problems may also occur at the sites of anastomoses, particularly the junction between the ureter and bladder.

The drugs used to suppress the immune response are extremely powerful and can produce several serious undesirable effects upon the body. Antimetabolites, such as azathioprine, depress the bone-marrow and may damage the liver. There is also some concern that they may be responsible for inducing malignancy. Steroids, such as prednisolone, increase the susceptibility to infection and may predispose to gastrointestinal bleeding.

Transplantation of almost every other organ and tissue has been attempted. So far, only the liver and the heart have been transplanted to any great extent. These organs are unpaired and therefore only cadaveric material is available. Moreover, there is no satisfactory method of keeping the recipient alive by artificial means until a suitable organ becomes available, nor of supporting the patient if the transplanted organ does not immediately function or is rejected. Despite such technical difficulties, many liver and heart transplants have been performed throughout the world and an increasing number of survivors is being reported. Transplantation of these organs should only be undertaken in highly specialised centres.

FURTHER READING

Dudley, H. A. F. (1981). Body water and electrolytes. In *Clinical Science for Surgeons*. Ed. Burnett, W. London: Butterworth.

Hill, G.L. (1981). *Nutrition and the Surgical patient*. Edinburgh: Churchill Livingstone.

Muir, I. F. K. and Barclay, T. L. (1974). *Burns and their Treatment*. 2nd ed. London: Lloyd-Luke.

Wardle, N. (1979). Bacteraemic and endotoxic shock. Brit. J. Hosp. Med.; 21, 223–228.

3

Skin

Sebaceous cyst

Obstruction to the duct of a sebaceous gland results in the formation of a retention cyst which contains white material with an unpleasant odour having the same consistency as toothpaste. Infection with abscess formation is a common complication. Incision or spontaneous discharge is not always followed by healing. An ulcer may form, which has a foul discharge, resembles an epithelioma and is often referred to as Cock's peculiar tumour. A sebaceous horn is an uncommon complication and is the result of sebaceous material escaping from the cyst and drying in successive layers to form a projection. An epithelioma may occasionally occur.

A familial tendency often exists. Single or multiple cysts occur, particularly on the scalp or neck, although they may be present wherever there are sebaceous glands. Each cyst is a spherical swelling, firm in consistency and with a regular margin. Skin attachment is an important feature, and a punctum may be seen at the apex. If infected, the cyst increases in size, becomes red and painful and there may be surrounding cellulitis with associated regional lymphadenitis.

Treatment

Excision should be undertaken to prevent complications and for cosmetic reasons. Infection should be treated initially by antibiotics and local heat, or incision of an abscess may become necessary. The cyst should be removed when the inflammation has subsided. Biopsy of a Cock's peculiar tumour may be necessary to exclude carcinoma.

Dermoid cysts

Fusion of adjacent skin processes occurs normally during foetal development, but occasionally a portion of skin becomes detached and buried at one of these sites giving rise to a dermoid cyst. Histologically the wall consists of all layers of the skin; hair follicles, hairs, sweat and sebaceous glands being present. Infection is the most important complication. Common sites are the scalp, neck and face; the external angular dermoid at the outer end of the eyebrow being the most frequent. The presentation is of a tense, painless swelling which lies deep to the skin. Excision should be undertaken.

Epidermoid cysts

Congenital and post-traumatic types are described. The former grows from an ectodermal cell nest which later forms a cyst. There is some doubt about the method of development of the post-traumatic kind. It has been suggested that a portion of the epidermis displaced at the time of injury later formed the cyst, the name 'implantation' epidermoid being given. More recent work has suggested that the lining epithelium comes from an adjacent sweat gland and that a breach of the epidermis is not essential. Macroscopically it differs from a dermoid cyst in not containing hair. Histology shows the cyst wall to consist of stratified squamous epithelium, but hair follicles, sweat and sebaceous glands are absent.

Clinically there is a cystic swelling deep to the epidermis, but it may be adherent to an overlying scar. The congenital lesion on the scalp may have a deep attachment which may include the dura. The post-traumatic type is often situated on exposed parts, particularly on the hands of manual workers. Treatment consists of excision for cosmetic reasons and also to prevent infection.

Keratoacanthoma

Pathology

This condition results from proliferation of the epithelium of hair follicles. In early lesions histology shows increased growth of the cells lining a hair follicle. At this stage there is great activity of the basal cells with many mitotic figures and apparent invasion of surrounding structures; only the superficial layers are keratinised and the hair itself has usually been destroyed. Differentiation from a squamous-cell carcinoma is difficult, but invasion of the dermis does not occur.

Clinical features

The lesion is uncommon and occurs in adults, particularly on the face, but also on other parts such as the head and neck. It begins as a papule which grows rapidly to attain maximum size in two or three months. This rapidity of growth is an important feature in distinguishing it from a squamous-cell carcinoma. When fully mature it is hemispherical with erythema around the base. The apex later becomes ulcerated and the crater filled with necrotic debris, presenting a similar appearance to a squamous-cell carcinoma. Inflammatory enlargement of the regional lymph nodes occurs and may suggest metastatic deposits.

Treatment

Biopsy should be undertaken in all cases to confirm the diagnosis. Most lesions heal without specific treatment. The best cosmetic results are achieved by excision of the superficial portion and curettage of the base, when rapid healing ensues.

TUMOURS

Tumours and hyperplasia occurring in the skin may be difficult to differentiate; both are therefore included in the following three groups. Melanoma is considered separately.

1. Epidermal origin.
   a. Innocent:
      Papilloma.
      Verruca vulgaris.
      Seborrhoeic keratosis.
   b. Premalignant:
      Bowen's disease.
      Leucoplakia (p. 62).
      Keratosis senilis.
   c. Malignant:
      Basal-cell carcinoma.
      Squamous-cell carcinoma.
      Paget's disease (p. 140).
2. Sweat and sebaceous gland origin.
   Innocent and malignant forms occur.
3. Dermal origin.
   Capillary angioma.
   Cavernous angioma.
   Sclerosing angioma.
   Glomus tumour.

INNOCENT TUMOURS

Papilloma is an innocent tumour of the epidermis, frequently situated on the head and neck or limb, although it may arise in squamous epithelium at any site. It presents as a pedunculated or sessile projection which is usually small, but if large may have a cauliflower appearance. Pigmentation may occur, particularly in the senile warts of the aged, and confusion with melanoma may arise. Histological examination shows hypertrophied cells, particularly of the basal layer, and the presence of horny 'pearls'. Malignant change with the development of a squamous epithelioma occurs in a small proportion.

Excision should be performed for cosmetic reasons and to establish the diagnosis. The senile variety, often multiple, requires no treatment unless irritation or bleeding becomes troublesome.

Verruca vulgaris (common wart). This probably results from a virus infection of the skin and is characterised by hyperplasia of the prickle cell layers of the epidermis with thickening of the superficial horny layer. Clinically it presents as an elevation of the skin, often situated on the finger, palm of the hand, forearm and perineum. It may be single or multiple, and may disappear spontaneously. Plantar warts occur on the sole of the foot, often in relation to the metatarsal heads, and cause pain on walking. Malignant change is unusual. The wart can be destroyed either by podophyllin, cryosurgery, liquid nitrogen or cautery; excision is sometimes necessary.

Seborrhoeic keratosis is characterised by hypertrophy of the skin and is not a true tumour. Hyperplasia of the prickle cell layer occurs, but the cells are of uniform type with no invasion of surrounding tissues. The lesion is often multiple. Raised pigmented areas which may be confused with melanomas occur, particularly in exposed sites. Malignancy does not supervene and differentiation should be made from senile keratosis, which is premalignant. Excision is usually necessary to establish the diagnosis.

PREMALIGNANT TUMOURS

Bowen's disease may be considered as a carcinoma *in situ* or a premalignant condition. It is often the site of a squamous-cell carcinoma and is hence described under premalignant lesions. Histology shows thickening of the epidermis with hyperkeratosis and hypertrophy of the papillary processes. Multinucleated cells, mitotic figures and hyperchromatic nuclei occur, and characteristic large round vacuolated cells are often seen. The lesions may be single or multiple, and each is an irregular brownish-red area which proceeds to ulceration or encrustation. Excision should be performed to prevent malignant change.

Keratosis senilis is a condition occurring in old people, particularly on the face and hand. Hyperchromasia and irregularity in the size of the basal cells are found with mitotic figures, but invasion of the surrounding structures does not occur. Superficially there is hyperkeratosis. Malignancy supervenes in 20 to 25 per cent of cases. Excision of the hard scaly areas should be undertaken to prevent malignancy.

MALIGNANT TUMOURS

Basal-cell carcinoma (rodent ulcer)

This disease is associated with prolonged exposure of the skin to the rays of the sun. It is prevalent in Australia and almost invariably occurs in uncovered skin. Histology shows clusters of cells of uniform type having origin in the basal layer of the epidermis. The epidermis at first intact later becomes ulcerated. The tumour invades surrounding structures, and fat, fascia, muscle, bone and cartilage may become involved in a slow but relentless process. Metastasis is very unusual.

Approximately 98 per cent occur on the head and neck, particularly on the face above a line joining the angle of the mouth and the lobe of the ear. A plaque is first formed in the epidermis, which may remain quiescent for years, later enlarging and eventually forming an ulcer, the edge of which is rolled. The central part may become encrusted, giving the appearance of temporary healing, to be followed by further and more extensive ulceration.

Treatment

Superficial radiotherapy is the method of choice with a cure rate of 99 per cent in suitable cases. It is contraindicated (*a*) if there is a risk of producing post-irradiation chondritis, which is extremely painful; (*b*) if the lesion is near the eye, as blindness can result if that organ is not adequately protected; (*c*) if muscle, bone or cartilage are directly invaded; (*d*) if there is recurrence after irradiation. Excision should be undertaken in these circumstances, skin graft cover often being necessary.

Squamous-cell carcinoma

Pathology

In many instances this lesion is the result of prolonged contact with the skin of certain agents which produce an initial chronic dermatitis and later carcinoma. The scrotal epithelioma in mule spinners and chimney-sweeps is now only of historical importance, but Khangri cancers still occur in Kashmir, where it is the practice to hold charcoal burners on the anterior abdominal wall as a source of heat. Exposure to excessive irradiation either from radiotherapy or from the sun may result in neoplastic change. An epithelioma occasionally develops at the site of a chronically discharging sinus, or chronic leg ulcer, or in a burn scar. Histologically the tumour consists of cells which invade the dermis and the adjacent structures, cell nests usually being present and characteristic. Spread is slow and mainly local. The draining lymph nodes are involved at a relatively late stage and blood stream spread is unusual.

Clinical features

The condition is more common in the elderly and the head and neck are typical sites. The lesion may at first be papillary, later becoming ulcerated, or it may commence as an indurated ulcer with an everted edge. The regional nodes may be enlarged, or occasionally more distant deposits encountered. Biopsy to confirm the diagnosis and a radiograph of the chest to exclude metastases are essential investigations.

Treatment

This is either by excision, with a skin graft if necessary, or radiotherapy. The contraindications to radiotherapy are similar to those listed under basal cell carcinoma. Palpable regional lymph nodes may be due to infection but if they persist or are discovered at follow-up examination, block dissection should be carried out. In those cases where the primary tumour and nodes are in close proximity, a monobloc dissection is undertaken.

SWEAT AND SEBACEOUS GLAND TUMOURS

Sub-epidermal basal-cell tumours

It is likely that the basal-cell proliferation originates from sweat or sebaceous gland epithelium. Histology shows an intact epidermis with sheets of cells of the basal type deep to it. Secondary deposits do not usually occur. Clinically the condition is often familial and multiple lesions are common, occurring on the head, neck and chest. When the tumour predominates on the scalp and becomes large it is known as a 'turban tumour'. Excision is usually necessary for cosmetic reasons and to establish diagnosis.

Sweat gland tumours

These are non-metastasising growths closely related to subepidermal tumours, but the cells have an acinar arrangement and resemble normal sweat glands. Occasionally an adenocarcinoma is present. The lesions are deep to the skin and may be single or multiple. Excision is required.

ANGIOMAS

Pathology

The majority of angiomas are due to abnormal development of vasoformative tissue. Venous, arterial and capillary elements are all present, but one usually predominates and determines the type. Spider angiomas are occasionally caused by severe liver damage, probably as a result of abnormal oestrogen metabolism. Malignant lesions are rare and the usual benign form may be divided into capillary and cavernous varieties.

The **capillary angioma** consists of a network of capillaries through which the circulation is slow. Proliferation of the endothelial cells occasionally results in obliteration of the lumen. Although mainly occurring in the skin, particularly the head and neck, it is also found in the mucosa of the alimentary tract. The **cavernous angioma** is less common, and although encountered in the skin the usual site is in the liver. It consists of large blood-filled sinuses lined by endothelium, and may infiltrate widely. Complications include haemorrhage, which in the cavernous angioma may be severe, thrombosis, ulceration and hyperkeratinisation of the overlying skin.

Clinical features

The **capillary** angioma consists of one of the following types:

1. *Spider naevus*. This lesion is usually situated on the face and is the type associated with liver disease. It is seen to consist of a central vessel with

a number of radiating capillaries deep to the epidermis.

2. *Salmon patch*. More frequent in the head and neck this type is pink and blanches on external pressure. It is not raised above the surface.

3. *Strawberry mark*. This occurs in infancy and is recognised as a lobulated growth, which may spread deeply or to the surrounding skin. The deep elements are often cavernous.

4. *Port-wine stain*. This consists of a flat mauve area which does not disappear with time but tends to grow with the child. Areas of hyperkeratosis appear later in the skin and facial lesions are often disfiguring.

5. *Campbell de Morgan spots* are small red areas situated on the thorax or abdomen, and occur particularly in the older age group. They are no longer considered to have an association with malignant disease.

6. *Osler's disease*, comprising multiple small angiomas, affects the mucosa of the gastro-intestinal tract. Haematemesis or melaena may result.

The **cavernous** angioma occurs mainly in the face and cheek as a soft compressible tumour which may produce considerable deformity. Ulceration or trauma may cause excessive haemorrhage.

Treatment

Spontaneous regression may occur in spider naevi or in a salmon patch. When persistent the former are better treated by diathermy and the latter by carbon-dioxide snow. Port-wine stains should be excised, the defect may require skin grafting. Active treatment is not indicated in the majority of cavernous angiomas and strawberry marks, since they often regress spontaneously. A small number will require surgery as a result of rapid growth, if they become large and liable to injury, and in the presence of complications. Excision is the method of choice but haemorrhage and sepsis can be controlled by pressure and antibiotics. Irradiation should not be used, particularly in children, as agenesis and malignant change may follow.

Sclerosing angioma (histiocytoma)

There is considerable doubt whether an angioma always precedes this lesion. Histology shows spindle cells in the dermis, and blood pigment is also present. The extremities are usually involved, and one or more nodules may be present in the skin. They are often yellowish-brown in colour and have been confused with melanoma. Excision should be performed.

Glomus tumour

It is probable that this tumour is derived from the glomus body or communication between arteriole and venule. Histology shows blood-vessels, smooth muscle, epithelial cells, myelinated and non-myelinated nerve fibres. The majority occur in the upper limb, particularly on the pulp of the finger and under the nail. Pain is a characteristic feature and is often severe, tending to come in attacks and radiate up the limb. The tumour is small in size (1 to 3 mm) and frequently difficult to locate. Excision undertaken for the relief of pain gives good results.

Multiple self-healing squamous-cell carcinoma

This condition is often familial and histology shows the typical appearance of a squamous-cell carcinoma, but metastases do not occur. The skin of the face and extremities is usually involved. Papules develop first; these become raised and then ulcerate, spontaneous healing eventually occurring. Treatment is unnecessary, though a lesion is often excised before the diagnosis is made.

Calcifying epithelioma

This is not a malignant condition. Histology shows masses of epithelial cells in the dermis, and this on superficial examination may suggest malignancy. There are often areas of calcification and many foreign body giant cells. The lesions tend to occur on the face and arms as small, firm areas deep to the epidermis. Excision is the treatment of choice.

MELANOMA

This tumour is derived from melanocytes and is almost always pigmented. Innocent and malignant forms occur.

Innocent melanoma

Pathology

There are five types of innocent melanoma, each with a characteristic histological picture.

1. *Junctional.* The principal feature of junctional activity refers to an accumulation of melanocytes in the junctional area of the skin. All the cells are similar in type and do not invade the underlying dermis. Mitotic figures may be seen and pigment is invariably present.

2. *Compound.* In addition to junctional activity melanocytes are also present in the dermis. A narrow band of connective tissue separates these two groups of cells. All cells are of similar type and pigment is always present.

3. *Intradermal.* Melanocytes are present in the dermis but junctional activity is absent.

4. *Halo naevus.* Usually occurring in adolescence, the central compound naevus is surrounded by an area in which the melanocytes are devoid of melanosomes.

5. *Blue naevus.* A mass of densely packed melanocytes is present in or just deep to the dermis. Junctional activity is absent and melanin always present.

Junctional activity is encountered more often in early life than in the adult and it is feasible that the first three types are stages in the development of an innocent melanoma. The compound form could be due to junctional cells becoming detached and entering the dermis, the intradermal type then resulting from the disappearance of junctional activity.

Clinical features

Most individuals possess a large number of innocent melanomas. In young persons 90 per cent are junctional, but this level falls to 10 per cent in adults. An increase in size and pigmentation often occurs with hormonal stress such as puberty and pregnancy. Junctional melanomas are usually small, dark, flat lesions, which tend to be situated peripherally on the limbs and on the perineum. Those occurring on the sole of the foot, palm of the hand and on the external genitalia are of this type. Intradermal and compound melanomas may be raised above the surface, and a number are hairy. The majority are small, but occasionally they may be extensive. Halo naevi have a circular or elliptical area of total depigmentation surrounding a pale brown central portion. They remain unchanged for many months or years and then regress without a scar. Blue naevi are flat and possess a characteristic slate-blue colour. They are most often seen on the face, dorsum of the hands and feet, and on the buttocks. Diagnosis of the various types of innocent melanoma can be uncertain on clinical grounds and essentially depends on the histological features.

Treatment

Although theoretically all innocent melanomas might be better removed, this is not a practical proposition. The potentially dangerous lesions lie in the following three groups and should be excised.

1. If *junctional activity* is likely to be present. It is probable that malignancy commences in areas of excessive junctional activity, this applying particularly to small flat lesions.

2. Lesions subject to *repeated irritation* as from clothes or shaving.

3. *Suspicion of malignancy.* This includes increase in size, itching, bleeding and deepening pigmentation. Increased elevation of the tumour may be apparent and surrounding cutaneous deposits are characteristic.

Malignant melanoma

Aetiology

This aggressive tumour may arise in the skin, mucous membranes of the nasal and oral cavities, the anal canal or the vagina, the conjunctiva, the choroid and the meninges. The incidence and mortality appear to be on the increase, possibly related to changes in dress and custom allowing more exposure to solar irradiation. Racial factors play a part, dark-skinned races having a lower incidence than whites.

While the tumour may arise *de novo* most patients give a long history of a pre-existing innocent melanoma. There is no proof that a benign melanoma turns malignant and it is more likely that the malignant form arises in association with a benign pre-existing naevus. Two varieties of benign pigmented naevus do carry a definite risk of malignant change, namely the congenital giant bathing trunk naevus and Hutchinson's melanotic freckle, and should be excised prophylactically. It is otherwise unrealistic to excise all moles and there is no definite evidence that repeated trauma of a benign naevus predisposes to malignant change.

Although moles enlarge and darken during pregnancy, malignancy does not supervene and as yet no definite hormonal relationship has been established.

Pathology

It may begin as a small, firm, elevated mass or more commonly appear as malignant change in an innocent melanoma. Histologically there is well-marked junctional activity and invasion of the dermis and deeper structures by direct extension. It thus differs from the compound melanoma where the cells in the junctional area and dermis are separate. There is an alveolar arrangement of cells which show marked metaplasia and numerous mitotic figures. Pigment granules are present in both cells and stroma in variable amounts. In the rare instances where blue naevi become malignant junctional activity is absent, but the histology is otherwise similar. Spread is initially by the lymphatics, later in a widespread manner by the blood stream; eye lesions are exceptional in only metastasising by a vascular route. An important feature is that the primary growth often remains small despite extensive dissemination. Secondary deposits are common in the skin, but most sites may be involved.

There are three main clinical types:

1. *Lentigomaligna melanoma* is usually preceded for many years by a slowly enlarging flat black patch, often with partial regressions appearing as pale areas and occurs on the face in elderly patients. Nodules appear when malignancy occurs but lymph node metastases occur only very late.

2. *Superficial spreading melanoma* develops over several years as a slowly growing, flat, darkly pigmented patch. Again nodules indicate malignancy and it occurs more often on the trunk in males and on the lower limb in females.

3. *Nodular melanoma* occurs as a pigmented or amelanotic tumour with no previous spreading pigmentation. It is invasive from the start and metastasises early.

A guide to the prognosis is given by the thickness of the tumour and the depth of tumour penetration of the skin. In levels I to V the tumour lies respectively entirely superficial to the basement membrane, penetrating the basement membrane into the papillary zone of the dermis, filling the papillary zone, invading the reticular dermis and invading the subcutaneous tissue. Level I is cured by excision biopsy and is really a malignancy in situ. Level II has 80–90 per cent five-year survival, levels III and IV 50 per cent, and level V 30 per cent.

Clinical features

There is a slight female preponderance with a peak age incidence between 20 and 40 years. The condition is more common in the peripheral portions of the limb, approximately one half in the lower and one eighth in the upper limb. The trunk, head and neck are less often affected, and the mucous membranes and perineum only occasionally. The features suggesting that an innocent melanoma has apparently become malignant are an increase in size, the onset of weeping or bleeding, particularly when this is spontaneous, and an increase in pigmentation. Occasionally depigmentation is seen. The presence of a dark 'halo' around a melanoma is characteristic of malignancy, and cutaneous deposits surrounding the primary tumour diagnostic. Enlarged lymph nodes and hepatomegaly may be found, and when the original growth is small may be the first indication of malignancy.

Treatment

Excision of the primary tumour should be undertaken but it is now accepted that wide excision and grafting is only required for thicker tumours. When the primary tumour lies close to the draining lymph nodes, an *en bloc* dissection to include the nodes may be carried out, especially for thicker tumours. Prophylactic excision of clinically negative regional lymph nodes is controversial and again a compromise would suggest it should only be carried out for thicker tumours such as in levels III to V described above. Full block dissection is required for clinically involved nodes. An alternative to block dissection is *endolymphatic therapy* where a radioactive isotope is introduced into lymphatics peripherally. Theoretically this is the ideal treatment for clinically negative nodes which may have minute metastases, but results have not been improved by this technique over delayed block dissection.

Amputation is required for digital and subungual lesions but only rarely in other instances. The most radical resections do not prolong survival and should only be used if palliation is required for large recurrences ulcerating through the skin.

External irradiation may be helpful in lentigo-maligna melanoma but most malignant melanomas are radio-resistant. It may have a place in palliating fixed node masses and painful bony deposits. Regional intra-arterial perfusion with melphalan can prove useful for the treatment of local recurrences and intransit disease where skin deposits have occurred between the primary site and the draining lymph nodes, and it is sometimes used as an adjuvant treatment to prevent these deposits. Systemic chemotherapy can prove helpful and the most effective agent so far found is dimethyl triazeno imidazole carboxamide (DTIC). This produces response rates of 20–30 per cent and is most effective in skin and node deposits.

Purely intradermal deposits can be destroyed by injection with vaccinia virus and BCG produces a similar effect but may cause persistent ulceration. There is no convincing evidence of any generalised immune reaction and immunotherapy has proved singularly ineffective so far. Neither systemic chemotherapy nor immunotherapy has any place as an adjuvant treatment.

PLASTIC SURGERY

Plastic surgery is concerned with the repair of congenital defects or those deficiencies which result from trauma, burns, infection or operative removal of tumours. Skin healing may result in the formation of contractures, which can lead to disfigurement or limitation of function if situated near a joint. Excision of the contracted scar and replacement by new skin will allow healing without contracture. The technical procedures involved include rotation or advancement of skin flaps (Fig. 3.1) or cover with a free or pedicle skin graft.

Skin grafts

Skin grafts are employed to cover defects in the surface epithelium thereby lessening infection, minimising the formation of granulation tissue and resulting in more rapid healing. The graft may be applied to a clean fresh wound or to a granulating area. Gross infection will not allow a graft to take;

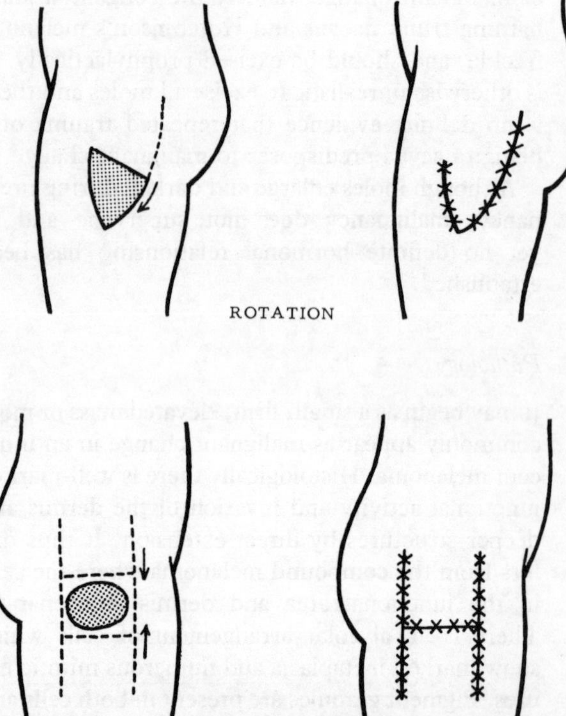

Fig. 3.1 Rotation and advancement flaps to cover a skin defect

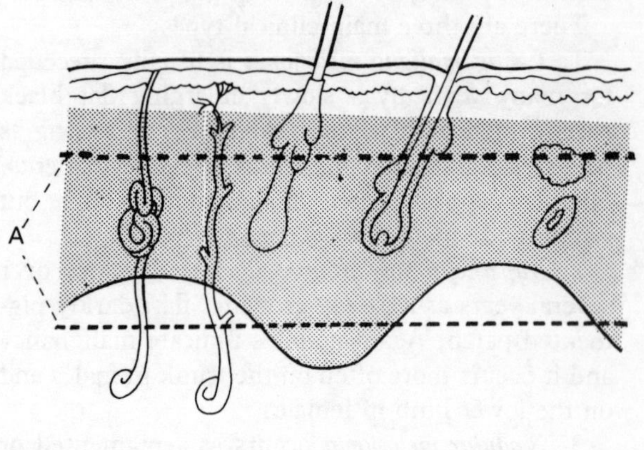

Fig. 3.2 **A.** Split thickness skin graft. **B.** Full thickness skin graft.

poor nutrition and anaemia are further factors which limit healing. Skin grafts are divided into three types.

1. **Split thickness** grafts are derived from part of the epithelial layer and range from 10 to 30 μ in thickness. The donor area contains islands of epithelium, hair follicles and sweat glands from which re-epithelialisation occurs (Fig. 3.2).

2. **Full thickness grafts** include the whole dermis but no subcutaneous fat. These two varieties are free grafts and maintain their viability in the first few days by permeation of the wound exudate. Capillary buds from the recipient area invade the graft after 48 hours and blood flow can be observed in a graft within five days.

3. **Pedicle grafts** are fashioned so that an area of skin retains an arterial blood supply when transferred to a new site. It may be shaped as a flap or formed into a tube and transferred in stages, acquiring an efficient circulation at each temporary halting place. In this way large areas of whole-thickness skin and subcutaneous fat may be moved from chest or abdomen to correct a deformed face or cover a denuded area of bone.

Skin grafts may only be transferred successfully in the same individual or between identical twins. The homograft reaction (p. 48) affects skin grafts from another individual. Nevertheless, homografts may be used in certain instances of large burns where temporary epithelial cover is required to restrain infection and fluid exudation. Alternate strips of autograft and homograft are laid on the burn. The homograft degenerates in about three weeks and this area can then be regrafted with further autografts.

FURTHER READING

McGregor, I. A. (1975). *Fundamental Techniques of Plastic Surgery and their Surgical Applications*, 6th ed. Edinburgh: Churchill Livingstone.

Milton, G. W. (1977). *Malignant Melanoma of the Skin and Mucous Membrane*. Edinburgh: Churchill Livingstone.

Westbury, G. (1979). Malignant Melanoma of the Skin. In *Surgical Review* I. Tunbridge Wells: Pitman Medical.

4

Mouth and tongue

CONGENITAL LESIONS

Failure of natural fusion of the maxillary and mandibular processes of the first branchial arch results in enlargement of the mouth or *macrostoma*; more extensive fusion than normal causes *microstoma*. Hypertrophy of the lip is known as *macrocheilia*, but it may also be due to tumour, such as lymphangioma or angioma, fibrosis following chronic infection, or associated with acromegaly.

Dermoid cysts occur in the floor of the mouth in the midline or to one side, and may lie above or below the mylohyoid. They contain sebaceous material and are recognisable as a swelling projecting into the mouth or protruding below the mandible. Distinction from a ranula may be obtained by their opaque appearance. Treatment is by excision.

Ankyloglossia or 'tongue-tie' is not uncommon in mild forms and is the result of shortening of the frenum. Treatment is usually unnecessary as there is seldom any interference with speech, but division of the tight frenum will release the tongue if required. *Macroglossia* or enlargement of the tongue may occur as a congenital deformity, but it is also secondary to tumour or infection or associated with acromegaly.

Hare-lip and cleft palate

The term *hare-lip* refers to a congenital cleft of the upper lip due to failure in fusion of its components. The central part of the upper lip is formed by the median nasal process and the lateral parts by the maxillary processes. As fusion occurs initially in the superior part and extends downwards, minor lesions involve only the inferior portion and are known as incomplete; where the lesion extends to involve the nostril it is known as a complete type. The deformity may be unilateral or, less commonly, bilateral, and may be associated with cleft palate or other congenital deformities. The unilateral type is more common on the left side. Although the aetiology is unknown, certain dietetic factors are responsible for the condition in animals, and similar lack of essential amino-acids and vitamins may also produce the condition in the human. A relationship between the occurrence of rubella in the mother during the first trimester and cleft palate in the child has been noted. A family history of cleft is not uncommon in affected children.

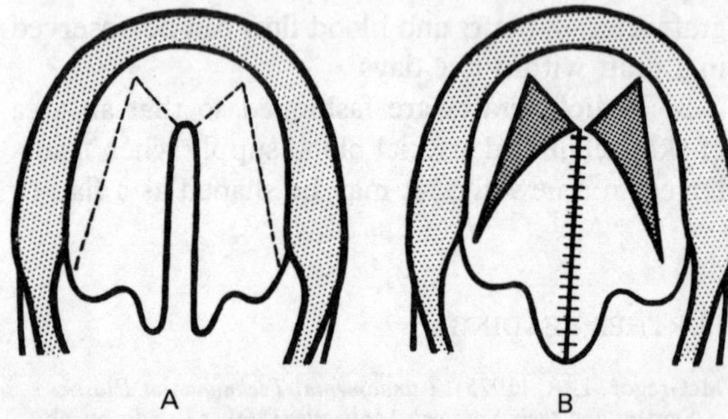

Fig. 4.1 Cleft palate. **A.** The common type involving the hard and soft portions. **B.** Operative closure of the defect after mobilisation of the palate. The lateral shaded areas are rapidly covered by ingrowth of epithelium.

The *palate* is formed by fusion of the central median nasal process which forms the premaxilla and the palatal processes of the maxillary processes which form the rest of the hard and soft palate. Fusion of this Y-shaped junction commences anteriorly, and minor degrees of cleft thus give rise to a bifid uvula, whilst more severe degrees may result in a free premaxilla. The common lesion is one involving the stem of the 'Y' with a defect in the hard and soft palate (Fig. 4.1, A).

Clinical features

The main problem in hare-lip is one of disfigurement. The alar cartilage on the affected side is flattened and adds to the cosmetic deformity. In severe cases difficulty in suckling may be apparent and special teats or spoon feeding may be required. The effects of cleft palate are of more serious consequence. In complete clefts dental abnormalities affecting the upper incisors are apparent and, as in the common form of incomplete cleft, the nasal and oral cavities are continuous. Rhinitis and sinusitis occur later, together with the typical disturbance of speech.

Treatment

In *hare-lip* repair is not urgent as the deformity is mainly cosmetic. Surgery should be postponed until the sixth month when the child is well established as a separate individual. The principles involved include freeing of the lip from the underlying maxilla, paring of the cleft and accurate suturing of the component parts of the lip. Normal development of the orbicularis oris muscle permits a satisfactory result. If surgery is undertaken earlier—in the first few weeks of life—a second operation is generally required later to improve the cosmetic appearance.

The aims in treating *cleft palate* are (*a*) to obtain closure of the cleft and thus to separate the nasal and oral cavities, and (*b*) to produce satisfactory approximation of soft palate and posterior pharyngeal wall thus allowing separation of nasal and oral pharynx on phonation. To this end relaxing palatal incisions with freeing of the soft palate are important steps in the operative procedure (Fig. 4.1, B).

Operation should be undertaken before speech commences and is advised at about 12 months. Before this the parts are small and there is considerable technical difficulty; if left longer than 18 months faults in talking may be difficult to eradicate. Spoon feeding may be required in the earlier stages of the more severe type, but it is unnecessary in the milder forms. Following operation oral feeding may be commenced within a few hours, and aided by the abundant vascular supply of the mouth, wounds heal quickly. Speech therapy forms an important part of the after-care, and in particular where the mother is already affected by the same condition. In older cases where the defect is confined to the hard palate an occlusive denture may be of value.

INFLAMMATION AND ULCERATION

Acute inflammation may affect both the tongue and buccal cavity and may follow excessive tobacco or spirits, be the result of allergic or drug reaction, or it may be caused by a specific infection such as Vincent's angina. Acute candida infection is more often seen at the extremes of life, but occurs in the debilitated or those on long-term antibiotics or chemotherapy for malignant disease. The lesion in the tongue is usually confined to the mucous membrane, is seldom of serious surgical significance, and generally responds to local hygiene directed towards the eradication of sepsis. Amphotericin B washouts are helpful in candidiasis. Occasionally the deeper portion becomes inflamed as the result of secondary infection of a traumatic lesion from dentures or teeth, or due to an insect bite. Diffuse oedema renders this form more dangerous due to respiratory embarrassment. Antibiotics, antihistamine drugs, incision or, rarely, tracheostomy may be required. Inflammation of the gums is considered on page 66.

Ulceration may follow stomatitis, may be a local manifestation of a general disturbance or occur as a purely local phenomenon.

General conditions encountered surgically which produce ulceration include excessive antibiotic therapy, particularly of the broad spectrum type. An acute attack of herpes may produce multiple vesicles more often on the lip than the tongue which break down to form shallow ulcers. Aphthous ulcers occur, particularly in children, due to a virus infection. They begin as small superficial vesicles with bright red margins and rupture within 24 hours. Pain is marked, but healing is rapid. Larger aphthae with indurated edges are occasionally seen in association with ulcerative colitis. Agranulocytosis due to overtreatment with toxic drugs in hyperthyroidism or from chemotherapy in malignant disease may cause ulceration.

Specific ulceration due to syphilis or tuberculosis is less frequently encountered but is of surgical significance in differential diagnosis. The chancre of the primary stage is rare on the tongue but the serpiginous ulceration of the secondary stage or the punched-out gumma of the tertiary stage may be observed, particularly on the dorsum. Tuberculous ulceration is indicative of advanced pulmonary or laryngeal disease. The characteristic undermined edge, shallow ulceration and anaemic granulations are generally situated at the tip of the tongue. The important carcinomatous ulcer requires exclusion and is described under carcinoma of the tongue.

All cases of persistent ulceration should be submitted to biopsy for histological confirmation of their nature. General causative factors require appropriate therapy, and local traumatic conditions should be removed. The management of carcinomatous ulceration is considered on page 64.

LEUCOPLAKIA

This is the most important form of chronic superficial glossitis. It is a precancerous lesion which may involve the tongue, buccal cavity or lip. It is caused by chronic irritation from such factors as smoking, particularly pipe smoking, carious teeth and ill-fitting dentures, betel and tobacco chewing and the drinking of hot fluids and spirits. Syphilis and vitamin deficiency may also play a part in the aetiology. Chronic hyperplastic candidiasis can resemble fissured leucoplakia and is precancerous.

The pathological changes include an initial redness and hyperaemia related to the area of irritation, followed by hyperkeratinisation of a localised or diffuse pattern. Papilliferous proliferation or mucosal atrophy may follow with later induration and fissure formation. Neoplasia usually takes place in the more extensive forms, either in the fissured areas or the hyperkeratotic zones. The histological appearance is one of hyperaemia and round-cell infiltration of the dermis with either hyperkeratinisation or atrophy of the epidermis.

Clinically there is a marked male preponderance. The tongue is mainly affected and the area is small when local trauma is responsible, the redness from contact with a pipe stem being characteristic. Thickened white patches are usual and the condition may remain stationary for years. With desquamation and exposure of the sensitive epithelium, the tongue presents a raw beef appearance. In advanced states the fissures are separated by areas of papillary formation which may simulate or become a malignant lesion.

The management is initially one of observation, any definite cause being removed. Although syphilis requires treatment, the general management of this disease seldom affects the local condition. Vitamin deficiency if present must be corrected. Cryosurgery in the form of a spray using liquid nitrogen may be used to remove extensive lesions, the new mucosa being free of leucoplakia. Biopsy of several fissured areas may be required to exclude neoplasia.

TUMOURS

The benign lesions include papilloma, fibroma, lipoma and angioma. When exposed to irritation or producing symptoms removal should be performed. A small proportion, about 5 per cent, of mucous and salivary gland tumours are found in the oral cavity (p. 71). The common benign lesion is a fibro-epithelial polyp which occurs on the mucosa of the tongue, lips or gums. It is pedunculated and is the result of chronic irritation from either a sharp tooth or a gap in the teeth. The mucosa is drawn into the latter and there is a fibrous tissue core. Removal of the cause is necessary after excision of the polyp. Other associated benign swellings include ranula, mucous cyst and lingual thyroid.

A *ranula* is a cystic swelling involving the under surface of the tongue or floor of the mouth, originating as an extravasation cyst, the wall of which is lined by granulation tissue. It is a bluish fluctuant swelling generally to one side of the midline, and appears in the first few years of life. It may increase in size and interfere with mastication and speech or embarrass respiration and should be excised together with the wedge of tissue in the floor of the mouth, which includes the gland responsible for the extravasation. *Mucous cysts* are common, particularly on the under surface of the tongue, are generally small, may be multiple and should be punctured or excised. A *lingual thyroid* is occasionally found on the dorsum of the posterior part of the tongue and is described under Thyroid Gland (p. 80).

Malignant tumours may be either sarcomatous or carcinomatous. The former are rare and are usually lymphosarcomas.

Carcinoma of the tongue

Pathology

Aetiological factors include dental trauma, smoking, alcohol, syphilis and other forms of chronic irritation. Leucoplakia is also a precancerous lesion.

The common site is at the edge of the tongue in its anterior two-thirds. The majority of lesions present as an ulcer although nodular, papillary or fissured forms later becoming ulcerative may be recognised (Fig. 4.2). The main histological type is a squamous-cell carcinoma, but in the posterior one-third it is more usual to find a transitional-cell carcinoma. Spread is both local and to the regional lymph nodes. The floor of the mouth, the alveolar margin and, in posterior growths, the tonsil and palate may be all directly affected. Lymphatic dissemination occurs to the submental, submandibular and deep cervical groups. Node involvement is generally ipsilateral, but in the posterior one-third tumours may be bilateral. Further lymphatic spread to the mediastinum or vascular spread is unusual and is a late finding.

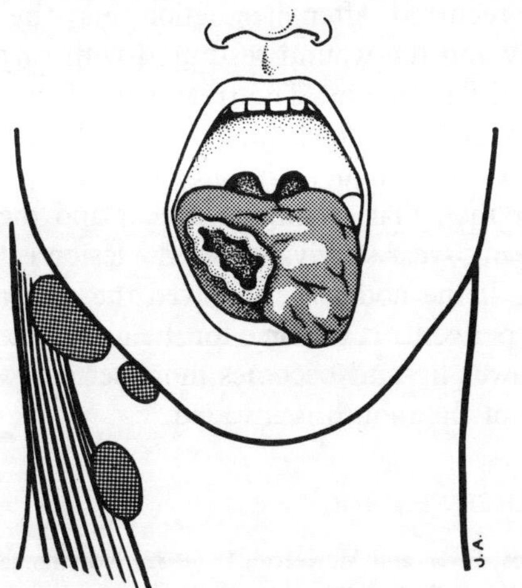

Fig. 4.2 Carcinoma of the lateral aspect of the tongue, with areas of leucoplakia and fissures. Metastatic spread occurs to deep cervical nodes.

Clinical features

The initial symptoms are of a swelling or ulcer with later superadded infection and pain. The latter may be localised to the site of the lesion, or be referred by the chorda tympani and auriculo-temporal nerve and cause earache. Excessive salivation and halitosis are noted, and dysphagia and slurring of speech from lingual immobility are later symptoms. The ulcer presents a typical everted edge with indurated base. Repeated minor haemorrhage from its surface and toxic absorption from the infected area may cause debility and anaemia. The neck must be examined for palpable lymph nodes which may be enlarged due to tumour or infection or both. In some instances, particularly in growths of the posterior one-third of the tongue, such glandular enlargement is the first indication of malignancy. Death may be due to inanition through refusal to eat because of severe pain, to bronchopneumonia from aspiration of infected material, or to sudden haemorrhage from involvement of the lingual vessels. The differential diagnosis includes the various lingual ulcers, but where the suspicion of malignancy is entertained confirmation by biopsy is imperative.

Treatment

This may be considered under the following headings:

1. Preliminary.
2. The primary lesion.
3. The cervical lymph nodes.

Preliminary treatment by antibiotics may be necessary for an infective focus in mouth, teeth or pharynx. Dental extractions or removal of badly infected tonsils may occasionally be required before any specific therapy is commenced.

The primary lesion. The treatment of choice is radiotherapy, which does not mutilate and preserves function. In the anterior two-thirds of the tongue this is best administered in the form of radium needles, which are implanted in the tumour under general anaesthesia according to a plan prepared before operation in collaboration with a physicist. The usual duration of treatment is about seven days. In the posterior one-third of the tongue it is more difficult to implant needles accurately, and telecobalt or supervoltage therapy is preferable. A larger amount of tissue has to be irradiated, and the duration of treatment is six to eight weeks.

Surgery is required under the following circumstances:

1. For radio-resistant growths.
2. For post-irradiation recurrence.
3. For growths producing excessive fibrosis associated with a poor blood supply.
4. In some cases where there is extensive bony involvement.

The operation is partial glossectomy. Preliminary ligation of the external carotid artery is often advisable to reduce haemorrhage. The disfigurement produced even when mandibular resection is required is well corrected by modern prostheses inserted either at the time of operation or at a later date. Palliative excision or diathermy coagulation may be worth while when radical removal is not feasible. Large necrotic tumours may be controlled by cryosurgery with considerable relief of pain. When the latter is severe and intractable, division of the lingual nerve in the third molar region under local anaesthesia produces permanent analgesia.

The cervical lymph nodes. Treatment may be conveniently considered under the following headings:

1. Nodes not palpable.
2. Nodes palpable and operable.
3. Nodes palpable but inoperable.

When the nodes are not palpable prophylactic surgical or radiotherapeutic treatment is unnecessary. Careful follow-up at regular intervals, initially of two months but later of six months, is required and the state of both primary lesion and cervical nodes noted.

When the nodes are both palpable and operable the treatment of choice is ipsilateral block dissection of the cervical lymph nodes to include the sternomastoid muscle, the internal jugular vein, the posterior belly of the digastric and the deep cervical fascia. In tumours of the posterior one-third of the tongue a unilateral or bilateral upper block dissection may be preferable. The primary lesion should be healed, appear to be remaining healed, and the general condition of the patient should be satisfactory.

When the glands are palpable but inoperable, surgery is contraindicated and palliation by radiotherapy is required.

In advanced cases local mouth hygiene to reduce sepsis, the avoidance of excessively hot or cold fluids, of irritant and spicy foods and the local insufflation of benzocaine powder may alleviate pain and permit an adequate calorie intake.

Carcinoma of the floor of the mouth and remainder of the buccal cavity presents the same pathological features and is managed in a similar manner, although when surgery is required a monobloc dissection removing primary lesion and cervical nodes may be necessary.

Carcinoma of the lip

Similar aetiological factors are at play as in carcinoma of the tongue, and its pathology and management follow the same lines. Spread is to the submental glands or to the submandibular group, later to the deep cervical chain. It is more slowly growing than lingual cancer, generally found in elderly males, more often on the lower lip and best treated by radiotherapy. Small lesions or those that have recurred after irradiation may be excised widely and the wound resutured with surprisingly little disfigurement. The treatment of the adjacent lymph nodes follows that described under carcinoma of the tongue. The prognosis of lip cancer is better than that of lingual cancer and there is 90 per cent 5-year survival when the lesion is less than 2 cm. If the nodes are involved the cure rate falls to 50 per cent. It is worse for the upper lip than for the lower lip and becomes more serious when the angle of the mouth is invaded.

FURTHER READING

Brookes, G. B. and McKelvie, P. (1982). Carcinoma of the tongue. *Brit. J. Hosp. Med.* 28, 6–21.

5

Jaws and salivary glands

JAWS

Trauma

Dislocation of the jaw may be anterior, posterior, unilateral or bilateral. Fracture more often involves the mandible than the maxilla.

Anterior dislocation

This is the most common type and is generally bilateral. It is caused by opening the mouth too widely in yawning or in dental extraction, particularly under anaesthesia. A blow on the jaw while the mouth is open may also be responsible. If severe trauma is applied the condyle may be driven upwards through the base of the skull with secondary brain damage—an anterosuperior dislocation. Clinically the mandible is displaced forward, or in unilateral dislocations to the unaffected side, and the jaw held open. Pain and inability to talk or swallow are prominent features. Treatment is manual reduction by downward traction and backward displacement with or without anaesthesia.

Posterior dislocation

Trauma to the closed jaw is generally responsible, and the condition is accompanied by fracture of the tympanic plate. The condyle enters the external auditory meatus and may be seen with an auriscope. Treatment is reduction of the deformity.

Clicking jaw

This condition is the result of an internal derangement of the meniscus of the temporo-mandibular joint. Laxity or a tear of the cartilage may cause the syndrome of pain, clicking and, in more severe instances, locking of the jaw. It may follow difficult dental extractions or trauma or be more insidious in its onset. Occasionally it is painless. The avoidance of excessive opening in speech or in mastication may control the condition, but when troublesome removal of the meniscus may be necessary.

Fracture of the mandible

This may follow a direct or indirect injury, the most common cause being fighting. The body, angle, ramus, condylar neck, or rarely the coronoid process, may all be affected (Fig. 5.1).

Fracture of the angle or ramus is usually the result of a direct blow, but fracture of the body may occur from an injury to the opposite side of the jaw. Fracture of the neck of the condyle often follows a blow on the chin. Multiple fractures such as those of the body and neck of condyle are not infrequent. All fractures of the body in front of the third molar

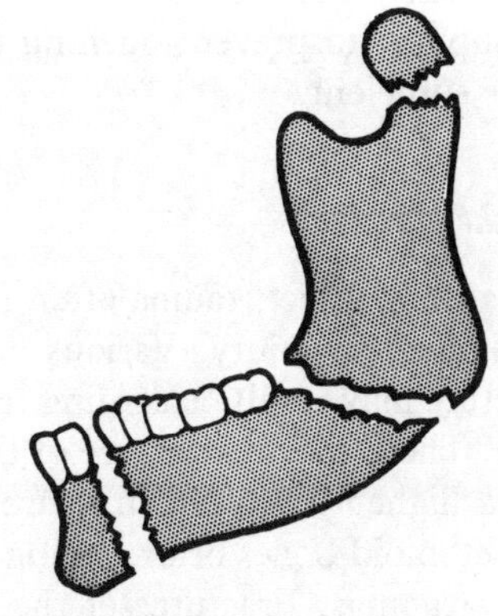

Fig. 5.1 Common sites of fracture of the mandible

tooth are compound. Displacement may occur as the direct result of injury, or be exaggerated by the upward pull of the temporalis and masseter muscles and the downward and backward pull of the genio-hyoid and genio-glossus.

The diagnosis is made from the history of injury and pain on moving the jaw. Local tenderness, swelling and perhaps crepitus and displacement, all of which are more easily recognised in fracture of the body, confirm the damage. Inability to close the mouth fully and anaesthesia over the distribution of the mental branch of the inferior dental nerve may be present. Radiography confirms the diagnosis. Complications include obstruction to the airway, haemorrhage and infection.

Treatment. Transportation with the patient on their side is essential. If allowed to lie on their back respiratory obstruction due to posterior displacement of the tongue may be fatal. The side position also permits free drainage of saliva. Portable suction apparatus should be available and in the unconscious patient a tongue suture and airway inserted. Careful oral hygiene, combined with antibiotics, help to prevent infection, and early reduction before the swelling is pronounced further diminishes this risk.

Definitive treatment of fractures of the body is best carried out in a maxillo-facial unit with special experience of such injuries. The principles include general anaesthesia, accurate reduction, and maintenance either by the fitting of a metal cap to the teeth around the fracture or by means of special type splintage or transosseous wiring in the edentulous; conservation of the teeth and bone is important. Fractures other than those of the body of the mandible seldom require operative treatment and temporary support to prevent opening the mouth too widely is sufficient.

Fracture of the maxilla

The usual cause is direct trauma often following a car accident or crush injury. Various degrees and types of fracture may result, according to the direction of force. There may be fracture of the alveolar margin, or a higher transverse fracture including the nasal or ethmoid bones or extending to include one or both zygomas. Fractures of the zygomatic arch may occur independently and follow direct trauma such as a blow with the fist.

The diagnosis is made from the history of injury and from the appearance of early swelling, discoloration, local tenderness, and in severe cases by extreme mobility. Accurate radiography is essential when the condition is suspected, and treatment is preferably carried out in a maxillo-facial unit. Following disimpaction and reduction a splint is fitted to the teeth, or in the edentulous to the alveolar margin, and then connected to a plaster head cap with the aid of transbuccal cheek wires and an anterior connecting bar. Immobilisation is generally required for five weeks and oral hygiene and correct feeding are important aspects of the post-operative care. Liquid meals of about 2000 calories per day supplemented by vitamin and protein preparations should be given at two-hourly intervals. A liquidiser is helpful in preparing food and feeding cups and flexible drinking straws are needed. Early treatment is essential if there is derangement of occlusion to prevent the deformity which follows fibrosis. In zygomatic arch fractures elevation with a lever is adequate.

INFECTIONS

The gums may be infected by a specific organism such as Vincent's spirochaete and the condition of *gingivitis* follows. More often the latter is due to an infection by non-specific streptococci and known as suppurative periodontitis or pyorrhoea. Mode of entry is often through a carious tooth and progression to a periapical abscess may occur. Oedema of the gums, a marked tendency to bleed and small pockets of pus around the teeth may be observed. Later fibrosis with gum recession and loosening of the teeth may take place. The treatment is by local antibiotic therapy in the acute stage followed by dental extractions where required. Untreated cases maintain a focus of infection which may spread throughout the body.

Infection may also spread from a carious tooth to form an *alveolar abscess*. Extension superficially to the outer alveolar margin may follow with the formation of a 'gum boil', or if it spreads above or below the buccinator it may discharge on to the skin of the face or neck. Orbital, palatal and nasal swellings may arise from upper dental inflammation. Occasionally such infection tracks deeply and involves the antrum or produces osteomyelitis. Treatment is by dental extraction or by incision and drainage of the pus followed by appropriate dental care.

Actinomycosis may follow a dental extraction and manifests itself three weeks later as a painless mass generally involving the lower jaw. Abscesses may form with marked induration of face and neck and multiple sinus formation. The pus may show the typical sulphur granules and sunray fungus. Treatment is generally conservative and is discussed on page 8.

Osteomyelitis

Pathology

Unlike osteomyelitis affecting the long bones, this condition is more common in adults, and the lower jaw is more frequently involved than the upper. The majority of cases are secondary to dental infection or fracture. Occasionally it may follow the irradiation of neoplasms, chronic metal poisoning with mercury or phosphorus, or infection of a bone cyst.

The commonly responsible organism is the staphylococcus or streptococcus, but infection with specific organisms as in tuberculosis, syphilis or actinomycosis may occur. The ensuing pathological changes resemble osteomyelitis in other sites with medullary infection, periosteal elevation, new bone formation and sequestration. The extent of the last named may vary from small localised areas to complete necrosis of mandible or maxilla. Involucrum formation is seldom pronounced in the maxilla and marked loss of substance may be apparent. In the specific infections a chronic and more indolent osteomyelitis occurs, whilst sinuses may be seen in either type.

Clinical features

Pain, swelling and trismus associated with general constitutional disturbance, such as pyrexia and malaise, are encountered in the acute infection. A recent history of dental extraction or compound fracture may be obtained. Localised bony tenderness is present and often associated with enlarged and tender cervical lymph nodes. Extension from the upper jaw to the adjacent nose, orbit or sinuses may take place. In the more chronic forms sinuses, frequently multiple, purulent discharge and repeated constitutional upsets are observed. Radiography in the early acute stage may confirm a dental lesion or fracture, but is of no value in the detection of osteomyelitis. In the chronic form cavitation, sequestration and new bone formation may all be apparent.

Treatment

Adequate treatment of any inflammatory dental state or compound fracture will help to prevent the development of osteomyelitis. In the established condition antibiotic therapy and the drainage of abscesses will be required. When sequestrectomy is necessary it should be deferred until new bone has formed to maintain the dental arch. In the upper jaw a prosthesis may be indicated.

TUMOURS

Tumours of the jaw may be divided into the following groups:

1. Alveolus—
   - Epulis: Fibrous; Giant cell
2. Dental origin—
   - Odontome: Epithelial; Mesoblastic; Mixed
3. Bone—
   - Mandible. Benign. Osteoclastoma
   - Malignant: Primary—osteogenic sarcoma; Secondary—direct spread
   - Maxilla—As above, plus carcinoma of the antrum.

Alveolar tumours

An *epulis* or tumour of the gum may be either fibrous or giant cell in type (Fig. 5.2).

The **fibrous epulis** arises as a small pedunculated fibroma from the periosteum and grows upwards between the teeth. It is more common in the lower jaw and is often associated with low-grade dental infection. Smooth in outline, slowly growing and painless, its presence is often considered unimportant until dental advice is sought. Treatment consists of removal of the tumour together with adjacent diseased teeth. Recurrence is unusual.

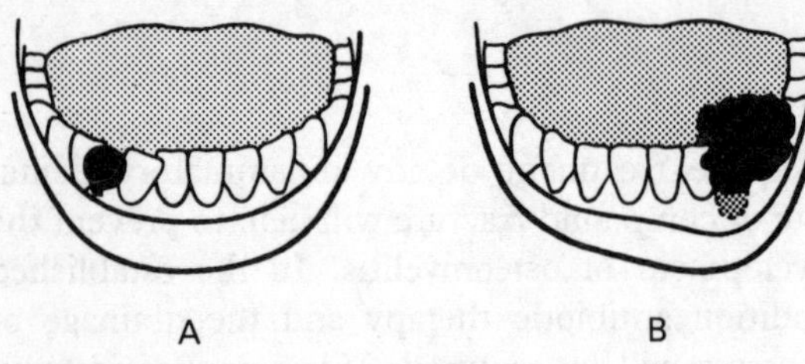

Fig. 5.2 Epulis. **A.** Fibrous. **B.** Giant cell with extension into bone.

The **giant cell epulis** is a larger and more sessile lesion. Lobulated and highly vascular, it grows more quickly than the fibrous epulis and is liable to ulceration and haemorrhage. It is composed of giant cells in a vascular stroma and may extend into the bone. Like the fibrous type, it is more common in the lower jaw and may disrupt the teeth. Treatment is wide excision and should include the adjacent teeth and bone.

The odontomes

Numerous varieties are described which are mainly of interest to the dental surgeon. Only the principal types will be mentioned.

The *epithelial odontomes* include dental cysts, dentigerous cysts and adamantinomas.

A **dental cyst** arises in a pulpless or infected tooth as a result of infection irritating epithelial cell rests in the periodontal membrane (Fig. 5.3, A). It is a single cyst containing serous or mucoid material and cholesterol crystals. Painless, unless infected, it is more common in adults and presents as a firm hard swelling usually in the outer and upper alveolar region, occasionally on the palate.

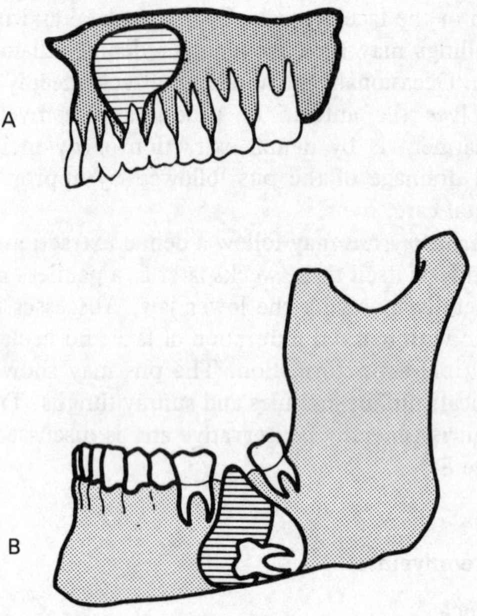

Fig. 5.3 **A.** Dental cyst arising in maxilla. **B.** Dentigerous cyst arising in mandible.

When large, crepitant fluctuation may be obtained. The diagnosis is confirmed by radiography. Treatment by initial clearance of other infected teeth is followed by removal of the causative tooth and the epithelial lining of the cyst. Primary closure is usual but it may be necessary to excise a wide window in the outer bony wall and allow adequate drainage into the oral cavity.

A **dentigerous cyst** forms around the crown of an unerupted tooth, and is generally seen in patients under the age of 15 years. It has a similar structure to a dental cyst, and on radiography the unerupted tooth may be demonstrated (Fig. 5.3, B). Excision of the cyst and dental extraction are required, it being seldom possible to save the unerupted tooth.

An adamantinoma, more commonly called an **ameloblastoma**, is a malignant tumour arising from the ameloblasts of the enamel organ. It is a unilocular or multilocular cystic lesion which is locally invasive, but a small percentage have metastasised. Generally encountered in the fourth decade, it is most common at the angle of the mandible in the region of the third molar tooth. It may reach a large size and exhibit egg-shell crackling. Radiography shows a characteristic multilocular soap-bubble appearance and differentiates it from a dentigerous cyst. Treatment is removal, together with an adjacent rim of bone to prevent recurrence.

The *mesoblastic odontomes* include the cementomas and fibrous odontomes. The former are composed of hyperplastic cement around the root of an erupted tooth; the latter are extremely rare and found only in rachitic subjects. Treatment in either case is removal.

The *mixed odontomes* are composed of a conglomeration of dental tissue, and associated with unerupted teeth. They may cause pain, become infected or interfere with normal dental development, and should be removed.

TUMOURS OF BONE

The mandible

Benign growths include fibroma, chondroma, osteoma and osteoclastoma which, although not common, is the most important.

The **osteoclastoma** is similar in appearance to that tumour elsewhere (p. 355) and is composed of large numbers of giant cells. A usual position near the angle of the jaw is often attributed to persistent osteoclastic activity associated with the excavation of the third molar tooth. It is a soft grey or haemorrhagic tumour, developing centrally within the bone and expanding its surface. In large lesions the classical egg-shell crackling may be elicited. Radiography demonstrates a soap bubble appearance. The differential diagnosis includes single or multiple bone cysts, such as those occurring in osteitis fibrosa cystica, and the presence of a general endocrine disease should be excluded. Treatment is by radiotherapy, or initial excision or curettage followed by radiotherapy.

Primary malignant tumours of the mandible are uncommon, but include osteogenic sarcoma and chondrosarcoma. They are recognised as a hard, irregular and progressive swelling, which may ulcerate into the buccal cavity or on to the exterior. Treatment is radical excision when feasible or radiotherapy for palliation.

Secondary malignant disease is seldom due to metastatic deposit, but more often caused by direct invasion from tumours of the buccal cavity, particularly carcinoma of the tongue. Modern techniques of radiotherapy allow it to be used in the management of early cases, but recurrences require surgical excision and the implantation of a prosthesis. Subsequent deformity is not marked.

The maxilla

In general similar lesions affect both jaws, but with some variation of frequency. The osteoclastoma is less often encountered in the maxilla; the osteogenic sarcoma more so than in the mandible.

The usual primary malignant lesion is **carcinoma of the antrum**. Generally squamous cell in nature, it begins within the maxilla and may extend in any direction to produce a characteristic syndrome. Growth medially may block the nose or cause a unilateral nasal discharge or epistaxis. Upward extension may displace the eye or produce ocular palsy. Backward growth into the pterygomaxillary fissure may give an atypical trigeminal neuralgia, whilst downward extension may produce a palatal swelling or loosen the teeth, and the first indication of malignancy may be the failure of a tooth socket to heal. A prominent facial swelling is a later symptom, but occasionally a cervical swelling due to glandular metastases may be the first sign of an occult primary growth.

Treatment is by supervoltage radiotherapy in the first instance. In the event of failure or recurrence, excision of the maxilla should be performed. Deformity may be prevented by the use of a prosthesis, particularly satisfactory when the floor of the orbit can be preserved. The cervical lymph nodes should be managed as outlined in the treatment of carcinoma of the tongue (p. 64).

SALIVARY GLANDS

Injury to one of the glands or ducts may occur as a result of a contusion or laceration or be secondary to a fracture of the mandible. An external fistula may be apparent and should be looked for in facial injuries in proximity to a gland or its duct. Failure to recognise such a salivary fistula results in persistent discharge and may lead to duct obstruction from scarring. If the opening is into the mouth the injury is not important, but when external, operative closure or transference of the tract into the mouth may be required. Irradiation of the gland to destroy its secretions is an alternative form of treatment.

Inflammation

Parotid gland

The common type of acute inflammatory state is mumps or epidemic parotitis.

Acute suppurative parotitis is less often seen today because of better understanding of its aetiology. It was formerly a frequent accompaniment of severe dehydration from intestinal obstruction or gastro-enteritis and often followed abdominal operations. It results from an ascending infection along the parotid duct from the oral cavity. Dental caries or a contaminated mouth provide the source of infection, the usual organism being the *Staph. aureus*. Initial oedema and congestion may progress to abscess and sinus formation.

The clinical picture is the sudden onset of pain and swelling in the parotid region in a middle-aged or elderly patient with imperfect oral hygiene a day or two after operation. General manifestations of malaise and pyrexia may follow. The gland is tender, and the overlying skin may be red; because of the rigidity of the overlying fascia fluctuation is a late sign. Examination of the mouth shows a pouting and inflamed duct orifice from which pus may be expressed. Cervical lymph node enlargement is common. In the untreated case rapid extension of infection with cellulitis, pyaemia and pulmonary infection with a fatal termination may occur.

Treatment includes the prevention of severe dehydration and careful attention to oral hygiene. In the established case any associated dryness or infection requires prompt correction by intravenous fluids, sialogogues and local mouth washes. Antibiotic therapy resolves the majority of infections, but incision and drainage may be required.

Chronic parotitis occurs more commonly and is due either to obstruction of the salivary flow, a stricture being more common than a calculus, or to diminution in the amount of saliva secreted. Infection, frequently caused by *Strept. viridans*, spreads easily from the mouth with recurring and persisting attacks of pain and swelling. A sialogram may demonstrate the presence of either stricture or calculus and may show any associated ductal dilatation.

Treatment is similar for both types. Antibiotics should be prescribed during an attack together with analgesics for the relief of pain. When the cause lies in the vicinity of the duct orifice dilatation with bougies may be beneficial. Intraoral operations aimed at removing a calculus or at enlarging the orifice are often followed by stricture. Exploration through an incision on the cheek with dilatation of any stricture present is to be preferred. An alternative is preliminary parotid irradiation to depress secretion with ligation of the parotid duct intraorally. This converts the gland into a non-functioning organ isolated from a potentially infected oral cavity. Where symptoms are very severe or other measures fail, parotidectomy with preservation of the facial nerve may be required.

Submandibular gland

Both acute and chronic inflammation occur and are often associated with calculi. In the former type spreading infection may result in Ludwig's angina. Treatment of the acute lesion is by antibiotics and local mouth hygiene. The chronic form often requires excision of the affected gland.

Mikulicz disease

This is an uncommon and chronic condition in which there is enlargement of one or more of the salivary and lacrimal glands. The normal parenchyma becomes replaced by lymphoid tissue. Enlargement may occur in leukaemia or lymphosarcoma, and is designated Mikulicz syndrome. Generally seen in young adults, the condition often responds to radiotherapy.

Calculus

A salivary gland calculus is composed mainly of calcium carbonate or calcium phosphate and follows infection. It is more common in the submandibular than the parotid gland, due to the less viscid secretion of the latter. Frequently encountered in the main duct it is usually single and pea-like, but may be elongated and resemble a date stone. Occasionally multiple calculi are present within the smaller ducts of the submandibular gland.

The effects are those of obstruction to the salivary flow and of infection. Periodic swelling of the gland, generally at meal-times, is characteristic, and persistent chronic enlargement particularly of the submandibular gland is not uncommon. A stone may be directly palpable in the duct or encountered by probing. Radiography often confirms the findings. Calculi may be removed from the submandibular duct through the floor of the mouth, but involvement of the gland requires its excision. The passage of small parotid calculi may be aided by dilatation of the ductal orifice, and more radical surgery is seldom necessary.

TUMOURS

The common benign tumour is the *mixed parotid tumour*. As this is not restricted to the parotid gland but may occur in the other salivary glands, the palate, lip or buccal mucosa, it is better named a mucous and salivary gland tumour. Less common benign tumours are the adenolymphoma, fibroma, lipoma and angioma.

Mucous and salivary gland tumour

('Mixed parotid tumour' or 'pleomorphic adenoma')

Pathology

Eighty-five per cent of these tumours occur in the parotid gland, 10 per cent in the submandibular gland, and the remainder elsewhere in the mouth, cheek or palate. They are of epithelial origin, although they may contain material which resembles cartilage, which accounts for their previously supposed mixed nature. Encapsulation is seldom complete, and either as a result of this or because of multicentric foci of origin, recurrences following removal are not infrequent. Histologically they are composed of epithelial cells arranged in acini or sheets with spindle cells lying in a mucoid matrix resembling cartilage. Sudden growth and a highly cellular structure indicate malignancy.

Clinical features

The majority of tumours appear in the third and fourth decade, two-thirds occurring before the age of 40 years. There is a slight preponderance in women. Presentation is in the form of a firm, painless swelling, generally in the parotid region, not altering with salivation and of long duration, at times 10 to 20 years. It may lie in the substance or on the surface of the gland and be extremely mobile. There is no involvement of the facial nerve and no evidence of metastases.

Treatment is removal of the tumour. Simple enucleation is inadequate and may be followed by recurrence. A surrounding margin of compressed normal tissue must be included. Radiotherapy may be used post-operatively. In the usual site of the parotid area, the facial nerve must be defined to avoid damage and removal of the superficial lobe, or in deep lesions total parotidectomy, is advocated. Temporary partial or complete facial palsy follows in about 30 per cent of operations but recovery generally takes place within six months. Recurrences following operation grow more rapidly and 25 per cent may become malignant. When the submandibular gland is involved total removal of the gland is simple and satisfactory.

Adenolymphoma

This is a rare lesion accounting for less than 10 per cent of salivary tumours. The majority appear in the parotid gland and grow very slowly. They are well encapsulated and seldom followed by recurrence. Generally solid, with a slightly lobulated surface, they are composed of a lymphoid stroma in which the epithelial parenchyma resembles the salivary gland ducts. They appear at a later age than the mucous and salivary gland tumours and are more common in men. Treatment is by excision of the tumour.

Malignant tumours of the salivary glands

The parotid gland is most frequently involved in primary malignant disease, the submandibular gland less often, and the sublingual gland only exceptionally. About 30 per cent of all parotid tumours are malignant, and in the submandibular gland the incidence is still higher. A considerable number of parotid carcinomas develop from mixed parotid tumours. The main types of growth are adenocarcinoma, malignant mixed tumour and squamous-cell carcinoma.

The adenocarcinoma may develop from the serous cells and present a glandular appearance or develop from the ducts, being highly cellular and known as a *cylindroma*. The malignant mixed tumour resembles an adenocarcinoma. The squamous-cell carcinoma is the least common and similar in structure to these tumours elsewhere. Growth in most salivary gland tumours is slow. Spread of all types is by local extension and by the lymphatics to the adjacent nodes. More distant metastases are uncommon. In addition to primary carcinoma the salivary glands may be involved in secondary tumour, particularly the submandibular gland from a lingual lesion.

Clinically, primary carcinoma occurs chiefly between 45 and 60 years and is recognised as a hard mass growing fairly rapidly and becoming attached to adjacent structures and to skin. In parotid lesions the facial nerve becomes involved producing palsy, and pain from local infiltration may be severe. Enlargement of cervical lymph nodes may be apparent. Treatment is total parotidectomy where the tumour is resectable, with sacrifice of the facial nerve. An alternative treatment is local excision of the growth followed by radiotherapy. The cervical nodes are managed as in carcinoma of the tongue (p. 64).

FURTHER READING

Hobsley, M. (1979). Swellings in the parotid region. In *Pathways in Surgical Management*. London: Arnold.

Moore, J. R. (1982). *Surgery of the Mouth and Jaws*. Oxford: Blackwell.

6

Neck

BRANCHIAL CYST

Pathology

The aetiology has not been precisely determined, but it is probable that development is from the second branchial cleft. This is suggested by the occasional presence of a track which passes upwards between the external and internal carotid arteries. The lining is generally of squamous epithelium, and the viscid fluid contents contain a high proportion of cholesterol crystals.

Clinical features

A branchial cyst is usually encountered in young adults of 20 to 25 years, and is more common in the female. Recognised as a smooth, rounded non-translucent swelling in the upper and lateral part of the neck below the angle of the jaw, it lies deep to sternomastoid protruding from its anterior border (Fig. 6.1). Growth is slow and the swelling often reaches 4 to 6 cm in diameter before advice is sought. Infection may lead to rupture, which is followed by a persistent fistula. The cyst should be excised through a transverse curved incision.

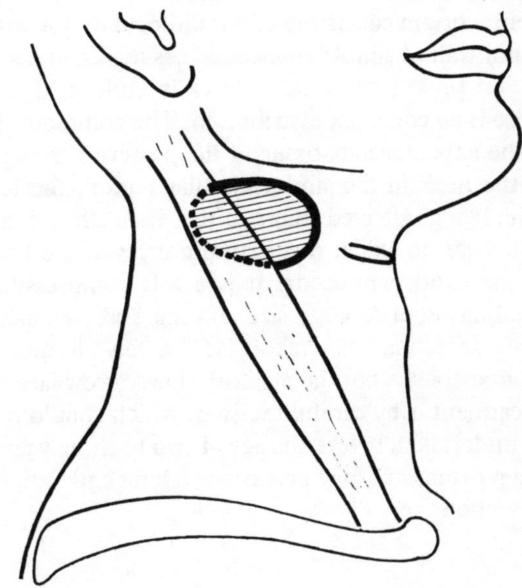

Fig. 6.1 Branchial cyst

BRANCHIAL FISTULA

Pathology

Congenital in origin it arises from the second branchial cleft. It may rarely follow rupture of a branchial cyst. The lower opening is at the anterior border of the sternomastoid muscle at the junction of the lower one-third and upper two-thirds. The track passes upwards between the internal and external carotid arteries, and may open into the supratonsillar fossa. Complete fistulae are unusual, and the majority are more accurately designated sinuses. The lining is of squamous or columnar epithelium, surrounded by lymphoid tissue and an outer connective tissue wall. Occasionally the lesion is bilateral.

Clinical features

Although the majority are present from birth, the external opening at that time may be difficult to detect. With growth of the child and perhaps associated infection the orifice becomes more prominent and the upper margin resembles the crescentic fold of a thyroglossal fistula. Intermittent discharge of clear thin fluid is common, but with infection pus may be present. It is unusual for a probe to pass the entire length of the fistula, but radiography after the introduction of radio-opaque dye may outline the extent. The track should be excised through two small transverse incisions over its course.

CYSTIC HYGROMA

This is a cavernous lymphangioma of developmental origin consisting of a multilocular cyst with a thin wall of simple connective tissue. The majority are present at birth or in early childhood and there is an equal sex distribution. The common site is the subcutaneous tissue of the posterior triangle of the neck in the supraclavicular region, the left side being affected more often than the right. Extension to axilla, mediastinum or even the base of the skull may occur. It is a soft compressible swelling often of large size and markedly translucent. Infection may take place, a few disappear spontaneously, but the majority slowly grow larger. Treatment is by careful excision, which should not be undertaken before the age of two to three years. Deep extensions may necessitate a long and tedious dissection.

TRAUMATIC LESIONS

Serious damage to the neck is often prevented by protective flexion, but penetrating injuries from the side are potentially more dangerous. **Cut throat**, which is usually self-inflicted, is the most frequent form of incised wound. Damage may occur to the respiratory or alimentary tracts, to the internal jugular vein, the carotid arteries or to the vagus nerve. On a more superficial plane the external jugular veins are prone to injury, and in the supraclavicular region the brachial plexus or apex of the lung may be involved. On the left side of the neck the thoracic duct may be divided and cause persistent lymphorrhoea. The main immediate dangers are haemorrhage and respiratory embarrassment; infection and occasionally aneurysm or arteriovenous fistula involving the carotid artery and internal jugular vein or the subclavian vessels may follow.

Haemorrhage is generally external and often profuse from injury to the external jugular vein; the internal jugular vein and carotid arteries are less liable to damage in the suicidal attempt when the head is characteristically thrown back. The straining and non-co-operation of a frightened patient also increases venous haemorrhage. Trauma to the main vessels or smaller veins in the absence of an incised wound may well result in a subfascial haematoma with the dual effect of blood loss and acute respiratory embarrassment. The latter may also occur from division of the mylohyoid and hyoglossus just above the hyoid bone, allowing the tongue to fall back, from bleeding into a divided larynx or trachea, or by division of the vagus or recurrent laryngeal nerves.

Infection may be introduced externally by wound contamination, but the more important route is spread from the pharynx or oesophagus. It may lead to the development of mediastinitis and cervical abscess.

Treatment

Immediate control of haemorrhage and relief of respiratory obstruction are essential. When the latter is not present venous haemorrhage may be lessened by transport in a slightly head-up position to diminish bleeding from the proximal cut end, and reassurance of the patient is important in decreasing back pressure due to struggling. An adequate airway must always be established, either by the aspiration of blood and secretions, intubation or tracheostomy. Blood transfusion may be indicated, and when the general condition permits, full exploration and repair should be performed.

INFECTIONS

Superficial lesions, such as boils and carbuncles, are common on the back of the neck, particularly in men where the rubbing of a collar causes minor abrasions. *Deep* infections are less common but more serious. They usually result as a spread from a primary focus in mouth, teeth, salivary glands, larynx, pharynx or oesophagus; occasionally external injury may be responsible. The common organism is the haemolytic streptococcus. The danger of deep infections lies in the spread of cellulitis beneath the ensheathing layer of deep cervical fascia with extension to the mediastinum, or in laryngeal obstruction from oedema. Ludwig's angina, now encountered less frequently, is caused by infection in the floor of the mouth in the region of the submandibular gland. It is often of dental origin and produces a cellulitis deep to mylohyoid. Spread deep to geniohyoid may occur with oedema of the floor of the mouth and upward and backward displacement of the tongue.

Clinical features

The history of previous inflammation, particularly in the mouth, pharynx or teeth, is usually present in deep infections, and Ludwig's angina can occur after a difficult dental extraction. Painful swelling of the floor of the mouth or suprahyoid region is common with severe constitutional upset. Difficulty in speech and swallowing occurs with protrusion of the tongue between the teeth in severe cases. Trismus and intrapharyngeal swelling may be pronounced, and progressive dyspnoea may follow in the absence of adequate treatment.

Treatment

Antibiotic therapy is generally sufficient, but when oedema persists with the risk of respiratory obstruction, drainage is essential. Only occasionally is tracheostomy required.

Acute lymphadenitis

The cervical lymph nodes are commonly affected from inflammatory lesions of the face and scalp, teeth, tonsils and pharynx. The upper deep cervical and submandibular glands are principally involved, and the organisms are usually the haemolytic streptococcus or staphylococcus. Resolution or abscess formation occurs, depending on host resistance and treatment.

The clinical picture is one of local pain, occasionally referred to the shoulder or ear. There is tenderness over the affected nodes, which increase in size and become closely adherent. Redness of the skin and a fluctuant swelling denote an abscess which may extend in the neck or discharge through the skin. The general state is reflected in anorexia, malaise and lassitude with tachycardia and pyrexia.

Initial treatment consists of antibiotic therapy and attention to the primary focus. Bed rest may be required if symptoms are severe, and abscesses should be drained.

Chronic lymphadenitis

Non-specific infection may occur from mildly inflamed lesions in similar sites to the acute form. Moderate enlargement with tenderness, particularly of the upper cervical group, is common. Treatment of the primary focus of infection is usually followed by resolution. Specific infection, due to syphilis, may occur in the primary or secondary stages, but is recognised by the other manifestations of the disease and treated accordingly. The more usual specific form is due to tuberculosis.

Tuberculous cervical lymphadenitis

Pathology

Although in common with the other manifestations of tuberculosis this variety is less often encountered at the present time, the cervical region is not infrequently involved. Infection may be of the human or bovine type, the latter being more common, but with the more widespread pasteurisation of milk the incidence has diminished. There are two main forms and a third less frequent type.

1. *Upper cervical*. This is the usual lesion in children and young adults. Infection enters through the tonsil or pharynx and spreads in the lymphatics to reach the jugulo-digastric (tonsillar) lymph nodes, extension often occurring later to other nodes of the anterior group of the deep cervical lymph chain. The importance of this type of lesion lies in its being a primary focus of infection and not secondary to tuberculosis elsewhere.

2. *Lower cervical*. This form occurs principally in adults, particularly the elderly, where a breakdown in resistance occurs through malnutrition or infirmity. It is always secondary to disease elsewhere, generally in the apex of the ipsilateral lung, and the cervical involvement results from upward extension from associated tuberculous mediastinal nodes. The nodes initially involved are those of the supraclavicular region.

3. *Diffuse*. This is an uncommon form in which all the cervical nodes may show moderate enlarge-

ment. It is also related to a tuberculous focus elsewhere and probably follows a bloodstream spread.

In all three forms the pathological changes are hyperaemia and inflammatory reaction in the affected node with tubercle formation. Periadenitis with the matting together of a number of nodes may follow. Resolution may occur or the lesion proceed to caseation. Necrotic tissue may extend to the surface, first perforating the ensheathing layer of deep cervical fascia and later involving the skin. A 'collar-stud' abscess may result from the small hole in the deep fascia. Calcification may occur in the node and wall off the lesion. Secondary infection may follow rupture or operative interference with the associated changes of an acute inflammation. More distant spread results in bone and joint involvement, meningitis or miliary tuberculosis.

Clinical features

The usual picture is one of a slowly progressive cervical swelling, present for many months, which proceeds to a typical 'cold abscess' with an overlying thin and bluish-red discoloured skin. In children and young adults this is situated in the upper part of the anterior triangle below the angle of the mandible, deep to sternomastoid. There are usually associated palpable nodes which are closely adherent. Occasionally this form may present as an acute non-specific infection which has failed to respond to antibiotics. The general disturbance is at times minimal.

In older patients the swelling is more commonly found in the posterior triangle, where the supraclavicular nodes become palpable, and a cold abscess may follow. The general disturbance from the underlying pulmonary lesion causes lassitude, anorexia, loss of weight and night sweats. In the less common diffuse form encountered in adults moderate enlargement, mainly of the nodes of the anterior triangle, without abscess formation, is present. The general constitutional effects may not be obvious.

Investigations.

In children a negative Mantoux test may be of value in excluding tuberculosis. Radiography will indicate any pulmonary lesion, or calcification may be noted in the neck, but node biopsy is often required.

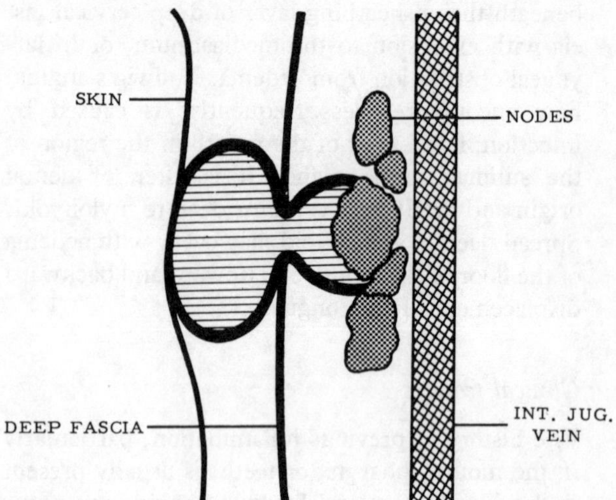

Fig. 6.2 Tuberculous 'collar-stud' abscess arising from caseating deep cervical lymph nodes

Treatment

General measures of antituberculous therapy with concentrated chemotherapy are essential (p. 13).

Local measures are directed towards any abscesses or to the lymph nodes. The former should be evacuated by aspiration or through a small incision, but the collar-stud variety requires adequate drainage of the deeper abscess and excision of the underlying affected glands (Fig. 6.2). Primary wound suture should be performed. Dissection of the nodes should only be undertaken for the upper cervical group because, being a primary focus, this permits total eradication of the disease. The optimum time is approximately three months after the commencement of therapy when there has been an initial response and before further breakdown occurs. The tonsils if grossly infected should be removed at a later date.

CAROTID BODY TUMOUR

This is a growth of the carotid body which lies at the bifurcation of the common carotid artery. Originally classed as a chromaffinoma, because on staining it shows a great affinity for chromic acid, it is now regarded as a 'chemodectoma' and is of similar type to the glomus jugulare tumour. It is a slowly growing, generally benign lesion with a slightly lobulated appearance. Histologically it resembles the normal structure of the carotid body. Although few are malignant, it is of potential danger because of adherence to the carotid vessels which it may occlude.

Clinically it is recognised in the age group 30 to 50 years as a slowly progressive swelling of several years duration, present deep to the sternomastoid at the level of the hyoid bone. Symptoms are few, but it may cause dysphagia or occasionally the carotid sinus syndrome of dizziness and syncope when handled. It does not move on deglutition, gives a transmitted pulsation and is easier to move in a horizontal than in a vertical direction.

Treatment is by removal, occasionally resection and grafting of the internal carotid artery being required. The cerebral circulation is maintained by a temporary by-pass.

DIFFERENTIAL DIAGNOSIS OF A CERVICAL SWELLING

History

The *age* of the patient should be first considered. Some congenital lesions, such as cystic hygroma or sternomastoid tumours, are encountered in the newborn, whilst others, such as branchial or thyroglossal cysts, are more frequent in young adults. Age is also helpful in lymphatic node enlargement; pyogenic and tuberculous lesions are more often seen in children and young adults; the reticuloses in young and middle-aged persons; secondary neoplastic nodes in the elderly. The *sex* of the patient may help; certain swellings, such as goitre, predominating among females. The *duration* of the swelling should be known. A short history suggests an acute inflammatory episode, whilst a long one is more likely to be due to chronic inflammation or neoplasia. Little change, associated with a long history, suggests a congenital lesion. *Pain* is indicative of pyogenic inflammation. Pressure symptoms, *dyspnoea* more than dysphagia, occur with a goitre, the reticuloses or new growth. Associated *general symptoms*, such as *fever*, suggest an inflammatory cause; high in pyogenic cases, lower in tubercle, and of an undulant nature (Pel-Ebstein) in Hodgkin's disease. Lassitude and malaise are suggestive of tuberculosis, the reticuloses or neoplasia.

Physical examination

Local considerations

The *situation* is important, and this may be in the midline or in a lateral position. The former is probably due to a swelling of the thyroid isthmus or thyroglossal cyst, but may be a subhyoid bursa or a dermoid. Lateral swellings in the anterior, or less commonly in the posterior triangle, may be lymph node enlargements (Fig. 6.3). Submandibular gland swellings are found below the body of the mandible, and parotid gland swellings behind the ramus. A branchial cyst lies below the angle of the jaw and a carotid body tumour at the bifurcation of the common carotid artery. Although *size* is important in measuring change, it may be difficult to assess correctly, as in retrotracheal thyroid enlargement. The *shape* of a swelling may suggest

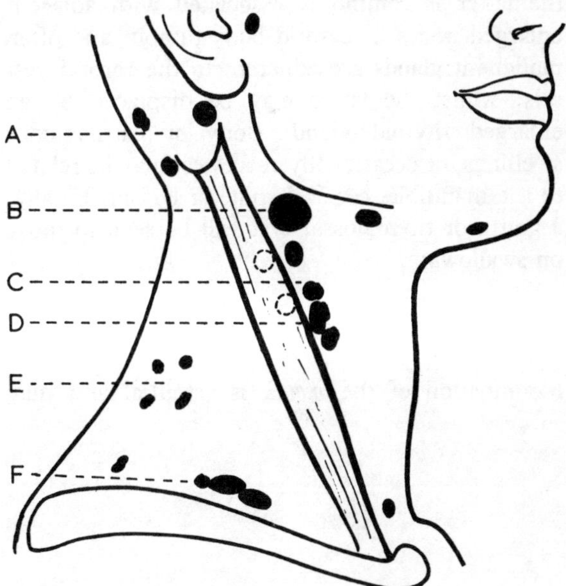

Fig. 6.3 The common sites of cervical lymph node enlargement. **A**. Chronic infection and glandular fever. **B**. Metastatic (mouth and pharynx). **C**. Chronic infection, non-specific or tuberculous (child). **D**. Reticulosis. **E**. Reticulosis. **F**. Metastatic (lung or breast, and stomach when left sided). Tuberculosis (secondary to pulmonary lesion in aged).

the rounded contour of a cyst or bear resemblance to the original structure, such as the thyroid gland. The *surface* may show the matting of adherent tuberculous nodes, the discreteness of Hodgkin's disease or the irregularity of some secondary deposits. The *consistency* must be ascertained for the tenseness of a cyst, the firmness of a goitre or the hardness of malignant disease or calcification. The nodes in Hodgkin's disease are rubbery and the pulsation of an aneurysm is characteristic. There may be an associated thrill or bruit in a carotid body tumour, and these findings may also suggest a primary toxic goitre. *Tenderness* indicates an acute pyogenic lesion and may be accompanied by other signs of local inflammation. Fluctuation may be found in a branchial or thyroglossal cyst unless it is tense, or in a tuberculous abscess. Transillumination is marked in a cystic hygroma. The *attachments* are an important aid in diagnosis. A swelling in the skin is likely to be a sebaceous cyst; one adherent to the skin, an abscess or neoplasm. The relation to the sternomastoid muscle should be determined. A branchial cyst and tuberculous abscess both lying deep to it may be confused, but the latter is commonly associated with adjacent enlarged nodes. A carotid body tumour and often malignant glands are adherent to the carotid vessels, whilst the latter may be displaced by an enlarged thyroid gland. Bony or cartilaginous swellings, or occasionally abscesses, may be related to the mandible, cervical spine or larynx. Finally, a goitre or thyroglossal cyst will be seen to move on swallowing.

General considerations

Examination of the *mouth* is essential and may reveal the primary cause of an infective or neoplastic lesion. Bimanual examination of a submandibular swelling should be performed, whilst protrusion of the tongue will cause upward movement of a thyroglosal cyst. Lesions of the *head* or *cervical spine* must be excluded as the primary cause of acute or chronic infection or malignancy. *Other sites* of possible lymph node enlargement must be carefully examined, and evidence of disease in other organs, such as pulmonary tuberculosis or neoplastic hepatomegaly, may suggest the diagnosis.

Investigations

A *blood examination* reveals the leucocytosis of a pyogenic infection, the changes of leukaemia, or the positive serological reaction of syphilis. A *plain radiograph* of the neck may demonstrate a bony or calcified mass or the relation of a soft tissue tumour to the trachea. *Tomography* and a *barium swallow* may further indicate the site of the swelling. A *radiograph* of the *chest* will show evidence of pulmonary or mediastinal disease supporting the diagnosis of tuberculosis, carcinoma or the reticuloses. Endoscopy of the upper respiratory or alimentary tracts may indicate the origin of a cervical swelling. Radioactive scanning may distinguish benign and malignant thyroid lesions and ultrasonography may demonstrate a thyroid cyst or other cystic lesion.

FURTHER READING

Stell, P. M. and Maran, A. G. D. (1982). Head and neck surgery. In *Essential Surgical Practice*. Eds. Cuschieri, A., Giles, G. R. and Moossa, A. R. Bristol: Wright.

7

Thyroid and parathyroid glands

THYROID GLAND

Physiology

Ingested iodine in the form of iodide ions is absorbed from the intestine into the bloodstream, from where it is selectively extracted by the thyroid gland. At periods of heightened physiological activity, such as childhood, puberty, menstruation and pregnancy, the iodine requirements of the gland are increased. The uptake of iodine by the thyroid is also greater than normal in hyperthyroidism. The extracted iodine is converted by the epithelial cells into *l*-thyroxine, a compound which contains four iodine atoms linked to the aminoacid thyronine. Storage of this compound in colloid is accomplished by a peptide linkage with globulin to form thyroglobulin. Both the storage and release of thyroxine into the bloodstream are under the control of the thyroid-stimulating hormone of the anterior pituitary gland (TSH or thyrotrophic hormone). Excess of circulating thyroxine depresses the formation of thyrotrophic hormone and vice versa, but whether this is a direct action of thyroxine or an indirect one through the hypothalamus is not known. Triiodothyronine is formed by the release of one iodine atom from thyroxine, is probably the active principle and is three to four times as potent as thyroxine.

Certain drugs may be used to prevent the synthesis or release of thyroxine, the most common being the thiocarbamides, such as carbimazole. These inhibit all the intracellular steps in the production of thyroxine, namely oxidation of iodine to ionic iodine, its binding to tyrosine, and the coupling of the iodotyrosines to triiodothyronine and thyroxine. Potassium perchlorate acts by interfering with the uptake of blood iodide into the gland. Iodine is used in the preparation of thyrotoxic patients for operation including those already treated with carbimazole and increases colloid storage, causes involutionary changes and reduces the vascularity of the gland. Clinical improvement with iodine is only temporary.

Several thyroid function tests are now available and the following are the most useful.

1. Serum thyroxine (T_4)

The total serum thyroxine can be measured by competitive protein binding or by radioimmunoassay. The normal range is 50 to 150 nmol per litre. As this test measures the total serum thyroxine, it cannot distinguish between hyperthyroidism and raised thyroxine-binding globulin states such as pregnancy, or between hypothyroidism and lowered thyroxine-binding globulin states such as renal failure, acromegaly and malnutrition. It is now possible to estimate the 'free' T_4 by radioimmunoassay and the normal range is 8–23 pmol per litre. This is a more accurate test than total serum thyroxine as it is not influenced by thyroxine binding globulin levels.

2. Serum triiodothyronine (T_3)

Radioimmunoassay of triiodothyronine is now available and is probably the most reliable single test for hyperthyroidism as in some patients with thyrotoxicosis the serum thyroxine may be normal (*T_3 thyrotoxicosis*). The normal range is 1 to 3 nmol per litre.

3. Serum thyroid stimulating hormone (TSH)

Serum TSH may be measured by radioimmunoassay with a normal range of less than 5 mU per litre. While TSH may be undetectable in some normal individuals without a stimulation test, it is almost always so in hyperthyroidism. In hypothyroidism raised levels are usually present and may be very high in long-standing cases.

4. Thyrotrophin releasing hormone test (TRH test)

In normal subjects intravenous injection of TRH is followed within a few minutes by release of TSH, the concentration reaching a peak within 15 to 20 minutes and returning to normal within one to two hours. The response is dose-dependent and a standard dose of 100 mg. TRH is usually given. The test is of most value as a test of exclusion, a positive response excluding hyperthyroidism and a negative one excluding hypothyroidism.

5. Radioactive isotope studies

Technetium (^{99m}Tc) is replacing the iodine isotopes, ^{132}I and ^{131}I, because of its low energy and short half-life. The radiation dose to the thyroid from a tracer dose is one-thousandth of that using ^{131}I. As technetium is not bound to tyrosine it gives a more accurate measure of the iodine uptake of the gland.

(a) *Uptake*. The best time to measure isotope uptake is 10 to 120 minutes after oral administration. This shows the greatest rate of accumulation in the thyroid gland and in general reflects the rate of secretion of thyroid hormone into the circulation. It is influenced by the amount of inorganic iodine in the serum and this depends on recently ingested iodine or iodine used in radiological techniques which may remain for several weeks.

(b) *Scanning*. Scanning the thyroid will distinguish between functioning and non-functioning nodules. It may also be used to detect metastatic deposits of functioning thyroid tissue. If ^{131}I is used, 20 to 40 microcuries (μCi) of sodium radioactive iodide is given orally 24 hours before the scan. If ^{99m}Tc is used, 1 to 2 mCi is given orally and the neck scanned 15 to 30 minutes later.

Ectopic thyroid

The thyroid gland may be situated in any part of the thyroglossal tract. Occasionally it is lingual and projects as a rounded or irregular swelling at the back of the tongue. The onset of symptoms of dysphagia, dysphonia, dyspnoea or haemorrhage necessitate glandular removal. A search for normally situated thyroid tissue should be made by radioactive tracer methods, and if none is found some of the excised gland should be transplanted into the sheath of the rectus abdominis muscle or permanent administration of *l*-thyroxine commenced. Rarely the whole thyroid tissue is in an aberrant position in the thorax.

THYROGLOSSAL CYST AND FISTULA

These anomalies, arising in the developmental remains of the thyroglossal tract, usually present in late childhood.

Thyroglossal cysts commonly occur as midline swellings below the hyoid bone (sub-hyoid), but are also found at the level of the thyroid cartilage to the left of the midline and in the suprahyoid position. A history of recurrent inflammation is often obtained. The cystic nature is often difficult to determine on palpation. Characteristically the swelling tends to rise on protrusion of the tongue.

Thyroglossal fistula is not congenital but follows rupture or incision of an infected cyst or the inadequate removal of a cyst. Recurrent inflammation occurs and the fistula intermittently discharges mucus.

Treatment of both these conditions involves complete excision of the fistula or cyst together with all the thyroglossal tract up to the foramen caecum. The middle portion of the hyoid bone should also be removed.

GOITRE

A morbid enlargement of the thyroid gland is known as a goitre (Fig. 7.1.). Metabolic disturbance may be absent or there may be signs of hyperthyroidism, less commonly hypothyroidism.

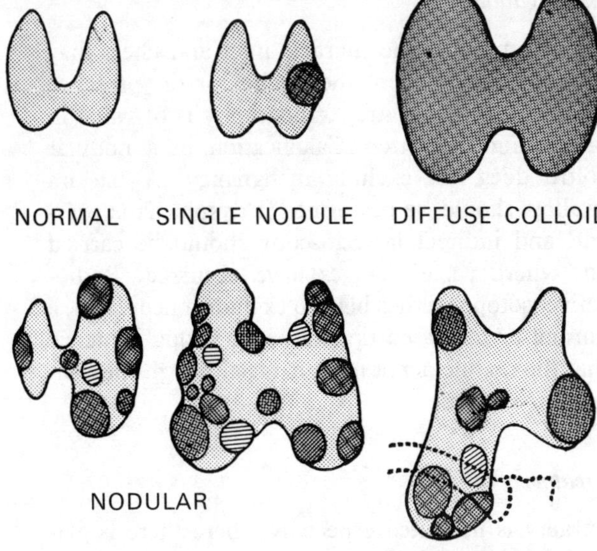

Fig. 7.1 The various types of goitre

Enlargement of the gland may be diffuse or nodular. The latter is usually multiple, but may be due to a single adenoma or malignant tumour.

A soft diffuse thyroid enlargement is frequently seen in females during periods of active growth, puberty, pregnancy and, to a lesser extent, during menstruation. The swelling, which is due to hyperplasia and some colloid retention, usually disappears without treatment but iodised salt in the diet may aid the regression. If hypothyroidism is present thyroid extract or thyroxine should be given. A few cases persist as colloid goitres after the cessation of the 'stimulus'.

Colloid goitre

This common cause of thyroid enlargement occurs both sporadically, and in large numbers in certain areas as endemic goitre.

Pathology

Certain geographical regions, such as Switzerland and Derbyshire, have been noted for endemic goitre. Iodine deficiency, either in the water or due to certain goitrogens interfering with iodine utilisation, is the factor generally responsible. The pituitary regulating mechanism may be at fault in some instances, and in certain congenital goitres an inability of the thyroid to synthesise thyroxine is assumed. As a result of an iodine deficiency inadequate amounts of thyroxine are produced, causing increased stimulation of the thyrotrophic hormone of the anterior pituitary gland. The thyroid responds by undergoing epithelial hyperplasia, which, if sufficient thyroxine is produced, results in the acini becoming distended with colloid and a less active gland. Histologically the epithelium lining the vesicles has a flattened appearance. Repeated phases of hyperplasia and involution result in a nodular goitre.

Clinical features

Young women over the age of 20 years are usually affected. Soft diffuse enlargement of the thyroid gland becomes noticeable, but disability only occurs from pressure symptoms, which are of gradual onset. Like all goitres, the enlarged gland moves upwards on swallowing.

Treatment

Prevention by the addition of iodised salt to the diet should be recommended where the disease is endemic. Thyroxine may be required if a hypothyroid state persists. Partial thyroidectomy is indicated only when the gland reaches exceptional size or where there are pressure effects, particularly in the mediastinum.

Nodular goitre

Pathology

Hyperplasia and involution occur irregularly in different parts of the same gland over many years and are responsible for the production of a nodular goitre. There is irregular enlargement of the thyroid with varying numbers of discrete nodules. The latter are not well encapsulated and differ in size, being scattered throughout the gland. Degenerative changes occur with cyst formation and haemorrhage. Microscopically there are areas showing both hypoplastic and hyperplastic changes. Distended vesicles containing watery colloid are present as cyst-like spaces. There is increased connective tissue between the nodules, and areas are present in which calcification, haemorrhage and lipoid deposits occur.

Nodular goitres are subject to a number of complications.

Pressure effects may be considerable on the adjacent trachea due to displacement or compression. The oesophagus may be subject to similar pressure, although less commonly, and in retrosternal goitre venous congestion of the neck and upper chest may be marked and associated with respiratory difficulties. *Haemorrhage* may occur into a cyst, and if sudden and large may markedly accentuate pressure symptoms or even lead to fatal respiratory obstruction. Secondary *thyrotoxicosis* is a common complication. *Follicular carcinoma* may arise in a nodular goitre as a result of persistent stimulation by thyrotrophic hormone but the evidence is not conclusive.

Clinical features

Cases occur sporadically and endemically, and the disorder is more common in females. Nodular goitre is most frequently seen over the age of 30 years, but in endemic areas it may be seen in children. A swelling in the neck is frequently noted, but symptoms mainly occur as complications arise. Cough, alteration in the voice and dyspnoea are common, and dysphagia may also be noted. In some instances evidence of toxicity is apparent. On examination there is an asymmetrical and multinodular thyroid swelling, varying in consistency from firm to tense or hard where a cyst or calcification is present. Displacement of the trachea may be detected, and there may be obvious stridor with alteration of neck posture. A retrosternal prolongation may become obvious in the suprasternal notch on swallowing or coughing. Rarely a Horner's syndrome may be present. In large goitres the jugular veins may become obstructed with dilatation of the superficial veins; cyanosis or oedema of the face and neck may also be found. Malignant change is suggested if there is rapid growth of the gland, by the development of pain or if there is involvement of a recurrent laryngeal nerve.

Investigations

A radiograph of the thoracic inlet and chest may show displacement of the trachea or the presence of a retrosternal goitre; tomography is of value in diagnosing the latter. Calcification in a nodular goitre does not exclude malignancy. A barium swallow should be performed if dysphagia is present, and indirect laryngoscopy should be carried out where voice changes have occurred. Radioactive isotope studies help to exclude a neoplasm, a normal or increased uptake being strong evidence that the nodule is not malignant, although the converse is not true.

Treatment

Surgery is indicated especially where there is evidence of pressure effects, when toxicity arises or where there is suspicion of malignancy. Surgical treatment may also be performed for cosmetic reasons.

Subtotal thyroidectomy is performed when the gland shows evidence of nodularity in both lobes. Resection of one lobe is adequate for the case when the contralateral lobe is not involved. Unless there is secondary thyrotoxicosis the operation should be less radical than for hyperthyroidism. Small nodules may be left in the remaining portion of the gland, and small doses of *l*-thyroxine should be administered post-operatively to inhibit further growth.

Solitary nodular goitre

The majority of suspected cases probably represent the first nodule in a gland which subsequently becomes multinodular.

A *benign adenoma* occurs only uncommonly. It is well encapsulated and the blood supply enters at one point. Another uncommon benign nodule is the *foetal adenoma* which contains primitive-looking cells and follicles and is functionless. The single nodule should be excised together with a covering of normal thyroid tissue. Enucleation is inadequate and a lobectomy may be performed in suitably placed tumours. It is often only on subsequent histology that malignancy can be excluded, particularly in a younger patient.

HYPERTHYROIDISM

Two main forms occur in which excessive secretion takes place:

(*a*) *Primary thyrotoxicosis*, where the thyroid gland was previously normal, and (*b*) *secondary thyrotoxicosis*, where the thyroid gland was previously abnormal (nodular goitre). In addition, hyperfunction of secondary deposits from a thyroid carcinoma may rarely occur.

PRIMARY THYROTOXICOSIS

Pathology

A frequent history of physical or emotional stress, such as accident, fright, illness or bereavement, tended to suggest that the cause might be hypothalamic stimulation of the adjacent pituitary, but it is now certain that the pituitary thyroid stimulating hormone (TSH) is not directly concerned in the pathogenesis of primary thyrotoxicosis. The goitre and hyperthyroidism are due to the action of a humoral agent acting on the thyroid gland. Previously thought to be the long-acting thyroid stimulator (LATS), it is now known that this immunoglobulin is not immunologically active in man. The responsibility is now thought to be with thyroid-stimulating immunoglobulin (TSI) antibodies which stimulate TSH receptors on the human thyroid cell. TSI is found in 70–90 per cent of patients with primary thyrotoxicosis and is also known as LATS-protector as it prevents LATS binding with human thyroid cell membranes. There is also probably an immunological deficit which allows the TSI antibodies to stimulate the thyroid.

The thyroid gland is slightly but diffusely enlarged, possesses a smooth surface and is very vascular. The cut surface is fleshy and homogeneous. Microscopically there is gross hyperplasia and irregular small acini into which projections of tall epithelium occur. Little or no colloid is seen, and there are often interacinar lymphoid aggregations. This appearance is altered by the administration of drugs; iodine produces a smaller, firmer, less vascular gland showing involution and colloid storage; thiouracil derivatives cause further hyperplasia and a friable and vascular gland with a histological picture similar to malignant disease.

The pathological change seen in exophthalmos is a deposition of water-binding mucopolysaccharides in all the tissues of the orbit. These changes, which are present in the extraocular muscles as well as connective tissue and eyelids, may later exist in other skeletal muscles producing 'thyrotoxic myasthenia'. Thyroid-stimulating immunoglobulin antibodies may be responsible for these changes seen in the orbital contents, and in pre-tibial myxoedema.

Clinical features

Women between the ages of 20 and 30 years are most commonly affected, and only 10 per cent of cases occur in men. Primary thyrotoxicosis is a disease with acute exacerbations and remissions, in which the onset may be insidious or rapid. Nervousness, irritability, restlessness and insomnia are frequent. In spite of a good appetite there may be weight loss and diarrhoea. Cold weather is preferred, and undue sweating is noticed in a warm atmosphere. Menstruation may be upset, usually in the form of oligomenorrhoea.

General nervousness is obvious on examination, and the outstretched hands and protruded tongue may exhibit a fine tremor. The skin, especially in the palms of the hands, is usually warm and moist. There is a moderate diffuse enlargement of the gland which is both firm and smooth, but occasionally there is no increase in size. The increased vascularity may produce a palpable thrill and a bruit, and the skin over the palpated area often remains red for some time after examination.

Various eye signs are frequently present. There may be a characteristic stare and one or both eyes may be prominent. This is due either to lid retraction or true proptosis (exophthalmos). Lid retraction allows the sclera to be seen around the cornea and is the basis of the 'lid-lag' sign; on looking down the lids do not follow the movement of the eye and a clear white space of sclera is noticeable. It may be difficult to converge the eyes and blinking tends to be infrequent. It varies in severity from a benign and moderate type, which may remain unchanged or improve after control of the disease, to a 'malignant' form in which extreme proptosis and oedema of the lids and conjunctiva are found.

Corneal ulceration and ophthalmitis may follow. Malignant exophthalmos may become obvious or progress after medical or surgical control of thyrotoxicosis has been obtained, and may even occur in patients without hyperthyroidism. Paralysis of the extra-ocular muscles may result, maximally affecting the inferior rectus and inferior oblique (exophthalmic ophthalmoplegia).

Tachycardia is usual, and a sleeping pulse rate of more than 80 per minute is reasonably diagnostic. There is no definite correlation between the rate and the degree of severity, but a return to normal on treatment is indicative of lessening toxicity. Extrasystoles also occur. The blood-pressure usually shows a raised pulse pressure and a 'water-hammer' pulse may be felt. The heart is not enlarged unless failure is present or hypertension co-exists, but a functional systolic murmur is often heard. Atrial fibrillation and congestive cardiac failure are infrequent in primary thyrotoxicosis, but hyperthyroidism must not be overlooked as a cause of heart failure. Paroxysmal atrial fibrillation or atrial flutter is occasionally encountered.

Pretibial oedema may be noted, either during the disease or following treatment. Initially of a pitting type, it later becomes solid, the overlying skin having a brown to red discoloration. It may be associated with exophthalmos, often of the malignant type.

Thyroid crises are now rare due to early and adequate management of hyperthyroidism. They represent an acute phase and occur post-operatively or during severe intercurrent infection. Mental symptoms, such as delirium, delusions or mania are evident, and fluid and electrolyte loss by diarrhoea and vomiting is marked. The pulse-rate is rapid, often being 200 per minute.

Investigations

Confirmation of toxicity is obtained by a raised serum thyroxine or triiodothyronine and an elevated radioactive isotope uptake. Radiography of the thoracic inlet may disclose tracheal shift or compression; the presence of a retrosternal goitre is demonstrated by a chest radiograph. Indirect laryngoscopy should be carried out pre-operatively to determine the position and movement of the vocal cords.

Differential diagnosis

An acute anxiety state is easily confused, and exclusion using the tests of thyroid function (p. 79) is necessary. Malignancy and pulmonary tuberculosis as a cause of weight loss and the causes of cardiac failure require consideration, particularly when the thyroid gland is not palpable. Other causes of unilateral exophthalmos, such as retro-orbital tumours and arteriovenous fistulae, must be excluded.

Treatment

The method of choice in the majority of cases is surgical, but medical measures may at times be employed as an alternative. They include the antithyroid drugs and radioactive iodine. The choice depends on a variety of factors, including medical, administrative and social ones. The aim is to prevent the consequence of over-stimulation of the thyroid gland until such time as a natural remission occurs.

Surgical management

Operative treatment possesses the advantage of immediate cure without the necessity for long term drug maintenance. It should be advised when tracheal compression exists or might be precipitated by the antithyroid drugs, which increase glandular vascularity and size. It is indicated for all toxic nodular goitres, for relapse after prolonged medical treatment, where there is non-co-operation by the patient in long term medical management, or where sensitivity to the antithyroid drugs exists. Operation should also be undertaken when malignant disease cannot be excluded.

Adequate pre-operative preparation is essential and varies with the degree of toxicity. When not severe Lugol's iodine, 0.6 ml t.d.s., should be given for 10 to 14 days or potassium iodide 30 mg t.d.s., the patient being admitted for surgery towards the end of this period. Severe cases require antithyroid drugs to ensure a euthyroid state, carbimazole 10 mg t.d.s. being usually employed for about four to six weeks. It should be discontinued one week before operation to decrease vascularity, iodine therapy being given for two weeks pre-operatively to produce a firm and smaller gland. More recently, beta-adrenergic blockade using propranolol with or without iodine, has been used as pre-operative preparation. Treatment time is much shorter than with carbimazole and the gland is much more pliable at operation.

Subtotal thyroidectomy is performed, involving the removal of the majority of both lateral lobes, the isthmus and the pyramidal lobe. Approximately one-eighth of the gland is left behind, this being sufficient to protect the parathyroids and maintain thyroid function. Ligature of both superior and inferior thyroid arteries diminishes the risk of recurrence.

Operative complications

Reactionary haemorrhage may occur within the first six hours, particularly where antithyroid drugs have been used pre-operatively. In most instances it is deep to the investing layer of deep cervical fascia and may not at first be recognised, but later produces acute respiratory embarrassment. Immediate re-opening of the wound may be required as an emergency measure to relieve tracheal compression. *Recurrent laryngeal nerve damage* is a serious hazard, as the nerve is intimately related to the inferior thyroid artery and bilateral injury may cause severe dyspnoea, necessitating tracheostomy. Hoarseness produced by mild trauma or oedema eventually recovers, but division of one nerve causes it to persist and speech therapy may be required. *Tetany* occasionally follows surgery, due to post-operative hypocalcaemia and not to damage to the parathyroid glands as was previously thought. Thyrotoxicosis induces gross skeletal decalcification and after surgery, especially if radical, the 'calcium hungry' bones produce rapid hypocalcaemia within a few hours. This is corrected by temporary calcium supplements until the negative calcium balance is restored. A *thyroid crisis* is very rare today with adequate pre-operative preparation, but is treated by immediate fluid and electrolyte replacement combined with Lugol's iodine intravenously in doses up to 5 ml per day. Heavy sedation and cooling with ice packs may be indicated. Sympathetic blockade with propranolol 80 to 120 mg four times a day is useful.

Late complications include *myxoedema*, which occurs in up to 30 per cent of cases, and for which replacement therapy is required. Pretibial oedema may also occur. *Cataract* and *epileptiform convulsions* may be observed later due to hypoparathyroidism but this is rare. It may occur in those cases developing tetany in the immediate post-operative period, when calcium is not continued after cessation of the symptoms. The serum calcium should be estimated three months after operation and calcium administered if it is low. Vitamin D may also be required. *Recurrent thyrotoxicosis* is encountered in up to 6 per cent of patients following adequate surgical excision. Further operation imposes considerable risk to the parathyroids and to the recurrent laryngeal nerves, and treatment should be with radioactive iodine. *Exophthalmos* becomes progressive in about one per cent of cases, the majority being men.

Medical management

Mild cases may respond satisfactorily to rest, sedation and a change in environment. More severe cases require the antithyroid drugs or radioactive iodine.

Antithyroid drugs. These are of particular value in young children and in those suffering from physiological stress at puberty, pregnancy and the menopause. Long-term therapy is required and may extend over a year or more, a plan not acceptable to many patients. The main disadvantages are a high relapse rate after treatment and toxic reactions from the drug. The most frequent of these include skin rashes and arthralgia, but the most serious is agranulocytosis. The usual drug employed is carbimazole. Potassium perchlorate is at times used, its action being slower than carbimazole.

Radioactive iodine. This is of considerable value, but because of the slight risk of producing carcinomatous changes it should only be used in patients over the age of 45 years. The main indication is recurrent toxicity after previous surgery. It is more effective in diffuse than in nodular goitres. The full effect of irradiation does not occur for about three months, and where marked toxicity exists supplementary antithyroid drugs may be required. Dosage is calculated from gland size and estimation is difficult. Hypothyroidism in the long term is very common, involving up to 80 per cent of cases after 15 years.

Management of exophthalmos. Minor degrees of exophthalmos usually regress or remain stationary when thyroid function returns to normal, and even early forms of ophthalmoplegia may recover. If hypothyroidism follows thyrotoxicosis, thyroid substitution therapy should be given to reduce the risk of exophthalmos developing or being accentuated. The chief risk in progressive exophthalmos is the development of infection with ultimate loss of the eye, and careful protection against trauma is essential. Radiotherapy to the orbit may be efficacious in the malignant forms of exophthalmos, and some benefit may be derived from thyroxine and cortisone. Major degrees of exophthalmos may require tarsorrhaphy or even orbital decompression.

SECONDARY THYROTOXICOSIS

Clinical features

As this form usually occurs in a previously nodular goitre, the age incidence is higher than in primary thyrotoxicosis, and most cases occur in females over the age of 40 years. Toxic effects are generally less severe in this form, the nervousness and psychogenic changes less pronounced and exophthalmos less noticeable. The cardiovascular system is mainly affected when irregularity of rhythm rather than sustained tachycardia is produced. Although secondary thyrotoxicosis is more commonly encountered in association with multiple nodular enlargement, occasionally it occurs with a single nodule and rarely has been observed in children.

Investigations

Thyroid function tests will establish the diagnosis although frequently the radioactive isotope uptake is within normal limits.

Treatment

Surgery is the treatment of choice as medical treatment may aggravate pressure symptoms by enlarging the goitre and radioactive iodine should be used only when the risk of surgery is prohibitive.

THYROIDITIS

Acute pyogenic thyroiditis is a very rare disorder following an upper respiratory tract infection and occasionally leads to suppuration.

Subacute thyroiditis is due to a virus infection and is more commonly encountered in the United States of America than in Great Britain. It occurs more frequently in women than in men, usually between 30 and 50 years of age. The onset is often abrupt with marked malaise and fever, together with local pain in the thyroid gland. Radiation of the pain to the back of the neck or to the ears is common. The thyroid is swollen and tender in the early stages, but may be hard and painless later. It rarely has a rising auto-antibody titre, and this forms a distinguishing feature from the more subacute 'auto-immune thyroiditis'. It does not respond to antibiotics, but steroids result in recovery within a few days and thyroxine will help to rest the gland.

Auto-immune thyroiditis

Pathology

Diseases formerly known as Hashimoto's disease and lymphadenoid goitre have now been shown to be due to an auto-immune process. For an unknown reason the patient develops an immune reaction to thyroglobulin which has leaked into the circulation. Auto-antibodies are formed and these can be demonstrated in the serum. Histologically there is a progressive change in the thyroid gland of diffuse infiltration by lymphocytes and plasma cells, degeneration of the epithelium and later fibrosis. There is glandular enlargement with a smooth lobulated capsular surface, which on cross-section shows a firm homogeneous white or pink tissue.

Clinical features

Typical auto-immune thyroiditis occurs in women about the age of 50 years. A moderate increase in the size of the thyroid gland is noted over a period of a few months to a year. Occasionally some pain or constitutional upset is present. Mildly toxic symptoms may be followed by those of myxoedema. The gland is firm to palpation, diffusely involved, and possesses an uneven surface. The association with macrocytic megaloblastic (Addisonian) anaemia is well established.

Investigations

Auto-antibody titres are high as measured by a complement-fixation test, and the gamma-globulin is raised on electrophoresis of the serum proteins.

Treatment

Hypothyroid or euthyroid auto-immune disease should be treated by 0.2 mg *l*-thyroxine daily. Substitution therapy is an important prophylaxis against myxoedema. Hyperthyroid forms of the disease respond to carbimazole. Therapy must be continued indefinitely, and over a period of months the gland becomes smaller and softer. If much fibrosis has occurred in the gland a firm remnant will be felt. Partial thyroidectomy followed by substitution therapy may be undertaken when the diagnosis is in doubt, if the gland is very large and for marked pressure symptoms.

Riedel's thyroiditis

This rare condition is of unknown aetiology and does not appear to be related to auto-immune disease. Massive fibrosis is found extending beneath the capsule of the thyroid gland to involve surrounding structures. Men are affected as often as women and the main complaint is of a painless hard mass in the region of the thyroid gland giving rise to pressure symptoms. The irregularity and stoniness of the lesion suggest advanced carcinoma. Surgical exploration is generally required to establish the diagnosis, and it is usually only possible to perform a biopsy or resect the isthmus to free the trachea.

CARCINOMA OF THE THYROID

Pathology

Various aetiological factros are known. Prolonged stimulation with thyrotrophic hormone plays a part in the initiation and maintenance of many thyroid carcinomas, especially the follicular type. Previous irradiation to the neck can initiate carcinoma in children and young adults but the evidence that radioactive iodine can do the same in adults is doubtful. Some cases of medullary carcinoma are familial and malignant lymphomas may develop in a previous auto-immune thyroiditis.

The pathological type depends on whether the parent cell is the follicular cell or the parafollicular (C) cell. Three types develop from the follicular cell (Fig. 7.2):

1. Papillary 2. Follicular 3. Anaplastic.

Medullary carcinoma develops from the parafollicular cell.

The *papillary* type probably commences in a young age group, although it may not manifest itself until later life, and then only by the presence of an enlarged lymph node. Circumscribed lesions are often seen in one lobe with other similar lesions

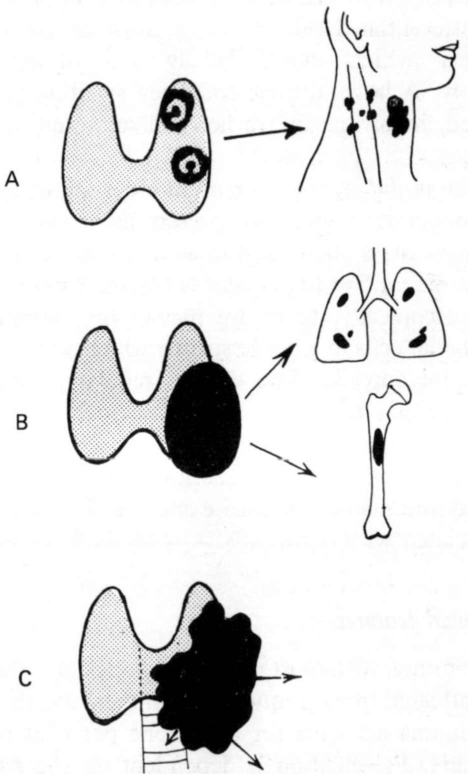

Fig. 7.2 Thyroid carcinoma developed from the follicular cell. **A.** Papillary, metastases to lymph nodes. **B.** Follicular, metastases to lungs and bones. **C.** Anaplastic, local infiltration.

scattered throughout both lobes. Large or small papilliferous processes, resembling normal thyroid cells on section, project into cystic spaces. Lymph node spread is common, but direct spread is late and venous involvement rare. The previously recognised 'lateral aberrant thyroid' is now known to be due to the presence of this slowly progressive lesion reproducing thyroid structure in involved lymph nodes.

The *follicular* form occurs in an older age group, usually between 40 and 50 years. Various degrees of differentiation occur, but commonly this type tends to reproduce thyroid follicles. A large greyish tumour is usual. Spread is more rapid than in the papillary form and is mainly by the blood stream to the lungs and bones. The osseous metastasis may be extremely vascular and even pulsate. Spread also takes place by the lymphatics.

The *anaplastic* variety is found more often in elderly patients and usually develops in a previously normal gland. It is composed of sheets of undifferentiated cells of the spindle or giant cell variety which spread locally and disseminate widely. A large, diffuse and fixed swelling is produced, involving the trachea and surrounding soft tissues.

The *medullary* type occurs in older adults and is of moderate malignancy presenting a very firm, invasive mass often fixed to adjacent structures. It accounts for 5 to 10 per cent of thyroid carcinomas. Microscopically, there are masses or columns of epithelial cells in a dense stroma which stains typically for amyloid. The tumour regularly contains and secretes calcitonin. Metastases occur in local lymph nodes and distantly.

Malignant lymphomas constitute up to 10 per cent of thyroid malignant disease and are almost always associated with thyroiditis.

Clinical features

In common with most other thyroid lesions women are affected more frequently than men and thyroid carcinoma accounts for about one per cent of all cancers. Presentation is dependent on the pathological type of lesion. The first indication of a papillary tumour may be a persistent lymph node in the neck or a small swelling in one lobe of the thyroid gland. Such a solitary nodule, particularly in children or young people, should be regarded with suspicion. In the follicular and anaplastic forms the chief symptom may be a rapidly increasing goitre, perhaps associated with pain in the neck or radiating to the ear. Medullary carcinomas present a slower growing hard enlargement of the gland which is fixed. Dyspnoea, cough, voice changes or dysphagia, indicative of local spread, may be prominent features. Distant spread is recognised by cough, haemoptysis, bone pain or fractures. Loss of weight occurs. A firm, soft, or even cystic mass of one lobe is found in younger patients, but in the more elderly a hard and fixed irregular swelling may be noted. Unilateral or bilateral lymph node enlargement occurs. Further invasion causes venous engorgement and oedema of the head and neck, and a Horner's syndrome may also be produced. Metastatic bony deposits are recognised as tender, palpable enlargements which may occasionally pulsate.

Investigations

Laryngoscopy should be undertaken to exclude vocal cord involvement, whilst chest and skeletal radiographs may reveal metastatic deposits. Thyroid function tests are usually normal and raised levels exclude a carcinoma. A radioactive scan of the gland is helpful as most malignant nodules do not take up the isotope. Ultrasound may be of use. An interesting feature of many thyroid carcinomas is the endocrine activity of the secondary tumours, and radioactive iodine studies may thus indicate the extent of spread. A serum calcitonin level of more than 0.1 mg per ml indicates medullary carcinoma and this test can be used to monitor the appearance of metastases after resection of the primary tumour.

Differential diagnosis

Non-toxic or toxic nodular goitre, subacute thyroiditis, auto-immune thyroiditis, haemorrhage into a cyst, Riedel's thyroiditis, other causes of cervical lymph node enlargement or a branchial cyst may all require exclusion. Osteolytic bone secondaries from the breast, lung, kidney, and occasionally the prostate, may need consideration.

Treatment

Papillary carcinoma should be treated by a hemithyroidectomy on the affected side. If the adjacent nodes are involved their dissection should also be performed. This type of tumour does not generally respond to radiotherapy. Thyroxine should be given post-operatively to diminish the likelihood of pituitary stimulation of further growth.

Follicular growths require total thyroidectomy for the removal of both tumour and functioning thyroid tissue. Two months later the radioactive iodine uptake of any functioning secondary lesions should be determined and the metastases then irradiated. The administration of anti-thyroid drugs, by increasing the circulating thyrotrophic hormone, may encourage the uptake of radioactive iodine by the metastases. Any affected cervical nodes require a block dissection.

Anaplastic tumours can seldom be adequately removed by surgery, show no response to radioactive iodine and should be treated by radiotherapy.

Medullary carcinoma requires total thyroidectomy and, if necessary, repeated surgical clearance of involved lymph nodes is worthwhile. It does not respond to radiotherapy.

The prognosis is good in papillary carcinoma, poor in the anaplastic form, whilst the follicular type occupies an intermediate position. Medullary carcinoma often pursues a low grade but progressive course and patients may survive for many years.

PARATHYROID GLANDS

Physiology

The hormone parathormone (PTH) secreted by the parathyroid gland exerts a profound effect on calcium and phosphorus metabolism by its vital role in deposition and resorption of these substances from bone. It modifies their excretion through the kidney and stimulates intestinal absorption. Active PTH appears in small quantities in the peripheral blood and is difficult to assay. The active hormone, in addition to increasing calcium absorption in the gut, acts by reabsorbing calcium in the renal tubules and from bone, and increasing phosphate loss in the urine. The overall effect of PTH is an increase in plasma calcium level and a reduction of plasma phosphate. A reduction in serum calcium concentration stimulates PTH secretion and hypercalcaemia suppresses it. The hormone calcitonin originates in the thyroid gland and has a hypocalcaemic action; hypercalcaemia leads to higher levels of calcitonin secretion which helps to correct this abnormality. The normal serum calcium is 2.2 to 2.6 mmol per litre and the serum phosphate 0.80 to 1.45 mmol per litre. Of 1000 mg of calcium in the diet some 850 mg is excreted in the faeces and although some 70 g of calcium may be presented to the kidneys daily, only 150 mg are finally excreted in the urine. The renal threshold for calcium is 1.75 mmol per litre and there is therefore a large amount of renal reabsorption of filtered calcium. Various forms of plasma calcium do exist, including some 45 per cent of free calcium ions, some 42 per cent bound to protein (e.g. albumin) and some 13 per cent having a complex with citrate. It is suggested that it is the calcium fraction bound as citrate which is finally excreted and the citrate excretion differs in cases of hyperparathyroidism with and without bone abnormality; often when bone disease is absent the serum calcium is at times normal.

Parathormone controls the ionised calcium level. Neuromuscular function is not disturbed if the ionised serum calcium is normal, even when the total serum calcium falls to tetanic levels. Raised serum alkaline phosphatase and hydroxyproline levels in the plasma and urine are indicative of increased bone metabolism in hyperparathyroidism.

The role of magnesium metabolism in relation to the parathyroid gland is more difficult to define. Magnesium deficiency with hypomagnesaemia has been found in some patients with hyperparathyroidism, and has also been found after removal of a parathyroid adenoma, more particularly when extensive remineralisation of bones has to take place. Tetany may be due to a low serum magnesium.

HYPOPARATHYROIDISM

Deficiency or absence of parathyroid hormone most commonly follows thyroidectomy and is due to the removal of one or more normal parathyroids, or direct trauma or vascular damage with delayed fibrosis in the glands. Congenital and idiopathic cases are only rarely encountered. Removal of a hypersecreting parathyroid will precipitate symptoms of hypoparathyroidism if adequate pre-operative preparation or post-operative maintenance therapy is omitted.

Clinical features

Hypocalcaemia in the first few days following thyroidectomy is no longer thought to be due to hypoparathyroidism (p. 85). The onset of true hypoparathyroidism may be delayed for a few weeks or months or remains latent, manifesting itself during menstruation or pregnancy. There may be tinglings or numbness of the extremities, lips and nose and a feeling of 'being distant'. Peculiar and unpleasant twitching of muscles and later actual spasm may be noted lasting from a few seconds to an hour or more. Blurring of vision and a feeling of suffocation due to spasm of the ocular and respiratory muscles respectively are occasionally present.

The classical features of fully developed hypoparathyroidism are mainly motor and produce tetany affecting forearm and hand muscles and those of the lower limb. The hand tends to assume the cramped 'obstetrical' position and the feet may go into equinus. Occasionally severe, generalised muscle spasms are evident. When hypocalcaemia persists for a prolonged period there is a risk of cataract formation. Children are prone to laryngismus stridulus and convulsions.

In latent tetany, evidence of neuromuscular irritability may be obtained in the following ways:

1. *Trousseau's sign*. A sphygmomanometer inflated to 200 mm of mercury around the upper arm for three or more minutes will cause fibrillation of the interossei muscles or even development of the 'obstetrical' hand. In this position the hand is contracted with the fingers extended at the interphalangeal joints and flexed at the metacarpophalangeal joints, the thumb being adducted.

2. *Chvostek's sign*. Tapping in front of the ear over the facial nerve in the parotid gland elicits a brisk contraction of facial muscles.

The serum calcium and phosphate should be estimated, the former rarely falling below 1.75 mmol per litre.

Differential diagnosis

Any disorder producing real or 'relative' hypocalcaemia can lead to a state of neuromuscular excitability and tetany. Real hypocalcaemia may be caused by a deficient intake of calcium and vitamin D, or poor absorption of calcium, as in rickets, osteomalacia and steatorrhoea. Idiopathic hypocalcaemia is seen in the newborn. Hypocalcaemia is a feature of renal failure, and is associated with hyperphosphataemia. The full explanation of this hypocalcaemia is linked with phosphate retention, metabolic responses and calcium absorption.

Relative hypocalcaemia occurs when the diffusible calcium falls in conditions of alkalosis, such as vomiting of gastric contents in congenital or acquired pyloric stenosis or following the excessive intake of alkalis. Hyperventilation in hysterical individuals raises the blood *p*H due to loss of carbon dioxide and tetany may occur.

Treatment

Care must be taken to avoid unnecessary damage to the parathyroids at operation. If one is removed unintentionally, and this is recognised, it should be transplanted into the neck muscles. When hypoparathyroidism becomes evident in the post-operative period, symptoms may be controlled by the slow intravenous injection of 20 ml of a 10 per cent solution of calcium gluconate. A more prolonged effect is obtained if the intramuscular route is used. If the onset of deficiency is anticipated by measuring the serum calcium level, therapy may be started early and calcium can be given intramuscularly or by mouth. Dosage may be reduced gradually, and if the symptoms abate and the serum chemistry remains stable maintenance therapy is discontinued. Patients with minimal symptoms do not require any therapy, but where severe spasms are present sedation becomes necessary. Persistent symptoms are an indication for treatment, usually with 1-alpha-hydroxycholecalciferol, an analogue of 1:25, dihydroxycholecalciferol. Other means include calciferol (vitamin D_2), 50 000 to 200 000 units (1.25 to 5.0 mg), and 5 to 15 g of calcium lactate per day, together with a low phosphorus diet. Parathyroid extract (parathormone) is potent, requires to be given by injection, and should only be used in cases difficult to control by other methods. Dihydrotachysterol (A.T.10), a vitamin D derivative which may be given orally, is less potent than parathormone but necessitates careful biochemical control. The majority of cases of hypoparathyroidism are not severe, and with or without medication settle over a period of weeks or months. Only a small proportion require maintenance therapy.

HYPERPARATHYROIDISM

Pathology

Adenomas are the usual cause of excess parathyroid hormone and are less uncommon than was previously supposed. Rarer causes include carcinoma and hyperplasia. The size of an adenoma varies from 0.5 to 2 cm. The tumour is reddish in colour with a tendency to become yellow with age. Large varieties may become cystic. Microscopically they resemble normal parathyroid tissue and the inferior parathyroids are more commonly involved.

Hyperplasia usually involves all four glands. Secondary hyperplasia is less marked than the primary variety and is seen in renal disease with acidosis and phosphate retention, and when steatorrhoea causes excess faecal loss of calcium. Macroscopically the enlargement resembles the normal parathyroid, but histologically there are many cells with water-clear cytoplasm. Occasionally multinodular hyperplasia may occur and this may prove to be a diagnostic difficulty for the pathologist, particularly at the time of frozen section during surgery.

Carcinoma produces a greater degree of hyperparathyroidism with considerable atrophy of the remaining parathyroid glands. It consists of sheets of cells resembling the 'principal' cells and metastasis occurs by both blood stream and the lymphatics.

Hyperparathyroidism mainly affects the urinary and skeletal systems (Fig. 7.3). Due to increased parathormone output decalcification of bones occurs with elevation of the blood calcium, the

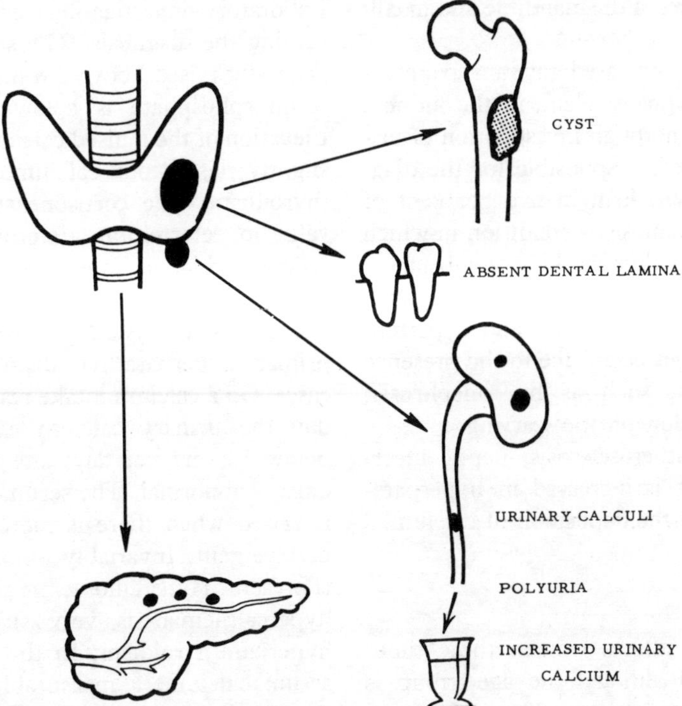

Fig. 7.3 The effects of a parathyroid tumour on bone, urinary tract and pancreas

excess being excreted by the kidneys. A correspondingly low serum phosphate is usually associated with a high renal clearance of phosphate, although at times a normal serum phosphate occurs with minimal hypercalcaemia and normal renal function. Direct simultaneous measurement of blood and urinary phosphate and creatinine concentration (tubular reabsorption of phosphate) may help to establish a diagnosis in these cases, as the T.R.P. is usually lowered. With impaired renal function the serum phosphate may be normal or even raised. Greater reliance is now placed on serum calcium and phosphate measurements coupled with estimation of parathyroid hormone in the serum.

Osteitis fibrosa cystica is the late result of hyperactivity of the parathyroids. A combination of decalcification, particularly of bone trabeculae, with fibrous tissue replacement and cyst and tumour formation is seen. The bones become broader and more spongy, granulation tissue filling the spaces. Osteoclasts are found in the vicinity of the cysts and a varying amount of osteoid tissue is formed. Pathological fractures result, and deformities of the long bones and vertebrae cause reduction in height and kyphosis. Tumours of the mandible and maxilla occur.

In the *urinary tract* increased calcium excretion leads to calcium phosphate calculi in the kidney, ureter and bladder. Thorough investigation of urinary calculous disease is responsible for the diagnosis of hyperparathyroidism in five per cent of such cases. Nephrocalcinosis, a condition in which calcium is deposited within the kidney substance, together with calculus formation may lead ultimately to permanent renal damage and hypertension. Secondary changes occur due to the presence of stones themselves, such as hydronephrosis, pyonephrosis and pyelonephritic scarring.

The incidence of atherosclerosis, peptic ulceration and pancreatitis is increased in hyperparathyroidism because of the deposition of calcium.

Clinical features

Hyperparathyroidism affects women three times more than men, and although no age group is exempt most cases occur between 40 and 60 years. The clinical picture is non-specific for several years unless symptoms due to renal and skeletal complications occur. Lassitude, easy fatiguability, nausea, vomiting, anorexia, constipation, abdominal cramps and polydipsia may precede the symptoms of urinary calculi, and are followed at a later stage by renal failure. Skeletal deformities include kyphosis, coxa vara, decreasing height and genu valgum and varum. Bones may be tender and tumours may be obvious, particularly in the mandible and maxilla. On occasions the occurrence of a pathological fracture leads to the correct diagnosis. There is a variation in muscle tone and reflex activity and in advanced cases hypertension is present. It is only seldom that the parathyroid tumour may be palpable in the neck. Rarely the chronic nature of the disorder may take an acute form which may be fatal unless treated promptly. Progressive weakness and drowsiness may lead to coma, hypotension and circulatory collapse or alternatively the acute symptoms may be predominantly gastro-intestinal, the vomiting and distension simulating subacute intestinal obstruction.

Investigations

Laboratory investigations are important in confirming the diagnosis. The serum calcium level is generally raised above 2.6 mmol per litre and the serum phosphate is below 0.8 mmol per litre. Elevation of the ionised calcium in a normal or only slightly raised total calcium occurs in hyperparathyroidism. The cortisone suppression test is of value in determining a steroid-resistant hypercalcaemia, which is indicative of hyperparathyroidism. The various tests of phosphate clearance have not proved consistently reliable in distinguishing primary hyperparathyroidism from many other diseases. On a calcium intake restricted to 200 mg per day the urinary calcium excretion is normally below 175 mg per day; any figure above 200 mg daily is abnormal. The serum alkaline phosphatase is raised when there is more than minimal bone involvement. Invariably a normochromic anaemia is present. Hyperchloraemic acidosis, together with hypercalcaemia, is very suggestive of primary hyperparathyroidism. In the presence of a raised serum calcium, a measurable or elevated serum parathormone level is generally diagnostic.

Radiography may show generalised bony decalcification or cyst formation. Subperiosteal bone resorption in the middle and terminal phalanges of the hands or at the ends of the clavicles should be sought. The skull may have a pepper-pot appearance in a lateral view, and deformities and pathological fractures of the long bones and vertebrae may be seen. Radiographs of the abdomen may show scattered opacities in the renal area or renal and ureteric stones, and rarely a barium swallow reveals the location of a parathyroid tumour indenting the oesophagus. Radioimmunoassay for PTH from venous blood obtained from the neck by passing a catheter via the femoral vein through the inferior and superior vena cava is helpful in localising a tumour.

Differential diagnosis

The hypercalcaemia of myelomatosis can usually be distinguished by examining the urine for Bence-Jones protein and by determining the electrophoretic pattern of blood proteins. Hypervitaminosis D improves on ceasing the administration of drugs, and the hypercalcaemia of metastatic malignant disease of bone is differentiated by skeletal radiographs. Sarcoidosis may occasionally be confused, but tends to resolve spontaneously or on the administration of cortisone. The milk-alkali syndrome follows the prolonged intake of milk and alkalis for peptic ulcer. Some carcinomas are sites of ectopic PTH production and may require exclusion.

Treatment

Surgical exploration of the neck should be undertaken. Pre-operative treatment is usually unnecessary unless acute hyperparathyroidism is present, when massive fluid and electrolyte replacement may reduce the hypercalcaemia present, but if not, then intravenous infusion of neutral phosphate should be given or calcitonin infused. An adenoma when present should be removed, but careful search should always be made for multiple tumours. Usually there are four parathyroid glands and all should be identified. They are ovoid yellow bodies related to the back of the thyroid gland. Superior parathyroids are more constant in position than the inferior pair and are found posterior to the thyroid gland at the junction of the upper third and lower two-thirds of the lateral lobes or within the thyroid substance. The inferior parathyroids are usually found near the lower part of the thyroid lobes, close to the branches of the inferior thyroid artery which supplies them, but because of their origin from the third branchial cleft they may migrate caudally with the thymus, or be placed in the superior mediastinum. Very occasionally a gland lies deep to the pretracheal and prevertebral fascia and thus the tumour may be related to the oesophagus. Frozen section of the tissue removed is of value but it is sometimes difficult to differentiate between adenoma and hyperplasia. If hyperplasia is present in all four glands three and a half glands should be removed. Parathyroid tumours may be difficult to find, and if not located in the neck or present in the thymic remnants which can be drawn into the neck, exploration of the mediastinum may be necessary. This should be undertaken two weeks later after radioimmunoassay of PTH in venous samples has helped localisation. There is a tendency to post-operative hypoparathyroidism, and this should be anticipated by regular serum estimations and medications according to the severity of the condition. Urinary and orthopaedic problems necessitate treatment as they arise. A low pre-operative serum magnesium level should be corrected by administration of magnesium hydroxide or by the infusion of magnesium chloride in severe cases. Severe chronic renal involvement is a contra-indication to operation.

FURTHER READING

Beaugié, J. M. (1975). *Principles of Thyroid Surgery*. Tunbridge Wells: Pitman Medical.
Evered, D. C. (1976). *Diseases of the Thyroid*. Tunbridge Wells: Pitman Medical.
Greenfield, L. D. Ed. (1978). *Thyroid Cancer*. Florida: C. R. C. Press Inc.
Taylor, G. W. (1979). *The Surgery of Hyperparathyroidism*. In Surgical Review I. Tunbridge Wells: Pitman Medical.
Various Authors (1981). Endocrine Disorders Part I and Metabolic Disorders Part 2. *International Medicine*, Vol. 1. Nos. 6 and 9.

8

Pharynx and larynx

PHARYNX

Inflammatory conditions

Acute infections are generally non-specific in type and may affect the whole or part of the pharynx or a particular structure, such as the tonsil. Less frequently they are due to the specific organisms, Vincent's spirochaete or the diphtheria bacillus. Pharyngitis may be the first clinical manifestation of agranulocytosis following drug administration, particularly chemotherapy. Surgical treatment is only required in the management of some of the complications.

Peritonsillar abscess occurs as a complication of acute tonsillitis, particularly in adults, and is recognised by pain and further signs of inflammation when the original infection would normally have regressed. Dysphagia and restricted jaw movements occur and a red oedematous swelling involving the soft palate and the pillars of the fauces may be seen. The condition is usually unilateral and gross displacement of the uvula may occur. Treatment is by incision and drainage of the abscess.

Retropharyngeal abscess. The *acute* form follows inflammation in the prevertebral lymph nodes secondary to an upper respiratory infection, and is more common in children. Both dysphagia and dyspnoea may be apparent, together with alteration in the voice. Treatment is drainage of the abscess through the mouth, with the child in the extended and head-down position to prevent aspiration.

Chronic retropharyngeal abscess may be secondary to tuberculous infection of the cervical spine. Clinical and radiological signs of bony disease will be evident. Drainage should be performed through the posterior triangle of the neck, the intra-oral route being avoided because of the increased risk of secondary infection.

Pharyngeal diverticulum

Pathology

This is not a true diverticulum containing all coats but a false acquired pulsion type. Its close proximity to the cervical oesophagus has previously given the erroneous impression of an oesophageal pouch. It arises in the posterior and lower part of the pharynx through a potentially weak area between the oblique and transverse fibres of the inferior constrictor (Fig. 8.1). The probable cause is inco-ordination of the cricopharyngeus with resultant raised intrapharyngeal pressure. The diverticulum, composed of mucosa and pharyngeal aponeurosis, gradually increases in size and descends initially posterior to the oesophagus, but

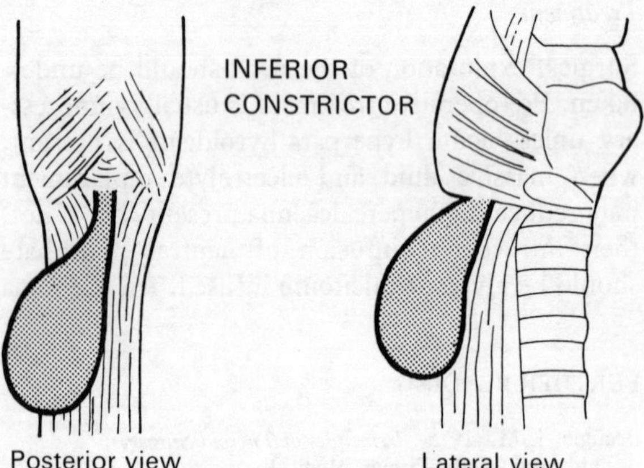

Fig. 8.1 Pharyngeal diverticulum, emerging through a weakness in the inferior constrictor

later to one side, generally the left. It may become large and extend as far as the mediastinum because food enters it more readily than the oesophageal opening on the anterior wall. Infection, perforation and malignant change may follow.

Clinical features

The condition is more common in men than in women and occurs in middle or old age. The main complaint is of longstanding difficulty in swallowing, often accompanied by a gurgling noise as food and fluid enter the sac. A swelling which can be emptied by compression later becomes apparent in the neck, usually on the left side. Regurgitation of undigested food and attacks of choking and coughing from overflow into the larynx may be noted. Respiratory symptoms due to an aspiration pneumonia may be a feature. In the late stages severe dysphagia and emaciation occur. The diagnosis is confirmed by a barium swallow which outlines the diverticulum and shows the characteristic teapot-spout deformity. In cases of haemorrhage or suspected malignant change direct pharyngoscopy is required.

Treatment

Small pouches discovered accidentally on radiological examination do not require treatment. When symptoms are present, particularly nutritional disturbances, excision should be undertakan. A myotomy of cricopharyngeus should be added. The operation is performed in one stage, but in large and infected pouches pre-operative lavage is of value. Care must be taken not to remove the diverticulum too close to the wall of the gullet as stenosis may follow. Post-operatively food should not be given by mouth for four to five days.

Tumours

Benign tumours include fibroma, lipoma and angioma, which may require removal because of obstruction or haemorrhage.

Malignant tumours are generally carcinomas, though a fibrosarcoma occasionally occurs in the nasopharynx. The carcinoma is epidermoid in type, but differs from the squamous cell lesion by the absence of cell nests or cornification. Two forms occur, the *transitional cell carcinoma*, composed of round or polyhedral cells, and the *lymphoepithelioma*, showing large numbers of lymphocytes and resembling a lymphosarcoma. Pharyngeal tumours are found in the following sites:

1. Nasopharynx.
2. Oropharynx.
3. Laryngopharynx—
   Epilaryngeal.
   Hypopharyngeal.

The primary lesion is often small, varying from a fine granular erosion, which may easily be overlooked, particularly in the nasopharynx, to a deep excavated ulcer. The majority of tumours are in the

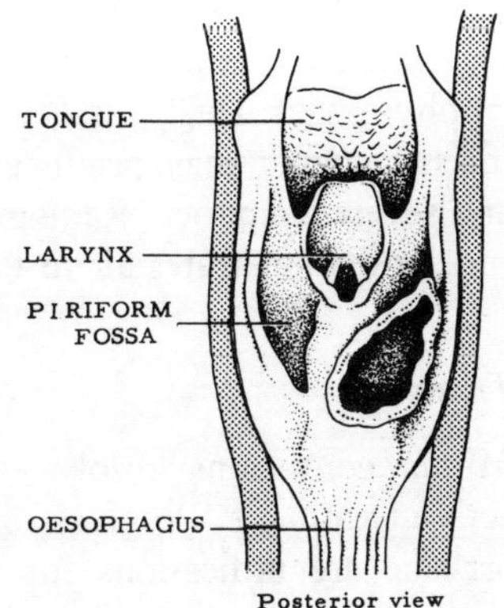

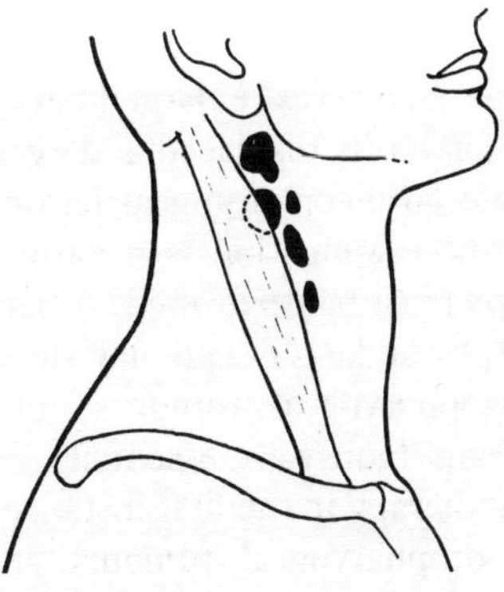

Fig. 8.2 Carcinoma of the hypopharynx. Metastasis occurs to many lymph nodes.

laryngopharynx, particularly the epilaryngeal region, which includes the piriform fossae and ary-epiglottic folds. Hypopharyngeal or post-cricoid growths begin on the lateral or posterior wall of the distal pharynx. Spread is both local and to adjacent lymph nodes, the latter often occurring early in the course of the disease (Fig.8.2). In later stages obstruction or laryngeal involvement with fistula and pulmonary infection may cause death.

Clinical features

With the exception of post-cricoid lesions pharyngeal tumours are more common in men. The primary lesion is notoriously silent, particularly in the piriform fossa, and the first indication is often a unilateral cervical swelling due to glandular metastatic growth. Although this also applies to nasopharyngeal tumours they may present with post-nasal discharge or bleeding, deafness from obstruction of the Eustachian tube, or cranial nerve palsies from infiltration of the skull foramina. Minimal symptoms such as a tickling sensation or a desire to clear the throat may be experienced with pain and dysphagia in the advanced case.

Hypopharyngeal tumours are distinctive in occurring almost exclusively in women and often associated with a clinical syndrome, first described by Paterson and Brown-Kelly, and usually referred to as the Plummer-Vinson syndrome. This is characterised by atrophic glossitis, koilonychia and dysphagia, with iron-deficiency anaemia and achlorhydria. This precancerous state may progress to post-cricoid carcinoma unless treated by the administration of iron and dilute hydrochloric acid, B.P.

Physical examination may reveal enlarged cervical lymph nodes or a forwardly displaced and even fixed larynx in the late laryngopharyngeal lesion. More commonly routine examination is negative. Indirect pharyngoscopy must be performed. A barium swallow, tomography and a CT scan may show the extent of laryngopharyngeal tumours, but direct pharyngoscopy and biopsy are essential.

Treatment is by radiotherapy in the first instance. Nasopharyngeal and oropharyngeal tumours are markedly radiosensitive, but spread is rapid and the prognosis poor. Laryngopharyngeal tumours respond less satisfactorily to such treatment, and in the event of failure total laryngopharyngectomy is required. A new pharynx and oesophagus is constructed either by mobilising the stomach or by using a skin or plastic tube, but the end results of phonation are not so satisfactory as those following total laryngectomy.

LARYNX

Traumatic lesions

Aetiology

Injury may occur from an external or internal force, the former being more common. Motor car accidents, war wounds and suicide attempts are the usual causative factors. Internal injury may be the result of impaction of a foreign body or instrumentation. Because of its mobility and partial protection by the mandible, fracture of the larynx is less common than contusion, and more often involves the thyroid than the cricoid cartilage. Oedema and extravasation of blood may follow contusion or fracture and lead to respiratory obstruction. Infection may later aggravate the condition. Incised wounds are of particular danger from aspiration of blood into the bronchial passages. Although foreign bodies are uncommon in the larynx, where coughing tends to expel them, they are an occasional cause of respiratory obstruction.

Clinical features

Local pain, bruising, hoarseness and dyspnoea may follow external injury. Swelling often makes palpation difficult but undue mobility, crepitus or displacement confirm a fracture with which surgical emphysema is usually associated. Bleeding from an incised wound may produce early exsanguination and severe dyspnoea. Radiography confirms a fracture or demonstrates air in the cervical tissues.

Treatment

Minor contusions resolve satisfactorily without active treatment. Progressive dyspnoea and haemorrhage are indications for urgent surgery. Tracheostomy to relieve the obstruction, the arrest of haemorrhage, the aspiration of inhaled material, particularly blood, and the removal of foreign bodies may all be required.

Inflammation

Both acute and chronic forms of laryngitis are common, but are only of surgical importance if they proceed to respiratory obstruction.

Acute lesions

These occur from a virulent haemolytic streptococcal infection. They may be associated with pharyngitis, or may follow one of the acute infectious fevers or Ludwig's angina. Injuries or burns of the larynx, perichondritis, or the lodgement of foreign bodies are occasional causes. Gross submucous oedema, abscess and even necrosis of cartilage may result. Dyspnoea, hoarseness and pain occur, and there may be dysphagia and a diffuse cervical swelling. Stridor, restlessness and tachycardia with suprasternal recession and cyanosis are seen in late cases. Indirect laryngoscopy reveals oedema of the larynx or, as in diphtheria, an obstructing membrane whilst radiography may indicate a foreign body or cartilage necrosis. Treatment in the milder case is conservative, and involves the use of antibiotics, steroids, local ice compresses, an oxygen mask or tent, and particularly reassurance. Only rarely is tracheostomy required, but foreign bodies should be removed.

Chronic lesions

These often follow an acute laryngitis or are associated with chronic pharyngitis. The *non-specific* type is commoner in the male, and related to overuse of the voice and excessive consumption of tobacco and alcohol. Hoarseness is the main symptom, but there may be pain and dysphagia. The condition may be confused with malignant change, but indirect laryngoscopy shows symmetrical mucosal thickening. Treatment is removal of the cause.

Perichondritis of the laryngeal cartilages is the result of chronic inflammatory change. It may follow injury, the acute infectious fevers, tuberculosis, syphilis, or excessive radiotherapy, and proceed to abscess formation and cartilage necrosis, with later laryngeal stenosis. Pain is often severe with hoarseness, aphonia and dyspnoea in advanced cases. Preventive measures include the careful employment of radiotherapy, but the established case may require antibiotics and drainage. Late laryngeal stenosis often necessitates a plastic repair.

Tuberculosis may produce a submucous infiltration of the larynx with secondary ulceration and perichondritis. It is a late manifestation of the disease and usually denotes an underlying advanced pulmonary lesion. Weakness of the voice and hoarseness are often associated with severe pain. An irritating cough is frequent and dyspnoea occurs later. Treatment consists of general antituberculous measures and chemotherapy. Local measures include a linctus or application of a local analgesic before food when pain is severe. Cauterisation of ulcers may be helpful. *Syphilitic* laryngitis is rare, generally of the tertiary stage and occurs two or three years after acquiring the infection.

Bilateral abductor palsy

This is of particular importance after bilateral recurrent nerve injury in thyroidectomy, but it may also occur in malignant lesions of the thyroid gland, the oesophagus or mediastinal lymph nodes, and in bulbar palsy. Both cords lie in the midline in a position of adduction. The voice is hoarse and weak and severe dyspnoea occurs on mild exertion. In non-malignant conditions preliminary tracheostomy should be followed by lateral fixation of the arytenoid cartilages.

Tumours

Benign. The usual growth is a papilloma, but fibroma, lipoma and angioma also occur. The common site is on the vocal cord where it appears as a single pedunculated tumour. More frequent in men than in women, it causes huskiness and a weakened voice with later dyspnoea. The lesion is easily seen on laryngoscopy and should be excised.

Malignant. These growths are usually carcinomas, but sarcomas also occur.

Carcinoma of the larynx

The usual lesion is a squamous-cell carcinoma arising from the mucous membrane of the vocal cord in the anterior half of the larynx. There is a higher incidence in smokers, bartenders, and others whose voice is in constant use, and a marked male

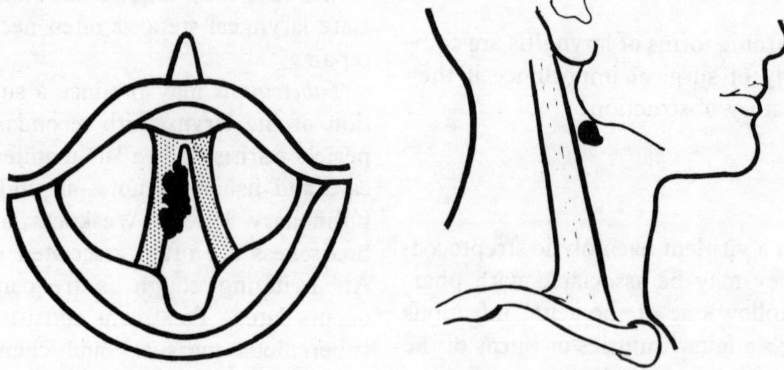

Fig. 8.3 Carcinoma of the larynx. Metastasis to one lymph node occurs late.

preponderance exists. Direct involvement of the whole of the cord, the sub-glottic region and the opposite cord is slow and, unlike carcinoma of the pharynx, lymphatic spread to the deep cervical glands is late (Fig. 8.3).

Clinical features

The predominant symptoms are hoarseness and loss of voice, and when they occur in a patient in the cancer age group they should arouse the suspicion of malignancy. Pain or the feeling of a lump in the throat, followed later by dyspnoea are indicative of advanced disease. Indirect laryngoscopy will reveal a nodular or infiltrating tumour and its extent should be assessed by CT scanning. Cervical lymphadenopathy may be present. Direct laryngoscopy and biopsy confirm the diagnosis.

Treatment is by radiotherapy in the early case. The majority of lesions respond satisfactorily with a 5-year survival rate of about 85 per cent, and the voice is restored. Small tumours may be locally excised by a laryngofissure with preservation of the voice. Failure of radiotherapy or recurrence necessitates laryngectomy, which is also preferable as a primary treatment for the advanced condition. Post-operative speech therapy is important in developing oesophageal speech, and reassurance from a patient who has developed the technique is invaluable in psychological readjustment.

FURTHER READING

Ballantyne, J. and Groves, J. (1979). In *Scott-Brown's Diseases of the Ear, Nose and Throat*. 4th ed. Vol 4. London: Butterworth.

Griffith, I. P. (1982). Tumours of the nasopharynx. Brit. J. Hosp. Med. 28, 32–37.

9

Oesophagus, mediastinum and diaphragm

OESOPHAGUS

Congenital atresia of the oesophagus

Pathology

This is the most common and important congenital lesion of the oesophagus. Various types occur, with or without a communication into the trachea. A fistula may exist between either upper or lower oesophageal pouch, or both, and the trachea, but in more than 90 per cent of cases the lower oesophagus communicates with the trachea near its bifurcation (Fig. 9.1). As with other congenital abnormalities, there may be associated anomalies.

Clinical features

Early diagnosis is essential and should be made by an alert midwife at the first feed. Overflow into the trachea produces an attack of coughing, choking and cyanosis which is sufficient evidence for a presumptive diagnosis. Frequently the significance of such symptoms is not realised and with further feeds bronchopneumonia soon follows.

The diagnosis is confirmed by the finding of a block to the gentle passage of a fine urethral catheter into the oesophagus. The level may be confirmed radiologically by a plain film or following the introduction of only 1 to 2 ml of radio-opaque medium. To prevent pulmonary damage in the presence of a fistula or overflow, a watery or oily (lipiodol) medium and not barium must be used. A radiograph of the abdomen will demonstrate air in the stomach and intestine when a fistula exists.

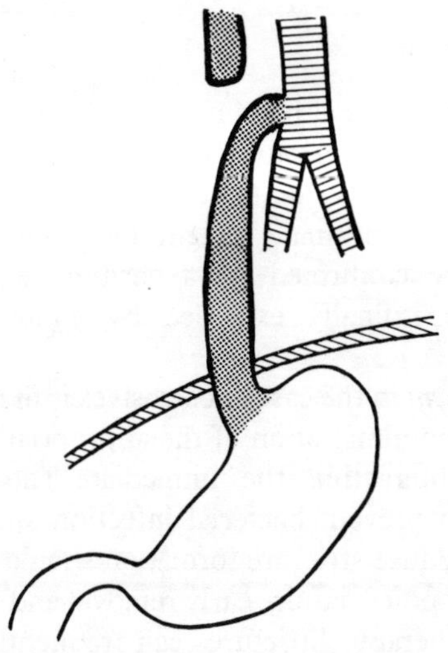

Fig. 9.1 The common form of congenital atresia of the oesophagus

Treatment

Adequate pre-operative preparation is essential prior to major surgical repair. All food and drink is withheld and continuous suction applied to the upper oesophagus by a small catheter. Antibiotics are administered both prophylactically and to counteract any existing infection. Fluid and electrolyte imbalance is corrected before operation. Through a transthoracic approach any fistula present is repaired and an end-to-end oesophageal anastomosis performed.

Traumatic lesions

Perforation of the oesophagus may follow instrumention with either oesophagoscope, gastroscope or bougie, the impaction of a foreign body, biopsy, particularly in the presence of carcinoma, or a penetrating wound.

Mucosal rupture at the oesophago-gastric junction may be caused by the physical strain of sudden distension of the lower oesophagus (Mallory-Weiss syndrome). It is usually due to vomiting, the highest incidence being in alcoholics, but it may result from prolonged coughing or follow epileptic convulsions.

In oesophagoscopy or gastroscopy rupture is most usual in the posterior cervical region, particularly in the presence of cervical osteophytes. Perforation may occur at the site of the primary lesion as a result of bouginage or biopsy, whilst spontaneous rupture occurs at the lower end. Foreign bodies perforate because they are sharp or from pressure necrosis. Surgical emphysema and mediastinitis result with later abscess formation and probable death in the untreated case.

Clinical features

A history of instrumentation, swallowed foreign body or penetrating wound is generally obtained. Following instrumentation many cases may not initially be recognised, but with subsequent food and drink there is pain in the neck or chest and dyspnoea. An early sign is tenderness in the suprasternal notch at the side of the oesophagus. Surgical emphysema with palpable and audible cervical crepitus may follow. A localised swelling denoting an abscess with signs of general malaise and fever may occur some days later. Severe toxaemia and the clinical picture of empyema may follow in the untreated case. In the Mallory-Weiss syndrome there is initial vomiting of food or liquid followed later by the bringing up of blood.

Radiography may show a radio-opaque foreign body when present or demonstrate air in the tissues. The exact site can be localised by ingesting a water-soluble radio-opaque medium. Oesophagoscopy is only required when the perforation is caused by a foreign body or in the Mallory-Weiss syndrome.

Treatment

Care in instrumentation is an important preventive measure and early and skilful removal of impacted foreign bodies by means of a fibreoptic oesophagoscope lessens the tendency to perforation.

In minor degrees of perforation and where the diagnosis is made early, conservative measures generally suffice. Oral intake is prohibited and antibiotics and intravenous fluids are administered for five days. Subsequent abscesses should be drained. In severe injuries and penetrating wounds thoracotomy and operative repair should be undertaken. In most cases of the Mallory-Weiss syndrome the bleeding ceases but occasionally ligation of the artery at the base of the laceration with suture of the mucosal tear is required.

Oesophagitis

The most common form is peptic oesophagitis due to reflux of gastric juice. This is associated with a hiatus hernia and is discussed under Diaphragmatic Hernia (p. 106). Less frequently the accidental or intentional swallowing of corrosives, acute infections, particularly monilial, an impacted foreign body or the prolonged use of a nasogastric tube for gastro-intestinal suction may produce oesophagitis. Specific lesions such as tuberculosis, syphilis or actinomycosis, or the non-specific conditions of Crohn's disease or scleroderma may rarely cause inflammatory changes. The most severe effects follow the ingestion of corrosives. Complete mucosal destruction at either end or throughout the oesophagus is followed by a stricture.

Clinical features

Severe retrosternal pain, shock and vomiting occur immediately after the swallowing of caustics. Later, dysphagia due to stenosis is the main complaint, with ultimate weight loss. The stricture should be confirmed by a barium swallow and malignancy finally excluded by endoscopy and biopsy.

Treatment in the case of corrosives is first directed towards administration of the appropriate antidote and counteracting the immediate shock. Antibiotics to prevent bacterial infection and steroids to help reduce stricture formation should be given. Foreign bodies require early removal and infections specific therapy. Strictures can frequently be prevented by the passage of bougies when the pain has disappeared. The timely repair of a hiatus hernia which is producing oesophagitis may also prevent the onset of a stricture. Once stenosis is established dilatation with bougies passed over a guide wire inserted through a fibreoptic oesophagoscope can be undertaken. Subsequent bouginage may be required, together with intensive medical management of the gastric reflux (p. 108). This will suffice in most cases, but vagotomy to lower gastric acidity may in addition be necessary. It is only rarely that excision of the stricture following peptic oesophagitis is required, together with restoration of continuity using stomach or jejunum.

Diverticula

Oesophageal diverticula are uncommon, usually small and not of major surgical importance. Two main types occur: (*a*) traction, (*b*) pulsion.

Traction diverticula are due to adhesion of the oesophageal wall to inflammatory lesions outside. The anterior wall near the bifurcation of the trachea is more often involved from the traction of tuberculous lymph nodes.

Pulsion diverticula are congenital, occur at the upper or lower end and develop as the result of increased intra-oesophageal tension.

The condition produces no manifestations except at the lower end, where dysphagia and retrosternal discomfort may occur, or perforation. The majority are noted as an incidental finding on barium swallow examination and few require excision.

ACHALASIA OF THE CARDIA

Pathology

The cause of this condition is unknown. Abnormalities in the myenteric plexus, in the dorsal nucleus of the vagus nerve and in the vagus nerve have been thought to be responsible. Primary peristalsis, which is the contraction occurring on swallowing and involving the whole length of oesophagus, is absent and the cardio-oesophageal sphincter fails to relax but there is no organic stenosis. Tertiary irregular contractions which are non-propulsive may be demonstrated by cineradiography and confirmed by manometry. There is hypertrophy of the circular muscle, the longitudinal muscle remaining normal. Oesophageal dilatation follows, the lower end having a smooth outline which ends abruptly, generally at the diaphragm.

Initially fusiform and flask-shaped, with lengthening of the oesophagus, it becomes tortuous and sigmoid in appearance. In late stages the lower portion may sag through the diaphragm to lie below the level of the cardia, allowing stagnation of the contents. Mucosal atrophy and even ulceration may follow. There is an increased tendency to carcinoma.

Clinical features

The condition occurs mainly in men between the ages of 30 and 40 years. Dysphagia is the main complaint, often present for many years, frequently worse with fluids, and generally accompanied by a good state of health. Loss of weight is late. Food ingested two to three hours earlier may be regurgitated. Acute spontaneous retrosternal pain of wide radiation may occur and last for several hours. Spill-over of oesophageal contents into the respiratory tract is common in late cases with attacks of upper respiratory tract infection. Death due to pneumonia or oesophageal perforation may eventually result.

Physical examination may be negative but chest radiography may show a megaoesophagus with a fluid level. Barium swallow examination shows absence of primary peristalsis with degrees of oesophageal dilatation and food retention. The tapering cone at the level of the sphincter differentiates it from carcinoma (Fig. 9.2, A) whilst scleroderma produces a rigid cardio-oesophageal junction and allows free reflux. Endoscopy should be performed to confirm the diagnosis when the instrument passes easily into the stomach. Biopsy and cytology should be undertaken and benign strictures excluded. Fluoroscopy and manometry are both helpful.

Treatment

The aim in treatment is the rupture or division of the muscular fibres at the lower end of the oesophagus. This may be achieved either by dilatation or operation.

The most satisfactory form of dilatation is an

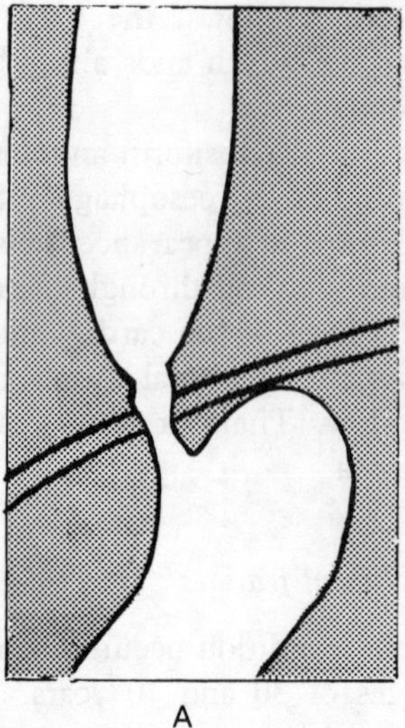

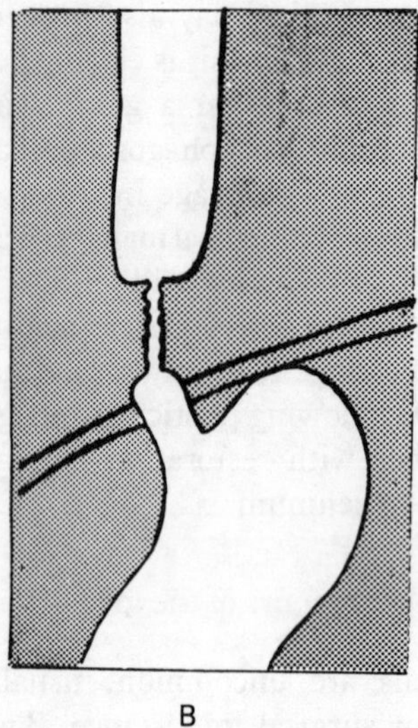

Fig. 9.2 The radiological appearances. **A.** Achalasia of the cardia. **B.** Carcinoma of the oesophagus.

inflatable bag placed at the lower end of the oesophagus under direct vision. Forcible rapid pneumatic dilatation ruptures the sphincter muscle and is successful in about 75 per cent of cases.

Operation is required where dilatation fails or is followed by relapse, and cardiomyotomy by the Heller technique is the method of choice. A longitudinal incision is made in the lower 10 cm of the oesophagus and upper part of stomach. All muscle fibres must be divided to obtain a cure. Reflux may occasionally follow.

TUMOURS

Benign

These are rare and usually either a leiomyoma or a lipoma, but papilloma,fibroma and angioma also occur. They may be intramural or pedunculated and produce dysphagia, although they are often symptomless and recognised incidentally on barium examination. The lesion should be confirmed endoscopically. Removal is required if gross symptoms are produced, and may be performed through an oesophagoscope or by thoracotomy.

Malignant

Sarcoma is rare and is usually a leiomyosarcoma. Dysphagia is the main symptom and treatment is directed towards surgical removal.

Carcinoma of the oesophagus

Pathology

The situation and male predominance of oesophageal cancer suggest the importance of tobacco, alcohol and other irritants as well as previous leucoplakia in its causation. It is common in the Far East, Iran and in the black population of South Africa. The greatest proportion of tumours are found in the middle one-third, particularly in the region of the bifurcation of the trachea; the least in the upper one-third. The majority of lower-third growths are gastric in origin. Macroscopically three main types are encountered:

1. Scirrhous
2. Ulcerative
3. Proliferative

The scirrhous form extends around the wall of the oesophagus as a hard, fibrous lesion, seldom involving more than 2 or 3 cm in length. The ulcerative type is similarly localised but has the typical everted edge of a malignant lesion and a similar tendency to penetrate. The proliferative form projects into the oesophagus, often with a narrow base, and grows intraluminally. The histological picture is generally a squamous-cell lesion without cell nests or keratinisation, but occasionally an adenocarcinoma is found at the lower end.

Spread is both direct and by the lymphatics,

bloodstream spread being rare. Local infiltration with penetration of the muscular coat is often advanced before the diagnosis is made. Surrounding perioesophagitis occurs and adjacent local structures such as the pleura, aorta, left bronchus, lung, diaphragm and pericardium, or thyroid in cervical growths, are frequently involved. Intramural spread in a proximal and distal direction is often considerable and necessitates extensive resection when surgery is employed. Lymphatic spread is initially to the deep cervical, para-oesophageal and tracheo-bronchial nodes. Later the nodes around the left gastric and coeliac arteries are invaded in 50 per cent of tumours of the lower third and in 30 per cent of the middle third.

Clinical features

Males are affected four times as frequently as females, generally between the ages of 50 and 70 years. The earliest and principal symptom is dysphagia, which may at first be intermittent. Difficulty is later experienced with soft food and finally with fluids. Localisation by the patient of the site of obstruction is often exact. Regurgitation and vomiting may occur. Deep boring pain in the neck or chest, in some instances extending to the back, indicates extra-oesophageal spread. Respiratory symptoms from the spill-over of stagnant oesophageal contents or fistulous communication are a late feature, as are cachexia, secondary anaemia and weight loss. There may be an accompanying brassy cough or laryngeal palsy from recurrent nerve involvement, and late extension may result in an empyema or a lung abscess. In the untreated patient the terminal stages are particularly distressing when even the saliva cannot be swallowed. Only the exceptional case is spared such suffering by immediate death due to haemorrhage from the erosion of a major vessel, such as the aorta.

Investigations

A barium swallow outlines the irregular deformity and defines the extent (Fig. 9.2, B). The absence of proximal dilatation and the irregular appearance of the stricture in carcinoma differentiate it from achalasia. Oesophagoscopy is essential, and the upper level of the lesion should be noted. A biopsy must be obtained in all cases and brush cytology is often valuable. Radiography of the chest may show pulmonary collapse from bronchial involvement or absent diaphragmatic movement from phrenic paralysis. Rarely secondary deposits are seen.

Treatment

The aim in all cases should be the restoration of alimentary continuity. Permanent cure may not be feasible, but palliative methods are fully justified to allow the passage of fluids.

Methods:

1. Surgery
2. Radiotherapy

Surgery may be employed at all sites; radiotherapy is unlikely to be curative in tumours of the lower one-third. Operative treatment may be (*a*) radical, (*b*) palliative.

Exploration with a view to radical treatment should be undertaken when the general condition is good and in the absence of distant metastases. Adequate resection with wide removal of regional lymph nodes, particularly in lower-third tumours, is often possible. Restoration of continuity by an oesophago-gastric or oesophago-jejunal anastomosis is performed. When palliation only is feasible, the insertion of a plastic tube through the tumour either by oesophagoscopy or following a gastrostomy, will allow normal eating. An alternative is a surgical by-pass using stomach or colon through a subcutaneous or mediastinal route. This procedure may also be preferable to intubation in the presence of a tracheo-oesophageal fistula. Gastrostomy should not be undertaken as a permanent measure. Adequate pre-operative preparation giving a high protein and high calorie intake with correction of anaemia and respiratory complications is essential. Post-operatively oral feeding is withheld until the fifth day, and physiotherapy and early ambulation are important in avoiding respiratory complications.

Radiotherapy can be curative in upper and middle third growths and may also be employed in palliation, either by external irradiation or by a radioactive element introduced in an oesophageal tube. It may also be used pre-operatively to permit removal of an otherwise inoperable tumour.

Approximately one-third of radically resected cases of tumours of the lower third of the oesophagus survive for five years, whilst results are less satisfactory for the remainder of the oesophagus.

MEDIASTINUM

Mediastinitis

Pathology

Infection may reach the mediastinum from the oesophagus, pharynx and neck or adjacent structures, such as lung, pleura, or vertebrae. The commonest cause is oesophageal perforation, generally as the result of endoscopy, but occasionally due to an impacted foreign body. Pharyngeal or cervical infection following dental extraction, retropharyngeal or cervical infection following dental extraction, retropharyngeal abscess or suppurative adenitis may spread along the planes to the mediastinum. Infection arising in the lung or pleura, formerly common, is infrequent today with widespread antibiotic use, and only occasionally is the primary focus in the vertebrae. The inflammation is seldom circumscribed and is characterised by a spreading cellulitis, often due to anaerobic organisms in a foreign body perforation or haemolytic streptococci when other causes exist. In the event of pus formation, discharge into the oesophagus, bronchus or pleura may occur, but if untreated the infection is fulminating and fatal.

Clinical features

A history of oesophagoscopy or gastroscopy is often present two or three days before the onset of characteristic symptoms of retrosternal pain, dysphagia and dyspnoea. Pyrexia is frequent, and there may be associated cervical tenderness, fullness and crepitus from surgical emphysema. A temporary improvement may be obtained followed by relapse. Radiographic findings include air in the tissues, widening of the mediastinum, and on lateral viewing an increased width between trachea and vertebrae.

Treatment

The prompt extraction of foreign bodies, adequate treatment of adjacent infections and the use of fibreoptic instruments has resulted in the present low incidence of this condition. The treatment following oesophageal perforation has already been described (p. 100), and the use of antibiotics controls the majority of mediastinal infections. When pus forms, drainage is essential, either through a lower cervical incision or transthoracic approach.

MEDIASTINAL TUMOURS

Benign

Dermoid and teratoma
Thymoma
Mesodermal fibroma, lipoma, leiomyoma, chondroma, lymphangioma
Neurofibroma
Ganglioneuroma.

Malignant

Primary
Malignant thymic tumours.
Neuroblastoma.
Glandular—the reticuloses.
Secondary
Lungs, oesophagus, breast and other sites.

Pathology

Dermoids are composed of two germinal layers, teratomas of all three. They originate in the anterior mediastinum, but may extend into other compartments. The dermoid tumour is often cystic and may contain hair, teeth, cartilage, bone and muscle. It may become infected and extend into the pleura with resultant empyema, or it may rupture into the respiratory tract. *Teratomas* are usually solid and may undergo malignancy in any of the three primary tissues. *Thymomas*, only 25 per cent of which are benign, are also found in the anterior mediastinum and have a similar structure to the normal gland. A *lipoma* is the commonest of the mesodermal tumours, and although slowly growing may, like the other lesions, produce obstructive effects from its position. Neurogenic tumours arise in the posterior mediastinum. The *neurofibroma*, arising from the spinal nerve roots, is described under spinal cord tumours (p. 327). The *ganglioneuroma* arises from the sympathetic ganglia and is composed of a similar type of ganglion cell; it may pass through all grades of malignancy to resemble a neuroblastoma. The pathology of the latter is described on page 271.

Lymph gland lesions are the commonest mediastinal tumours. They may be primary malignant swellings, such as the reticuloses—Hodgkin's disease, lymphosarcoma or reticulum-cell sarcoma—or more usually secondary glandular deposits from a primary growth in the lung, oesophagus or breast. Circumscribed and well defined they may mimic primary non-malignant lesions. Malignant thymic tumours include (1) *malignant thymoma*, characterised by rapid growth, necrosis and lymphosarcomatous cells, and (2) *thymic carcinoma*, less infiltrative, with flat cells arranged in concentric layers.

Other benign lesions which may present a similar picture include a goitre and oesophageal, bronchial, pericardial and thymic cysts. A *retrosternal thyroid* adenoma is a not uncommon mediastinal tumour and may or may not be associated with a cervical goitre. The various cysts are rare and developmental in origin. Oesophageal and bronchial lesions are found in the posterior mediastinum, the pericardial and thymic in the anterior mediastinum. Their lining resembles that of the parent organ.

Clinical features

Benign lesions may be asymptomatic and diagnosed only on routine radiography, or by expansion produce pressure effects. Dyspnoea or dysphagia may occur or the rupture of a dermoid cyst be diagnosed by the coughing up of hair. Infection produces the picture of mediastinitis. Symptoms of myasthenia gravis with incipient or pronounced weakness may be present with thymic tumours. Malignant growths give a short history of rapid extension with both pressure effects and nerve involvement—hoarseness from the recurrent laryngeal or a Horner's syndrome (ptosis, myosis, anidrosis and enophthalmos) from cervical sympathetic paralysis. Evidence of a primary neoplasm may be noted when enquiry is directed towards possible sites. In later cases obstruction of the superior vena cava may occur with dilated veins on the anterior chest wall, oedema and cyanosis of the head, neck and upper limbs, chemosis and prominence of eyes and tongue.

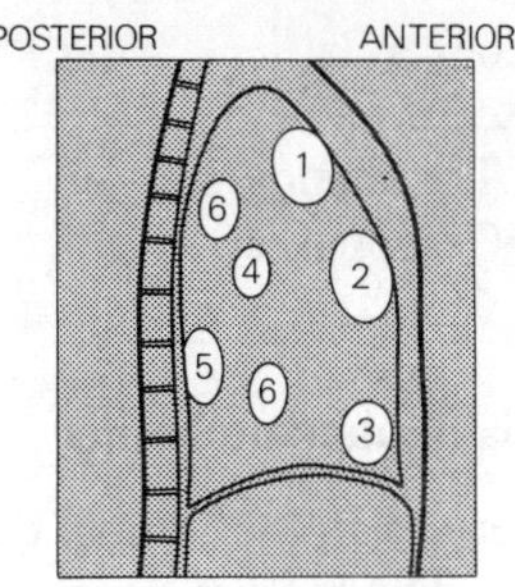

Fig. 9.3 Lateral radiograph of the chest. 1 = Retrosternal goitre; 2 = Thymus; 3 = Pleuropericardial cyst; 4 = Lymph nodes; 5 = Neurogenic tumour; 6 = Bronchogenic or foregut cyst.

Anteroposterior and lateral radiographs are essential (Fig. 9.3): Ultrasonography or CT scanning confirm the diagnosis and add further information on localisation. A spherical swelling with broadening of the mediastinal shadow is usual, but there may also be evidence of primary or metastatic pulmonary disease. Elevation of the diaphragm will be noted in phrenic nerve involvement.

Treatment

In the absence of other primary or metastatic disease, and without evidence of gross local spread, the lesion should be explored by thoracotomy. Where feasible, excision should be undertaken. Radiotherapy should be employed as a palliative measure in lymph gland lesions and neuroblastomas. Chemotherapy may be used as an adjunct in the superior vena caval syndrome.

DIAPHRAGM

DIAPHRAGMATIC HERNIA

This may be defined as a weakness in the structure of the diaphragm, allowing the abdominal contents to protrude into the thorax. It should not be confused with eventration of the diaphragm where paralysis, usually of the left phrenic nerve, results in raising of the dome.

Types: 1. Congenital
2. Acquired:
Traumatic
Oesophageal

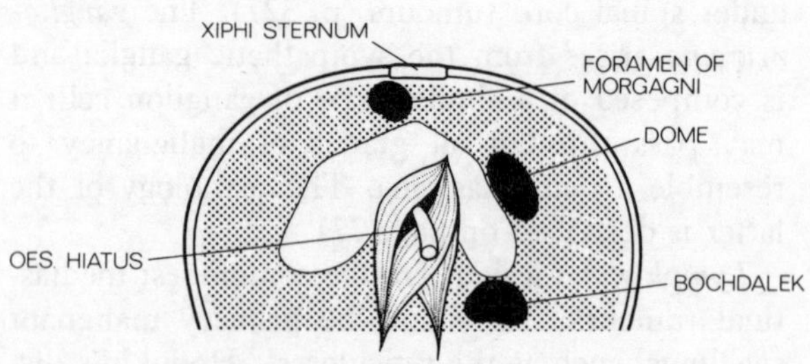

Fig. 9.4 Sites of diaphragmatic hernia viewed from below

Congenital diaphragmatic hernia

This follows errors in the normal development of the diaphragm. The septum transversum descends to form the central tendon of the diaphragm and fuses with the developing crura posteriorly and the anterolateral muscular portions arising from the ribs to constitute the complete diaphragm. A failure in fusion of the individual parts is responsible for herniation. It is more common on the left side, due to the protective presence of the liver on the right side (Fig. 9.4). There may be a complete communication between the pleural and peritoneal cavities or a deficiency may exist in the anterior and posterior portions of the diaphragm. The most common form is the para-oesophageal hernia.

A true congenital 'short oesophagus' is rare, the majority being produced by a 'sliding oesophageal' hernia. The lower part of the oesophagus may occasionally be lined by a gastric type of mucosa in which there are no oxyntic or pepsin-secreting cells.

Acquired diaphragmatic hernia

Traumatic

The usual cause is a penetrating wound, less commonly a crush injury. Sepsis, mainly subphrenic, has been cited occasionally as the responsible agent.

Oesophageal

This is the commonest form of diaphragmatic hernia and occurs through the oesophageal hiatus (Fig. 9.5). Two main types are recognised:

1. Para-oesophageal
2. Sliding.

1. Para-oesophageal hernia. A congenital widening of the oesophageal hiatus permits part of the

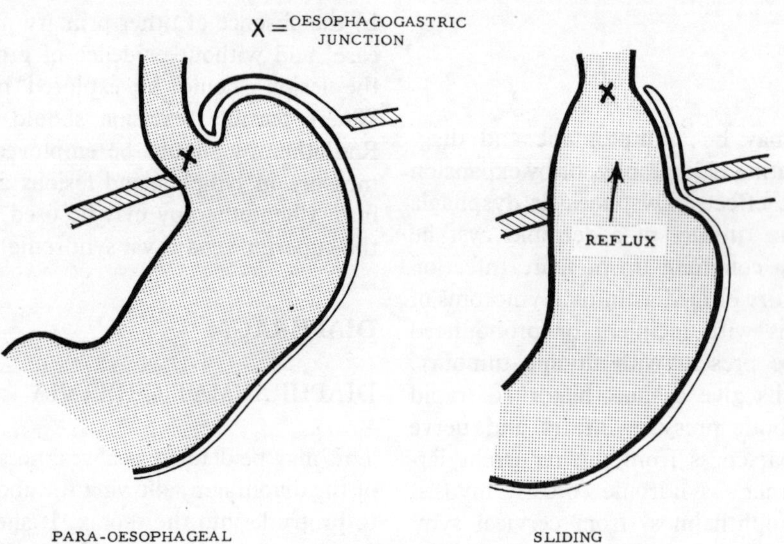

Fig. 9.5 Hiatus hernia

stomach to enter the posterior mediastinum. The important feature is that the oesophago-gastric junction remains at the normal level below the diaphragm and there is no incompetence at the cardia. A portion of the greater curvature enters the oesophageal hiatus to lie alongside the lower end of the oesophagus carrying with it a sac of peritoneum. When large, obstruction, strangulation and perforation may occur, but are rare.

2. *Sliding hernia*. This is the most common form of diaphragmatic herniation. Weakness of the oesophageal hiatus permits the abdominal oesophagus and upper part of stomach to enter the thorax. The oesophago-gastric junction may thus lie in the posterior mediastinum, when incompetence of the cardia and reflux oesophagitis may follow.

A number of aetiological factors are important. It is most frequent in the middle-aged and elderly and, like other direct herniae, is often associated with obesity. In addition an intra-oesophageal physiological sphincter appears to operate at the gastro-oesophageal junction and incompetence of this is probably a major factor in reflux oesophagitis. A stretched phreno-oesophageal ligament appears to be a further factor in its aetiology. An alteration in the power of sphincteric action of the right crus at the oesophageal opening or of the acute angulation of oesophagus and stomach may have some significance. It is further accentuated by increased intra-abdominal pressure, such as pregnancy or the wearing of tight corsets. The condition is at times found in young children with a large hiatus, and negative pressure within the chest cannot be discounted.

Although initially mobile, subsequent fibrosis results in fixity of the gullet with the appearance of a short oesophagus. Reflux oesophagitis may proceed to ulceration, haemorrhage or stricture, whilst carcinoma may develop in a hiatal hernia, as in the normally placed fundus.

3. *Mixed hernia*. A combination of the sliding and para-oesophageal types is present.

Clinical features

1. Congenital

Large apertures are recognised in the newborn by signs of respiratory distress and cyanosis. Dullness to percussion, usually on the left side of the chest, mediastinal shift and a scaphoid abdomen may all be apparent. Small apertures may be symptomless and recognised only on incidental chest radiography or at autopsy. Others produce symptoms of dyspnoea, flatulence or retrosternal discomfort in adult life. Acute intestinal obstruction may occur from bands or adhesions and provide difficulties in diagnosis because of the absence of abdominal signs.

2. Traumatic

A history of a penetrating injury is sometimes elicited. It may be recent and followed by acute respiratory distress and cyanosis, or the aperture may be temporarily sealed with omentum or other abdominal contents. The clinical picture is then similar to the small congenital hernia.

3. Oesophageal

(*a*) *Para-oesophageal*. Flatulent dyspepsia, retrosternal discomfort and fullness, particularly after meals, are common, though symptoms often may be absent. Reflex cardiac irregularities, such as tachycardia, and extrasystoles may be noted. Occasionally dysphagia is the main complaint. Physical signs are usually absent.

(*b*) *Sliding*. The main symptom of peptic oesophagitis, due to the regurgitation of gastric juice or of bile, is heartburn, which is aggravated by bending forwards or lying down. Common in pregnancy, it disappears dramatically after delivery. In newborn infants there may be evidence of dysphagia and of stricture. Retrosternal pain, at times radiating to the remainder of the chest, back, arms, or even occipital region, may be pronounced. Dyspepsia may occur, relieved by food and alkalis, and often characterised by its periodicity. Peptic ulcer and biliary disease may both be simulated but the most serious differentiation is from coronary artery ischaemia. Oesophagitis may also produce a secondary anaemia from chronic blood loss, or frank haematemesis may occur in about 15 per cent of patients. Chest infection varying from mild bronchitis to lung abscess, due to incomplete emptying of the oesophagus may also be apparent. Dysphagia due to stricture may result in weight loss and inanition. Perforation of the oesophageal ulceration is rare, but gastric perforation into mediastinum and pleura may be difficult to recognise. In the uncomplicated case physical signs are not apparent.

(*c*) *Mixed*. A similar syndrome to the sliding hernia is usually present.

Investigations

In the congenital and traumatic varieties radiography of the chest may show gas in stomach and intestine, but in the early congenital form a radio-opaque meal may be necessary. Eventration may be differentiated by screening when the dome is observed to be intact but high. A barium swallow and meal with the patient in the Trendelenburg position outlines an oesophageal hernia and shows the degree of reflux but the size of the hernia is not related to the severity of the symptoms. A blood count is required to exclude or confirm a secondary anaemia. Oesophagoscopy may demonstrate oesophagitis and when a stricture is present biopsy should be undertaken.

Treatment

Asymptomatic cases discovered incidentally do not generally require treatment. The acute congenital and traumatic types require immediate repair through an abdominal or thoracic approach.

Oesophageal herniae may respond to medical measures alone or these may be required pre-operatively. They include (1) posture, with the avoidance of stooping and the adoption of a semi-sitting position for sleep; (2) the administration of antacids, particularly a surface coating substance, to diminish gastric acidity; (3) the avoidance of constricting agents, such as tight belts and corsets; (4) weight reduction.

Surgery is to be preferred when such conservative measures fail in the presence of oesophagitis, in associated upper gastro-intestinal haemorrhage or in most instances when a para-oesophageal hernia exists. The oesophago-gastric junction is returned below the diaphragm in a sliding hernia and repair of the hiatus performed. The abdominal route is commonly used, as more sinister causes of dyspepsia are not infrequently present and would remain unrecognised in a thoracic approach. The treatment of stricture is discussed on p. 101.

FURTHER READING

Atkinson, M. (1980). The oesophagus. In *Recent Advances in Gastroenterology*. Ed. Bouchier, I. A. D. Edinburgh: Churchill Livingstone.

Earlam, R. and Cunha-Melo, J. R. (1980). Oesophageal squamous cell carcinoma: a critical review of surgery. Brit. J. Surg. 67, 381–390.

Harley, H. R. S. (1978). *Achalasia of the Cardia*. Bristol: Wright.

10

Chest and heart

CHEST

Patho-physiology

Ventilation is mediated via the phrenic nerves acting on the diaphragm. The intercostal and abdominal muscles also play a part as do occasionally the accessory muscles of respiration. Gas exchange occurs by diffusion across the alveolar and capillary walls and perfusion of the lungs with blood. Intrathoracic pathology may impair these physiological mechanisms in various ways. Disturbance of ventilation may occur by external pressure on the large airways, either by tumours or stenosis of the walls, clinically resulting in stridor and breathlessness. An obstructed bronchus may also cause marked hypoxia as perfusion of non-ventilated lung will allow shunting of venous blood to the systemic circulation. Obstruction of the smaller airways is common in chronic bronchitis and asthma, and may make lung resection hazardous.

Impaired pulmonary perfusion follows pulmonary embolisation with clot, tumour or fat; the impaction site being related to the size of the embolus. Trauma may cause diffuse intravascular coagulation with microthrombo-embolism of the lung capillaries producing '*shock lung*' (adult respiratory distress syndrome). This can also occur in septicaemia, after massive transfusions (particularly of unfiltered blood) and during open heart procedures ('*pump lung*'). A collection of fluid or air within the pleural space causes a loss of volume of functioning lung reflected in decreased vital capacity and total lung capacity. A similar effect may be achieved by trauma to the chest wall, which may produce a mobile, flail segment that moves paradoxically with respiration.

Thoracic pain emanates from three main sites: the chest wall, the pleural surfaces and the tracheal lining. All are important in that they may draw attention to intrathoracic pathology. Post-operatively such pain may be severe and prevent expectoration of secretions by inadequate coughing. This should be counteracted by sufficient analgesia and physiotherapy but excessive medication may depress respiration. Damage to the intrathoracic part of the left recurrent laryngeal nerve also impairs explosive coughing essential to expectoration. Pre-operative assessment of lung function is necessary, particularly where resection of functioning lung is being contemplated. The ability to exercise may provide a reasonable guide to fitness, such as measuring the distance that can be walked in 8 or 12 minutes. In most cases such information is sufficient, but in addition simple measurement using a peak flow meter will give an indication of airway obstruction. The forced expiratory volume in one second ($F.E.V._{1.0}$) and forced vital capacity (F.V.C.) can be measured with a spirometer and provide a measure of both obstruction and loss of useful lung tissue. In difficult cases more sophisticated assessment may be required.

Chest wall disorders

Sternal deformities are relatively common and are sometimes associated with spinal kyphoscoliosis or connective tissue disorders such as Marfan's syndrome. Occasionally congenital heart disorders co-exist. The deformities may present as depression or protrusion defects. Funnel chest (pectus excavatum) is the commonest variety. The sternum is concave from side to side and above downwards, often asymmetrically. The cause is unknown, although several theories of over- or undergrowth are postulated. The condition may be familial, is usually symptomless and requires only reassurance. Effort intolerance may result. The cosmetic defect is sometimes considered unacceptable, particularly in boys, and surgery may be advised. Pigeon chest (pectus carinatum) is more rare with similar sequelae. Correction is occasionally indicated.

DISEASES OF THE PLEURA

Spontaneous pneumothorax

Spontaneous rupture of the visceral pleura and lung with escape of air into the pleural space occurs in two main groups, and in both, males predominate. It may be primary or secondary. A congenital subpleural bleb may rupture spontaneously, particularly in tall and thin young adults. In the secondary type emphysema may be present; or less commonly pneumothorax may follow infections such as tuberculosis or pneumonia. Spontaneous rupture during artificial ventilation is particularly hazardous as rapid deterioration can occur without recognition due to an absence of symptoms. The effect of rupture is dependent on the underlying lung function and the size of the pneumothorax. If the rent is valved, air passes into, but not out of, the pleural space and results in *tension pneumothorax*. This may cause pressure on the mediastinum which can develop rapidly and may prove fatal (Fig. 10.1). Clinically there is pain and dyspnoea which often starts suddenly. Examination of the chest reveals absent breath sounds with resonant percussion over the affected lung. Mediastinal shift to the opposite side indicates tension. Air in the tissues (*surgical emphysema*) is often apparent and may be gross, affecting the chest wall, neck and face. Chest radiography, particularly on expiration, is diagnostic although small pneumothoraces may be overlooked.

Treatment

Active treatment is unnecessary when the pneumothorax is small and not progressive. In a large pneumothorax a drain should be inserted in the second intercostal space in the mid-clavicular line under local anaesthesia and connected to an underwater seal (Fig. 10.2). Urgent relief is essential, often before chest radiography, if a tension pneumothorax exists, either by the above method or even with the aid of a wide bore needle or stab drain. Where the pleura is appropriately drained with an underwater seal catheter, full lung re-

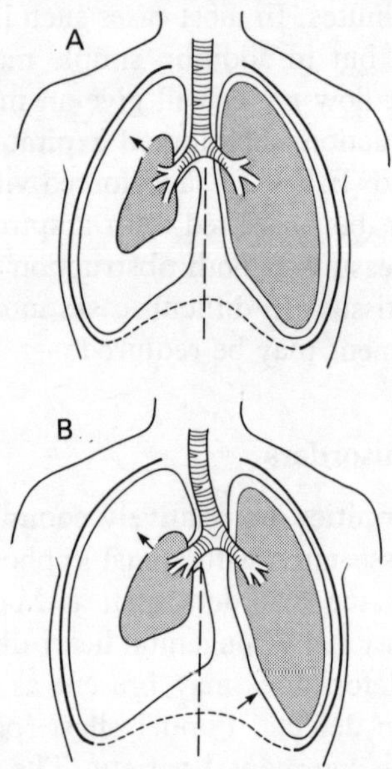

Fig. 10.1 Types of pneumothorax. **A.** Closed. **B.** Tension with mediastinal displacement compressing contralateral lung.

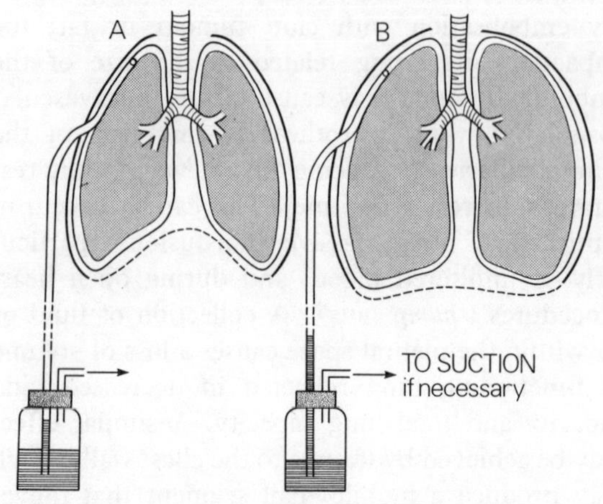

Fig. 10.2 Pleural drainage with underwater seal. **A.** Expiration. **B.** Inspiration.

expansion usually occurs within hours; failure to do so may be corrected by connecting to a low pressure suction pump. If this does not succeed after several days, surgery is advisable due to the risk of infection of the collapsed lung or pleural space, the dangers being greater in the presence of impaired lung function. Infection may cause rapid deterioration whilst a confused patient may withdraw or kink the chest drain and cause respiratory arrest. Thoracotomy should be undertaken, the site of air leak being sutured and the parietal pleura stripped. Obliteration of the pleural cavity by inducing adhesions with instillation of silver nitrate or iodised talc through a chest drain is useful. It obviates thoracotomy but is less effective in preventing recurrence and often is painful.

Pleural effusion

Fluid within the pleural space may be an exudate with a high protein content (greater than 30 g/litre) or a transudate with a low protein content (less than 30 g/litre). The latter occurs in cardiac failure or in association with hypoproteinaemia. About 500 ml is the smallest clinically detectable volume and about half this produces evidence on a plain radiograph. Common causes of exudates include:

1. *Cancer*. The effusion may be bloodstained and contain neoplastic cells.
2. *Tuberculosis*. Lymphocytes predominate in a clear fluid.
3. *Post-pneumonic and subphrenic abscess*. Polymorphs predominate in a clear fluid which may become purulent.
4. *Pulmonary embolus*. The fluid is often bloodstained.

Investigations are directed towards determining any underlying condition, but the fluid should also be aspirated and analysed bacteriologically, cytologically and biochemically. Failure to establish a diagnosis is an indication for closed pleural biopsy using a punch to remove a small piece of pleura. If this fails, an open pleural biopsy is necessary.

Treatment of the underlying cause is essential. Improvement in lung function follows aspiration but if the effusion is due to neoplasm then rapid recurrence will occur. This may be controlled temporarily by intrapleural instillation of radioactive or chemotherapeutic agents. Pleurectomy is rarely indicated.

Haemothorax

Blood may be present in the pleural cavity under the following circumstances:

1. Penetrating and non-penetrating wounds.
2. Post-operative.
3. Pulmonary embolus.
4. Tumour of lung and chest wall.

The blood generally remains fluid, but clotting may occur and also it may become infected.

Clinically the symptoms and signs of the underlying condition will be evident and fluid can be detected in the chest. The diagnosis is established by aspiration.

Treatment should be directed at the underlying cause, but aspiration of blood may be required urgently if there is any respiratory distress. The aspiration of any sizeable collection will also prevent infection. Thoracotomy is required when clotting has occurred or when there is continuous haemorrhage. If infected, repeated aspiration with instillation of antibiotics is necessary, but later drainage or decortication may be required.

Pleural tumours

Pleural metastases are commoner than primary tumours and can arise from a wide variety of sources. There may be a bloodstained exudate.

Mesothelioma. This primary pleural tumour is increasing in frequency; it may occur many years after exposure to asbestos. The diagnosis is generally established by either closed or open pleural biopsy. Treatment is largely unsatisfactory and the majority die within two years of diagnosis. Pleural resection is seldom successful and may even lead to rapid progression.

CHEST INFECTION

The three main forms of intrathoracic pus are empyema, lung abscess and bronchiectasis. They are now less common due to earlier and more effective antibiotic and physiotherapy treatment, and the complications of cerebral abscess and amyloid disease are rare.

Empyema

Pathology

An empyema is a collection of pus in the pleural cavity. The infection may originate in several ways: (Fig. 10.3).

1. *Lung*. Pneumonia, lung abscess or bronchiectasis may involve the pleural cavity. Bronchial obstruction by tumours or inhaled foreign bodies can produce atelectasis which may become infected.
2. *External sources* due to penetrating wounds or surgical procedures.
3. *Oesophageal rupture*, either spontaneous or due to tumours or instrumentation.
4. *Intra-abdominal infections*, particularly subphrenic abscess. The bacterial organisms are related to the source of infection. Previously common ones such as pneumococci and streptococci are now infrequent. Inadequate or inappropriate chemotherapy may leave unusual organisms, whilst the pus is at times sterile following treatment. Gram negative organisms such as *Esch.coli*, *Pseudomonas* and *Proteus* may be present when the origin is abdominal. Staphylococci may complicate a primary infection.

The empyema becomes localised due to adherence of the pleura which rapidly thickens. This can result in fibrosis of the chest wall which, if gross, leads to deformity and immobility of the surround-

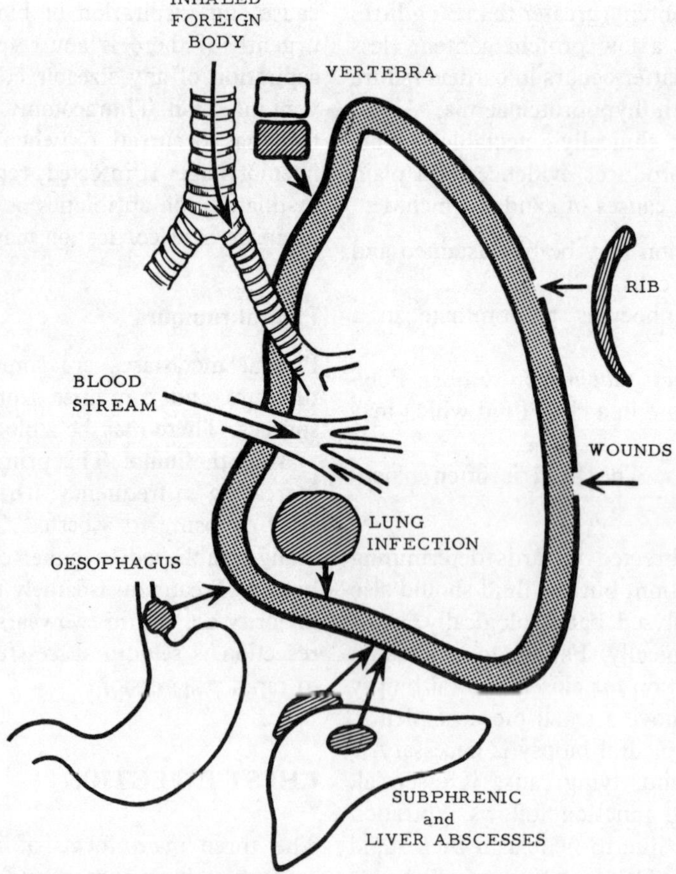

Fig. 10.3 The sources of infection of the pleural cavity

ing structures and scoliosis may occur. The empyema cavity may spread inwards, perforating a bronchus, to form a broncho-pleural fistula, or outwards through the chest wall, producing an empyema necessitans.

Clinical features

Those of the underlying cause may be apparent. In the *acute* form the symptoms and signs of acute inflammatory disease, often with pleuritic pain, coupled with clinical and radiological evidence of fluid in the pleural space, provide circumstantial evidence. In the *chronic* form the features are similar but less dramatic. The acute type slowly becomes chronic with the development of digital clubbing and chronic ill health. Malaise, lethargy, weight loss, anaemia and fever become evident.

Investigations

Postero-anterior and lateral chest radiographs demonstrate the empyema, but diagnosis depends on the aspiration of pus from the pleural cavity. The specimen is sent for bacteriological culture and sensitivities. An underlying cause, if not readily apparent, should be sought; bronchoscopy is essential to exclude any underlying pulmonary disease. Where surgery is contemplated radio-opaque contrast medium should be injected into the pleural cavity (*pleurogram*) to determine the extent of the empyema.

Treatment

Repeated aspiration of the pus with large doses of appropriate systemic and local antibiotics may be advised in early acute cases before gross thickening and fibrosis has occurred, but such management should not be unduly prolonged before *surgical drainage* is undertaken, as spontaneous discharge may occur, producing a broncho-pleural fistula or chest wall sinus. A section of rib overlying the lowest part of the empyema is removed and a large drain inserted, attached to the chest wall and thence to closed underwater seal drainage. Open drainage may later be allowed as further lung collapse cannot occur due to pleural adhesions

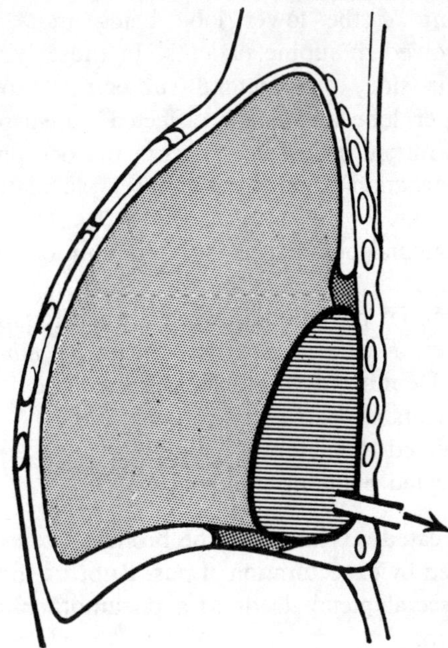

Fig. 10.4 Drainage of empyema by rib resection. The abscess cavity is walled off from the remainder of the pleural space by dense adhesions.

(Fig. 10.4). The cavity gradually becomes smaller, its size being checked with radio-opaque medium. In tuberculous empyema prolonged chemotherapy will be required. In chronic conditions thoracotomy, with removal of the cavity and surrounding fibrotic wall, releasing the lung and chest wall (*decortication*) may be necessary. Diseased functionless lung may require removal.

Lung abscess

Pathology

An abscess may result from lung necrosis following a localised infection which may occur in a number of ways.

1. Inhalation of fluid or vomitus in cases of head injuries in anaesthetised patients; this should be preventable. The right lung is more frequently involved than the left due to the straighter course of the right main bronchus. Dependent segments are more susceptible, the posterior segment of the upper lobe and the apical seg-

ment of the lower lobe being more often involved in supine patients. In those lying on their side, the pectoral subsegments of the upper lobe are usually affected. Unsuspected aspiration may also occur in oesophageal obstruction due to stricture, achalasia or tumour.
2. Bronchial obstruction by a tumour or foreign body.
3. Bacterial pneumonia, especially with staphylococci, *Klebsiella* and *Mycobacterium tuberculosis*. Debilitated, immunosuppressed and diabetic patients are particularly susceptible.
4. Infected haematoma of the lung.
5. Infected pulmonary infarct.

If untreated, extension to the bronchus can occur followed by expectoration of pus. Rupture through the visceral pleura leads to a pneumothorax and empyema.

Clinical features

These are generally those of an acute lung infection; more chronic forms with digital clubbing, halitosis and systemic ill-health are rare. The diagnosis is made by chest radiography, when an opacity or fluid level may be noted. Bacteriological examination of the sputum may reveal an underlying organism but is often unhelpful. Needle aspiration may assist but is rarely indicated. Where there is no obvious cause, bronchoscopy should be undertaken to exclude an occluded bronchus or inhaled foreign body. If an obstructive oesphageal cause is likely, barium swallow or endoscopy is indicated.

Treatment

The majority respond to antibiotics and physiotherapy. Where organisms are detected the appropriate antibiotic is administered, otherwise large doses of benzyl penicillin or metronidazole are given. Vigorous physiotherapy with postural drainage and coughing facilitates expectoration and expansion of the lung. Surgery is rarely indicated unless an underlying lesion such as a tumour or foreign body needs resection. Where part of the lung is irrevocably destroyed it may require excision.

Bronchiectasis

Pathology

Permanent dilatation of the bronchi with associated damage to their walls and infiltration with inflammatory cells can follow bronchial obstruction or severe infection such as measles, whooping cough (where the lymph nodes enlarge) or tuberculosis. Bronchial tumours are an increasingly common cause. Cystic fibrosis accounts for some cases. The extent of bronchial damage varies but is often widespread. Abnormally dilated and tortuous bronchial arteries are an associated finding.

Clinical features

Chronic copious expectoration of foetid sputum with exacerbations is typical and digital clubbing is frequent. Haemoptysis is common and occasionally massive. Investigations include identifying the bacteriological flora, common organisms being *H. influenzae*, staphylococci or mixed organisms. The anatomical distribution of disease is ascertained by bronchography. Bronchoscopy may exclude a foreign body or tumour and may help to localise the site of haemoptysis.

Treatment

The condition is now less frequent and surgery is rarely indicated. Management is by physiotherapy and postural drainage, together with appropriate antibiotic therapy. The latter is more effective if given on an intermittent basis during exacerbations; continuous therapy alters the flora and resistant organisms then colonise. Surgery may be indicated in the rare instance where severe symptoms occur in localised disease, demonstrated by bronchography. Uncontrollable severe haemoptysis may respond only to resection of the affected part of lung and may be required urgently. Occasionally an alternative is ligation of the related bronchial arteries. Where bronchiectasis is secondary to local bronchial occlusion, removal of the affected part of the lung is required.

Pulmonary tuberculosis

Such is the efficacy of modern antituberculous chemotherapy that surgery is very rarely required and the extensive and often complex procedures previously performed are of historical interest only. *Pulmonary resection* is occasionally indicated for drug resistance, and where chronic failure of compliance with prescribed medication exists with localised disease. Destroyed and functionless lung may require resection, especially when colonised by fungi, such as aspergillus, producing solid aspergillomata. Tuberculous empyema is now rare but may require decortication with removal of part or all functionless underlying lung tissue.

CHEST INJURIES

In the United Kingdom most chest injuries are 'closed' or non-penetrating and follow road traffic accidents. The resulting mortality rate is about 10 per cent and may be higher when other parts of the body are involved. The combination of head injury plus chest injury is particularly lethal. Chest injuries are often only part of a complex clinical traumatic problem and care must be taken to prevent them being overlooked. Penetrating wounds from knife or gunshot injury are increasing in frequency.

Anoxia and haemorrhage are the main causes of death. Hypoxia follows with airway obstruction due to blood, fluid or vomitus; or the lungs may be compressed by pleural collections of air (*pneumothorax*) (p. 110) or blood (*haemothorax*) (p. 111). The lung may be contused or lacerated whilst haemorrhage decreases the circulating blood volume and if occurring within the pericardium can cause tamponade (p. 130).

Management

Immediate first-aid resuscitative measures at the site of injury are often essential for recovery. Investigation and treatment in an intensive care unit is preferable, where facilities for bronchoscopy, intubation, ventilation and thoracotomy can be immediately available, because the clinical picture may undergo rapid change. Chest radiography may need frequent repetition. Contrast studies and angiography may be indicated. All intrathoracic viscera are at risk in open and closed chest injuries but some which are particularly vulnerable are discussed in the following section.

Rib fractures are painful, particularly on coughing, and thus prevent expectoration. Sharp ends may penetrate intrathoracic viscera, commonly the lung. When two or more ribs are fractured in two or more places or in association with sternochondral dislocation, paradoxical chest wall movement occurs on respiration which, if severe, produces hypoxia. The diagnosis is usually made where there is localised tenderness or deformity in association with an appropriate history. Chest radiography often underestimates the extent of injury.

At the accident site paradoxical respiration may be treated by external pressure from a roll of clothing. If the blood gases are abnormal, intermittent positive pressure ventilation is carried out in the intensive care unit until the chest wall becomes stable, which may take several weeks. Rarely in extensive injuries thoracotomy and stabilisation of the chest wall with pins and wire may be indicated. Sternal fractures due to steering wheels are often associated with tracheal or aortic injuries and have a high mortality. Relief of pain with analgesic drugs may be difficult due to associated respiratory depression and is best obtained using local anaesthesia infiltration or intercostal nerve block. Short term ventilation by nitrous oxide/oxygen mixtures is also valuable. Surgical emphysema is an important indicator of damage to air-containing viscera, the localisation of which is essential.

Pneumothorax is generally due to damage of the lung or major airways or to a penetrating wound. When small, it frequently does not cause symptoms and may not require treatment. Treatment of large pneumothorax is discussed on p. 110.

Haemothorax is easily overlooked but should be diagnosed by aspiration and treated by insertion of an intercostal drain. Continued excessive bleeding is an indication for urgent thoracotomy to achieve haemostasis (p. 111). Lung injury may be due to lacerations, contusions, 'shock lung' or embolisation by fat or thrombus.

Ruptured diaphragm may be unrecognised as other injuries can obscure the diagnosis. It may follow closed or penetrating injuries and surgical repair is required.

The heart and pericardium are liable to both closed and penetrating injuries. Tears of the pericardium may cause cardiac herniation but are less important than cardiac injuries. Closed injuries mimic myocardial infarction and occasionally lead to myocardial rupture. Septal defects (p. 122) and valvular lesions (p. 125) are described later. Penetrating cardiac wounds produce tamponade, where cardiac output falls due to inability of the compressed heart to fill. Associated haemorrhage may complicate the picture and urgent surgery is indicated.

Traumatic rupture of the thoracic aorta may follow a car or aircraft crash. The commonest site, just below the subclavian artery, is probably due to the difference in mobility between the arch and the descending aorta during sudden deceleration. The intima and media usually tear while a sheath of adventitia persists. This may later rupture or become the site of aneurysm formation. Chest radiography often reveals mediastinal widening but aortography is essential to confirm the diagnosis. Urgent surgical repair is indicated using a dacron graft whilst preserving the blood supply of the lower half of the body by an arterial shunt or partial by-pass.

Oesophageal injuries are most commonly due to instrumentation and seldom follow closed or open injuries (p. 99).

LUNG CYSTS

Congenital cysts

These follow abnormal development of the lung bud. The cyst, which may be large and solitary or small and multiple, is lined with respiratory epithelium, and may contain air or fluid or both. Infection is common, resulting in a lung abscess; numerous abscesses simulate the picture of bronchiectasis. Pneumothorax is rare. The clinical features are those of pressure especially from a large cyst in a small child. Often a routine radiograph reveals the lesion in an asymptomatic individual.

Treatment

Where symptoms exist resection should be undertaken. Where infection is present antibiotics often cause resolution but recurrence is frequent and is an indication for excision.

Emphysematous cysts

Most follow degeneration of the lung with alveolar wall rupture. The space then distends with air causing pressure effects on the remainder of the lung. These cysts have no epithelial lining and vary considerably in size. Although usually associated with chronic bronchitis, infection of these cysts is rare while spontaneous pneumothorax is common. Dyspnoea is the main symptom.

Treatment

Removal or obliteration is rarely indicated except when the cyst causes pressure effects on the remainder of the lung. In most cases overall lung function is impaired by loss of functioning tissue and surgery does not improve the condition. If a pneumothorax develops it may be fatal, hence it requires urgent treatment.

Hydatid cyst

This condition, caused by the *Taenia echinococcus*, occurs more frequently in the liver than in the lung, and the pathological aspects are described on p. 238. It is an uncommon entity in the United Kingdom.

Clinical features

In many instances the cyst is symptomless, and the diagnosis made as a result of incidental radiography, but when the cyst is large there may be cough, dyspnoea and occasionally blood-stained sputum. If the cyst ruptures into the bronchial tree, clear salty fluid is expectorated and small portions of membrane, which resemble grape skins, may also be present in the sputum. Rarely the membrane is sufficiently large to obstruct the trachea or bronchus and cause asphyxia. At the time of rupture there is often a severe generalised anaphylactic reaction. When infection has supervened the condition resembles a lung abscess with profuse purulent sputum, pyrexia and chronic ill-health.

Chest radiographs usually demonstrate the cysts as oval shadows with a sharp demarcation between cyst and lung. The haemagglutination test should be performed for confirmation (p. 238).

Treatment

Excision of the cyst should be undertaken to prevent complications. Spillage is to be avoided as this produces daughter cysts, and aspiration is contraindicated for a similar reason. When the cyst is small it can be removed safely without rupture by making an incision through the adventitia but leaving the laminated membrane intact. The anaesthetist then gradually delivers the cyst by increasing the pressure in the lung. Large cysts require dissection. If the cyst has become infected or the diagnosis is in doubt or a portion of lung has been destroyed, lobectomy should be performed.

TUMOURS OF THE LUNG

Bronchial adenoma and hamartoma are rare tumours, but carcinoma of the lung is common.

Bronchial adenomas are usually benign but may be of low-grade malignancy, and there are two main types. Cylindroma involves the larger bronchi and trachea, and invades locally or may metastasise to lymph nodes or liver. Carcinoid adenomas occur in larger bronchi and may cause atelectasis and distal infection; haemoptysis is common. Hormone production includes ACTH and 5-hydroxytryptamine and serotonin; the latter may produce the carcinoid syndrome.

Hamartoma may arise anywhere in the lung as an overgrowth of normal tissue elements in disorganised form, and histologically fibrous tissue, fat, cartilage or vascular cells predominate.

Carcinoma of the lung

Pathology

One-quarter of the total annual death rate of 125 000 from cancer in England and Wales is due to lung cancer. Three-quarters occur in males but the incidence in females is rapidly increasing; most are middle-aged or older. Cigarette smoking is the most important aetiological factor except in adenocarcinoma, but other causes include exposure to asbestos, radioactive minerals and to some metals such as nickel and chromium. Atmospheric pollution may be a causative factor whilst old lung scars may be the site of adenocarcinoma.

Four histopathological varieties occur. One-third are squamous-cell carcinoma, one-quarter are small oat-cell carcinoma and the remainder are equally distributed between adenocarcinoma and large cell undifferentiated tumours. The prognosis and management depend on the histopathological type. Most tumours occur centrally and affect the larger airways. Spread may take place by direct extension, through the lymphatics or by the bloodstream. Metastases are often early. Direct extension occurs to the mediastinum, chest wall, phrenic nerve, paricardium and pleura. When serous surfaces are involved blood-stained malignant effusions may develop. When the tumour is situated at the apex of the lung, the brachial plexus, sympathetic nervous system and upper ribs may be involved. On the right side the growth or its metastases may obstruct the superior vena cava, whilst the recurrent laryngeal nerve may be involved on the left side. Lymphatic spread is to bronchopulmonary, tracheobronchial, paratracheal and finally supraclavicular nodes. Axillary node involvement results from chest wall invasion. Distant blood-borne metastases commonly involve bone, brain, liver, skin and adrenals.

Clinical features

Males are affected more often than females. The greatest age incidence is 50–70 years. Symptoms may be produced by the effects of the carcinoma on the respiratory system, by the invasion of structures in or near the chest and by the general effects of the tumour (Fig. 10.5).

Respiratory system. The common presenting symptom is a persistent non-productive cough. A small amount of blood-stained sputum is frequently observed; rarely a brisk haemoptysis. Dyspnoea or pain in the chest may occur or there may be recurrent pulmonary infection believed to be an incompletely resolved pneumonia. A lung

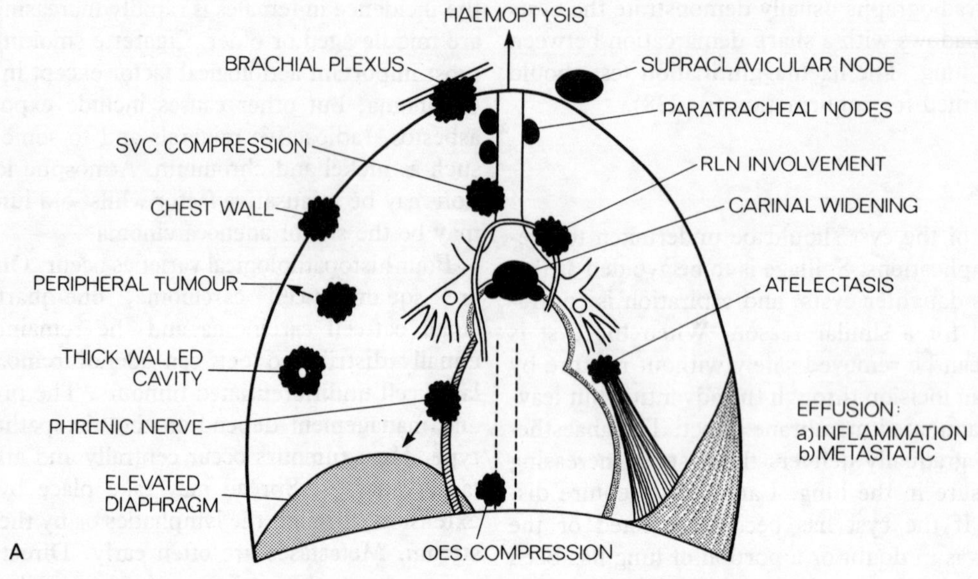

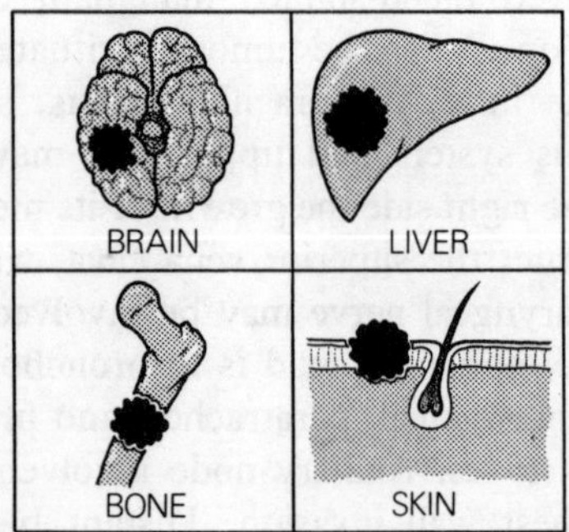

Fig. 10.5 Carcinoma of the lung. **A.** Involvement of adjacent structures by direct spread. **B.** Distant metastases.

abscess, a pleural effusion or an empyema may be the presenting manifestation or occur late in the disease.

Invasion of structures in or near the chest. Radiating arm pain or a Horner's syndrome (p. 105) may be caused by the extension of apical tumours. Hoarseness can arise from recurrent laryngeal nerve involvement. Swelling of the head, neck and upper limbs with turgid veins and prominent eyes is the clinical picture of superior vena caval obstruction. Pericardial invasion produces evidence of an effusion, whilst chest wall extension results in local pain.

General effects. A small and symptomless primary tumour can metastasise to the central nervous system and resemble a primary brain or spinal cord lesion. Hepatomegaly or cervical and axillary lymphadenopathy may at times be the presenting signs. Clubbing of the digits is seen at an early stage and hypertrophic pulmonary osteoarthropathy sometimes occurs when joints and surrounding structures become swollen. The joint symptoms may be the first manifestation of the disease. Anaemia, lassitude and weight loss can be apparent in late cases. Hormonal manifestations from a small bronchial primary may occur and be misleading. Cushing's syndrome with a low serum potassium may be noted early and is often of bad prognosis. An increased secretion of 5-hydroxytryptamine may be detected with symptoms suggestive of a carcinoid tumour. Hypercalcaemia, hypoglycaemia, thyrotoxicosis and gynaecomastia may on occasions be encountered as well as neuropathy and myopathy.

Investigations

A radiograph of the chest is essential and will demonstrate an opacity in the lung field. Tomography gives additional information. A pleural effusion or lung abscess may be noted. Diaphragmatic elevation suggests paralysis, which should be confirmed by screening. Sputum cytology is of particular

Table 4 Malignant tumours

Histological type	Smoking	Main sex incidence	Finger clubbing	Surgery	Radiotherapy
Squamous	Related	Male	+	Valuable	Valuable
Oat	Related	Male	–	Rarely valuable	Valuable
Adeno	Not related	Female	+	Valuable	Not valuable
Undifferentiated	Related	Male	+	Occasionally valuable	Valuable

value and bone, brain and liver scans may give additional information of distant spread. When surgery is contemplated assessment of lung function is important to prevent an operation where undue dyspnoea would follow resection.

Treatment

Surgery. The best results are obtained in localised squamous-cell carcinoma; adenocarcinoma and peripheral oat-cell tumours are less satisfactory. Distant spread precludes surgical resection. Most instances of local spread are signs of non-resectability, an exception being where chest wall invasion can be removed with the tumour. Extensive lymph node involvement is a poor sign but affected localised nodes may be removed. Surgical excision aims to remove all the tumour with its related lymphatic drainage whilst preserving as much lung function as possible. In most instances this means removal of a lobe (*lobectomy*) or the whole lung (*pneumonectomy*). A significant proportion of cases submitted to surgery as being operable are non-resectable when the full extent of spread is determined at operation. After lobectomy the remaining lobe or lobes expand to fill the available space whilst the contiguous structures such as the mediastinum, chest wall and diaphragm move towards it. After a pneumonectomy the space fills with fluid which absorbs and completely obliterates the cavity. Approximately one-third of patients are alive five years after lobectomy and a quarter after pneumonectomy.

Radiotherapy. The main use is for palliation, particularly for oat-cell carcinomas. Relief of superior vena caval obstruction and bone pain from direct or metastatic spread is also important. Other indications include severe haemoptysis and dyspnoea due to airway obstruction. Adenocarcinomas are radio-resistant.

Chemotherapy. This is presently only of value in prolonging the life of some patients with oat-cell carcinomas by months.

In many cases of advanced carcinoma of the lung specific chemotherapy should not be undertaken. Careful attention to nursing either at home or in hospital, with adequate control of pain and cough with analgesic drugs, is required (p. 445).

Secondary carcinoma of the lung

Metastatic pulmonary deposits are common, and their detection is important before embarking on the treatment of a primary tumour. Occasionally, as in hypernephroma or testicular tumour, a single secondary growth in the lung is amenable to operation and good results can follow resection.

TRACHEAL INTUBATION AND TRACHEOSTOMY

Respiratory failure may follow a wide spectrum of pathological conditions; many of these are not of primary pulmonary origin but restrict the availability of air to the lungs. Such conditions respond to intubation of the trachea combined in most instances with intermittent positive pressure ventilation by a respirator. In most cases intubation via the mouth or nose can be performed without difficulty; rarely is emergency tracheostomy necessary. If intubation becomes necessary for more than several days, elective tracheostomy is indicated, otherwise granulomata of the vocal cords or tracheal stricture may develop from pressure of the endotracheal tube.

Indications

1. *Neurological defects*
   (a) Central, such as deep coma from any cause. Head injuries, drug overdose or cardio-respiratory arrest.
   (b) Peripheral. Poliomyelitis, bulbar palsy, myasthenia gravis or tetanus.
2. *Obstructed upper airways*
   (a) Infections, particularly in children (viral and bacterial)
   (b) Tumours of the larynx or trachea, intrinsic or extrinsic
   (c) Inhaled foreign bodies, vomitus or excessive sputum production
   (d) Bilateral recurrent nerve palsy causing abductor paralysis
   (e) Glottic oedema and other allergic states, such as insect stings
   (f) Trauma, either facio-maxillary injury or burns
3. *Chest wall instability* such as flail chest from multiple fractures

Management

When the endotracheal tube is in position, bronchial toilet, oxygen therapy and positive pressure ventilation are possible. The aftercare of a tracheostomy requires careful management and meticulous attention to detail. The importance of keeping the airway clear must be emphasised. The latter may be lost if the tracheostomy tube becomes displaced from the opening in the trachea and enters the tissue planes. It is difficult to replace soon after operation, and a tracheal dilator, good light and spare tube should always be available. The tube tends to become blocked by sputum, which must be removed by coughing, suction or cleaning. Plastic tubes are in common use and can be changed completely. Suction should be carried out with a catheter, angulated at the end to prevent it always entering the right bronchus, and frequent aspirations are performed. Strict sterile precautions with the use of a new sterile catheter on each occasion are essential to prevent secondary infection of the lung.

Inhaled air no longer passes through the nose, pharynx and larynx where moisture is normally added; the sputum is thus hard and tends to form crusts. The latter may obstruct the airway either at the tube or in the trachea and a humidifier is of value in preventing their formation. Where a cuffed endotracheal tube is being used, as in poliomyelitis, the balloon should be deflated for two minutes in every hour to prevent sloughing of the trachea from pressure. Prior aspiration of fluid lying above the cuff should be carried out. Mechanical ventilation by positive pressure may be required in some instances, and a pencil and paper or bell should be available as a means of communication.

TRACHEA

Tracheal stenosis may be caused by external compression or by damage or disease of the wall. The former is seen in an extreme form due to retrosternal goitre where the trachea is reduced to a narrow slit. Other causes include aortic aneurysm or enlarged lymph nodes. Damage from intubation is now the commonest cause and occurs following pressure by the cuff or end of an endotracheal or tracheostomy tube, and can often be prevented. Tuberculosis is a rare cause. Tracheal tumours are unusual and are either adenoma or primary carcinoma. The latter occasionally originate in the trachea but more often the tracheal wall is involved by secondary spread from the bronchus or oesophagus. The principal symptom is stridor associated with breathlessness and an irritating cough. Sudden death is not uncommon due to anoxia precipitated by exacerbation of the narrowing by oedema or sputum.

Primary tumours and stenoses may be resected with direct anastomosis provided that only a short length is removed. Malignant extrinsic compression may sometimes be palliated by radiotherapy.

Inhaled foreign bodies

A wide variety of foreign bodies may be inhaled, particularly by children, and include bones, peanuts, metallic and plastic objects. The right main bronchus pursues a more direct course and lodgement is usually on this side. Following inhalation, atelectasis and infection are common. Peanuts generally produce an acute inflammatory reaction at the site of impaction, making removal difficult.

Clinical features

Luminal obstruction produces a cough and wheezing whilst distal infection produces the symptoms and signs of atelectasis or suppuration. Chest radiography may reveal atelectasis with compensatory emphysema or demonstrate a radio-opaque foreign body.

Treatment

The foreign body should be removed at bronchoscopy, but if this fails, thoracotomy is indicated. Bronchotomy may be sufficient, but if the distal lung is destroyed, resection may be necessary. Antibiotics should be given where infection has occurred.

Bronchoscopy

Bronchoscopy may be performed using a rigid instrument, but only the main airways are seen and general anaesthesia is usually required. The fibreoptic bronchoscope is preferable as it can enter the second and third order bronchi, giving more distal information, and requires only local anaesthesia. The mucosa of the airways may be inspected directly and vocal cord movement noted. Narrowing or rigidity of the airways may be seen. Widening of the carina between the main bronchi provides strong circumstantial evidence of lymph node enlargement. The site of origin of haemoptysis may be identified. Abnormal appearing epithelium may be biopsied and secretions aspirated for bacteriological or cytological investigations. Transbronchial lung biopsy using a fibreoptic endoscope is now the procedure of choice to obtain specimens of lung tissue for pathological investigation.

Therapeutic aspiration of secretion or inhaled material may be a life-saving measure where severe hypoxia exists and where physiotherapy or tracheal suction has failed. Such patients are frequently unconscious or semi-conscious.

HEART

CONGENITAL HEART DISEASE

Between 0.5 and 1 per cent of babies born alive have a congenital cardiac anomaly. Several aetiological factors have been identified; others are strongly suspected. These include:

a) Maternal infections such as rubella, particularly in the first trimester of pregnancy.
b) Drugs in the first trimester.
c) Heredity and chromosomal abnormalities, as in Down's syndrome.
d) Maternal illnesses: diabetic mothers have a higher incidence of babies with transposition of the great arteries and ventricular septal defect.
e) Maternal age: very young and very old mothers appear to have a higher susceptibility.

In the majority of cases the cause is unknown. Although about a third present with dyspnoea due to cardiac failure or cyanosis, many are diagnosed on either routine medical examination or chest radiography. Over one hundred different types of congenital lesions have been described and many patients have more than one anomaly. Only eight are common and comprise 90 per cent of the total.

The commoner types of congenital heart lesions

Left to right shunts

1. Persistent ductus arteriosus
2. Atrial septal defect
3. Ventricular septal defect

Left ventricular outflow obstruction

1. Aortic stenosis
2. Coarctation of the aorta

Right ventricular outflow obstruction

Pulmonary valve stenosis

Cyanotic congenital heart disease

1. Fallot's tetralogy
2. Transposition of the great arteries

Clinical features

Some clinical features are common to most congenital lesions. Cardiac failure may occur at an early stage in infancy when urgent treatment is required. This is usually a feature of more severe or complex lesions. In many cases the extra burden on the heart is tolerated well for many years and the onset of cardiac failure may be delayed. Most cases of congenital heart disease are susceptible to subacute bacterial endocarditis, though this is rare in the case of atrial septal defect. Surgical treatment is available for most varieties of congenital anomaly, either in the form of palliation or total correction. The decision as to which treatment to adopt depends largely on the clinical condition at the time. An accurate anatomical diagnosis is essential before embarking on surgery and this generally involves cardiac catheterisation. Only the salient features of a typical case will be described in each instance.

Left to right shunts

As the pressure on the left side of the heart is higher than on the right side a shunt of oxygenated blood occurs from left to right. The chambers carrying this extra load enlarge and the blood flow through the lungs is considerably increased (pulmonary plethora) which can be seen as increased vascular markings on radiography. This damages the small vessels and the pulmonary vascular resistance may increase with the production of pulmonary hypertension which, if severe enough, leads to shunt reversal and central cyanosis.

Persistent ductus arteriosus

In-utero short-circuiting of blood from the pulmonary artery to the aorta occurs through the ductus as the lungs are not ventilated. Soon after birth this communication becomes obliterated with the formation of the ligamentum arteriosum in most instances, but in some the duct persists with consequent haemodynamic problems. The pressure in the aorta is higher than that in the pulmonary artery and thus the shunt is from left to right with increase in the pulmonary blood flow. Left ventricular strain and failure are generally late features but may occur in infancy.

Clinical features. In small babies where the shunt is large cardiac failure may result but in most children there are no symptoms. The physical signs are those of a machinery murmur best heard in the left second space associated with left ventricular enlargement. An electrocardiograph usually shows sinus rhythm often with evidence of left ventricular enlargement. Cardiac catheterisation confirms a left to right shunt at the level of the great arteries. The duct may be traversed by the catheter.

Treatment. Closure of the ductus either by ligation or by division and over-sewing the ends is indicated. This is occasionally necessary in small babies but is more often performed in childhood.

Atrial septal defect

Several varieties occur. The ostium secundum defect is situated in the middle of the septum. Ostium primum defects occur close to the mitral and tricuspid valves and may be associated with abnormalities of these. Sinus venosus defect occurs higher up close to the superior vena cava. Persistent foramen ovale is a common abnormality and a small defect lies in the middle of the septum. The pressure in the left atrium is higher than in the right, leading to shunting from left to right. Usually the larger the septal defect the larger the shunt. Atrial fibrillation and right heart failure occur late.

Clinical features. Most cases of atrial septal defect are asymptomatic until the patient gets older, when the association of atrial fibrillation and a low cardiac output leads to congestive cardiac failure. There is usually clinical evidence of right ventricular enlargement; an ejection systolic murmur caused by excessive flow through the pulmonary valve and a widely split second sound which does not move with respiration. An electrocardiograph initially shows sinus rhythm with later atrial fibrillation. Right axis deviation and right bundle branch block are common. Cardiac catheterisation confirms a shunt at atrial level. Primum defects may also show atrio-ventricular valve abnormalities. The septal defect should be closed and although this may be done directly, where distortion of the atrio-ventricular valves is likely a patch is necessary.

Ventricular septal defect

Ventricular septal defect is the commonest congenital cardiac anomaly, most of the defects being in the membranous septum just below the aortic valve. Some occur lower down and occasionally multiple defects are present. The shunt from left to right causes overloading of both ventricles. The volume of blood transferred usually depends on the size of the defect as does the consequent liability to develop pulmonary hypertension.

Clinical features. Typically there is a pansystolic murmur at the fourth left interspace with an associated thrill. Additional signs of biventricular enlargement may be evident on the electrocardiograph. Cardiac catheterisation confirms a shunt at ventricular level.

Treatment. Many small ventricular septal defects close spontaneously and do not require any therapy. Palliation by banding the pulmonary artery is sometimes indicated in infancy where the shunt is large and there is danger of flooding the pulmonary vasculature. Total correction should be carried out where the shunt is large and when there is a danger of endocarditis.

Left ventricular outflow obstruction

Aortic stenosis

This is due to a bicuspid aortic valve. Obstruction of the outflow of blood from the left ventricle may cause problems in infancy but is often well tolerated and signs of left ventricular dysfunction do not occur until later (p. 126). Left ventricular failure produces breathlessness. Poor coronary perfusion of an enlarged left ventricle causes ischaemic pain and poor cerebral perfusion causes syncope. Sudden death is not uncommon.

Clinical features. The peripheral pulse is characteristically of low volume. An ejection systolic murmur is best heard in the second right interspace associated with an ejection click. Initially the electrocardiograph is unchanged but later shows signs of left ventricular hypertrophy and strain. Cardiac catheterisation confirms a systolic gradient across the aortic valve. Often there is also mild regurgitation due to poor cusp approximation.

Treatment. In young patients valvotomy is the treatment of choice as there is usually no suitable prosthetic device for valve replacement. In older patients where the annulus is large enough valve replacement is advisable in symptomatic patients with evidence of ventricular strain.

Coarctation of the aorta

The commonest form of coarctation of the aorta is the adult type where the ductus arteriosus is obliterated (Fig. 10.6). Less frequently the duct remains open in the so-called infantile type. In the adult type hypertension occurs particularly proximal to the coarctation site. Cerebral vascular accidents of various forms, including subarachnoid haemorrhage from aneurysms, may occur as well as aortic rupture. Left ventricular failure is usually a late development. Perfusion of the lower half of the body is achieved through a collateral circulation involving the superior intercostal and internal mammary arteries and also the anastomosis around the scapula and chest wall. These link up with intercostal branches of the descending aorta and with the inferior epigastric branches of the femoral arteries. Uncommon associated abnormalities include an abnormal aortic valve and hypoplasia of the aorta.

Clinical features. Hypertension and any of its sequelae in a young patient should always raise the possibility of coarctation of the aorta. A systolic murmur may be heard over the front or back of the chest. Absent or delayed femoral pulsation is common. Cardiac failure is a late event except in infancy. There may be evidence of collateral vessels. Chest radiography shows rib notching due to pressure by the intercostal collaterals. The aortic arch outline frequently looks abnormal. An electrocardiograph may show signs of left ventricular hypertrophy and strain, whilst cardiac catheterisation and angiography will confirm the diagnosis.

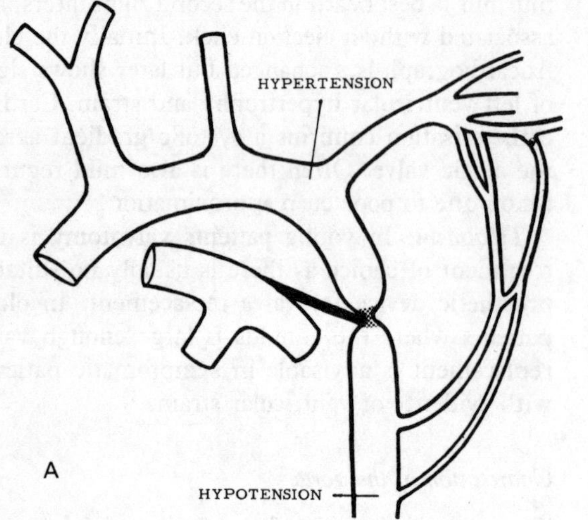

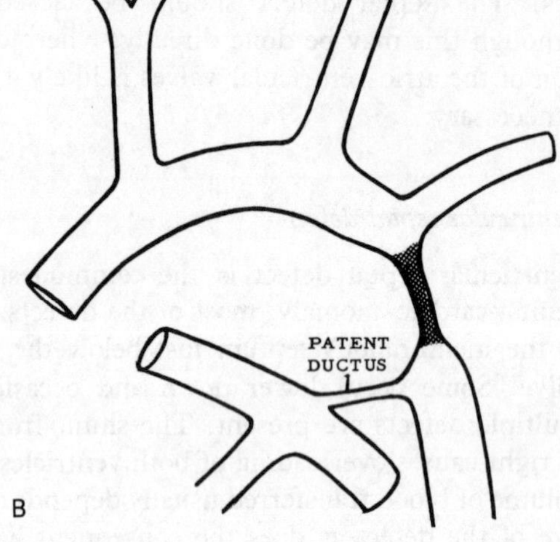

Fig. 10.6 Coarctation of aorta. **A.** Adult type. **B.** Infantile type.

Treatment. Relief of the obstruction is important. This may be achieved by resection of the coarctation with direct anastomosis or by a Dacron graft. Patch angioplasty is also being used as a more satisfactory procedure. Not all patients become normotensive following surgery and antihypertensive therapy may be necessary on a long-term basis.

Right ventricular outflow obstruction

Pulmonary valve stenosis

In this condition the valve is dome-shaped with a small orifice at its apex and the commissures are adherent to the walls of the pulmonary artery; a wide range of severity of stenosis occurs. A systolic gradient occurs across the valve with increased right ventricular pressure and right ventricular hypertrophy. Right atrial pressure and the jugular venous pressure may thus be raised.

Clinical features. Most patients are asymptomatic but on auscultation an ejection systolic murmur is audible in the second left interspace. Right ventricular enlargement may also be present. Right ventricular hypertrophy is seen on the electrocardiograph. Cardiac catheterisation confirms the pressure gradient across the pulmonary valve. Open pulmonary valvotomy will relieve the right ventricular outflow obstruction.

Cyanotic congenital heart disease

The two main causes of this condition are Fallot's tetralogy and transposition of the great arteries. The latter is the commonest cause of cyanotic heart disease but as most babies with this condition died within the first year of birth, it was wrongly assumed that Fallot's was the commonest cause. Both have many features in common. In the typical case the patient is frequently underdeveloped. Central cyanosis, digital clubbing and compensatory polycythaemia are evident and the patient is breathless and susceptible to syncopal attacks and sudden death.

Fallot's tetralogy

In this condition there are four abnormalities. Right ventricular outflow obstruction is due to valvular or infundibular obstruction or both. A ventricular septal defect is present. The aorta overrides the ventricular septal defect and right ventricular enlargement occurs. Desaturated blood crosses the septum into the systemic circulation, producing cyanosis. In addition infected material normally filtered out of the blood stream by the lungs may also cross the defect and cause a brain abscess. Polycythaemia may lead to the development of thrombosis.

Clinical features. An ejection systolic murmur is audible at the left sternal edge with a single second sound, in association with right ventricular enlargement. Cardiac catheterisation confirms a right to left shunt at ventricular level with systemic desaturation and right ventricular outflow obstruction.

Treatment. Palliation to increase pulmonary blood flow produces symptomatic improvement. This may be achieved by relief of the right ventricular outflow obstruction by dilating the pulmonary valve or a systemic-pulmonary shunt procedure will increase pulmonary blood flow. Anastomosis of the subclavian artery to the pulmonary artery is suitable in older children but where the vessels are very small it may better to anastomose the aorta directly to the pulmonary artery. Radical correction should be the main objective and is being increasingly carried out in small infants. Basically, two of the four anomalies are corrected during an open heart operation. The ventricular septal defect is closed with a patch and the right ventricular outflow obstruction is relieved either by valvotomy or resection of the infundibular muscle or by both.

Transposition of the great arteries

There are several varieties which come under this general heading and depend on the relationships of the atria, ventricles and great vessels. In the commonest form the atria and ventricles are normally related but the aorta comes off the right ventricle and is incompatible with life unless mixing of blood can occur, so that venous blood can reach the lungs and saturated blood the systemic circulation. This generally occurs at atrial or ventricular levels or both. Most patients die within two years of birth if the situation is uncorrected. The clinical features are those of a cyanotic baby with few abnormal physical signs in the cardiovascular system.

Treatment. Palliation can be achieved by enlarging the atrial septal defect using a balloon catheter. This often results in clinical improvement and allows definitive surgery to be postponed. Total correction of the physiological situation is achieved by an intra-atrial patch. This directs the systemic venous blood to the left ventricle and thus to the pulmonary artery and lungs, which then allows the pulmonary venous return to go to the right ventricle, the aorta and the systemic circulation.

VALVULAR HEART DISEASE

Valves may become stenotic or incompetent. The former is either due to congenital abnormalities or rheumatic involvement. Valve regurgitation may result from many pathological processes. The incidence of rheumatic heart disease is declining in the western world but it is still common in many countries. It is the sequel of acute rheumatic fever caused by an allergic response to a throat infection with β-haemolytic streptococcus group A type 12 (and rarely other types). Joint involvement also occurs but is less important. Pancarditis results with inflammation of the pericardium, myocardium and endocardium. It affects those valves subjected to greatest stress, which in order of frequency are the mitral, aortic and tricuspid valves: pulmonary valve involvement is rare. Often more than one valve is affected.

Mitral valve disease

Mitral stenosis

This is caused by fusion of the valve cusps over a period of several years resulting in an orifice measuring approximately 1 cm in diameter, which leads to the development of several haemodynamic changes. The pressure in the left atrium is raised and is transmitted to the lungs where it may exceed the osmotic pressure of the plasma proteins resulting in pulmonary oedema. The pressure in the atria and pulmonary capillaries is increased by exercise producing effort dyspnoea. The symptoms are accentuated in conditions associated with a raised cardiac output such as pregnancy or fluid retention. Increased pulmonary vascular resistance causes elevation of pressure in the pulmonary artery and eventually results in right heart failure and occasionally functional tricuspid regurgitation. Stagnation of blood in the left atrium, particularly when atrial fibrillation supervenes, causes thrombus formation usually in the left atrial appendage. The thrombus may remain within the left atrium but often it becomes detached, passes through the stenotic valve and forms an embolus. The effects of impaction include cerebral infarction, femoral artery occlusion and mesenteric obstruction. An abnormal valve is susceptible to bacterial endocarditis which may follow dental treatment or genito-urinary tract instrumentation without the cover of antibiotics. This infection further damages the valve, producing regurgitation. Deterioration in effort tolerance follows and the patient becomes bed-ridden, developing venous thromboses and pulmonary embolic episodes which may prove fatal. If untreated, most patients die in middle life.

Clinical features. Initially there is sinus rhythm but atrial fibrillation develops later which is usually associated with a decrease in cardiac output and clinical deterioration. Pulmonary oedema occurs relatively early whereas congestive cardiac failure is usually a late manifestation. The right ventricle may show signs of enlargement, the left ventricle remaining small. The typical auscultatory features, particularly when the valve is mobile are of a loud first heart sound due to closure and an opening snap. Flow of blood in diastole causes a rumbling diastolic murmur, which in the presence of sinus rhythm shows pre-systolic accentuation due to atrial contraction. The murmur is often localised to the apex of the heart. The clinical picture may be modified by embolic complications and sub-acute bacterial endocarditis. The electrocardiograph may show sinus rhythm with a P mitralae; atrial fibrillation later supervenes and there may be evidence of right heart strain.

Treatment. Mitral valvotomy is indicated where the valve condition is reasonable with non-calcified and mobile cusps. It may be performed by closed dilatation, either digitally or by using a dilator inserted through the apex of the left ventricle. This method has the advantage that it does not require open heart facilities, but the risk of dislodging an atrial clot into the systemic circulation exists. The degree of dilatation is difficult to control and the result may be under- or over-dilatation, which may be difficult to correct. An open operation on cardiac by-pass is preferable, the operation being carried out under direct vision. If the valve is not suitable for conservative treatment valve replacement is performed.

Mitral regurgitation

Rheumatic heart disease is the commonest cause of mitral regurgitation, but it may be due to valve destruction following endocarditis, ruptured chordae tendineae or ischaemic heart disease which may damage the mitral sub-valvular apparatus. Other causes are associated with redundant cusp tissue of obscure origin and occasionally collagen disease. The haemodynamic features are similar to those of mitral stenosis except that in systole some of the stroke volume of the left ventricle is ejected through the mitral valve. The left atrium is commonly larger with mitral regurgitation than with mitral stenosis. In patients with ruptured chordae the heart often remains in sinus rhythm. The clinical features are also similar in many aspects except that there is a pansystolic murmur at the apex which radiates to the axilla and sometimes into the back. The left ventricle shows signs of enlargement. Left ventricular angiography confirms ejection of blood into the left atrium in systole and the left atrium often shows a marked systolic 'V' wave. Occasionally it is possible to repair a regurgitant valve, particularly in the case of chordal rupture, but valve replacement is frequently necessary.

Aortic valve disease

Aortic stenosis

Rheumatic heart disease and congenital heart disease are the two main causes. The latter is discussed in the congenital section. It is common for a developmentally abnormal valve to be symptomless until middle or later life when it calcifies and produces calcific aortic stenosis. Often the valves are so abnormal that it is impossible to identify correctly the exact cause at operation. Stenosis at supravalvular or subvalvular level is much less common but produces a similar clinical picture.

Clinical features. The left ventricle hypertrophies to overcome the outflow obstruction. Eventually the left ventricle fails, causing elevation in left atrial and pulmonary venous pressures, producing pulmonary congestion and oedema. Decreased cardiac output causes poor visceral perfusion manifested in the brain by syncope and in the heart by angina. The classic symptomatic triad is shortness of breath, syncope and angina. The heart is generally in sinus rhythm with a small volume pulse. As the ventricle is hypertrophied ventricular enlargement is frequently not detectable but a basal thrill radiating to the neck is common.

Investigations. An electrocardiograph in well-established cases shows evidence of left ventricular hypertrophy and strain. Chest radiography usually shows a small heart; calcification of the aortic valve is common and is best seen on lateral views. Catheterisation reveals a small, thick-walled left ventricle with a systolic gradient of 50–100 mmHg or more across the aortic valve. When symptoms are present urgent treatment is required. Conservative valvotomy is rarely feasible, particularly in children, and in most cases aortic valve replacement is necessary.

Aortic regurgitation

This may be caused by dilatation of the aortic annulus from syphilis, Marfan's syndrome, dissecting aneurysm of the ascending aorta or by regurgitation from damaged cusps, due to rheumatic heart disease, endocarditis and rarely trauma. Some of the stroke volume is regurgitated into the left ventricle which becomes dilated. The pulse pressure is increased with rise in systolic pressure and fall in diastolic pressure. The symptoms are similar to those of aortic stenosis. Physical signs are those of left ventricular enlargement, water-hammer pulse and carotid pulsation in the neck. The auscultatory features are mainly those of a diastolic murmur heard at the base and along the left sternal edge. This increases with the severity of the regurgitation but disappears if extremely severe, associated with low cardiac output. A systolic murmur is often present due to the large stroke volume injected into the aorta. An electrocardiograph shows signs of left ventricular hypertrophy and strain. Catheterisation reveals regurgitation through the aortic valve, a large left ventricle and frequently a dilated aorta. Aortic regurgitation is initially well tolerated but cardiac enlargement leads to irreversible myocardial damage and valve replacement is advised.

Tricuspid valve disease

Tricuspid stenosis is generally a manifestation of chronic rheumatic heart disease. The right atrial pressure rises and is transmitted to the jugular venous pressure. Increased pressure in the inferior vena cava causes hepatomegaly, peripheral oedema and ascites. The condition is often associated with disease of other valves. Dyspnoea is not a marked feature as the lungs are 'protected'. A diastolic murmur similar to that heard in mitral stenosis is often heard at the left sternal edge. Investigation is difficult but stenosis may be diagnosed by demonstrating a pressure gradient across the valve in diastole. It is preferable to repair the valve rather than replace it but occasionally this is required.

Tricuspid regurgitation may be due to organic rheumatic disease. Many cases are 'functional' due to mitral valve disease and pulmonary hypertension causing right heart failure. The clinical features are similar to those of tricuspid stenosis but a marked systolic 'V' wave is seen in the jugular vein. Minor degrees of tricuspid valve disease are well tolerated, but if severe valve repair by reconstruction of the annulus is preferable to valve replacement.

ARTIFICIAL VALVES

The replacement of diseased valves may be achieved by the use of mechanical prostheses or by biological tissue. Consideration of several factors is required before determining which valve is more appropriate to each individual case.

Mechanical valves. These are constructed partly of a rigid frame and central occluder with a fabric sewing ring. In the cage variety the occluder is either a metal or plastic ball, while in the low profile variety the occluder is a disc. These valves are durable and haemodynamically adequate. Their main disadvantage is that all have a tendency to cause thromboembolism, which is decreased but not abolished by anticoagulants or by agents affecting the stickiness of platelets.

Tissue valves. These are homografts from cadavers or heterografts from animals. They may be inserted 'free' or sewn on to a semi-rigid frame. The advantages include good central flow haemodynamics and usually freedom from the complication of thromboembolism, making anticoagulation unnecessary, but their long-term durability is doubtful and gradual failure may necessitate further replacement.

Tissue valves are preferable where there is any contra-indication to anticoagulation, such as peptic ulceration, bleeding diatheses, pregnancy or failure to comply with regular drug therapy. The elderly, unlikely to live longer than the estimated valve durability, would probably be better managed with a tissue valve.

ISCHAEMIC HEART DISEASE

This is the cause of about one quarter of the annual mortality in Western countries and in the United Kingdom 130 000 people die per annum from ischaemic heart disease.

Two coronary arteries arise from the aorta above the aortic valve. The right, arising from the right coronary sinus, appears anteriorly, descends in the interventricular groove giving off branches along its course, then continues along the diaphragmatic aspect of the heart. The left coronary artery arises posteriorly from the left coronary sinus, runs to the left behind the pulmonary artery and then appears anterior to the left atrial appendage. It there divides into two main branches, the anterior descending coronary artery which descends along the anterior interventricular septum, and the circumflex coronary artery, which proceeds around the back of the heart giving off branches. Atheroma occurs in a patchy manner most frequently in a proximal distribution and sparing the distal parts of the vessel to a large extent. Complete occlusion of a coronary artery generally leads to myocardial infarction and either death or the development of a scar.

Clinical features. The symptoms of angina pectoris are those of central chest pain radiating to the arms, neck, back and epigastrium, provoked by exercise and emotion and relieved by rest and sublingual glyceryl trinitrate. Occasionally the symptoms increase in frequency and severity compared with the normal pattern—without evidence of actual infarction—and then the condition is called 'unstable' or 'pre-infarction' angina.

Investigations. Electrocardiography is of much value but the most important investigation is left ventriculography and coronary arteriography by means of a cardiac catheter. This gives information as to the contractility of the ventricle and the exact distribution of the coronary arterial disease, both factors having an important bearing on prognosis. Increasing use is now being made of nuclear angiography which provides similar data for the ventricle without the need for cardiac catheterisation. Blood flow in the coronary arteries becomes significantly impaired when the lumen is reduced by three-quarters of its normal diameter.

Treatment. Surgery has a fairly well-defined place in the treatment of such conditions through a) re-vascularisation operations designed to improve the myocardial blood flow and b) operations designed to treat the complications of myocardial infarction.

Chronic stable angina pectoris which does not respond to medical therapy provides the main indication for *re-vascularisation*. Unstable angina, where there is a strong likelihood that infarction may occur, provides another indication but is more controversial. Attempts to treat acute infarction by re-vascularisation are largely unsatisfactory. In general, the less the extent of established myocardial damage prior to surgery the more favourable the outlook. The operation involves placing a saphenous vein graft from the side of the ascending aorta to the side of the coronary artery distal to a significant stenosis or occlusion (Fig. 10.7). Implantation of the internal mammary artery provides an alternative method; it is already conditioned to the systemic blood pressure and obviates the need for a proximal anastomosis, but multiple distal anastomoses cannot be achieved. In the case of a very diseased coronary artery, endarterectomy over several centimetres can be carried out and the

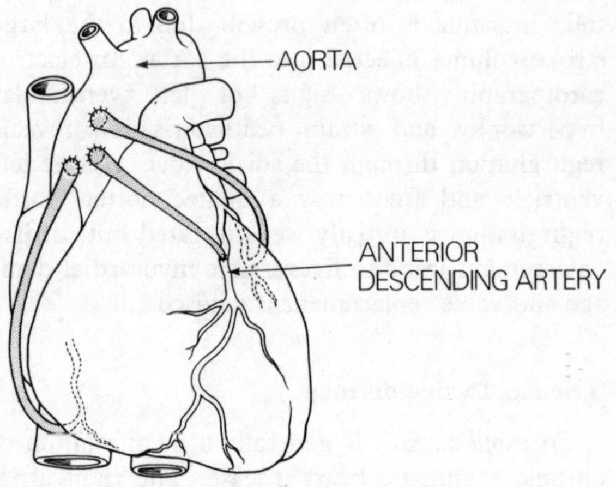

Fig. 10.7 Anastomosis of saphenous vein grafts from the ascending aorta to the distal right and circumflex coronary arteries (behind heart) and to the anterior descending artery

vein graft anastomosed to the arteriotomy. The revascularisation operation is performed during cardiopulmonary by-pass with a resting heart to facilitate careful surgery. The operative mortality is 1–2 per cent and depends mainly on ventricular function or the presence of associated cardiac defects which need treatment. Following vein by-pass surgery there is over 80 per cent relief of pain or marked improvement and good correlation exists with the graft patency. Initially this is 85–90 per cent but a steady attrition rate leads to about a third of the grafts being occluded within a year or two. Grafts patent at this stage tend to remain open subsequently. Life expectancy following coronary artery surgery may be increased but final analysis awaits the results of long-term trials. There is good evidence that patients with left main coronary artery stenosis survive longer after surgery than with medical treatment and this may also be true of multiple vessel disease.

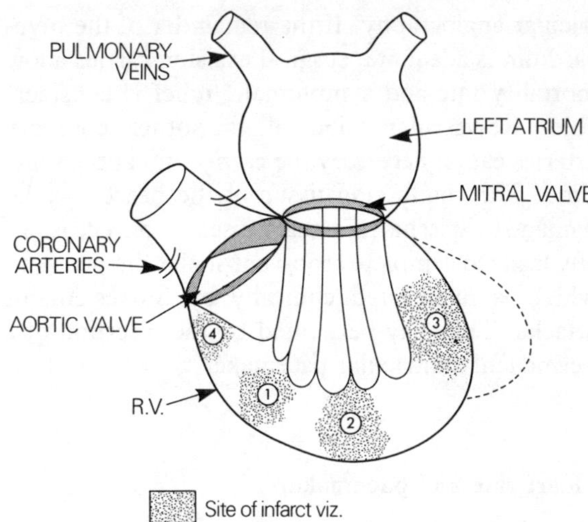

Fig. 10.8 The effect of myocardial infarction on left ventricle and relations (1 = Septal, causing ventricular septal defect; 2 = Papillary muscle, causing mitral dysfunction; 3 = Full thickness anterior wall, causing aneurysm; 4 = Septal, causing conduction defects)

Complications of myocardial infarction

Infarction of certain parts of the left ventricle usually adds a further serious haemodynamic burden (Fig. 10.8). Necrosis of the inter-ventricular septum may cause a ventricular septal defect with a left to right shunt. Damage to the papillary muscles may lead to rupture or mitral sub-valve dysfunction causing mitral regurgitation. A full-thickness infarct of the free wall of the left ventricle produces an aneurysm. Damage to the ventricular conduction pathways may cause complete heart block.

Ventricular septal defect and *mitral regurgitation* have a similar presentation and complicate about 2 per cent of infarcts. The onset is often 7–10 days after the initial infarct due to muscle necrosis and is accompanied by sudden clinical deterioration and signs of low cardiac output. Auscultation reveals a pansystolic murmur. The conditions are difficult to differentiate clinically and may even co-exist. The diagnosis may only be established by cardiac catheterisation and angiography, when radio-opaque medium injected into the left ventricle passes into either the left atrium or the right ventricle in mitral regurgitation or ventricular septal defect respectively. If untreated, the prognosis is grave. Mitral regurgitation requires prompt valve replacement if regurgitation is severe. Ventricular septal defect is more difficult to treat in the early stage because of the difficulties of suturing friable tissue. Preferably surgery is postponed by supporting the circulation by medical means and counter-pulsation by intra-aortic balloon pumping, until sutures can be placed in well-healed fibrous tissue.

Ventricular aneurysms

Full-thickness infarction of the left ventricular wall usually leads to adherence of the pericardium and clot formation within the ventricle. Rupture of a ventricular aneurysm is rare. Death usually occurs from ventricular failure and pulmonary oedema or from a systemic embolus from the ventricular clot. Occasionally death is caused by dysrhythmia.

Clinical features. Typically a left ventricular aneurysm takes several weeks to form following myocardial infarction. Increasing dyspnoea some time after a myocardial infarction should suggest the possibility of a left ventricular aneurysm. An electrocardiograph often shows persistent ST elevation, whilst the cardiac outline on chest radiographs does not generally correspond to the classical 'boot-shaped' image, but is more likely to show generalised cardiomegaly. The diagnosis can be made by cardiac catheterisation and left ventricular angiography. If the remainder of the myocardium is adequate, surgical excision carries a low mortality rate and symptomatic relief is considerable. Re-vascularisation of the other coronary arteries can, if necessary, be carried out at the same time. The conduction tissue of the heart may be damaged by ischaemic heart disease and occasionally leads to complete atrio-ventricular dissociation, which is manifested clinically by Stokes-Adams attacks. This may be treated by the insertion of a permanent ventricular pacemaker.

Heart-rate and pacemakers

The atrioventricular bundle carries impulses from the atria to the ventricles and synchronises the action of the four chambers. The bundle may not function due to congenital deformity, surgical repair of congenital heart disease, cardiac infarction or idiopathic fibrosis. Complete heart block may result when the ventricle contracts at the idioventricular rate of 25 to 45 beats a minute. This change of rhythm is often associated with fainting due to periods of asystole—Stokes-Adams attacks.

A normal cardiac rate can be achieved by using electrical stimulation. Direct stimulation of the heart can be carried out by the passage of an electrode into the ventricle through an upper limb vein. This method is particularly useful as initial treatment before the implanting of an internal pacemaker. The disadvantages include sepsis, penetration of the ventricle and the lack of an independent existence.

Prolonged pacemaking with freedom of movement is best achieved by using an internal pacemaker. The lead may be attached to the surface of the heart (epicardial pacing) or to the inside of the heart (endocardial pacing). The latter is more frequently used. The electric impulse is supplied by a battery buried in a suitable site and this requires to be changed at intervals. When the heart block is complete and permanent the pacemaker is required to work at a fixed rate, but when there are periods of normal rhythm it is preferable to use a type of pacemaker which supplies impulses 'on demand' with periods of inactivity during normal rhythm.

PERICARDIAL DISEASE

Pericardial effusion

This may be a transudate, with low specific gravity and protein content, related to cardiac failure or low protein states. Alternatively exudates occur with higher protein content and a high specific gravity. They can follow infections, infarction or malignant disease. A large effusion may compress the heart and prevent filling in diastole. There is systemic venous congestion with raised jugular pressure, hepatomegaly, ascites, ankle oedema and a low cardiac output. Chest radiography reveals an enlarged cardiac silhouette whilst echocardiography confirms the site. The cause may be obvious but occasionally aspiration of fluid is necessary for biochemical, bacteriological and cytological analysis. Treatment is often unnecessary but repeated aspiration of fluid or formation of a pericardial opening (fenestration) may be required, allowing excess fluid to drain into the pleural space.

Tamponade

This may follow open or closed thoracic injuries from knife or bullet wounds or blunt trauma, or it may follow cardiac surgery. Failure of the heart to fill in diastole leads to a rapidly falling cardiac output, manifested by its effect on various organs and viscera. The skin is cold, pale and clammy. Poor brain perfusion produces confusion and eventually coma. Inadequate renal perfusion leads to dysuria and anuria. Compensatory haemodynamic responses include tachycardia and hypotension, which is a late sign. The jugular venous or central venous pressure is raised. Urgent relief of pressure is essential. While pericardial aspiration may be occasionally helpful, thoracotomy and pericardial incision is required at an early stage, followed by measures to control the source of haemorrhage.

Chronic constrictive pericarditis

Tuberculosis is the main cause of this condition. Collagen diseases also produce constriction occasionally as do the sequelae of acute infections. It is often difficult to determine the original cause at surgery years later. The pericardium thickens, often grossly compressing the heart, particularly near the great veins and the atrio-ventricular grooves. Calcification commonly occurs later. The haemodynamics consist of a lowered cardiac output caused by failure of the heart to fill and evidence of peripheral venous congestion, with elevated jugular venous pressure, hepatomegaly, ascites and peripheral oedema. Persistent sinus tachycardia or atrial fibrillation are common. Electrocardiography shows low voltages and may confirm atrial fibrillation. Chest radiography demonstrates a small heart; calcification in the pericardium is best seen on oblique views. The main clinical differentiation is a form of cardiomyopathy, where muscle damage alters compliance and produces a similar clinical picture. Rarely an exploratory operation is required to distinguish them. Removal of the diseased pericardium is the only effective treatment.

FURTHER READING

Collis, J. L., Clarke, D. B. and Abbey Smith, R. (1976). In D'Abreu's *Practice of Cardiothoracic Surgery*. 4th ed. London: Arnold.

Holden, M. P. (1982). *A Practice of Cardiothoracic Surgery*. Bristol: Wright.

11

Breast

Anatomy

The main anatomical features are concerned with the lobular arrangement, the attachments and the lymphatic drainage. The disposition of 16 to 20 lobules, each with a lactiferous duct terminating at the nipple, is important, because certain affections may remain confined to one segment. Incisions in the breast should preferably be placed in a radial direction from the nipple, thereby lessening the risk of damage to a lactiferous duct. The presence of the axillary prolongation should be remembered because tumours of this part of the breast can be confused with axillary lymph nodes. The perilobular fibrous tissue of the breast is attached to the skin by several fibrous strands. Irregular pitting of the skin, termed *peau d'orange*, may result either from oedema of the skin between these attachments or by their invasion with carcinoma. The gland is only loosely attached to the pectoral fascia, and increased fixity, demonstrated by elevation of the arm, should arouse the suspicion of cancer.

The breast has a profuse arterial supply from the lateral thoracic branch of the axillary artery and from the perforating branches of the intercostal vessels and internal mammary artery. The lymphatics, which surround the lobules of the breast, drain through its substance principally to the lateral thoracic group of lymph nodes, which pass from axillary tail to the apex of axilla (Fig. 11.1); some communication exists with the subscapular group of nodes. The main lymphatics accompany the major blood-vessels, namely the lateral thoracic artery to the axilla, the intercostal arteries to the internal mammary lymph chain, extending from the second to the fifth intercostal space, and the acromiothoracic artery to the infraclavicular region. The supraclavicular lymph nodes receive lymphatics which pass behind the clavicle from the apex of the axilla. Communication with lymphatics of the contralateral breast and axilla is not significant in the normal subject.

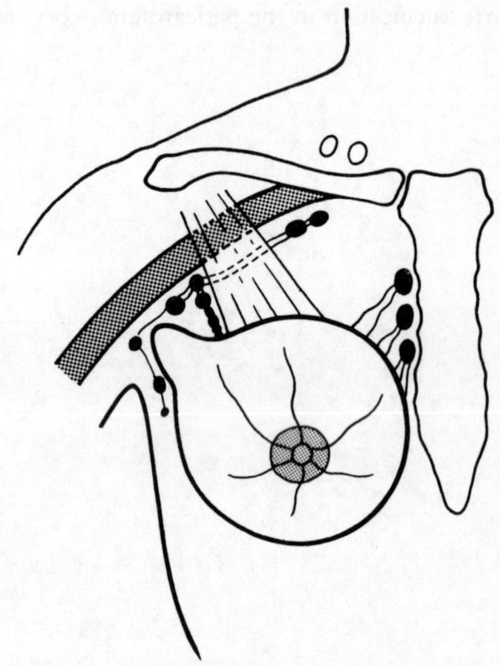

Fig. 11.1 The principal lymphatic drainage of the breast through the lateral pectoral lymphatics to axillary nodes and medially to internal mammary nodes

Functional abnormalities

Swelling of the infant breast after delivery is not uncommon. It occurs in response to hormones secreted in the maternal milk and usually subsides rapidly.

Enlargement of the male breast at puberty is commonly encountered, but only in rare instances is it a sign of an adrenal or testicular endocrine tumour, when it may be accompanied by a rise in the urinary 17-ketosteroids and oestrogen excretion. Excessive hypertrophy of the female breast warrants plastic reconstruction in some instances.

Fibro-adenosis is probably the result of alterations in hormonal control of breast function.

INFECTION

Acute mastitis and abscess

Acute mastitis occurs most commonly during lactation, when it results from infection of stagnant milk in the lactiferous ducts. The staphylococcus is usually the causative organism, but occasionally the streptococcus may be responsible. The portal of entry is either through an abrasion or crack in the nipple or through a main milk duct. The condition is particularly common after hospital confinement, when the infecting organism is often resistant to the majority of antibiotics. Retromammary abscess may be pyogenic, but is usually tuberculous, and arises from a rib or intercostal lymph node.

Clinical features

The infection generally occurs in the first few weeks of lactation. One segment of the breast becomes hard and tender, the overlying skin is reddened and oedema develops as inflammation proceeds. Extension into other segments of the breast may follow. Pus formation may occur after an interval of three or four days, but with early treatment resolution is frequently obtained. The general features of an acute inflammatory process are usually in evidence.

Treatment

Prophylaxis is important. Cleanliness and the early treatment of cracked skin of the nipple must be emphasised to every nursing mother. Massage of the nipple with bland creams and the application of gentian violet to broken skin are simple remedies. Accumulation of milk should not be allowed, and manual expression from the hard areas, though painful, is beneficial. Breast-feeding is permitted, but should be discontinued with the formation of pus. Antibiotic therapy should be commenced at an early stage. Penicillin or a broad spectrum antibiotic should be given for at least five days.

Pus formation, indicated by the presence of a localised, tender and red area, necessitates incision and drainage. Fluctuation may not be apparent in some cases of deep-seated abscess, and delay of incision until this sign develops may result in infection breaking into adjacent lobules, leading to unnecessary destruction of breast tissue. Wide incision and breakdown of loculi are essential for the neglected case with a large abscess. Identification of the organism and its antibiotic sensitivity facilitates appropriate therapy.

Chronic breast abscess is important as it may cause confusion with carcinoma. It may develop initially during lactation or result from infection of a haematoma. The swelling is often painless and hard, though softening may be detected in the centre. Attachment to the skin and the development of peau d'orange are common. Enlarged axillary lymph nodes may be present. Surgical exploration is often necessary to establish the diagnosis. Shortwave diathermy is useful in accelerating resolution.

FIBRO-ADENOSIS

This disease has received many confusing names, such as chronic mastitis, epithelial hyperplasia and cystic disease of the breast. The cause is unknown, but fluctuation of hormonal stimulation, in particular with excess of oestrogen, undoubtedly plays a part. It certainly does not have an infective origin.

Pathology

Three principal changes are present; interstitial fibrosis, cyst formation and epithelial hyperplasia (Fig. 11.2, A). The affected area of breast has ill-defined boundaries, is rubbery in consistency and is of grey colour. It contains bluish cysts, varying in size from 1 mm to 2 cm in diameter, the contents usually being clear fluid, but they may be creamy. Papillary proliferations may occur within

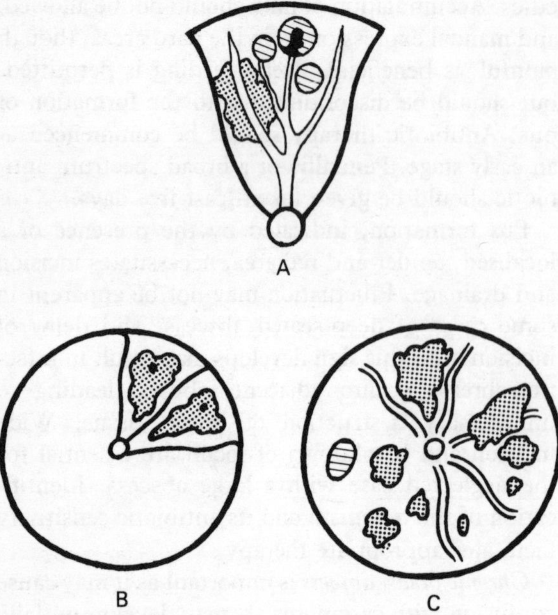

Fig. 11.2 Fibro-adenosis of the breast. **A**. The pathological changes consist of fibrosis, cyst formation and intracystic proliferation affecting (**B**) one or two breast segments or (**C**) the whole breast.

the cyst. Histological examination shows dense fibrosis surrounding the acini, enlargement and tortuosity of the ducts and desquamation of duct epithelium. Lymphocytic infiltration may be seen.

Clinical features

Fibro-adenosis is a common condition in the female between the ages of 20 and 45 years. The principal symptom is dull, aching pain in the breast, often worse prior to the menstrual period and more severe in the young patient. One or both breasts may be affected and the presence of a swelling may be noticed. Inspection rarely shows any abnormality, though a large cyst may be visible. A diffuse granularity is palpable in the younger patient, the nodules being up to 5 mm in diameter and tender. Larger swellings are present in the older patient, and one segment or the whole breast may be involved with ill-defined masses of rubbery consistency (Fig. 11.2, B and C). Attachment to the skin or deep fascia does not occur. A discrete swelling indicates the presence of a cyst, but although fluctuation is difficult to elicit, transillumination may be feasible. The axillary lymph nodes may be palpably enlarged, but this is not common.

The course of the condition is variable, frequent remissions being common, and pregnancy may bring relief. The relationship to carcinoma is variously expressed, statistical evidence in some cases indicating a slightly increased incidence when fibro-adenosis pre-exists. The histological appearance of intraduct papillary projections has also been considered precancerous, but bilateral local mastectomy is not justified as a means of cancer prevention.

Differential diagnosis mainly concerns fibroadenoma and carcinoma. The former is characterised by a mobile, clearly defined swelling, the surrounding breast often being normal. The distinction from carcinoma may be clinically difficult. The malignant mass is harder and readily palpable with the flat of the fingers; fibro-adenosis is more easily felt with the finger tips. Skin or deep fascial attachment and nipple retraction are indicative of carcinoma. The presence of hard lymph nodes suggests neoplasia. Mammography is helpful in diagnosis but must not be relied on absolutely (p. 138).

Treatment

Reassurance of the younger patient is important. The wearing of a well-fitting brassiere is beneficial, and by support gives relief in many cases. Hormonal therapy with the synthetic androgen danazol or the prolactin inhibitor bromocriptine is effective in relieving pain and swelling and is indicated when symptoms are severe. The presence of a cyst can be confirmed by needle aspiration and after complete evacuation of the cyst it rarely recurs. Cytological examination of the fluid may be undertaken to exclude malignancy and it is necessary to examine the patient three weeks later to confirm that the swelling has not recurred. The presence of a solid swelling requires excision or biopsy for accurate histological diagnosis and this procedure removes a source of worry and relieves symptoms. Total mastectomy is to be preferred in the older patient when the whole of the breast is involved by widespread fibro-adenosis with multiple cyst formation.

Serocystic disease of Brodie

This occurs in middle-aged women, who present with a large multicystic swelling of the breast. It is slowly growing and often becomes 25 to 30 cm diameter, the cysts being 5 to 8 cm across. Intracystic papillary growths occur and carcinomatous change can follow, though more commonly sarcomatous degeneration of fibrous tissue takes place. Local excision of the breast is required, skin graft replacement often being necessary.

Galactocele

Galactocele is an uncommon type of breast cyst. It develops during or after lactation as a result of the blockage of a lactiferous duct. The contents are at first fluid, but later become inspissated. It presents as a smooth swelling near the nipple. Excision is required if the mass persists.

TUMOURS

The common benign tumours are fibro-adenoma and duct papilloma, a lipoma being rare. Carcinoma is the important malignant tumour, sarcoma being unusual.

Fibro-adenoma

Two types of fibro-adenoma occur.

Pericanalicular fibro-adenoma is encountered most commonly between 20 and 30 years. The tumour is small, firm and well encapsulated, the cut surface bulging, of grey-white colour and whorled appearance. Histological examination shows proliferation of fibrous tissue with round or oval acini lined by cubical epithelium. The condition appears as a symptom-free slowly growing swelling, usually oval in shape and seldom more than 2 cm in length. It is firm in consistency, not tender, and characteristically is freely mobile. Multiple tumours are uncommon. Treatment consists of removal of the mass through a small radial or submammary incision. Recurrence is infrequent.

Intracanalicular fibro-adenoma arises between the years 30 and 50. It forms a soft or partly cystic tumour, often 5 to 10 cm in diameter. Histological appearance is of slit-like spaces between masses of connective tissue. Sarcomatous change may take place. The swelling usually grows rapidly and is generally mobile. Occasionally it becomes adherent to the skin as a consequence of impending necrosis due to pressure. Simple excision will usually suffice, though the suspicion of neoplastic change requires frozen-section histology, the result of which may be an indication for removal of the breast.

Duct papilloma

The tumour is situated in the ampullary dilatation of a lactiferous duct and varies in size from about 1 to 5 mm in length. It has a typical papilliferous structure surrounding a central stalk. Histological examination shows columnar cells which at times have a glandular arrangement. Malignant change may occur.

Bleeding from the nipple is the principal symp-

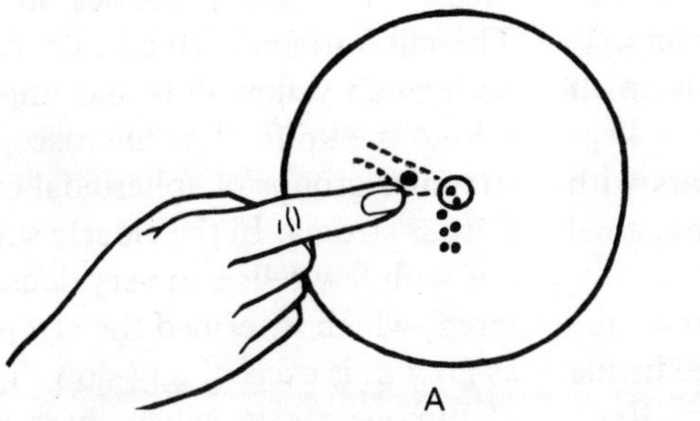

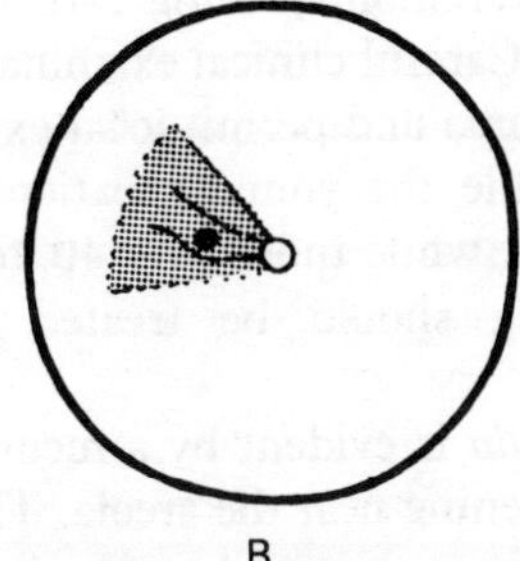

Fig. 11.3 Duct papilloma of the breast. **A.** Pressure on the lactiferous duct containing the papilloma results in bleeding from the nipple. **B.** Excision of the affected breast segment is performed.

tom, which occurs sporadically and is usually of small amount. A palpable tumour is seldom present, but pressure applied systematically at intervals around the areola often promotes a blood-stained discharge from the nipple (Fig. 11.3). Localisation by this method permits excision of the affected segment of breast. Total mastectomy may be required for the recurrent case because of the tendency to malignant change.

Traumatic fat necrosis

Traumatic fat necrosis is a benign condition often confused with tumour. It results from a severe blow on a fatty breast. The injury leads to direct damage of the fat lobules and also produces haemorrhage. Lymphocytic and giant-cell infiltration occurs, small cystic collections of fat form and subsequently considerable fibrosis develops.

The clinical resemblance to carcinoma often makes the diagnosis difficult; the mass is hard and skin attachment is common. The history of injury followed by bruising of the skin may serve to make a differentiation, but doubt will only be resolved by excision and histological examination.

Nipple discharge

The occurrence of a clear or whitish-green discharge from the nipple is often associated with fibro-adenosis; it varies in amount and duration and is of no great significance.

Blood-stained discharge or frank bleeding is a sign of considerable importance and should not be neglected. It occurs most commonly with duct papilloma and duct carcinoma, being rare in a scirrhous carcinoma. Careful clinical examination may localise the papilloma and permit local excision. If no mass is palpable the younger patient is kept under observation, while those over 40 years with recurrent bleeding should be treated by total mastectomy.

Mammillary fistula is evident by a recurrent discharge from an opening near the areola. The fistula communicates with an enlarged major duct. Excision of the affected part of the areola and lactiferous duct is necessary to effect a cure.

CARCINOMA

Carcinoma of the breast is the most common malignant tumour in women, occurring slightly more frequently than carcinoma of the uterus.

Aetiology

Experimental work in mice, whilst having no direct relationship to the human, suggests that a special factor is present in the milk of certain strains which are highly susceptible to breast cancer. Large dosage of oestrogen also stimulates a cancerous growth in some strains. In the human it is probable that the hormonal changes of pregnancy and lactation lessen the risk of the development of cancer, it being clearly established that nulliparous women have a higher incidence of the disease. The rate of occurrence in Japan is extremely low, a fact which is thought to be explained by the custom of prolonging lactation for several years. There is a definite alteration with the hormonal changes of the menopause as the incidence is greatest in the fifth decade, then declines slightly and is followed by a further increase up to the age of 60 years. The relationship to fibro-adenosis has been discussed on page 134.

Pathology

Two principal varieties occur. Spheroidal-cell carcinoma with fibrous stroma (scirrhous) and the papillary (duct) carcinoma. The former is more common and more invasive.

Scirrhous carcinoma varies considerably in size from a half to several centimetres; it infiltrates breast tissue and possesses an ill-defined margin. The cut surface is rough, concave, grey in colour with small yellow dots and imparts a gritty sensation to the knife. The microscopic appearance is of irregular groups of spheroidal cells in an abundant fibrous stroma. In the elderly subject a type of tumour with few cells and very dense stroma is encountered, which is termed the atrophic scirrhous type, as growth is exceedingly slow. The *encephaloid* type of tumour results when there is little stroma and many cells. The resulting tumour is soft and fleshy and usually rapidly growing. *Duct carcinoma* produces less stroma than the scirrhous variety, resulting in a softer tumour with areas of necrosis, the edge being well defined. It is characterised by a papillary structure of cells and little stroma. Mucoid change is seen in a small proportion of all types of tumour.

Spread

This may be by direct invasion, by lymphatics or by the bloodstream (Fig. 11.4). *Direct* invasion will involve surrounding breast, skin or chest wall. *Lymphatic* spread is important and occurs through the perilobular lymphatics to the axilla or anterior mediastinum. The axillary nodes are affected most commonly, though involvement of the internal mammary nodes occurs most frequently with medially situated tumours, but can also occur with those in the outer quadrants. Spread to the supraclavicular nodes is a late development. *Haematogenous spread* may result in deposits in distant sites, though these may also occur by lymphatic permeation. The lungs and pleura are principally affected, followed by the skeleton, liver and brain. Skeletal metastasis occurs mainly in the spine, pelvis, femur, ribs and skull.

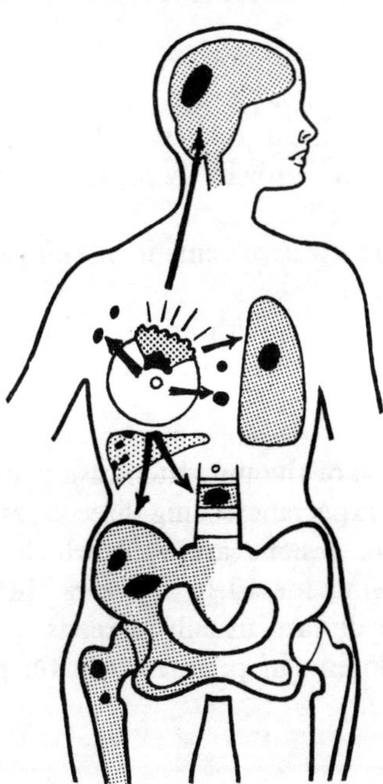

Fig. 11.4 Spread of carcinoma of the breast occurs locally and to regional lymph nodes, bones, lungs, liver and brain

Hormone dependency

The results of surgical extirpation of the ovary, adrenal cortex and hypophysis suggest that certain types of breast carcinoma are dependent on hormones for their development (Fig. 11.5). Growth hormone and prolactin from the pituitary, ovarian oestrogen and progesterone and adrenal corticosteroids are concerned in the full development of a normal breast. It is thought that these hormones play some part in the control of breast carcinoma, though their deprivation will lead to regression of tumour growth in only about 50 per cent of cases.

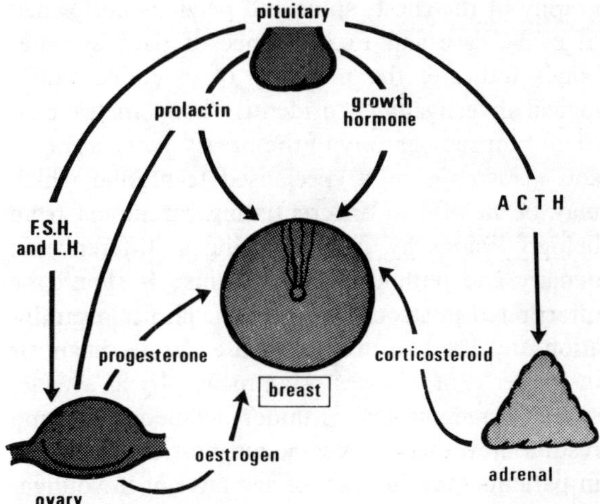

Fig. 11.5 Breast carcinoma is under hormonal control from the pituitary, adrenal and ovary

Clinical features

The history is frequently one of accidental discovery of a lump in the breast. Pain is often present but is not a prominent feature. Blood-stained nipple discharge and evidence of skin involvement may be first noted. Secondary deposits may occasionally be responsible for the initial symptoms, which may include pain in the back, paraplegia, bladder dysfunction, dyspnoea, headache and vomiting or a pathological fracture.

The lesion occurs most commonly in the outer

and upper quadrant of the breast. Slight puckering of the skin may be observed and is accentuated by elevation of the arm, whilst nipple retraction and alteration in contour or level of the breast become evident at a later stage. Extensive involvement of skin by multiple nodules or a continuous layer of cancerous tissue with resulting ulceration indicates advanced disease. A *hard* mass is evident on palpation and is the *earliest sign* of breast carcinoma. The margins are indefinite and irregular and firm pressure may cause pain. Attachment to skin or pectoral fascia should be determined. Axillary and supraclavicular lymph node enlargement may be present and any fixity is noted. Occasionally the opposite breast may be involved. More distant dissemination may be demonstrated by the finding of a pleural effusion, hepatomegaly or ascites. Radiography of the chest, spine and pelvis is performed in every case and the presence of pain in other bones indicates the necessity of extended radiological investigations to identify bony metastases. Plain film radiography of the breast (*mammography* and *xerography*) is a specialised technique which may be helpful in differentiating carcinoma from benign lesions by demonstrating a difference in density and outline of the swelling. It should be interpreted in association with the clinical examination and the two may give an accurate diagnosis in 97 per cent of cases. Mammography as a widespread screening test is under detailed study and results show that it has some diagnostic significance in patients over 50 years of age but not in younger age groups.

Clinical staging of breast carcinoma

Accurate description and the recording of clinical findings are important, the T.N.M. classification being recommended (p. 436). Difficulty arises in correct pre-operative assessment of axillary node involvement and it may not be feasible to distinguish between N0 and N1 in certain cases. The following clinical staging is still in use and therefore described.

Stage 1

The primary tumour is freely movable on the pectoral muscle. Skin involvement, including ulceration, may be present, but such involvement must be in direct continuity with the tumour and there must not be any extension into the skin wide of the tumour itself.

Stage 2

As Stage 1, but there are palpable mobile lymph nodes in the axilla of the same side.

Stage 3

The primary growth is more extensive than Stage 1 as shown by:

(*a*) The skin invaded or fixed over an area wide of the tumour itself, but still limited to the breast.
(*b*) The tumour fixed to underlying muscle but not to chest wall. Axillary lymph nodes may or may not be palpable, but if lymph nodes are present, they must be mobile.

Stage 4

The growth has extended beyond the breast area, as shown by:

(*a*) Fixation of axillary lymph nodes
(*b*) Tumour fixed to chest wall
(*c*) Secondary growth in supraclavicular lymph nodes
(*d*) Secondary involvement in skin wide of the breast
(e) Secondary growth in the opposite breast
(*f*) Distant metastases, such as bone, liver, lung.

The course of the untreated case is variable, the average life expectancy being three years, but in the older patient lesions are seen which have been slowly growing for 10 to 15 years. In the young woman the disease usually spreads quickly, and when developing in pregnancy has a particularly rapid course.

Differential diagnosis

This most frequently includes fibro-adenosis (p. 133) and fibro-adenoma (p. 135). The former has a softer consistency and is often widespread in the breast, while the latter is characteristically well defined and mobile. It is to be emphasised that the presence of a hard lump palpable with the flat of the hand is highly suspicious of carcinoma. Other conditions to be considered are chronic breast abscess and galactocele, which may be related to pregnancy, and fat necrosis where there is a history of trauma.

Treatment

Early diagnosis is of prime importance and education of the public with emphasis on medical consultation at the first suspicion of a breast lump should be a feature of preventive medicine. The discovery of a doubtful swelling in the breast should be followed by early removal to establish the exact diagnosis. Excision should be complete and include surrounding normal breast tissue. Inspection and palpation of the gross specimen is usually diagnostic, but frozen section histology should be performed for confirmation. Alternatively a needle or trucut biopsy can be undertaken and following bone scanning the management can be planned prior to admission.

The extent of the disease influences the form of therapy and may be varied to suit individual circumstances. Considerable research and discussion is being undertaken to evaluate the best form of treatment for the early case and widely divergent views are held. The more commonly accepted forms of therapy are summarised as follows.

Stage 1

Total mastectomy, *or*
Total mastectomy plus irradiation of lymph node area, *or*
Radical mastectomy *or* modified radical mastectomy.

Stage 2

Total mastectomy plus irradiation of lymph node areas, *or*
Radical mastectomy *or* modified radical mastectomy.

Stage 3

Irradiation of breast and lymph node area.

Stage 4

Irradiation of breast, lymph node area and solitary metastases, *or* irradiation of breast plus hormonal therapy, *or* hormonal therapy alone.
Quadruple chemotherapy.

Total mastectomy removes the tumour intact and also any other areas of malignant or premalignant change in the breast. Local removal of the carcinomatous lump is feasible in selected cases with small tumours and must be followed by a course of radical radiotherapy to the breast.

Radical mastectomy is designed to remove the breast, pectoral muscles with the lymphatics passing to the axilla, the axillary lymph nodes and fat. The nerves to the serratus anterior and latissimus dorsi muscles are normally preserved. Skin graft replacement may be needed in closure of the wound. The operation carries a low mortality but may be followed by oedema of the upper limb and some limitation of shoulder movement. The *modified radical operation* which entails removal of the breast and axillary lymph nodes but preserves the pectoral muscles is more commonly undertaken. The long-term follow-up results indicate that there is little to choose between these procedures and current opinion tends to favour more conservative surgical measures. The percentage of involved axillary nodes can be correlated with prognosis: if more than four contain tumour deposits it is highly likely that the tumour has metastasised widely and this may be considered an indication for adjuvant chemotherapy (p. 140). Total mastectomy is not satisfactory where there is severe local involvement (T3 or T4) or general dissemination (N2, N3 or M1) but it may be of value in the treatment of severe bleeding from a fungating lesion. A portion of the tumour should be assayed for the presence of oestrogen-receptors (p. 140).

Irradiation is given by a high-voltage machine, a linear accelerator or by a cobalt unit. In Stages 1 and 2 it is directed to the lymph node areas of axilla and anterior mediastinum. It is not given as a routine after radical mastectomy but may be used later to treat an isolated recurrence or metastasis.

Irradiation of the primary site in Stages 3 and 4 may lead to considerable regression of the tumour. Treatment of an isolated osseous metastasis may relieve pain, or if situated in the spine treatment may prevent the development of paraplegia. Radiotherapy to pulmonary secondaries produces excessive fibrosis of the lung and should not be adopted.

Hormonal therapy is employed for advanced disease with widespread metastases.

Tamoxifen is an anti-oestrogen which may act by blocking receptor sites, and is useful in the treatment of skin lesions and enlarged lymph nodes. Oestrogen in the form of ethinyl oestradiol is of benefit in some elderly patients.

Surgical hormonal management includes bilateral oophorectomy, bilateral adrenalectomy and hypophysectomy, and is usually employed when control with medical measures ceases. **Oophorectomy** is the best treatment for advanced disease in the pre-menopausal patient and may be beneficial for two to three years after the menopause. Adrenalectomy and hypophysectomy are now rarely performed but may benefit patients with painful osseous metastases. The results of hypophysectomy appear slightly better than adrenalectomy, but it necessitates the attention of specialised centres.

Remission after oophorectomy, adrenalectomy and hypophysectomy occurs in about 50 per cent of cases. The average duration of remission with these operations is 9 to 18 months and only a small proportion survive five years after recurrence. The interval between initial treatment and the appearance of a recurrence has some bearing on prognosis; the longer the period the better is the response to endocrine surgery. Measurement of the oestradiol receptors in breast tumour tissue gives an indication for the use of either endocrine therapy or chemotherapy. It seems that oestrogen receptor positive tumours may have a better prognosis and respond better to oophorectomy, while oestrogen negative results indicate treatment by chemotherapy. Further, oestrogen negative results indicate a lower response rate to hormonal treatment and chemotherapy may be considered at an earlier stage.

Metastatic lesions in special sites involve specific therapy. A pleural effusion may require aspiration, and instillation of bleomycin solution diminishes the rate of recurrence. Laminectomy may be necessary to relieve spinal cord pressure and aid paraplegia. Fixation of pathological fractures is required in some instances and may be followed by subsequent union of the bone. Extensive osseous metastases with bone destruction may cause hypercalcaemia.

The effect of the contraceptive pill containing oestrogen is uncertain but although present evidence is inconclusive it should not be given to a patient under treatment for mammary carcinoma as it may accelerate tumour growth. Pregnancy is better avoided for two years following mastectomy but probably does not produce adverse effects after this period. Carcinoma of the breast appearing in the first half of pregnancy should be treated by the appropriate surgical measures without termination of pregnancy. In the second half of pregnancy it is probably wiser to delay treatment until the early post-partum period. Oestrogens should not be given to suppress lactation in a patient who has had mammary cancer.

Chemotherapy using combination drug therapy of methotrexate, 5-fluorouracil, vincristine and cyclophosphamide may be given for advanced disease. Toxic effects may be troublesome and involve marrow suppression and alopecia. Doxorubicin (Adriamycin) is also used but may be cardio-toxic.

Adjuvant chemotherapy given at the time of mastectomy and for variable periods thereafter is the subject of extensive clinical trials. The results indicate that slight improvement in survival can be expected, but the toxic effects of long-term treatment cannot be ignored.

Paget's disease of the nipple

This is an eczematous condition associated with carcinoma of the breast. A red, granular eruption of the skin of nipple and areola exudes a watery discharge and slowly increases in size. The carcinomatous mass may not be evident until a later date.

The deeper layers of epidermis contain clear, rounded 'Paget cells', which may either be cancer cells or oedematous epidermal cells. The precise relationship to the carcinoma is not clear. One theory suggests that the underlying tumour causes blockage of the skin lymphatics resulting in oedema; another that there is an intraduct carcinoma near the nipple.

In cases of doubtful diagnosis local applications of hydrocortisone over a period of three weeks usually improve a simple eczematous condition. Histological examination of surface scrapings may show the presence of 'Paget cells'. Treatment involves removal of the breast if there is no contraindication.

FURTHER READING

Baum, M. (1980). Carcinoma of the breast. In *Recent Advances in Surgery*. 10. Ed. Taylor, S. Edinburgh: Churchill Livingstone.

Coombe, R. C., Powles, T. J., Ford, H. T. and Gazet, J. C. (1981). *Breast Cancer Management*. London: Academic Press.

Forrest, A. P. M., Roberts, M., Hughes, L. E., Webster, D. J.T., Baum, M. and Bonnadonna, G. (1980). Breast cancer. *Brit. J. Hosp. Med.* 23, 8–53.

Gravelle, I. H. (1982). Diagnostic imaging in breast cancer. In *Clinics in Oncology*. Vol. 1, No. 3. Eastbourne: Saunders.

12

Hernia

The word hernia probably comes from the Greek word *ernos*, which means a sprout, and hence a protrusion. Usually this refers to protrusions from the peritoneal cavity, such as inguinal and femoral herniae, but also included are diaphragmatic and internal herniae.

GENERAL FEATURES

Pathology

Abdominal herniae have a complete peritoneal protrusion or sac into which are extruded the contents. The sac has a fundus, body, neck and mouth. The neck is usually well defined and tends to be the narrowest portion of the sac, a notable exception being found in direct inguinal hernia. In children the sac of an indirect inguinal hernia is thin and tears easily, whereas the adult form is much stronger. The contents of a hernia (Fig. 12.1) are most commonly: (1) Omentum (omentocele, epiplocele). (2) Intestine (enterocele), usually the small bowel, occasionally the large bowel, and rarely the appendix. When only a portion of the circumference of the intestine is present in the sac it is called a 'Richter's hernia'. (3) Bladder in the medial wall of a direct inguinal hernia or femoral hernia. (4) Meckel's diverticulum (Littré's hernia).

A hernia may be congenital or acquired. A *congenital* hernia develops in a peritoneal sac, which may be of sufficient size to give rise to a hernia in early life, or it may be present as a potential channel which becomes filled at a later date. These sacs, such as the processus vaginalis or the umbilicus, are the result of persistent embryological channels. An *acquired* hernia occurs as the result of muscular weakness following obesity, pregnancy, advancing

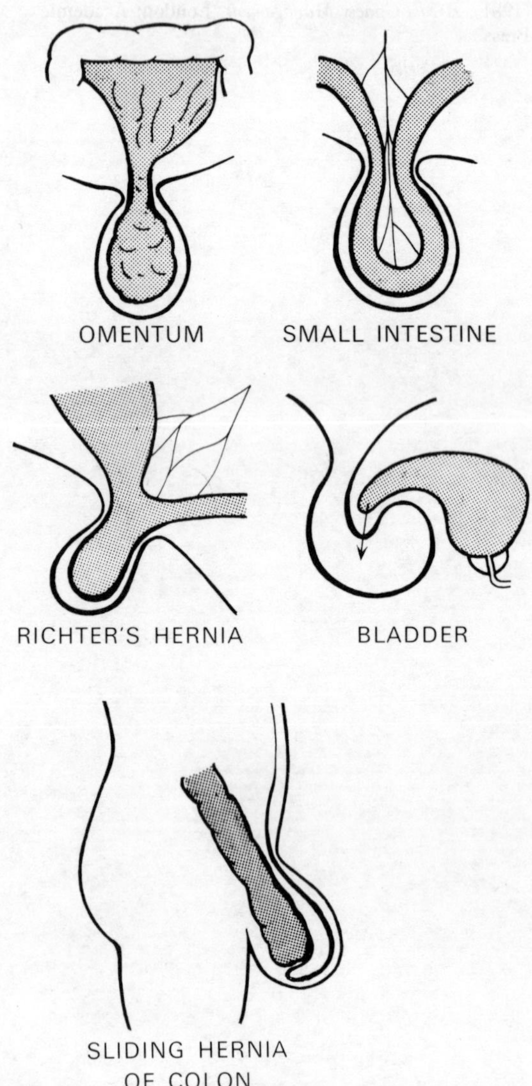

Fig. 12.1 Contents of a hernial sac. The bladder invaginates the medial wall of the sac. The peritoneal covering is absent from the posterior aspect of the colon in a sliding hernia.

years and poliomyelitis, whilst nerve injury, a wound haematoma or infection may lead to post-operative herniation. Straining to lift heavy objects, chronic cough, constipation and difficulty in micturition may all lead to the development of a hernia in the presence of the above predisposing factors.

A hernia is said to be *reducible* when it can be emptied of its contents by pressure or posture. *Irreducibility* results from the contents becoming swollen or adherent to the sac. Omentum is particularly liable to adhesion formation, notably in para-umbilical herniae.

Intestinal *obstruction* may occur in most varieties of hernia, the common causative factor being the neck of the sac. Small intestine is more usually involved, although colon may be found in umbilical and left inguinal herniae, and the stomach in the diaphragmatic type. Interference with the blood supply leads to *strangulation* (Fig. 12.2). The venous return is first obstructed producing congestion and oedema, followed by arterial obstruction. Gangrene may occur either at the site of constriction or on the antimesenteric border, and in extreme cases necrosis of all the contained bowel occurs. Free fluid, at first colourless then blood-stained, collects within the hernial sac. Initially sterile, it later becomes highly infected with organisms from the bowel. The peritoneal coat becomes dull, and with loss of viability the intestinal wall becomes black and later green. In the final stages rupture occurs into the sac and may lead to general peritonitis. Strangulation of omentum is less serious as this structure is better able to withstand ischaemia, but eventually infection and peritonitis result.

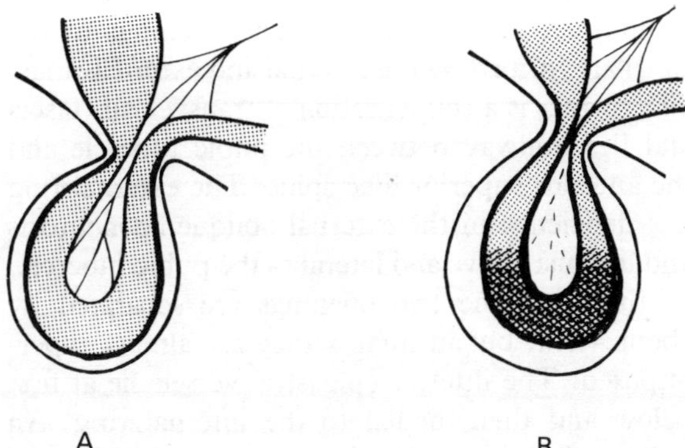

Fig. 12.2 The complications of a hernia. **A.** Intestinal obstruction. **B.** Intestinal strangulation.

Incarceration is often described as synonymous with irreducibility, but the word incarcerate means 'imprison,' and when applied to a hernia its meaning should be restricted to imprisonment of faeces within the contained large intestine.

Clinical features

The most common complaint is of a swelling which may or may not be painful. Occasionally localised pain following an unusual strain may precede the swelling. Disturbances of micturition may be present if the hernia contains bladder.

Examination of the patient in a standing position or after coughing may be necessary to detect a hernia which is not initially obvious. Careful inspection and palpation of anatomical landmarks are of help in establishing the type of hernia, particular attention being given to the direction of the cough impulse and of the reduction. The nature of the contents should also be determined; intestine gurgles on reduction whilst omentum does not. Initial difficulty in reduction suggests that intestine is present, the reverse occurring with omentum. The general health of the patient and the state of abdominal musculature should be assessed. Obesity leads to difficulties in repair and produces a tendency to post-operative respiratory complications. The presence of chronic bronchitis or persistent urinary obstruction makes post-operative recurrences more likely.

In an irreducible hernia there is usually no other symptom than that of a persistent swelling, but when intestinal obstruction and strangulation are present colicky abdominal pain and local discomfort or pain are constant features. The presence of a tense, tender, irreducible mass over which the skin may be red or oedematous is characteristic of strangulated bowel, and if involving small intestine is usually accompanied by vomiting, abdominal distension and increased bowel sounds. Omental strangulation is notable for local pain and tenderness. A strangulated Richter's hernia may have no signs of intestinal obstruction although local tenderness is present.

Treatment

This may be either operative or conservative. Preliminary treatment should be directed towards any aggravating factors. Obese patients are encouraged to lose weight and weak abdominal musculature is strengthened by exercises. Breathing exercises should also be instituted and smoking abandoned if a cough is present. Where serious pulmonary disease exists operation should be deferred until the summer period. Urinary obstruction should be treated before a hernia repair is contemplated or the two operations can be combined in certain circumstances. In the pre-operative and post-operative period the help of a physiotherapist is invaluable, particularly in the elderly, when early ambulation and exercises are essential to avoid venous thrombosis and pulmonary complications. A conservative approach is indicated in unfit patients or those unwilling to undergo an operation.

General operative principles include adequate exposure, reduction of the contents and excision of the sac (**herniotomy**). The deficiency may in addition require a repair to diminish the risk of recurrence. Where living material such as fascia is used the procedure is termed a *hernioplasty*, but more commonly absorbable or non-absorbable foreign material is employed (**herniorrhaphy**).

Recurrence of a hernia after operation may be due to inadequate excision of the sac or sacs, incomplete repair, or weakening of tissues by post-operative haematoma formation and infection. Obesity and persistent straining, as with a chronic cough, are further factors. Active physiotherapy, early ambulation and breathing exercises diminish the risk of recurrence by improving muscle tone and decreasing post-operative complications.

TYPES OF ABDOMINAL HERNIA

External herniae

1. Inguinal—indirect or direct.
2. Femoral—including prevascular.
3. Umbilical and para-umbilical.
4. Epigastric.
5. Incisional.
6. Rare forms such as lumbar, obturator, interparietal (interstitial), Spigelian, gluteal and sciatic.

Internal herniae

Apart from diaphragmatic hernia (p. 105), this type is rare and is only seen during operations for intestinal obstruction. Herniation of a loop of intestine may occur into or through natural or pathological openings. The former include (1) the lesser sac—through the epiploic foramen, (2) paraduodenal, (3) paracaecal and (4) intersigmoid—at the apex of the attachment of the sigmoid colon. Pathological foramina may be due to mesenteric openings following intestinal resection or partial gastrectomy, or to the unclosed lateral space after a colostomy or ileostomy. Intraperitoneal adhesions may also be responsible for an abnormal opening.

INGUINAL HERNIA

This is the most common variety of 'rupture', and can be of indirect or direct type. The former traverses the whole length of the inguinal canal, whilst the latter protrudes only through the medial portion.

Anatomy

The inguinal canal is the oblique passage in the lower part of the anterior abdominal wall through which the spermatic cord passes to the testis, or in the female the round ligament to the labium majus. The processus vaginalis traversing the canal is normally obliterated at birth, but persistence in whole or in part presents an anatomical predisposition to an indirect inguinal hernia. The openings of the canal are formed by the internal and external rings. The former is a condensation of transversalis fascia and lies midway between the pubic tubercle and the anterior superior iliac spine. The external ring is a deficiency in the external oblique aponeurosis and lies just above and lateral to the pubic tubercle. In the adult the two openings are separated by about 4 cm, but in infants they are almost superimposed. The inferior epigastric vessels lie at first below and then medial to the internal ring. An indirect hernia commences above and lateral to these vessels.

The internal oblique forms part of the anterior wall as it takes origin from the outer two-thirds of the inguinal ligament, and then arches over the spermatic cord to help form the roof (Fig. 12.3, A). Medially, part of it joins the transversus abdominis muscle to form the conjoint tendon, a structure variable in width and strength, which goes behind the cord to its insertion on the pubic crest and pectineal line. The outer two-thirds of the posterior wall of the inguinal canal is formed by the transversalis fascia, which may be thickened to form the 'interfoveolar ligament'. Behind these structures are the extraperitoneal fat and peritoneum. The anterior wall is formed largely by the external oblique aponeurosis with, in addition, a small portion of the internal oblique muscle laterally. The floor in the lateral two-thirds is formed by the union of transversalis fascia and the inguinal ligament, and medially by the pectineal part of the inguinal ligament. From a surgical point of view it must be realised that the femoral vessels are directly under the floor and are in imminent danger of being pierced by an ill-placed needle during a hernia repair. The ilio-inguinal nerve passes down the canal and may be damaged during hernia operations, as may also the ilio-hypogastric nerve, which lies 2 cm above it on the internal oblique.

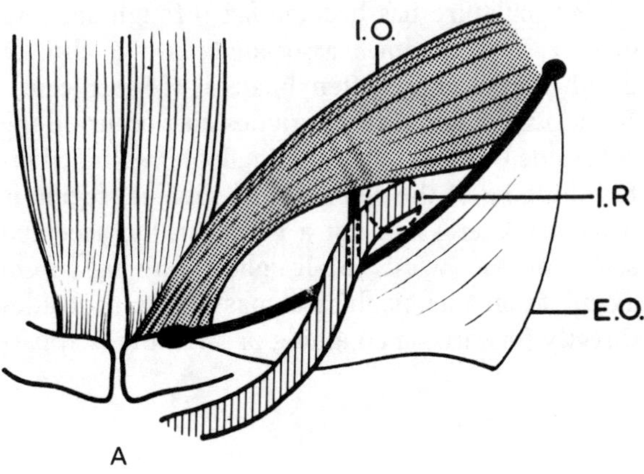

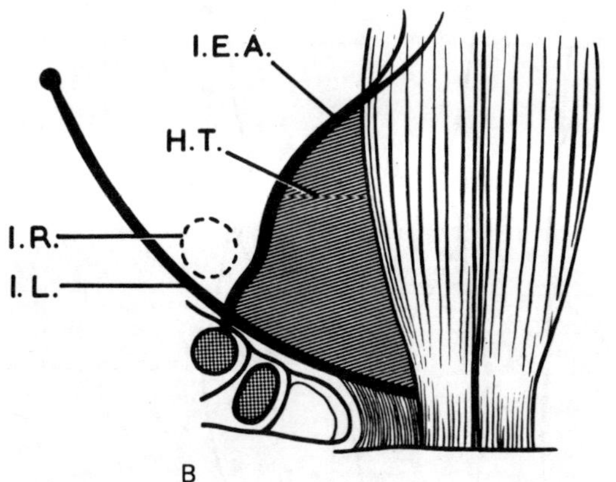

Fig. 12.3 Anatomy of the inguinal canal. **A.** Anterior view: I.O., internal oblique; I.R., internal ring; E.O., reflected aponeurosis of external oblique. **B.** Posterior view: I.E.A., inferior epigastric artery; H.T., Hesselbach's triangle; I.R., internal ring; I.L., inguinal ligament in front of femoral vessels.

A direct hernia protrudes through the posterior wall of the inguinal canal through Hesselbach's triangle, the boundaries of which are the lateral border of the rectus on the medial side, the inferior epigastric vessels on the lateral side and the inguinal ligament below (Fig. 12.3, B). The 'floor' of the triangle is formed medially by the conjoint tendon and laterally by the transversalis fascia, the obliterated hypogastric artery separating the two.

The coverings of an indirect inguinal hernia are the external spermatic fascia from the external oblique, the cremasteric fascia from the internal oblique and the internal spermatic fascia from the transversalis fascia; a direct hernia is covered by the external spermatic fascia, the conjoint tendon or its prolongations and the transversalis fascia.

The inguinal mechanism

The muscles of this region react to strain in the following manner; (1) Contraction of the external oblique narrows the gap in the external ring. (2) Associated tightening of the rectus sheath and underlying muscle forms a firm foundation for the remaining actions. (3) Straightening of the arched conjoint diminishes the interval between it and the inguinal ligament, but a weakened triangular area persists with its base in the region of the emerging cord at the external ring, due to the tendinous segment of conjoint tendon. Recurrent herniae are common at this site and care should be taken at operation to repair this portion adequately. (4) Lateral and upward movement of the U-shaped internal ring tightens the fascia transversalis. (5) Finally there is blockage of the inguinal canal by the bulk of the cremaster muscle which is pulled upwards on contraction.

The failure of this mechanism, of which the tightening of the fascia transversalis is the most important part, is responsible for the development of an indirect inguinal hernia. A congenital sac may not be obvious for some years until breakdown occurs in the inguinal mechanism. Similarly failure of the mechanism may permit the development of an acquired indirect sac.

Clinical features

Indirect hernia occurs at all ages. It is more common in males and in about 30 per cent of cases is bilateral. Three types are recognised.

1. Bubonocele. The hernia is limited to the inguinal canal.
2. Funicular. The hernia extends down to the top of the testis.
3. Complete or scrotal. The hernia extends into the scrotum, and the tunica vaginalis of the testis communicates with the general peritoneal cavity through the processus vaginalis.

The general clinical features of any hernia are apparent (p. 143), but the origin of the swelling above the inguinal ligament is important. When reducible the direction of return of the sac and contents is upwards and outwards, appearing with an impulse on coughing in the reverse manner. After reduction, pressure over the internal ring controls the hernia in the majority of cases (Fig. 12.4, A). Occasionally it may be necessary to invaginate the skin of the scrotum with the little finger which is then passed through the external ring in order to detect a small hernia, but the procedure is uncomfortable and should not be routinely employed.

Direct hernia occurs mainly in middle-aged and elderly men. It is always acquired, occurs where the musculature has become lax through age and obesity, is sometimes associated with a chronic cough and is more often bilateral (55 per cent). Both indirect and direct varieties may occur on the same side ('saddle-bag' or 'pantaloon' hernia). Diffuse bulging of the whole of the inguinal region is usually bilateral and not a hernia in the accepted sense of the word (Malgaigne's bulgings). On examination a hemispherical mass which protrudes directly forward on coughing or straining is appar-

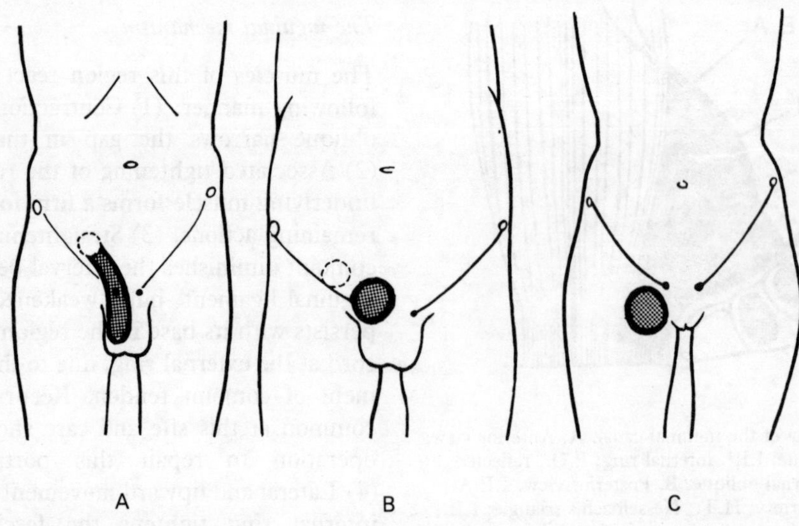

Fig. 12.4 Types of herniation in the groin. **A.** Indirect inguinal in young man. **B.** Direct inguinal in older man. **C.** Femoral in female.

ent in the medial part of the inguinal region. Digital pressure over the internal ring does not control reduction (Fig. 12.4, B). The hernia is seldom of large size and only occasionally does it enter the scrotum. Complications are rare.

Differential diagnosis

Femoral hernia. The relationship of the neck of the sac to the pubic tubercle is important. A femoral hernia arises below and lateral to this structure, whilst an inguinal hernia emerges through the external ring above and medial to the tubercle. If a swelling arises or is situated entirely below the inguinal ligament it cannot be an inguinal hernia and may be a femoral hernia.

Encysted hydrocele of the cord produces a tense spherical swelling which cannot be reduced. It may be differentiated from a hernia by a downward movement on traction of the testis. In the female a cyst of the canal of Nuck produces a similar picture.

Undescended or ectopic testis. In both conditions a hernial sac may be present, but the absence of the testis from the usual position indicates maldescent.

Hydrocele of the tunica vaginalis may cause confusion by extending up to the neck of the scrotum; careful palpation of the upper limit differentiates it from a hernia. It is also translucent and has no cough impulse.

Inguinal lymphadenitis produces a tender firm swelling which may be confused with an irreducible hernia, but the precise position and characteristics should lead to the correct diagnosis.

Treatment

Conservative measures are indicated when the patient refuses operation or is unfit for surgery because of a cardiac or pulmonary condition. Old age is not necessarily a contra-indication to operative treatment, although small direct herniae in elderly patients should be treated conservatively. In babies the majority of surgeons prefer to wait until the child is at least three months old before advising surgery.

A *truss* can be employed in the conservative management of a reducible hernia but, except occasionally in infants, it is not curative. Some degree of intelligence and perseverance by the patient is required. The hernia must be reduced by lying down before applying the truss and to be satisfactory pressure must be exerted directly over the inguinal canal. The rupture should then be controlled when the patient stands with the legs apart. Measurements are normally made by the appliance firm, but they may easily be undertaken by the surgeon. A tape measure is placed around the patient just below the iliac crests and the circumference is recorded at the pubic tubercle on the side of the hernia. The most effective form of truss has a pad joined to a leather-covered steel spring which encircles the patient below the iliac crest. A strap joins the two ends anteriorly, and a perineal strap joining the posterior circle of the spring to the pad helps to keep the truss in position. In infants a rubber truss which can be washed is preferable. Careful attention to cleanliness and powdering of the skin, although essential in all cases, is even more important in an infant.

Operative treatment is advisable whenever possible. The procedure adopted varies with the preference of the individual surgeon. Herniotomy is indicated in infants and children up to the age of about 14 years. The sac is a congenital one, and as the musculature of the posterior wall is satisfactory removal of the sac alone is usually adequate. In children under the age of three years the external oblique does not require to be opened as the external and internal rings are superimposed, but structures are small and great care must be exercised.

In adults some form of repair to strengthen the posterior wall of the canal must be carried out in addition. This assumes greater importance in the direct variety. The Bassini operation in which the conjoint tendon is sutured to the inguinal ligament behind the spermatic cord or round ligament is a commonly performed herniorrhaphy (Fig. 12.5). Where tension exists the Tanner slide modification of a relieving incision in the deeper portion of the rectus sheath allows the conjoint tendon to descend. In the direct variety, or in large indirect herniae, despite the slide a gap may exist in the posterior wall of the canal and to close this a darn may be necessary. Various materials may be used in the repair, but nylon, stainless steel, linen thread and floss nylon or silk all have their advocates, whilst fascia from the external oblique, rectus

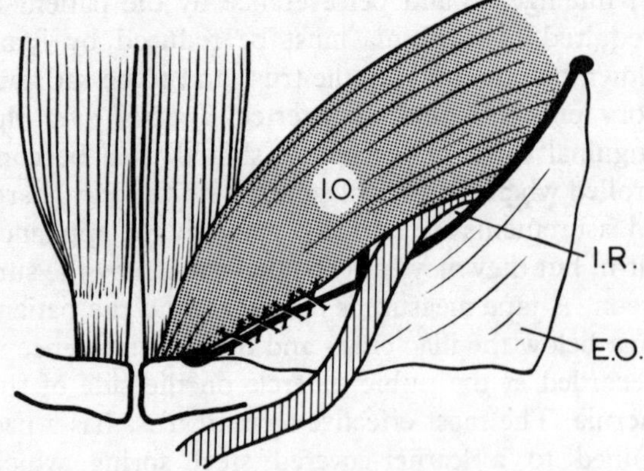

Fig. 12.5 Bassini repair of inguinal hernia. The conjoint tendon is sutured behind the spermatic cord to the inguinal ligament.

sheath or thigh may be employed. Post-operative recurrence is less likely when the canal can be completely closed as in the female, whilst orchidectomy in the elderly may be advantageous. Recurrence takes place in some instances irrespective of the method employed in repair, and the majority occur within 12 months. The rate is higher in the direct variety than in the indirect type.

Sliding hernia (hernie-en-glissade)

In this condition the pelvic colon on the left side, or less commonly the caecum on the right side, slides downwards extraperitoneally to enter the inguinal canal; occasionally the process may involve the bladder. The posterior wall of the sac is formed by visceral peritoneum covering bladder or bowel. These lesions begin as simple herniae, but with gradual stretching of the tissues enlargement of the internal ring follows and the sliding process is initiated.

Clinically it affects mainly men over the age of 40 years in whom obesity and weak musculature are prominent features. A large globular swelling is apparent, particularly on the left side, and when difficult to control with a truss, a sliding hernia should be suspected. Treatment is by herniorrhaphy, but no attempt should be made to strip the offending structures from the posterior wall of the sac or the blood supply will be imperilled. The recurrence rate is higher than in the simple form.

Complicated inguinal hernia

Obstruction and strangulation are serious and more common in the indirect variety. Neither sex nor age group is exempt, though strangulation is uncommon in infants. The pathological features have been previously considered (p. 143). The usual constricting agent is the neck of the sac, but it may be the external ring or adhesions within the sac.

Clinically there is often a long history of a groin swelling which may not have been fully reducible, but the sudden onset of the obstructive symptoms of abdominal pain, vomiting and distension may be the first indication that a hernia is responsible. Local pain and tenderness are important signs in strangulation and are soon followed by other evidence of intestinal obstruction.

Treatment

Early and mild obstruction may be managed conservatively by sedation, cold compresses and elevation of the foot of the bed. More severe cases require adequate fluid and electrolyte replacement followed by surgical exploration. Non-operative measures should not be continued in obstructive cases for more than two hours without evidence of relief, and should not be employed where there is strangulation. Any attempts at manual reduction (taxis) should be avoided where the possibility of strangulation exists, or gangrenous bowel may be returned to the abdomen with fatal results. Operative treatment involves division of the constricting agent through an inguinal incision, with inspection and liberation of the bowel. If signs of non-viability exist (p. 143) resection must be undertaken, if necessary through a separate lower paramedian incision.

FEMORAL HERNIA

A femoral hernia descends through the femoral canal, which is the medial compartment of the femoral sheath, containing fat, a few lymph vessels and a lymph node of the deep inguinal group (Fig. 12.6, A). In its passage the sac lies medial to the femoral vein and lateral to the rigid Gimber-

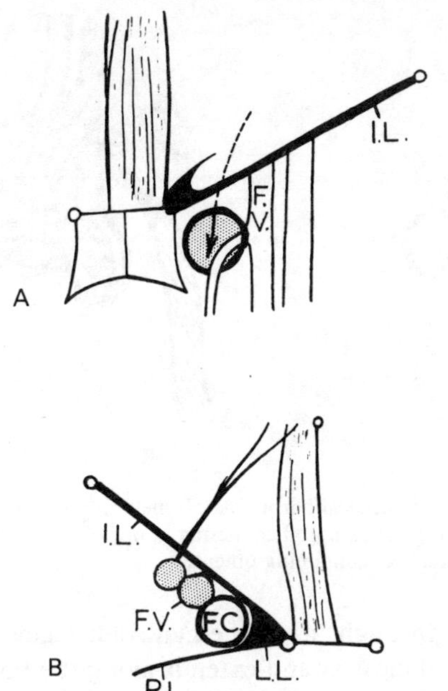

Fig. 12.6 Anatomy of femoral hernia. **A.** Anterior view, the arrow indicates the course of the hernia behind the inguinal ligament and through the saphenous opening. **B.** Superior view of the femoral canal (F.C.) indicating the boundaries; I.L., inguinal ligament; P.L., pectineal ligament; L.L., lacunar ligament; F.V., femoral vein.

nat's or lacunar ligament. Anteriorly is situated the inguinal ligament, and posteriorly the hernia is related to the pectineal ligament (Astley Cooper), the pubic bone and the pectineus muscle and fascia (Fig. 12.6, B). Rarer types of femoral hernia occur in front and behind the femoral vessels. The former is known as a prevascular hernia; the latter is rare and has only been described in congenital dislocation of the hip (Narath's hernia).

The majority of femoral herniae are acquired. The sac is generally small and often surrounded by extraperitoneal fat giving it a globular shape, whilst the neck may become plugged with omentum resulting in the formation of a hydrocele. As the hernia enlarges it passes through the cribriform fascia and is then directed upwards in front of the inguinal ligament. The narrowness of the neck of the sac and the unyielding nature of Gimbernat's ligament make strangulation ten times more common than in inguinal hernia. Small intestine generally enters the sac and a Richter's hernia often results.

Clinical features

Femoral hernia is more common in parous women than in men. Increased intra-abdominal pressure in pregnancy is a major causative factor as the incidence is not greater in nullipara than in men. It is rare in children, but accounts for 20 per cent of all herniae in women, although less common than inguinal hernia. It is recognised as a swelling originating below the inguinal ligament and lateral to the pubic tubercle, is apparent on standing or straining, but may disappear on lying down (Fig. 12.4, C). It is seldom large and in obese subjects may easily be overlooked. Often globular in shape it may be soft in consistency or tense if a hydrocele is present. A cough impulse may be seen or felt and if it continues laterally over the femoral vessels is suggestive of a prevascular component. The firm mass of an irreducible hernia and the pain, vomiting and abdominal distension of strangulation may develop later.

Differential diagnosis

Inguinal hernia may be excluded by careful attention to the anatomical landmarks. In a *saphena varix* the majority of patients have varicosities of the long saphenous system further down the limb. This swelling, like some femoral herniae, disappears on lying down, but a varix is softer and more compressible. Coughing gives rise not only to an impulse but to a palpable fluid thrill in the saphena varix. If the veins lower down the limb are tapped with the patient in the standing position an impulse is transmitted to the groin swelling. In *inguinal lymphadenitis* it is uncommon for one gland alone to be involved, but where this is the case an active or healed focus of infection should be present on the limb, perineum, buttock or lower abdomen on the affected side. With a *lipoma* of the femoral triangle differentiation may be difficult, but there will be no extension into the femoral canal. Other conditions, such as a psoas abscess presenting below the inguinal ligament, or a haematoma in the adductor longus muscle, may occasionally be confused with a femoral hernia.

Treatment

No satisfactory truss has been devised that will control a femoral hernia and because of the risk of strangulation surgery should be advocated.

Operation may be undertaken from below the inguinal ligament or via the abdomen. The lower approach is technically more difficult regarding the closure of the femoral canal, but the absence of an abdominal incision permits fuller respiration and produces less pain post-operatively thereby allowing freer movement, which is of advantage in the elderly patient. The trans-inguinal approach allows better access to the upper end of the femoral canal and any abnormal obturator vessel present on the free edge of Gimbernat's ligament can be more easily detected before the latter is divided, but this artery is not common and the operation may weaken the posterior wall of the inguinal canal. The McEvedy approach in which a lower paramedian incision is made with retraction medially of the rectus abdominis allows good extraperitoneal exposure of the upper end of the femoral canal. It is a satisfactory procedure for strangulated hernia as resection of gangrenous bowel can easily be undertaken. The mode of repair in each approach, following excision of the sac, is suture of the inguinal ligament to the pectineal ligament. Damage or constriction of the femoral vein must be avoided. Recurrence is not common, but may require a darn to obliterate the femoral space.

UMBILICAL HERNIA

Congenital and acquired forms exist. The former occurs in babies and young children, whilst the latter appears in the adult and is more correctly designated a para-umbilical hernia.

Congenital umbilical hernia

The most extreme form of congenital herniation is known as *exomphalos* in which the midgut fails to return to the abdominal cavity during foetal life. The condition is rare, and in 50 per cent of cases a considerable portion of the abdominal contents protrude. Immediate surgical replacement and repair is preferable to prevent infection in most instances, although conservative management by the application of sterile protective dressings is gaining popularity.

In the majority of cases a small peritoneal sac

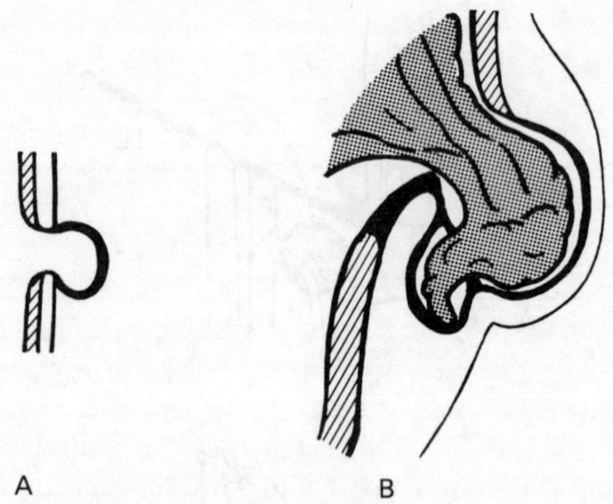

Fig. 12.7 Umbilical hernia. **A.** Herniation through umbilicus in a child. **B.** Para-umbilical hernia in obese adult with multilocular sac containing omentum.

passes through a congenital deficiency in the umbilical cicatrix and extends along the line of the umbilical vessels (Fig. 12.7A). Males are affected more often than females. The swelling is recognised as a subcutaneous protrusion of the navel, normally present at birth, but which may appear with intense crying, coughing or through muscular weakness in conditions such as cretinism or rickets. Most herniae are reducible through an easily palpable deficiency in the linea alba measuring about 0.25 cm in diameter. Obstruction and strangulation are rare occurrences.

Treatment

The majority of true umbilical herniae disappear within a year without any treatment as the child grows and the recti develop. Reassurance of the parents on this point is important. The application of a rubber umbilical pad and truss may encourage this process when a large hernia is present. Where a sac persists beyond this period, or if the hernia is large or complicated, herniotomy may be advised. The sac should be excised through a semicircular subumbilical incision preserving the umbilicus, and the edges of the fibrous defect closed.

PARA-UMBILICAL HERNIA

Weakness of the interlacing fibres of the linea alba in the region of the umbilicus due to increased intra-abdominal pressure, particularly from obesity and pregnancy, is responsible for this type of hernia. The neck is often narrow, but the main hernia may reach a large size and becomes progressively more pronounced. There may be more than one opening into the sac from the peritoneal cavity, and secondary projections often occur at different levels in the coverings (Fig. 12.7, B). The contents generally include omentum and transverse colon, but small intestine and even stomach may be contained in the protrusion. Numerous adhesions form between the sac and its contents, particularly the omentum, converting it into a multilocular cavity. The coverings, which include skin, superficial fascia, rectus sheath and transversalis fascia in advanced cases, become thin and attenuated. Excoriation, ulceration and gangrene may be followed by a faecal fistula. Irreducibility is common, whilst obstruction and strangulation are important and frequent complications.

Clinical features

The majority of patients are obese, middle-aged women who have borne a number of children, and in some there is a history of chronic bronchitis. Pain, due to a complication, may be the first indication in an obese subject who has mistaken the swelling for adiposity. Flatulence and constipation may be associated with incarceration of faeces in the transverse colon. In the early stages a cough impulse and a reducible swelling, usually below but often including the umbilicus, is apparent. With irreducibility the firm omentum and a tympanitic note over the contained bowel may be observed. An area of intertrigo is common on the under surface of the skin. The signs of strangulation may be present.

Treatment

Operative repair is indicated in most instances at an early stage because of the risk of strangulation which in these patients carries a high mortality. Pre-operative weight reduction and treatment of any respiratory infection is beneficial. The operation entails excision of the umbilicus and the hernial sac through a transverse elliptical incision, with careful reduction of the contents. Repair is performed by Mayo's method of overlapping the upper and lower portions of the rectus sheath which bound the hernial opening.

EPIGASTRIC HERNIA

This form of midline hernia of the abdominal wall occurs through the interlacing fibres of the linea alba. Extraperitoneal fat protrudes initially, in some instances drawing a portion of the peritoneum with it to form a small sac. The weakness occurs at the site at which blood-vessels perforate the linea alba. The probable cause is strain followed by tearing of the linea alba fibres.

The majority of cases occur in well-built muscular men. Pain may attract attention to the mass, which may range from the size and shape of a pea to a discoid swelling 2 cm or more in diameter. Many are asymptomatic, but tenderness may occur and suggest a diagnosis of peptic ulceration. Treatment is by excision of the hernia with repair of the underlying deficiency.

INCISIONAL HERNIA

An incisional hernia occurs through a previous operation scar; the majority are encountered in the midline, when the condition is known as a 'ventral hernia'. Predisposing causes in development are as follows:

1. Site of incision—a lower midline wound is weakened by the absence of the posterior rectus sheath.
2. Factors influencing healing of the wounds:
   a. Infection plays a major part in delaying healing. Fibrous tissue resulting from infection is not strong and stretches in later years.
   b. Haematoma formation similarly delays healing, produces fibrosis and may become infected.
   c. Drainage tubes in the wound leave a track which is a source of potential weakness.
   d. Post-operative cough or distension places extra strain on sutures and healing tissues.
   e. Poor operative technique, with rough handling and inaccurate apposition of the tissues.

3. Damage to motor nerves by the incision is occasionally seen after a subcostal or lower pararectal incision.

Clinical features

Variation in size of the swelling is in part related to aetiology, but in the common midline position a large and diffuse bulge is usual. Dull aching pain may be noted. Complications may follow, but are uncommon in the large ventral type. The small aperture related to a drainage tube is a potentially dangerous site for the inclusion of small intestine and subsequent strangulation.

Treatment

If the hernia is reducible it may be controlled by an abdominal belt and pad. Surgical treatment is preferable for small herniae liable to become strangulated, for those which cannot be adequately controlled because of their position, such as suprapubic lesions, and for the complicated variety. At operation the edges of the sac are defined, and if large the latter should be excised before closure of the defect. When a gap exists a darn or plastic mesh implant may be necessary.

RARE EXTERNAL HERNIAE

Lumbar hernia

The majority follow operations on the kidney, but two sites exist through which a lumbar hernia may appear. (1) *Lower* variety through Petit's triangle, which is bounded by the iliac crest inferiorly, the external oblique laterally and latissimus dorsi medially. (2) *Upper* type through the space formed by the twelfth rib superiorly, the internal oblique laterally and sacrospinalis medially. The hernia is generally diffuse and reducible and can usually be controlled by a belt.

Obturator hernia

In this variety the hernia occurs along the line of the obturator canal and it may accompany the obturator vessels and nerve into the thigh. It is more common in women than in men, and the majority of cases occur after the age of 50 years.

Clinically it may be recognised by a swelling in the upper and medial part of the thigh or by pain referred to the inner side of the knee along the geniculate branch of the obturator nerve. This pain is aggravated by coughing or straining but not by movements of the hip. The majority of cases are unsuspected until laparotomy is undertaken for intestinal obstruction. Treatment is operative reduction by an abdominal approach.

Interstitial hernia

In this form the hernial sac passes between one or other layers of the anterior abdominal wall. It may lie between the peritoneum and the muscles (*properitoneal*), between the muscles, usually the internal and external oblique (*intermuscular*), or pass through the external ring to reach the superficial fascia (*extraparietal*). The condition may be associated with imperfect descent of the testis or be the result of incorrectly applied pressure from a truss. It is commonly related to an inguinal hernia. Obstruction and strangulation occur. Surgical treatment is to be preferred.

Spigelian hernia

This hernia originates at a point lateral to the rectus muscle and emerges through the linea semilunaris, generally in the lower half of the abdomen. The sac extends between the muscle layers as an interstitial hernia. Middle-aged obese patients are usually affected and strangulation may take place. Treatment is operative.

Gluteal hernia

This type occurs through the greater sciatic foramen either above or below piriformis. Recognition is difficult because of the mass of muscle overlying it, but a gluteal swelling may be palpable. Strangulation may occur and the diagnosis not be established until laparotomy is performed. Treatment is removal of the sac.

Sciatic hernia

A hernia of this form protrudes through the lesser sciatic foramen and presents the clinical picture of a gluteal hernia. Pain may also be referred along the distribution of the sciatic nerve. If recognised, the sac should be excised.

Perineal hernia

The usual cause of a perineal (sacral) hernia is giving way of scar tissue in the newly constructed pelvic floor after an abdomino-perineal excision of the rectum. It is more common in women because of the wider pelvis in this sex, and it may be associated with a chronic cough during the healing of the wound. Discomfort on standing but relieved by lying down is the main complaint. Management is generally conservative by means of a perineal pad support, but occasionally surgical excision of the sac is required.

FURTHER READING

Nyhus, L. M. and Harkins, H. N. (1978). *Hernia*. 2nd ed. New York: Lippincott.

13

Stomach and duodenum

Physiology

The function of the stomach is of importance in understanding the aetiology and treatment of peptic ulceration. It may be grossly altered in obstructive lesions. Absorption is mainly limited to water, alcohol and glucose from hypertonic solutions. The chief functions are secretion of gastric juices and peristaltic activity of the muscular wall, both of which aid the early stages of digestion. Two or three litres of gastric juice are produced daily and effect the peptic digestion of proteins. Intermittent emptying of the stomach occurs when the intragastric pressure overcomes the resistance of the pyloric sphincter, and at the end of a meal small amounts of bile regurgitae into the stomach. Emptying is normally complete within six hours.

Gastric juice is mainly composed of hydrochloric acid and pepsin together with mucus which, containing the intrinsic anti-anaemic factor, also protects the mucosa against trauma. The hydrochloric acid secreted by the oxyntic cells converts the enzyme pepsinogen into active pepsin. Small amounts of the latter enter the blood and are excreted as uropepsinogen. The main stimulus to pepsinogen secretion is the vagus nerve, whilst histamine acts locally on the oxyntic cells to liberate hydrochloric acid.

Gastric secretion has three main phases. First there is the night secretion, vagal in origin but seldom of great amount; it is responsible for the nocturnal pain which awakens a patient with a duodenal ulcer. The second phase results from reflex vagal stimulation by the thought, sight or smell of food and produces a profuse secretion rich in pepsinogen and acid. The third phase is the most important and due to the entry of food into the stomach. Gastrin is released from the antral mucosa and absorbed by the bloodstream, stimulating the oxyntic cells to liberate hydrochloric acid. It may also stimulate the lower oesophageal sphincter.

The *basal secretion test* is commonly performed but, due to vagal and psychic stimuli and to alteration with the entrance of saliva and bile, is known to be variable. In the Zollinger-Ellison syndrome (p. 267) it is valuable, being markedly raised in quantity and acidity. *Maximal stimulation* of the oxyntic cells can be obtained using pentagastrin, but only one-third of duodenal ulcer patients hypersecrete gastric juices. Complete achlorhydria during the test is found in pernicious anaemia or global atrophic gastritis; two-thirds of patients with carcinoma of the stomach secrete acid. *Insulin hypoglycaemia* stimulates gastric secretion through the vagus nerve and it is used following vagotomy as a test of completeness. The blood sugar must fall below 2 mmol per litre but some rise in acid output does not necessarily indicate failure of treatment. Immunoassay of fasting *plasma gastrin* levels is helpful in the Zollinger-Ellison syndrome where it is raised.

CONGENITAL PYLORIC STENOSIS

Pathology

This condition is considered to be due to neuromuscular inco-ordination at the pylorus. The sphincter itself is not affected, but immediately proximal there is localised muscular hypertrophy, producing a well-circumscribed tumour (Fig. 13.1). This swelling is about 2 cm long, terminates abruptly distally, but tapers gradually to normal stomach at the incisura angularis. It is firm and

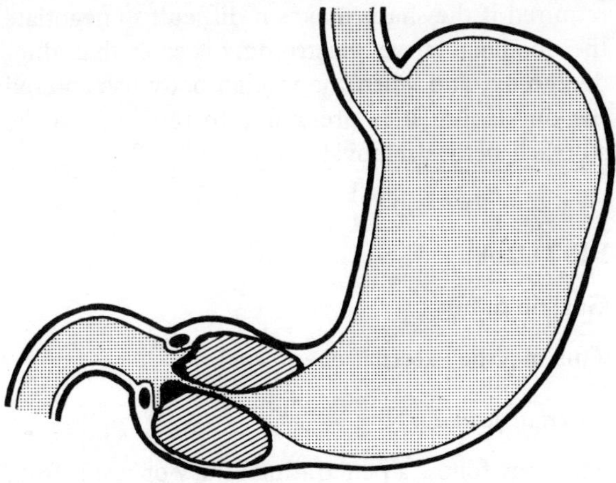

Fig. 13.1 Congenital hypertrophic pyloric stenosis

almost cartilaginous, pale in colour and mainly due to an overgrowth of circular muscle, although hypertrophy of longitudinal muscle is also present. The submucosa is thickened and the lumen further narrowed by folds of mucosa. Hypertrophy of the remaining stomach wall and dilatation occur later with secondary catarrhal and atrophic changes in the gastric mucosa.

Clinical features

Male children and often the first born are most frequently involved. Symptoms seldom arise until the second or third week and are projectile vomiting, constipation and failure to gain weight. The vomit does not contain bile. In severe and untreated cases dehydration, cachexia and death may follow, but such sequelae are rare today. Visible gastric peristalsis and a palpable pyloric tumour, most easily felt during or shortly after a feed, confirm the diagnosis and a barium meal is seldom necessary. Overfeeding and gastro-enteritis may cause confusion in diagnosis, but in these cases a tumour cannot be felt. Other rare causes of vomiting, such as duodenal obstruction, commence soon after birth and the vomit is usually bile-stained.

Treatment

Mild forms where pylorospasm is prominent may respond to conservative measures, with small frequent feeds, and the administration of an antispasmodic, such as Eumydrin, 15 minutes beforehand. Medical treatment should only be continued whilst the child is gaining weight.

Surgical treatment is required in the majority of cases; results are both satisfactory and dramatic. In severely ill and dehydrated children pre-operative fluid replacement is the first consideration and controlled amounts should be administered. Ramstedt pyloro-myotomy, which involves the longitudinal splitting of the muscle of the pyloric tumour, allows herniation of the underlying mucosa. The mortality from cross infection has been greatly reduced by post-operative isolation.

Duodenal atresia

Pathology

The aetiology has not been fully established. It is often considered due to a failure about the tenth week of intra-uterine life of re-canalisation of the duodenum which, with the remainder of the small intestine, is filled by a solid mass of epithelial cells during its early development. Obliteration of the vascular supply to a duodenal segment *in utero* is a more probable explanation. The extent of diminished vascularity determines the degree of atresia, which may vary from a diaphragm of mucosa to several centimetres length of duodenal wall. In some instances stenosis without atresia is produced. The second or third part of the duodenum is most often involved with either the common bile duct or an accessory duct entering proximal to the obstruction. Dilatation is found above the lesion and collapse below.

Clinical features

The predominant feature is vomiting, usually bile-stained, occurring 24 hours after birth. There may be signs of pain and discomfort, and in complete atresia there is absolute constipation. Dehydration occurs rapidly, there is little distension but marked loss of weight and death follows within a few days. Radiography of the abdomen confirms the level of obstruction by outlining the gas-filled stomach and proximal duodenum. Under no circumstances should a barium meal be given because of the risk of precipitating complete obstruction or blocking the stoma following surgery.

Treatment

Pre-operative correction of fluid and electrolyte imbalance should be followed by a short-circuiting procedure. This should be as near to the site of obstruction as possible by anastomosing duodenum proximal to the block to more distal duodenum (duodeno-duodenostomy) or to jejunum (duodenojejunostomy).

INJURIES

These may occur from without or within. The former is more common and may result from a bullet or stab wound, the latter from a foreign body or endoscopy. The stomach is more frequently involved than the duodenum. Injury is followed by signs of shock and peritoneal irritation, which may be accompanied by haematemesis. The diagnosis can be confirmed by the radiological evidence of intraperitoneal gas. Laparotomy and repair of the lesion with removal of any foreign body is indicated.

FOREIGN BODIES

A large number and variety of foreign bodies may enter the stomach. They are particularly liable to do so in children and mental patients, occasionally accidentally in dressmakers and carpenters during their work, and rarely in criminals with intent to avoid punishment.

The majority of foreign bodies that pass the oesophago-gastric junction will eventually traverse the alimentary tract. Symptoms result from obstruction, ulceration, perforation or haemorrhage. The diagnosis may be confirmed by radiography as the majority of foreign bodies are radio-opaque.

Treatment is conservative unless complications ensue or there is a grave risk of perforation. A bulky diet such as porridge and cotton-wool sandwiches may aid the passage of sharp objects and render them less dangerous. Removal may be feasible with special forceps passed down a fibreoptic gastroscope but if this fails surgery should be undertaken when there is more than a seven-to-ten-day hold-up of a sharp object unless pain and tenderness develop. Earlier operation may also be required if the shape makes it difficult to negotiate the duodenal curve. Gastrotomy is safer than duodenotomy, and when the foreign body has entered the duodenum it is preferable to return it to the stomach before removal.

FISTULA

Gastric fistula

This may be external or internal.

External fistula

This may follow a penetrating injury or result from leakage of the suture line after gastric operations or repair of a gastric perforation, particularly if this is due to carcinoma. Gastrostomy, occasionally performed as a temporary measure in upper alimentary tract obstruction or in preference to nasogastric suction post-operatively, is a surgically induced external fistula.

Clinical features. Leakage of the irritant fluid may be apparent either shortly after a history of upper abdominal injury or five to ten days after gastric surgery. The gastric origin of the discharge is suggested by the presence of acid on analysis and by the immediate appearance in the wound of methylene blue when this substance is given orally.

Treatment is conservative except for cases of injury which require immediate surgical repair. Oral feeding is withheld to diminish the amount of gastric secretion and careful fluid and electrolyte balance maintaned. The skin is protected with aluminium paste or barrier cream and continuous suction of the fistula maintained through a well-fitting tube until healing occurs.

Internal fistula

A communication may exist with duodenum, jejunum, colon or gall-bladder and may arise from disease in either the stomach or other part affected. The most common form is gastro-enterostomy following surgical intervention.

Gastroduodenal fistula, which is rare, may follow severe duodenal ulceration and produce symptoms only of the underlying disease. Treatment is directed to the cause.

Gastrobiliary fistula, usually secondary to cholelithiasis, is also rare, and recognition follows the presence of air in the biliary tree. Cholecystectomy may be required.

Gastrojejuno-colic fistula is of serious significance and generally follows anastomotic ulceration as a late result of gastro-enterostomy or partial gastrectomy for duodenal ulcer. Cancer of the stomach or colon may occasionally be responsible.

The clinical picture is one of severe diarrhoea and marked loss of weight with occasional true faecal vomiting. The cachexia and diarrhoea, which may prove fatal in a few months, are not due to the direct entry of food into the colon but to gastroenteritis resulting from the presence of colonic contents in the small intestine. The lesion is demonstrated most satisfactorily by a barium enema. Treatment necessitates excision of the fistula together with an adequate gastrectomy and closure of the colonic opening. In severely ill patients a preliminary proximal colostomy may be necessary to halt the diarrhoea. If the fistula is due to a malignant lesion, gastric and colonic resection as a curative or palliative procedure may be performed.

Gastrocolic fistula is usually due to malignant disease in the stomach or colon, more rarely to inflammation such as diverticulitis, or gastric ulcer. The clinical features and management are similar to those of a gastrojejuno-colic fistula.

Duodenal fistula. This may also be external or internal.

An *external duodenal fistula* is more common than a gastric one. It may result from injury to the intestine in cholecystectomy, right hemicolectomy or nephrectomy, but is more likely to occur from rupture of the duodenal stump five to ten days after a Polya type partial gastrectomy and is the commonest cause of death after this operation. Imperfect closure of the divided duodenum or afferent loop obstruction is responsible. The clinical picture and management follow the principles outlined under external gastric fistula.

An *internal duodenal fistula* may communicate with stomach, jejunum, colon or gall-bladder, the latter being the most common and caused by cholelithiasis. A gall-stone may pass through a fistula into the first part of the duodenum and obstruct the intestine distally—the condition of gall-stone ileus. Treatment of such fistulae is not generally necessary but may be that of the underlying cause.

INFLAMMATION

Acute gastritis

This occurs commonly after the ingestion of irritant food or drink, particularly alcohol and aspirin. It may follow the accidental or purposeful swallowing of corrosives, and if not immediately fatal from perforation or haemorrhage may be followed by stricture formation. Occasionally blood-borne infection from disease elsewhere, such as pneumonia, may be responsible, and rarely an acute *phlegmonous* type, due to streptococcal, staphylococcal or coliform organisms, may occur with abscess formation.

The clinical picture of anorexia, epigastric pain and vomiting may be confused with other acute abdominal disease and diagnosis depends on an accurate history. The simple forms are self-limiting and respond to initial fasting followed by a bland diet. Gentle gastric lavage may be of value in the corrosive form but caution must be exercised. In the infectious and phelgmonous types antibiotics should be used.

Chronic gastritis

The *non-specific* form is more often encountered and may be primary or secondary. The former may exhibit an atrophic or hypertrophic gastric mucosa and is frequently only diagnosed on gastroscopy. It is more usual in older patients whose symptoms resemble those of a peptic ulcer. Haemorrhage may occur and be severe enough to require emergency surgery. The uncomplicated case should be treated with antacids and a gastric regime. The secondary type occurs in conjuction with benign or malignant ulcer and may be associated with pernicious anaemia; the atrophic form may be a precancerous lesion.

The *specific* forms of chronic gastritis are extremely rare. A gumma or a tuberculous ulcer may resemble radiologically a peptic or cancerous ulcer; the diagnosis may be confirmed by biopsy at endoscopy.

Acute dilatation of the stomach

Improved pre-operative and post-operative management has rendered this condition uncommon. It is a localised form of paralytic ileus which occasionally occurs after pelvic or biliary operations—seldom those on the stomach—and also may follow spinal injuries, the application of plaster casts and urinary retention. The stomach, which contains air and gastric secretions, may become very large and occupy most of the peritoneal cavity.

Clinically it is recognised a day or two after operation or other trauma by abdominal distension, hiccup, vomiting and the signs of shock. If untreated, progression to severe dehydration and death is fairly rapid. Treatment is by immediate gastric aspiration with fluid and electrolyte replacement.

Chronic duodenal ileus

This is an uncommon condition of recurrent dilatation of the duodenum thought, in some instances, to be caused by compression by the superior mesenteric artery. The symptoms of upper abdominal distension and bilious vomiting may be relieved by the prone position. A barium meal demonstrates a dilated duodenum without a definite cause of obstruction. Treatment is mainly conservative by gastric aspiration, and only occasionally, is surgery indicated, a duodeno-jejunostomy then being performed.

Volvulus of the stomach

This may be partial or complete, and usually occurs in a direction at right angles to the long axis of the organ. The partial form is associated with an hour-glass stomach or extragastric adhesions, and may occasionally be caused by a tumour. In either form a diaphragmatic hernia may accompany the condition.

The clinical picture is one of upper abdominal colicky pain, vomiting and distension. The diagnosis is confirmed by a barium meal. Treatment should be directed to the underlying cause. Fixation of an excessively mobile stomach by temporary gastrostomy is only rarely necessary.

Diverticula

Gastric. These are occasionally found on the lesser or greater curvature and seldom give rise to any symptoms or complications. Recognised radiologically their importance lies in simulating an ulcer crater, and final diagnosis may depend on gastroscopy. Excision is seldom required.

Duodenal. *Primary duodenal diverticula* occur on the mesenteric border as a protrusion of mucosa and submucosa through the muscle wall at the point of entry of the blood-vessels and are probably the result of a congenital weakness. The second portion of the duodenum is most commonly affected, particularly adjacent to the ampulla of Vater. The opening is wide and complications are few.

Usually they are symptomless and recognised only on radiological examination. It is unwise to ascribe dyspeptic symptoms to their presence as co-existing peptic ulceration or cholelithiasis may easily be overlooked. Occasionally they may become infected or enlarge to produce biliary or pancreatic duct obstruction. In general, surgical treatment should be avoided, but rarely excision may be indicated. *Secondary duodenal diverticula* are more common than the primary variety and are found in relation to the scarring of a chronic duodenal ulcer in the first portion of the duodenum. They seldom become large and treatment is directed to the underlying disease.

PEPTIC ULCER

Both acute and chronic forms occur, the latter being more common.

Aetiology

Acute

This type of ulcer may arise in the course of general infections through a blood stream spread, may be associated with toxic states, such as uraemia, or may follow acute stress as in severe burns where an increase in the adrenocorticotrophic hormone occurs with a raised uropepsin and hydrochloric acid output. This may be responsible for a stress ulcer in the second part of the duodenum or, more commonly, for acute lesions. Vascular thrombosis and emboli involving the submucosal vessels have been suggested as possible causes, and gastric irritants, such as aspirin and alcohol, have been clearly indicated as being responsible.

Chronic

The exact aetiology is unknown, but the following factors are important:

1. Hyperacidity
2. Size of parietal cell mass
3. Atrophic gastritis
4. Genetic factors
5. Pancreatic tumour and multiple endocrine syndrome.

There is an increased number of parietal cells in many individuals with duodenal ulceration and excessive stimulation of these cells can occur with resultant hyperacidity. The latter may be neurogenic in origin or the parietal cells may be stimulated to produce excess acid by activity of the antral hormone gastrin. Fried and spicy food, spirits, irregular meals and long periods of fasting result in hyperacidity from this source. Genetic factors play a limited role in aetiology and it has been demonstrated that those with blood group O are more liable to duodenal ulceration than individuals in other groups. In addition a mucopolysaccharide may be missing from the gastric juice and saliva in patients with a duodenal ulcer. The relapse rate is also greater after medical or surgical management in those with blood group O who are non-secretors. The rare non-insulin-secreting islet-cell tumour of the pancreas may be responsible for excess hyperacidity and severe recurrent ulceration (p. 267). In addition to the Zollinger-Ellison syndrome a cause of duodenal ulcer may lie in an adenoma in more than one gland, such as in the pituitary, thyroid, parathyroid or adrenal cortex—the 'multiple endocrine syndrome'.

In gastric ulcer there is usually diminished acidity and a decrease in the size of the parietal cell mass. The state of the gastric mucosa is important in the aetiology of gastric ulceration. Diminished mucosal resistance may be followed by a spreading gastritis. The situation of most craters along the main food pathway in the stomach suggests that mechanical trauma to this atrophic mucosa may cause ulceration. Pyloric obstruction has been suggested as a possible cause of gastric ulcer and an alternative view postulates that there is a reflux of duodenal juices with antral gastritis and subsequent ulceration. In some instances hepatic cirrhosis is associated with both gastric and duodenal ulcer. Drug therapy with phenylbutazone and indomethacin can also cause gastric ulcers.

Pathology

Acute

The majority occur in the stomach and are less commonly encountered surgically than the chronic form. The whole stomach may be affected and the lesions are usually multiple. In the duodenum the first part is mainly involved. The ulcers are frequently small in outline, involve only mucosa and submucosa, and usually heal without any obvious scarring.

Chronic

The site is remarkably constant, more than 90 per cent being found on the lesser curvature of the stomach from the gastro-oesophageal junction to within 3 cm of the pylorus, or in the first part of the duodenum. Extension to anterior and posterior gastric surfaces may occur, but benign ulceration of the greater curvature of the stomach is less usual. Gastric ulcers are generally solitary, but duodenal ulcers may be situated on both anterior and posterior walls.

The *gross appearance* varies in stomach and duodenum. The gastric ulcer is round, or if extending to the anterior and posterior walls may be saddle-shaped. It is usually 0.5 to 1.5 cm in diameter, although ulcers 5 cm in width are occasionally seen. It is larger than the duodenal ulcer, which is rarely more than 1 cm across and often oval. Both present a punched-out appearance in the fully active state, with surrounding indurated and oedematous margins and a sloughing base. Thickening of the subserous layer over the lesion occurs, and at operation red stippling may be produced by rubbing the peritoneum. The adjacent lymph nodes are often enlarged.

The *histological picture* is one of chronic inflammatory change. Destruction of the muscle coat is usual and the wall contains a surrounding zone of fibrous tissue infiltrated with polymorphs and lymphocytes in which the vessels exhibit endarteritis obliterans. The cavity contains necrotic material, which forms the floor of the ulcer, and considerable distortion of epithelium is apparent at the ulcer margin.

End result

Chronic *gastric* ulcers may heal with adequate therapy. Scarring may follow and occasionally produces an hour-glass deformity. Large ulcers on the lesser curvature either fail to heal or easily break down because of the close attachment of the mucosa to the stomach wall at this site, unlike the loosely attached and abundant folds of the greater curvature. Posterior ulcers may become adherent to the pancreas with subsequent **penetration** of that organ. **Perforation** occurs more commonly with anterior ulcers although this may take place into the lesser sac from a posterior ulcer. **Haemorrhage** results from erosion of the wall of a blood-vessel lying in the ulcer bed; this may be a small intra-

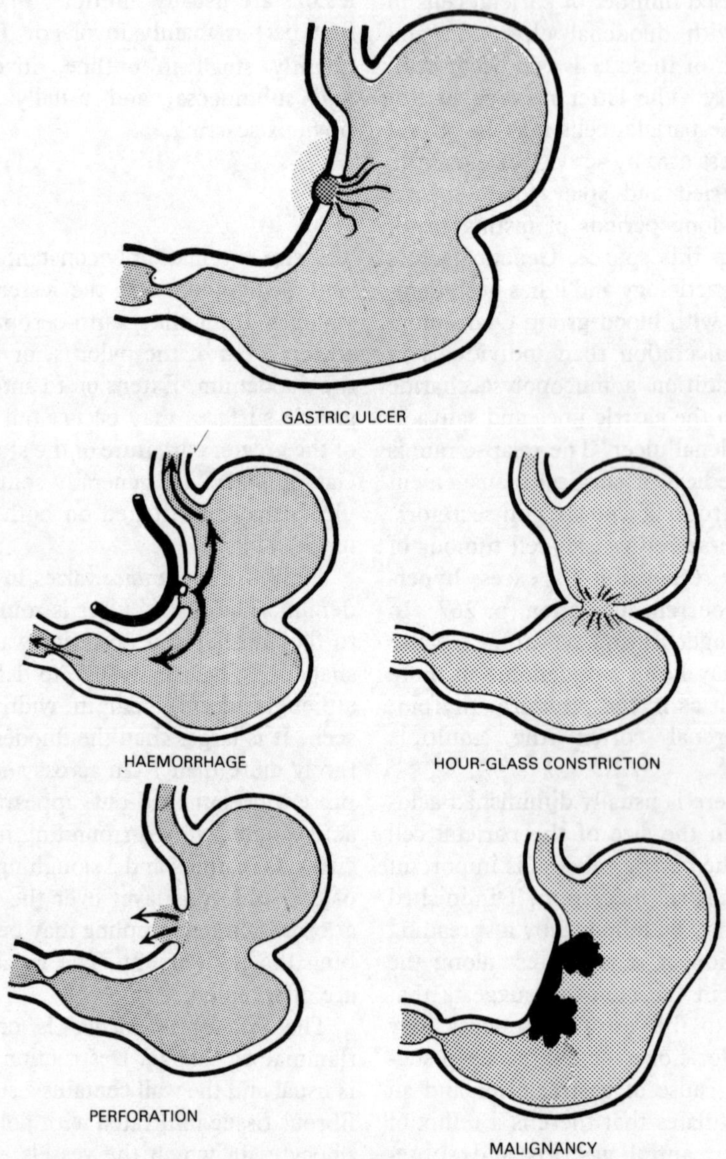

Fig. 13.2 Gastric ulcer and complications

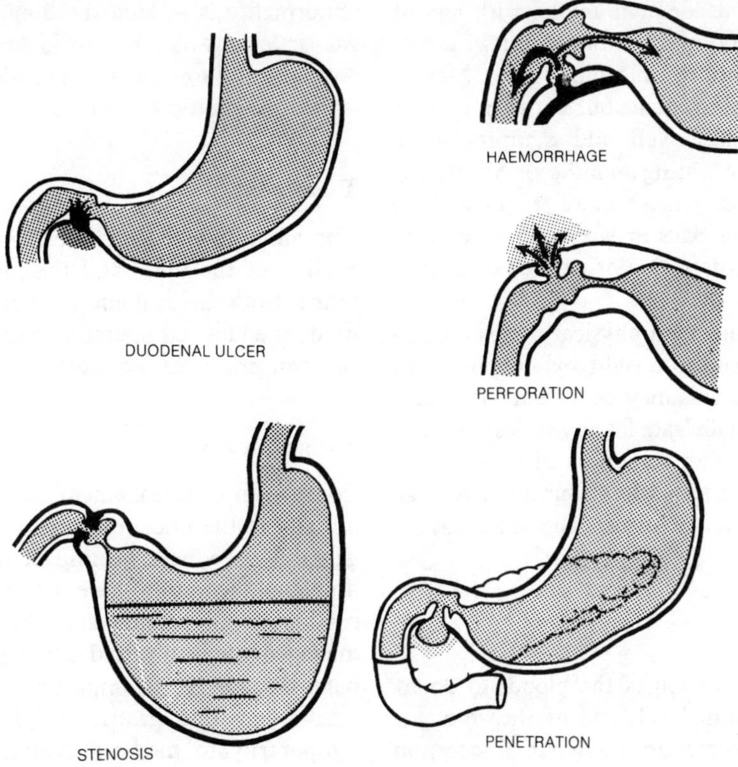

Fig. 13.3 Duodenal ulcer and complications

mural vessel or an adjacent larger artery such as the left gastric or splenic. Gastric ulcers may undergo malignant change (Fig. 13.2).

Chronic *duodenal* ulcers differ in one important respect; malignant change never occurs. Severe haemorrhage sometimes follows erosion of the gastroduodenal artery in a posterior ulcer which can also penetrate the pancreas. Anterior ulcers may perforate, and either type may produce **duodenal stenosis** by their subsequent healing (Fig. 13.3).

Clinical features

Approximately 10 per cent of the adult male population are affected by peptic ulceration. The male incidence is higher, the proportion being 3:2 for gastric ulcer and 10:1 for duodenal ulcer. Duodenal ulcers are three to four times as common as gastric ulcers and most occur between the ages of 30 and 40 years, a decade or so earlier than gastric ulcers. In about 20 per cent of the latter a duodenal ulcer is or has been present, and in almost all instances it precedes the gastric lesion.

The history is very important and the diagnosis may often be made on it alone. Periodic epigastric pain occurs after meals, discomfort from a gastric ulcer being noted half to one hour after food whilst the stomach is still full, gradually passing off as the organ empties, or relieved by vomiting. In a duodenal ulcer a longer post-prandial interval of two to three hours often exists before pain is apparent, and it may then occur immediately before the next meal. Both food and alkalis relieve the pain initially, although relief is greater in a duodenal than in a gastric ulcer. Involvement of the pancreas may produce backache which can mistakenly be attributed to an orthopaedic lesion. Nocturnal pain, at times sufficient to wake the patient from sleep, is often a feature of a duodenal ulcer. Flatulent dyspepsia may be the main symptom and aggravation by a fatty diet will simulate gall-bladder disease. The appetite generally remains good, but fear of the pain may prevent adequate intake with loss of weight. Lassitude and malaise may occur with secondary anaemia from chronic blood loss. Mental irritability is often prominent, but between attacks the patient is usually well and symptom-free. Remissions, initially lasting months or years, become shorter and the attacks more frequent. The latter may persist for days or weeks and are often related to dietary indiscretion or periods of intense worry or strain.

On examination the main physical sign is tenderness in the epigastrium or right hypochondrium, but between attacks this may be absent. The general condition is usually satisfactory unless complications ensue. Although some loss of weight may be apparent the reverse is often found when large quantities of milk have formed the mainstay of treatment.

Investigations

These include examination of the blood, to determine the haemoglobin level, and of the stool for occult blood. Basal secretion and maximal secretion tests (p. 154) are not required in all patients with peptic ulcer, but should be undertaken if a Zollinger-Ellison syndrome is suspected or in recurrent ulceration following previous ulcer surger. Gastrin assay is performed for a suspected Zollinger-Ellison syndrome or where there is concomitant hyperparathyroidism or other endocrine tumour.

Barium meal examination may establish the diagnosis. In a gastric ulcer a definite niche or crater may be apparent with localised tenderness, perhaps an associated notch on the greater curvature due to spasm, or the organic obstruction of an hour-glass stomach seen. In early or healing ulcers distortion of the mucosal pattern may be the only sign. The lesion may at times be best demonstrated by the persistence of a flake of barium when the stomach has emptied. Duodenal ulcers are generally more difficult to outline, but increased peristalsis and rapid emptying of the stomach are usual. A small crater may occasionally be demonstrated. Other typical changes include failure of filling of the duodenal bulb, or a trefoil deformity produced by pre-and post-stenotic diverticula.

Fibreoptic endoscopy is essential if a gastric ulcer is present and is also advisable if the duodenal abnormality is of long-standing duration, as small gastric lesions may be overlooked radiologically. A 4-quadrant biopsy of a gastric ulcer and cytological brushings should be obtained.

Treatment

The aims involved include the relief of pain, the healing of the ulcer and the prevention of recurrence. Both medical and surgical measures may be used, and close co-operation between physician and surgeon produces the most satisfactory results.

Medical treatment

Conservative management should be employed initially in the uncomplicated case and if adequate generally produces healing of the acute ulcer. In duodenal ulceration there is usually a natural clinical history of healing and chronic ulcers can be managed medically without the danger of malignant disease. It is important to remember that small ulcerating gastric neoplasms may respond temporarily to medical treatment and that their diagnosis must be established. Mild cases of duodenal ulceration may be adequately treated by antacids, regular meals and the avoidance of inappropriate food, alcohol and smoking. More severe symptoms can be abated and chronic ulcers healed by a course of H_2-receptor antagonist treatment such as cimetidine. The usual dosage is 400 mg b.d. for a period of six to eight weeks. A similar regime may be employed in the treatment of gastric ulcer. Alternatively carbenoxolone 50–100 mg t.d.s. for four to six weeks is a well-recognised method of treating the latter condition. Fluid retention may occur with the higher dosage and the drug should be prescribed with care when hypertension or cardiac failure are present. Potassium loss may follow and potassium supplements may be required. Radiological or endoscopic follow up of treatment is unnecessary in duodenal ulceration, but should be undertaken at monthly intervals until healing is complete in gastric lesions.

Surgical treatment

A number of large chronic gastric ulcers fail to heal, or break down fairly rapidly despite adequate therapy, and it is unwise to persist in medical treatment unless surgery is contraindicated for other general reasons. Although duodenal ulcers heal with proper care, failure to relieve the underlying stress may result in recurrence and the choice lies between long-term H_2-receptor therapy or surgery. The effects of such prolonged medical treatment are not yet fully known and surgery is usually to be preferred.

Patients with multiple chronic gastric ulcers or combined gastric and duodenal ulcers are best treated surgically. Ulcers in the prepyloric region and on the greater curvature are likely to be malignant, and for these and others where malignancy cannot be satisfactorily excluded operation should be advised. Both gastric and duodenal ulcers are liable to the complications of haemorrhage, perforation and stenosis, and in the case of gastric ulcer to malignancy, and surgery is then required.

The most satisfactory surgical treatment of a *gastric* ulcer is partial gastrectomy by the Billroth I type in which a gastro-duodenal anastomosis is performed (Fig. 13.5). Partial gastrectomy distal to the ulcer, when the latter is high and penetrating, may be employed and will usually result in healing. Prepyloric ulcers often being associated with gastric hyperacidity may be treated by vagotomy. The latter operation is also performed for more proximal lesions, but the ulcer requires careful biopsy both at surgery and endoscopically on follow-up as it is not removed. The results are not as good as after partial gastrectomy, but the poor-risk patient might gain sufficient benefit to justify the simpler procedure.

The procedure of choice in the surgical treatment of a duodenal ulcer is vagotomy. Division of the vagus nerve abolishes the neurogenic production of acid and slows gastric motility. The night acid secretion is abolished and food is retained for a longer period in the stomach, further reducing the hyperchlorhydria. Truncal or selective vagotomy may be performed, the latter retaining the hepatic branch of the anterior vagus and the coeliac branch of the posterior vagus. Both operations require a drainage procedure, either pyloroplasty or gastro-enterostomy to prevent stasis. Pyloroplasty preserves the duodenal inhibitory mechanism and avoids some of the nutritional problems of protein and fat malabsorption associated with a

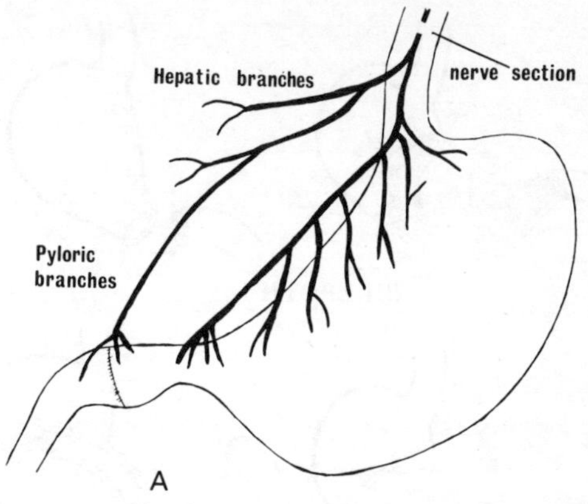

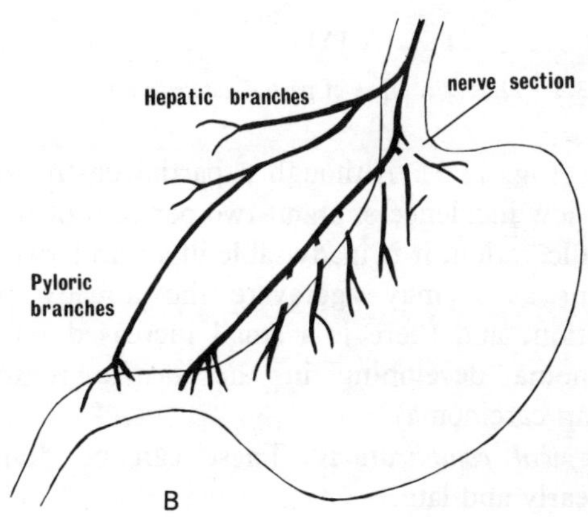

Fig. 13.4 **A.** Truncal vagotomy. **B.** Proximal gastric vagotomy (highly selective vagotomy).

blind loop. Proximal gastric vagotomy (Fig. 13.4) preserves the antral nerve supply and obviates the need for drainage in the absence of pyloric obstruction. The incidence of dumping, vomiting and diarrhoea is greatly reduced in this operation, which is to be preferred at the present time, but a small risk of lesser curve necrosis exists. Following vagotomy a recurrent ulcer rate of about 6–10 per cent is encountered. The efficacy of a vagotomy can be ascertained post-operatively by the insulin test meal, whereby there is a complete lack of acid response to the injection of insulin. Persistent diarrhoea can be helped by the elimination of roughage in the diet, the restriction of fluids and the administration of antispasmodics, sedatives and codeine phosphate. Alternative operations, usually with a lower recurrent ulcer rate, are truncal vagotomy and antrectomy, and a Polya type partial gastrec-

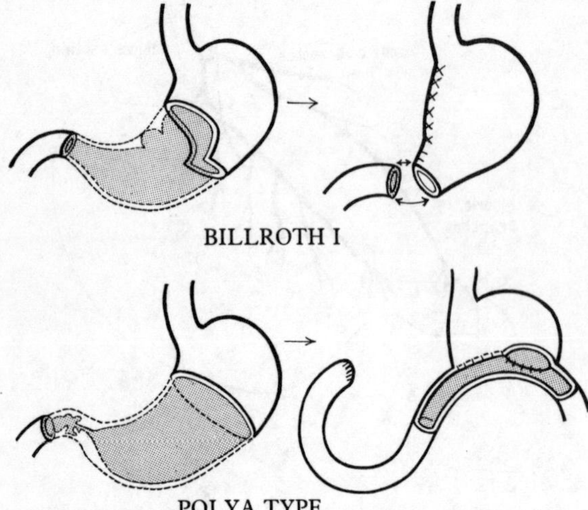

Fig. 13.5 The main types of partial gastrectomy

tomy (Fig. 13.5). Although a partial gastrectomy has a low incidence of about two per cent of recurrent ulceration, it is inadvisable in an underweight patient as it may aggravate the already poor nutrition, and there is a small increased risk of carcinoma developing in the gastric remnant (stump carcinoma)

Surgical complications. These can be divided into early and late.

Early problems include gastric and duodenal fistulae, gastric retention, haemorrhage and pancreatitis, the last being due to injury to the gland in operating on a deep penetrating ulcer. It is not common. The most important complication is a *duodenal fistula* due to leakage of the stump after a Polya type gastrectomy. It can be prevented by expert technique but is the commonest cause of mortality after a gastrectomy. Careful duodenal closure and avoidance of afferent loop obstruction are important. Clinically there is severe pain in the right hypochondrium several days post-operatively, associated with rigidity and pyrexia. Re-exploration is essential for adequate drainage and suction is applied. Intravenous support is required and spontaneous closure usually results.

Gastric retention with nausea and fullness four to five days post-operatively may be noted. It may be caused by oedema of the stoma and aggravated by atony following vagotomy. An organic lesion may be present due to an anastomotic leak or a haematoma and this can be differentiated from a functional one by a gastrografin swallow.

Continued naso-gastric suction and supportive treatment usually suffice but may take several weeks to resolve. Post-operative *haemorrhage* may occur within 24 hours or after several days, usually from a technical error. Blood replacement is generally sufficient.

Late complications include recurrent ulceration, the dumping syndrome, anaemia, malnutrition and diarrhoea. *Recurrent ulceration* is found in about 10 per cent of patients following a vagotomy and drainage, but in only about two per cent who have had a partial gastrectomy for a duodenal ulcer; it seldom occurs when the original lesion was a gastric ulcer. It resembles the original chronic peptic ulcer and is usually situated in the efferent jejunal loop about 1 cm. from the anastomosis. It is subject to the same complications as peptic ulcer elsewhere and may perforate into the colon, producing a gastro-jejuno-colic fistula. The majority occur within two years of operation and the diagnosis may be deduced from the history of pain which is often more severe than that of the original ulcer and less liable to remission. Vomiting is common and haemorrhage not infrequent. A localised tender area is often present just below and to the left of the umbilicus. Endoscopy usually demonstrates the lesion. Radiology is less reliable due to previous operative scarring. Healing can be obtained in most cases with cimetidine but recurrence is frequent and further surgery often necessary. If vagotomy had previously been performed, antrectomy or a partial gastrectomy should be undertaken, but if partial gastrectomy had been carried out, vagotomy is the correct treatment. The possibility of the Zollinger-Ellison syndrome (p. 267) should be considered, and serum gastrin levels determined if necessary.

The **post-gastrectomy syndrome** includes both dumping and bilious vomiting and is found in 5 to 10 per cent of patients. Dumping may be either of the early or of the late type. *Late dumping* occurs two or three hours after a meal. The quick emptying of the stomach and the large absorptive area of the jejunum produce a rapid rise in blood sugar which over-stimulates the islet cells of the pancreas producing over-correction and hypoglycaemia.

Hunger, tremor, weakness and giddiness occur, which respond rapidly to glucose. The patient should be instructed to carry sweets or chocolate, which will cut short an attack if taken when symptoms arise.

Early dumping is more common and important. It occurs with or shortly after a meal and produces epigastric distension, weakness, faintness, palpitations, sweating and sometimes diarrhoea. Each attack may last half to three-quarters of an hour and be exaggerated by the erect position. The majority disappear in 12 to 18 months, but severe cases may persist with loss or failure to gain weight.

The cause is unknown, but is probably associated with the rapid entry of food into the jejunum, and is more pronounced after a Polya type gastrectomy. It may be related to jejunal tension exciting sympathetic reflexes or to a reflex hypoglycaemia secondary to the entry of a hypertonic solution into the jejunum. Other theories include a fall in the plasma volume as a result of a fluid shift into the jejunum, due to a hypertonic solution, and hypokalaemia.

The incidence may be lowered by a return to normal meals before leaving hospital. It may be aggravated by certain articles of diet, such as sweet dishes and milk which should be avoided at the main meal, whilst fluids should be withheld during meals and for thirty minutes before and afterwards. It is also of value to limit the amount of carbohydrates and to administer anticholinergics before meals. Symptoms can generally be controlled by dietary means.

Bilious vomiting is secondary to chronic obstruction involving the afferent loop. Distension may result in nausea, weakness, palpitations and sweating, and copious amounts of bile may be vomited. The condition may be relieved by lying down. The most satisfactory treatment in severe cases is to convert the Polya type anastomosis, in which this is generally seen, to a Billroth I type or to insert a jejunal loop between stomach and duodenum.

Acute afferent or efferent loop obstructions are occasional complications and are often related to technical faults at the time of the original operation. Steatorrhoea is rare after a Billroth I procedure but occurs after a Polya gastrectomy or vagotomy and gastro-enterostomy. Changes in pancreatic function result in malabsorption of protein and fat. Hypochromic anaemia, due to impaired iron absorption as a result of a loss of gastric acidity, is more common after a Polya type gastrectomy where the site of absorption in the duodenum is bypassed, but seldom occurs within two years of operation. It should be corrected by adequate amounts of ferrous gluconate which should be continued indefinitely and an improved diet which includes extra meat. In a small number of cases megaloblastic anaemia may follow gastrectomy. The complication of osteomalacia due to diminished calcium absorption may also be apparent in about three per cent of cases, but seldom shows within five years of operation. It is more common after a Polya procedure, is probably due to vitamin D deficiency and responds to 1000 i.u. per week of vitamin D with calcium supplements (1 to 2 g per day). Osteoporosis also occurs for unknown reasons and should be treated with 1 to 2 g calcium per day. Retrograde intussusception of jejunum into stomach may rarely follow any type of gastro-enterostomy and provides a picture of acute or chronic intestinal obstruction requiring surgical reduction.

COMPLICATIONS OF PEPTIC ULCER

1. Haemorrhage:
   - Haematemesis
   - Melaena.
2. Perforation or penetration.
3. Obstruction:
   - Duodenal stenosis
   - Hour-glass stomach.
4. Malignant change:
   - Gastric ulcers only.

Haemorrhage

Pathology

Approximately 15 to 20 per cent of peptic ulcers bleed. Haemorrhage occurs with both acute and chronic lesions and may involve the vessels of the stomach or duodenum or, in deep and penetrating ulcers, those which lie outside. Bleeding from acute ulcers is due to erosion of the gastric mucosa with exposure of the vessels in that layer. In chronic ulcers the exposed vessels are often larger and deeper, and from fixation in fibrous tissue may fail to retract. Haemorrhage is then more persistent and the prognosis more grave. Occasionally a penetrating gastric ulcer may erode the splenic artery, or a duodenal ulcer the gastroduodenal artery, causing profuse and severe bleeding unless adequately treated, and lead to rapid exsanguination and death.

Clinical features

Haemorrhage may manifest itself as *haematemesis*, that is the vomiting of blood, occasionally bright red but usually 'coffee-grounds', or by *melaena*. The former is more likely to occur in gastric ulcers, the latter in duodenal ulcers, but in severe haemorrhage even bright red blood may be passed per rectum.

A previous ulcer history is not invariable and an absence of symptoms or only mild dyspepsia may precede the attack. The clinical picture varies with the degree of blood loss. Repeated small haemorrhages are more common than a single large one and may induce a false sense of security. Minor haemorrhage in a patient whose ulcer has been bleeding occultly for several months is sometimes more serious than a major loss in a previously fit subject. In older individuals blood loss is more pronounced because atherosclerotic changes prevent contraction of the vessel and the arrest of bleeding. Pallor is generally obvious with a cold and clammy skin, and in severe cases there are signs of shock and fluid loss. Tachycardia and hypotension are important in assessing the severity of bleeding, and a diastolic pressure of 60 to 65 mm Hg indicates a moderately severe haemorrhage. Delirium due to hypoxia or dehydration may follow a major loss, whilst in the elderly signs of cardiac ischaemia may be produced. Pain, tenderness and rigidity are absent, but auscultation often reveals sounds of intestinal hurry due to the presence of blood. In the absence of obvious melaena blood may be detected on the examining finger.

Investigations

The haemoglobin level should be estimated as it may reveal the presence of a previous anaemia, but it does not immediately reflect the amount of blood loss. It may even remain normal in dehydration and, if falling, does not necessarily indicate further bleeding but merely haemodilution. In severe cases the blood urea is raised, partly due to digestion of blood and partly due to lowered glomerular filtration from hypotension. The most important investigation is fibreoptic endoscopy which will demonstrate the cause in over 90 per cent of patients. Initial saline gastric lavage may be necessary when blood clot is present. Endoscopy is more valuable than barium meal examination in superficial erosions and in the Mallory-Weiss gastric mucosal tears. It is even helpful when a known cause of bleeding may exist such as oesophageal varices, as in more than half of such patients with an acute haemorrhage the cause will lie in gastritis or in a peptic ulcer. Double contrast barium meal examination can be performed later.

Differential diagnosis

Vomiting of swallowed blood from an epistaxis or haemoptysis must be excluded. Chronic peptic ulcer is responsible in about 80 per cent of cases, but other important causes are gastric erosions due to aspirin, alcohol, prednisolone, butazolidine or indomethacin, carcinoma of the stomach, oesophageal varices, oesophagitis from a hiatus hernia and the Mallory-Weiss syndrome. Stress ulceration or multiple erosions may follow major surgical operations, trauma or grave sepsis and cause bleeding. Less common conditions include the blood dyscrasias, polyposis, ruptured aneurysm, regional enteritis, and peptic ulceration in a Meckel's diverticulum.

Treatment

Accurate diagnosis is important and should be obtained as early as possible. Hospital observation and bed rest are advisable even in minor haemorrhage. Nasogastric intubation allows assessment of continued bleeding and lavage of blood clot may be required. In severe haemorrhage, rapid blood replacement, monitored by a central venous pressure line and with a urinary catheter in position to measure output, is essential. The majority of patients can be managed by conservative medical measures which include cimetidine. Within 24 hours a light diet may be tolerated, but a careful watch should be maintained for further bleeding.

Where haemorrhage is not controlled, particularly in older patients with atherosclerotic vessels or where severe or persistent re-bleeding occurs in hospital, surgery is advisable. Concomitant perforation although uncommon is a certain indication for operation. The exact procedure will be determined by the cause. In duodenal ulceration, pyloroplasty and vagotomy with under-running of the bleeding vessel is more often performed than partial gastrectomy but in bleeding from gastric ulceration a Billroth I gastrectomy may be preferred. An alternative is to under-run the vessels leading to the ulcer and perform vagotomy and pyloroplasty. The latter may also be carried out for superficial erosions. In the Mallory-Weiss syndrome, suture of the upper gastric mucosal tear should be performed through a high gastrotomy.

Perforation

Approximately 15 per cent of chronic ulcers perforate, the majority being duodenal, and over 90 per cent are in males who are generally between the ages of 30 and 45 years. Although acute ulcers may perforate, most are chronic lesions where there is a previous dyspeptic history. Rupture is more likely at times of individual or national stress, in winter when the general health is lower, or when associated with excessive physical or mental fatigue.

The base of the ulcer, usually an anterior one, sloughs and the perforation appears. There is rapid escape of air, acid gastric contents and perhaps food with resultant peritonitis. Initially a chemical peritonitis with severe local reaction, the acid contents become neutralised within six to twelve hours by the alkaline peritoneal fluid with diminished reaction. If untreated, bacterial peritonitis follows with paralytic ileus, toxaemia, fluid and electrolyte imbalance and death. The severity and rapidity of pathological changes vary with the size of the opening, being more pronounced in gastric than in duodenal ulcers. A natural attempt may be made in some instances to seal off the opening by omentum. This is more likely to be successful in a small duodenal perforation than in a large gastric one. Rupture may occur into the lesser sac or between the layers of the lesser omentum. Temporary sealing off may be followed by infection and a subphrenic abcess with subsequent rupture into the pleura, lung or general peritoneal cavity.

Penetration usually occurs in posterior ulcers. The stomach or duodenal wall is slowly destroyed and the floor of the ulcer is then formed by adjacent structures, such as pancreas, liver, diaphragm or bowel.

Clinical features

The majority of patients give a previous history of dyspepsia, but with the onset of acute perforation are gripped with sudden epigastric pain of great severity spreading over the whole abdomen. This may be accompanied by vomiting, which is seldom frequent. Pain in one or both shoulders due to irritation of the under-surface of the diaphragm may be present. Immediate collapse is unusual and the pulse may initially be slow and the blood-pressure normal.

The patient lies supine with knees drawn up and is afraid to move. There is an anxious expression, pallor, sweating, shallow respirations, which are thoracic in type, and a characteristic scaphoid appearance of the abdomen. There is deep tenderness in the epigastrium or right iliac fossa from the tracking of fluid into the paracolic gutter, but the most important physical sign is board-like rigidity. Diminution in liver dullness due to escaped gas may be elicited. After several hours the pain decreases in severity and the general condition improves, due to neutralisation of the leaked acid. If first seen at this stage the diagnosis may be missed, but abdominal rigidity always persists and should be detected. There may also be tenderness on rectal examination. Tachycardia, pyrexia and signs of shock become apparent later with the onset of bacterial peritonitis. Vomiting and distension occur with loss of bowel sounds as a result of paralytic ileus.

In the subacute form symptoms are less severe, often of a more local nature, and accompanied by less guarding and rigidity. Symptoms of the subsequent abscess become manifest later. A penetrating ulcer most commonly involves the pancreas, the main complaint being of backache.

Investigations

Intraperitoneal gas may be demonstrated by radiography in about 70 per cent of cases, the air shadow being under the diaphragm in the sitting position or in the flank with the lateral position. Bowel distension is seen in the later stages of paralytic ileus. A mild leucocytosis is found in the early stages but with a marked rise later.

Differential diagnosis

The following conditions might initially be confused with a perforated peptic ulcer:

1. Acute gastritis.
2. Acute pancreatitis.
3. Acute high intestinal obstruction.
4. Biliary disease:
   Acute cholecystitis.
   Biliary colic.
5. Acute appendicitis.
6. Colonic perforation:
   Diverticulitis.
   Carcinoma.
7. Intrathoracic lesions:
   Cardiac infarction.
   Diaphragmatic pleurisy.
8. Referred pain:
   Tabetic crisis.
   Spinal tumour.
   Herpes zoster.

In acute gastritis, there may be a history of an ingested irritant, vomiting is marked and guarding and tenderness are slight. Acute pancreatitis is more difficult to differentiate. Pronounced and repeated vomiting, cyanosis and profound collapse may suggest the cause together with an excessively raised serum amylase although a high level may occur in perforated peptic ulcer and in cholecystitis. Acute high intestinal obstruction presents difficulties due to the absence of distension, but the colicky pains and repeated vomiting are not accompanied by abdominal rigidity; a plain radiograph may confirm an obstruction. Acute cholecystitis or biliary colic may be diagnosed by the localisation of signs to the gall-bladder region. Acute appendicitis may be simulated by a perforated duodenal ulcer, and in the absence of an ulcer history the diagnosis depends upon the site of maximum tenderness. A colonic perforation generally produces lower abdominal signs, although if the transverse colon or hepatic flexure is involved a similar picture to peptic ulcer perforation may be obtained, but the patient is generally older, dyspepsia is less marked and large bowel symptoms predominate. Cardiac infarction may be distinguished by precordial or brachial pain and pulse irregularities and should be confirmed by an electrocardiograph and laboratory enzyme studies; in diaphragmatic pleurisy pulmonary disease may be apparent and the pain and tenderness remain in the upper abdomen. Referred pain due to a spinal tumour, herpes zoster or tabetic crisis requires exclusion by careful neurological examination but is infrequent.

Prognosis

The following are the main factors concerned:

1. Age and general condition.
2. Size of perforation.
3. Duration before treatment.
4. Associated complication of haemorrhage or malignancy.

The elderly and those in poor general condition carry a worse prognosis. Gastric ulcer perforations, generally of larger diameter than duodenal ulcer perforations, are more serious due to extensive peritoneal soiling and carry twice the mortality. The duration of the perforation before treatment is the most important factor in assessing prognosis. Under 12 hours it remains good, over 24 hours it is poor. The presence of an additional complication such as haemorrhage or malignancy materially affects the gravity of the situation.

Treatment

When the diagnosis has been established analgesics can be given and gastric aspiration performed to prevent further peritoneal contamination. The latter also prevents inhalation of vomitus when anaesthesia is required. Intravenous fluids should be given when shock exists and a broad spectrum antibiotic to counteract bacterial peritonitis. *Simple closure* of the perforation is the standard treatment having the merit of speed and simplicity. *Definitive surgery* for the ulcer can be performed in fit patients with an early perforation where operation would be otherwise indicated, as in those with a long ulcer history, recurrent perforation, associated haemorrhage or malignancy. Vagotomy with or without gastric drainage following closure of the perforation is the usual procedure. Partial gastrectomy is an alternative. *Non-operative* treatment by gastric aspiration, intravenous fluids and antibiotic therapy is reserved for those who are too ill for surgery due to other causes or late diagnosis. This may be followed by an increased incidence of subphrenic or peritoneal collections, often requiring later drainage.

Duodenal (pyloric) stenosis

Pathology

The usual cause is a duodenal ulcer which has healed with cicatricial contraction but pyloric stenosis may also occur from carcinoma of the stomach. Benign tumours, pyloric hypertrophy of adults and foreign bodies are an occasional cause and rarely conditions outside the stomach such as tumours in neighbouring organs, chronic pancreatitis or perigastric adhesions. There is retention of gastric contents, gastritis, and dilatation of the stomach which may occupy most of the peritoneal cavity. The less common causes seldom produce the same degree of long-standing obstruction. The effects produced are related (*a*) to obstruction and chronic starvation and (*b*) to vomiting of gastric secretions with fluid and electrolyte imbalance. Both sodium and chloride are lost in large amounts and dehydration and metabolic alkalosis follow. Potassium depletion may also occur although the serum level may remain normal.

Clinical features

A long history of dyspepsia is generally present but pain has usually ceased; recent vomiting is the main symptom, often accompanied by anorexia and a feeling of fullness which is worse towards the end of the day. With progression of the condition the amount vomited greatly increases and large quantities of food and drink taken many hours and even days earlier are returned. Constipation is noted, and weakness, drowsiness and even tetany may follow severe biochemical changes. Gross loss of weight may show a marked resemblance to advanced malignant disease, and dehydration is evident in an inelastic skin and dry, coated tongue. Abdominal distension may be in sharp contrast to the contracted appearance, and visible peristalsis and a succussion splash may be detected. In the untreated case death follows from starvation and biochemical abnormalities.

Investigations

Plain abdominal radiography may show a large gastric fluid level but the diagnosis can be confirmed by a double contrast barium meal. Gross retention after six hours or persistence of barium in the stomach after 24 hours is indicative of duodenal stenosis. Fibreoptic endoscopy should be performed and a biopsy taken. The serum electrolytes show hypochloraemia, hypokalaemia, hyponatraemia and increased bicarbonate. A low gastric acidity is usually present due to associated gastritis. In some instances a marked anaemia may be present.

Treatment

Gastric aspiration reduces pyloric oedema and spasm, and improves both gastritis and muscle tone. Retained food debris may require gastric lavage but this should be minimal. Improvement usually takes several days. Intravenous therapy is commenced with sodium chloride and water, but when a satisfactory urinary output is obtained potassium chloride may be given. The serum electrolytes and blood urea must be monitored daily until normality is reached. Severe cases usually require control with a central venous pressure line. In most cases surgery is necessary, generally within three to four days of initial treatment. When the obstruction is removed the stomach will return to normal size and partial gastrectomy is thus generally not required. Proximal gastric vagotomy with digital dilatation of the obstruction through a gastrotomy is now practised, but truncal vagotomy and drainage is an alternative.

Hour-glass stomach

Pathology

In 90 per cent of cases a healed gastric ulcer is responsible. Other rare causes include a congenital form with constriction at the incisura, and stenosis following corrosives or resulting from a slowly growing neoplasm. Fibrosis in the submucous and mucous layers produces two pouches, the proximal usually being the larger. In about one-third of cases there is associated duodenal stenosis.

Clinical features

Women are affected 10 times as frequently as men, the majority being between 50 and 70 years. A history of previous dyspepsia is obtained but pain is absent unless the ulcer remains unhealed. The main features are repeated and copious vomiting with emaciation and loss of weight. Malignancy may be suspected, but in hour-glass stomach the course is more protracted. The diagnosis is obtained by a barium meal which demonstrates the constant contracture and typical teapot-spout deformity but endoscopy and biopsy are mandatory.

Treatment is surgical following adequate pre-operative preparation and restoration of fluid and electrolyte balance. Billroth I partial gastrectomy removes the lesion and relieves the obstruction.

TUMOURS OF THE STOMACH

Benign

Non-malignant tumours are relatively uncommon. The most usual is a *leiomyoma* arising from smooth muscle and projecting as a single swelling into the gastric lumen. Generally small, it occasionally assumes large proportions and rarely may undergo malignant change. An *adenoma* may arise from the submucous region; it has a central fibrous core and presents as a gastric polyp. Such polypi may be single or multiple, the latter requiring to be differentiated from the gastric polyposis of hypertrophic gastritis. Malignant change may supervene but is less likely than in the colon or rectum. Other less common benign tumours include lipomas, fibromas and angiomas.

Benign tumours present with bleeding or obstruction, or an intussuscepting tumour may cause intermittent pain. The diagnosis may be noted on a double contrast barium meal but must be confirmed by endoscopy and biopsy. Adequate local removal of the tumour is sufficent when the benign nature is ascertained by immediate histology. Partial gastrectomy is preferable for tumours of the antrum.

CARCINOMA OF THE STOMACH

Pathology

This is one of the most common malignant tumours in the body with a marked tendency to early spread and dissemination. The aetiology is unknown, but the following are important predisposing factors:

1. Gastric ulcer.
2. Atrophic gastritis.
3. Genetic factors.

The number of malignant lesions preceded by a benign gastric ulcer is not fully established, but a small number appear to undergo neoplastic change. Cancer is believed to develop more commonly in association with atrophic gastritis, both conditions being accompanied by achlorhydria. The latter is also a feature of pernicious anaemia, where the incidence of gastric carcinoma is three times greater than in normal individuals of the same age. Benign polypi arising in an atrophic mucosa associated with achlorhydria appear to have a cancerous relationship. Genetic factors have been considered important; a higher frequency of gastric malignancy has been demonstrated in those possessing blood group A. It is particularly common in Japan and the Far East.

Carcinoma is sited predominantly in the prepyloric region of the lesser curvature. A small proportion arise higher on the lesser curvature or in the fundus, whilst 70 per cent of ulcers on the greater curvature are malignant. Three main macroscopic forms occur: (1) ulcerative, (2) polypoidal and (3) infiltrative (Fig. 13.6).

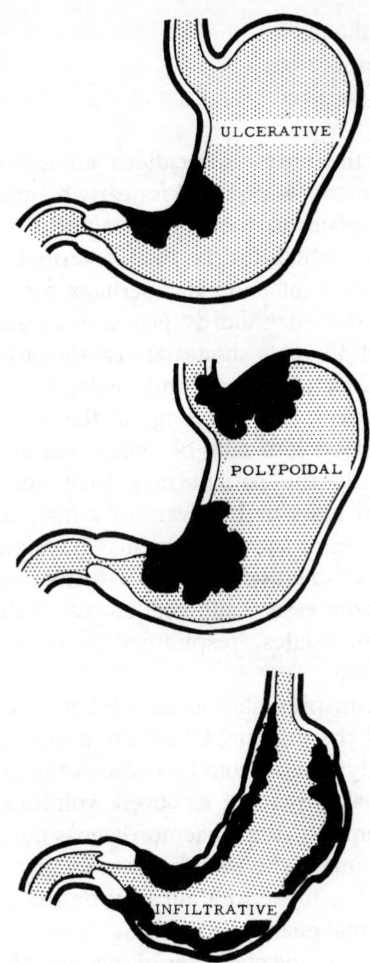

Fig. 13.6 The types of gastric carcinoma

The *ulcerative* lesion is the commonest, and has the typical heaped-up edge of a malignant ulcer. Although it may spread in both submucous and subserous layers, it is prone to penetrate deeply and involve the serosa at an early stage.

The *polypoidal* type is a proliferative tumour arising from the mucosa and forming a bulky projection into the gastric lumen. It may reach a large size before necrosis and ulceration of the mucous membrane occurs. Colloid degeneration is particularly liable to take place, but lymphatic spread is later than in the other two forms.

The *infiltrative* form has a marked tendency to extend throughout the stomach with thickening of the whole of the wall. The mucosa is only involved at a later stage, but the capacity of the organ is considerably reduced, the condition being known as a 'leather-bottle stomach'.

The main histological picture is of an adenocarcinoma with some glandular formation. Colloid degeneration may be observed. Anaplasia is a feature of the infiltrative tumour, but some forms of leather-bottle stomach may be accompanied by marked fibrosis.

Spread

Spread of the disease occurs by the following routes:

1. Local
2. Lymphatic
3. Transperitoneal
4. Blood stream.

Local spread occurs in the stomach wall, particularly in the submucous layer. The gastro-oesophageal junction is no bar to extension and invasion of the oesophagus from fundal tumours is common. Direct spread distally is less common, but the first centimetre of the duodenum may be involved. Penetration through the wall and involvement of adjacent structures such as peritoneum, pancreas, omentum, spleen, liver, small and large intestine is frequent.

Lymphatic spread in general follows the line of the main blood-vessels (Fig. 13.7,A). Pyloric tumours spread to glands at the gastro-duodenal junction, whilst lesser curvature growths involve the left gastric group. Fundal tumours and those of the upper part of the greater curvature spread to glands in the hilum of the spleen. Growths of the lower part of the greater curvature metastasise to the right gastro-epiploic and subpyloric groups. Glands in the porta hepatis may also be involved from pyloric lesions, and in all cases the coeliac nodes may be affected. Extension by the thoracic duct to the left supraclavicular group may follow.

Transperitoneal spread occurs when the serous coat of the stomach becomes involved and results in seedling metastatic deposits on visceral and parietal peritoneum. Ascites may follow in which malignant cells may be found. In about 3 per cent of cases involvement of the ovaries either by direct implantation or through the peritoneal lymphatics

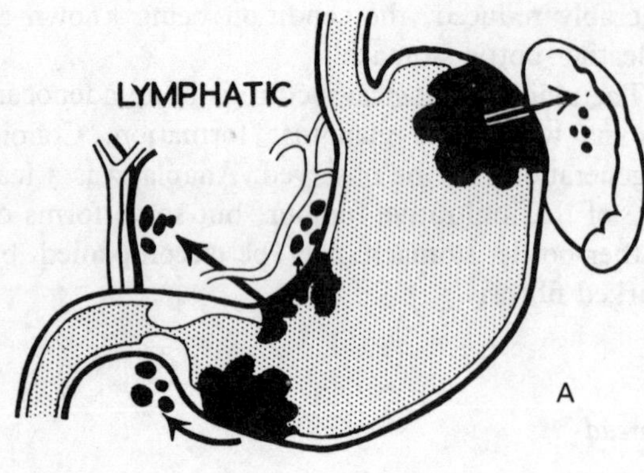

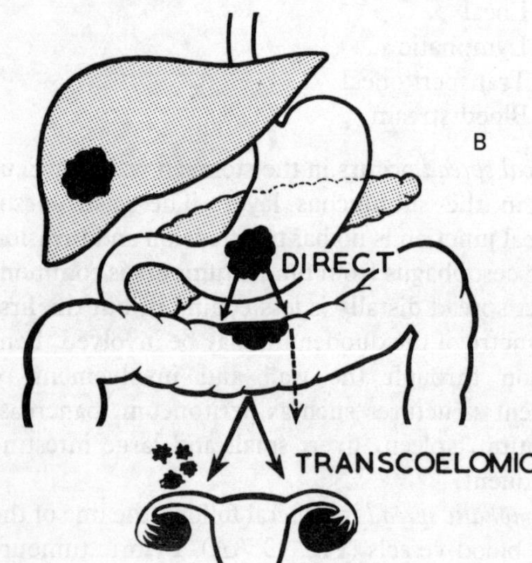

Fig. 13.7 The spread of gastric carcinoma. **A.** Lymphatic to lesser curvature, pancreatico-duodenal and splenic nodes. **B.** Intra-abdominal to liver, colon and pelvic organs.

produces a large tumour, often considered the primary lesion —Krukenberg tumour (Fig. 13.7,B).

Bloodstream spread via the portal system to the liver may take place with later involvement of other sites such as lungs, brain and bone.

Clinical features

Men are affected more frequently than women in the proportion of 3 to 1, and the commonest age group is between 40 and 70 years. It may present in the following ways:

1. Insidious.
2. Complicated.
3. Peptic ulcer.

When the onset is insidious an accurate and detailed history is essential for early diagnosis. The main complaint may be due to minor disturbances of function which can be easily overlooked, but a recent history of anorexia, perhaps for a specific article of diet, or mild dyspepsia in a patient over the age of 40 years should arouse the suspicion of cancer. General malaise and lassitude, or pallor, breathlessness and swelling of the ankles from chronic blood loss may be presenting symptoms. Occasionally the patient may have observed an abdominal mass or be aware of a marked loss in weight. The initial symptoms may be related to the presence of metastases with a history of recent painless progressive jaundice, increased abdominal girth from ascites, respiratory or even cerebral secondaries.

The main presentation may follow the complications of the tumour. Obstruction may be recognised by dysphagia from blockage of the cardia due to a fundal growth or as severe vomiting from a pyloric tumour. Acute haemorrhage is not common in carcinoma of the stomach, but sudden abdominal pain due to perforation may be the first indication of malignancy.

A change in the character of the pain of a patient with a known or suspected gastric ulcer is suspicious. It may become more constant, no longer relieved by food or alkali and remissions may be lost.

Physical examination may reveal nothing abnormal in the early stages. With more advanced disease pallor or an irregular abdominal mass due to the primary tumour or metastases may be evident. Visible peristalsis may be seen in pyloric obstruction, but seldom a succussion splash because of the rapidity of the disease. Gross cachexia and dehydration are late signs, whilst jaundice and ascites are indicative of disseminated disease. Palpable ovarian tumours (Krukenberg), metastatic deposits around the umbilicus through retrograde spread along the lymphatics of the ligamentum teres, an enlarged left supraclavicular node (Troisier's sign), or unilateral lower limb oedema from deep thrombosis (Trousseau's sign) are other late manifestations. Rectal examination may reveal nodular deposits in the rectovesical or recto-uterine pouch.

Investigations

Estimation of the haemoglobin level may indicate a secondary anaemia, and examination of the stools show the presence of occult blood. Barium meal examination may show a filling defect or ulcer crater and the double-contrast method often detects early mucosal lesions. Gastroscopy confirms the radiological findings and allows biopsy and brush cytology. Gastric acid studies generally reveal achlorhydria and perhaps blood and gastric retention. Radiography of the chest should be performed to exclude pulmonary metastases. Malignant cells may be discovered on examination of the ascitic fluid, whilst laparoscopy may reveal widespread dissemination.

Treatment

Surgical removal is the main form of treatment; radiotherapy only offers doubtful palliation. Treatment may be considered as follows:

1. Radical:
   - Gastrectomy.
   - Oesophago-gastrectomy.
2. Palliative:
   - Short-circuit or gastrectomy.
   - Radiotherapy.
   - Symptomatic.

A laparotomy should be undertaken unless there is definite evidence of widespread dissemination; many tumours deemed inoperable from their bulk can be removed.

The *radical* procedure is only feasible when the disease is localised with or without adjacent glandular involvement. Lesions of the pylorus require partial gastrectomy with removal of the omenta and draining lymph nodes. Involvement of the body of the stomach is treated by total gastrectomy and splenectomy to allow *en-bloc* removal of the hilar nodes. Fundal lesions necessitate an oesophago-gastrectomy. Vitamin B_{12} therapy is required when total gastrectomy is performed.

Palliative surgical measures are often of value. Obstruction may be relieved by gastro-enterostomy or oesophago-jejunostomy or by the insertion of a tube for fundal growths. Partial gastrectomy by removing most of the lesion may allow a further few months of comfort with a less unpleasant demise from metastases. Radiotherapy in the form of radioactive implants or external high-voltage therapy may palliate fundal tumours obstructing the cardia, but is of no value more distally. Gastrostomy should be avoided. Combination chemotherapy using 5-fluorouracil, Adriamycin and mitomycin C offers palliation in some cases, but its value has to be balanced against the toxic side effects.

The prognosis varies with the depth of penetration of the gastric wall. Superficial or early gastric cancer, confined to the mucosa and submucosa, may carry a 70–75 per cent five-year survival. This figure falls to 25 per cent when there is diffuse gastric involvement and is no better than 10 per cent when the nodes are implicated.

SARCOMA OF THE STOMACH

This is rare compared with carcinoma and constitutes about 1 per cent of all gastric neoplasms. There are two main types: (1) lymphosarcoma and (2) leiomyosarcoma.

Lymphosarcomas arise from lymphoid tissue in the submucous layer and may represent a local form of a more generalised reticulosis. They infiltrate locally and are composed of small round cells with little stroma.

Leiomyosarcoma arise from the smooth muscle of the muscularis, are composed of spindle-shaped cells, and grow more slowly. Metastases in both instances are by the bloodstream and lymphatics.

Clinically there is close resemblance to carcinoma, symptoms being produced when superficial necrosis and ulceration of the lesion takes place. Treatment consists of radical excision, the prognosis in leiomyosarcomas being more favourable than in carcinoma.

TUMOURS OF THE DUODENUM

Both benign and malignant tumours are rare. The **adenoma** is the least uncommon of the former and is usually recognised as a polyp on barium meal examination or on endoscopy. The main primary malignant tumour is an **adenocarcinoma** which may block the alimentary or biliary tracts, perforate or bleed. Diagnosis may be suspected by a barium meal which demonstrates a narrow stricture and confirmed by endoscopy and biopsy. Treatment is directed towards radical removal or palliative short-circuit.

FURTHER READING

Dykes, P. W. and Keighley, M. R. B. (1981). *Gastrointestinal Haemorrhage*. Bristol: Wright.

Johnson, D. (1980). Treatment of peptic ulcer and its complications. In *Recent Advances in Surgery*. 10. Ed. Taylor, S. Edinburgh: Churchill Livingstone.

14

Small intestine and appendix

SMALL INTESTINE

Developmental anomalies

Intestinal atresia

Congenital atresia of the intestine is an uncommon abnormality which results in complete obstruction in the majority of instances. In 40 per cent of cases the lesion lies in the duodenum (p. 155). The bowel may be occluded by a diaphragm or be represented by a fibrous cord of varying length; the segments are often multiple. The defect was originally attributed to failure of the stage of vacuolation whereby a solid mass of epithelial cells was formed into a tube. Recent investigation strongly supports the view that fibrosis develops as the result of ischaemia due to mesenteric vascular occlusion occuring *in utero*.

Symptoms commence soon after birth, vomiting of bile-stained fluid being a prominent feature. The passage of meconium is delayed, and the absence from it of swallowed epithelial cells indicate complete obstruction. The abdomen becomes progressively distended and this in the later stages may be gross. Radiographs of the abdomen show distended loops of bowel, with fluid levels, the colon being free of air.

Treatment involves replacement of fluid and electrolyte loss, which may be severe, and aspiration of the stomach by a naso-gastric tube. Early laparotomy is required, single areas of atresia are resected and anastomosis performed; multiple areas may require a short-circuiting procedure. Paralytic ileus is the most serious post-operative complication, but chest infection from aspiration of vomitus may be troublesome.

Meckel's diverticulum

Persistence of the intestinal end of the vitello-intestinal tract leads to the development of Meckel's diverticulum. It occurs in two per cent of the population and is present as a blind pouch, 2 to 6 cm in length situated on the free border of ileum nearly 1 metre proximal to the ileocaecal valve. The opening is wide and bowel contents normally enter and leave freely. The apex of the diverticulum is occasionally connected to the umbilicus by a fibrous band, and on rare occasions the duct may persist from bowel to umbilicus. Persistence of the umbilical extremity results in the formation of a red nodule of mucous membrane called a 'raspberry tumour'.

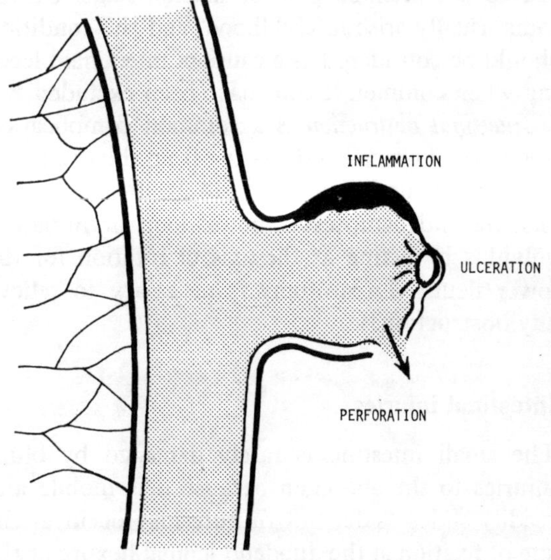

Fig. 14.1 Complications of Meckel's diverticulum. Inflammation, peptic ulceration and perforation.

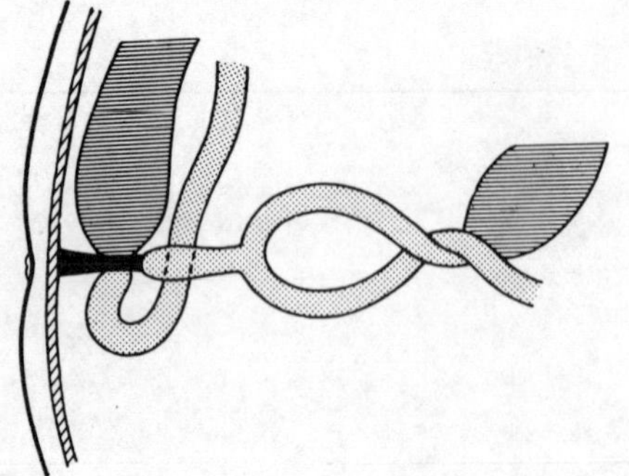

Fig. 14.2 Complications of Meckel's diverticulum. Intestinal obstruction.

The majority are asymptomatic, but complications may be related to the diverticulum or to the fibrous band (Figs. 14.1 and 14.2).

Inflammation of the diverticulum may be the result of impaction or stagnation of its contents. Perforation and peritonitis may follow, or be the result of penetration of the wall by foreign bodies or hard food particles. The condition simulates acute appendicitis, but the site of tenderness is usually more medial. Laparotomy is indicated and excision of the diverticulum and repair of the bowel should be undertaken.

Peptic ulceration of heterotopic gastric mucosa occurs in 15 per cent of diverticula and may give rise to postprandial pain or haemorrhage. Symptoms usually arise in childhood, and the condition should be considered as a cause of intestinal bleeding when common lesions have been excluded.

Intestinal obstruction is a common complication due to the fibrous band passing from the diverticulum to the umbilicus (Fig. 14.2). It may either ensnare and compress a bowel loop or initiate a volvulus by acting as the axis of rotation for the lower ileum. Laparotomy is necessary to relieve any obstruction.

Intestinal injuries

The small intestine is rarely damaged by blunt injuries to the abdomen because it is mobile and readily slides aside, but rupture may occur at the site of fixation at the duodeno-jejunal flexure or the caecal region. Peritoneal contamination is often delayed for many hours and may be a misleading feature. Intraperitoneal haemorrhage from rupture of the mesentery may be severe and lead to collapse. Damage to the mesenteric vessels may also lead to ischaemic necrosis of the bowel resulting in delayed peritonitis. It must be emphasised that careful repeated examination is necessary in all cases of abdominal injury. Tenderness, rigidity and a rising pulse-rate are indications for laparotomy, which should be performed whenever there is suspicion of a perforated viscus. With penetrating wounds doubt often exists as to the precise nature of the lesion and laparotomy is therefore advisable as early as possible for the diagnosis and treatment of any visceral injury. Irradiation given in therapy of abdominal and pelvic malignant disease may cause arteritis of bowel vessels leading to fibrosis or necrosis. Dense adhesions or perforation of the bowel may result, leading to obstruction, abscess formation or fistula between loops of bowel. Surgery may be required to treat these lesions.

Inflammation

Acute gastro-enteritis, due to food poisoning, dysentery, typhoid, paratyphoid and virus infections, may provide difficulty in diagnosis, especially in the young child. This may be resolved by attention to the history of central abdominal colicky pain, often severe in degree, accompanied by profuse vomiting and diarrhoea. There is diffuse tenderness, but a notable absence of localised tenderness and the bowel sounds are unduly active. The temperature may be elevated, but the pulse-rate does not rise until later in the course of the disease when dehydration is a marked feature. The white cell count shows a leucopenia in typhoid infection. Stool cultures and serum agglutination tests should be performed in all suspected cases.

Typhoid fever becomes a surgical problem when the bowel perforates or haemorrhage occurs from an ulcerating Peyer's patch. The patient shows signs of severe shock and toxaemia, which may mask the signs of peritonitis. If it is suspected early laparotomy and closure of the perforated bowel is required.

Acute ulcerative—obstructive lesions of the small intestine may result from the combined administration of thiazide diuretics and enteric coated potassium chloride, the latter drug appearing to be the main causative factor. Perforation of an ulcer is uncommon, but it will cause peritonitis. Closure of the perforation is usually required. Obstruction from fibrosis is more frequent; resolution on withdrawal of the drug can occur, but operation may be necessary to relieve the obstruction when conservative measures have failed.

Acute necrotising enterocolitis

This condition occurs in patients undergoing treatment with oral antibiotics, lincomycin being the principal drug, but many other antibiotics are implicated. The causative organism is *Cl. difficile*, which may normally be present in the bowel; it is resistant to antibiotics and rapidly overgrows. A powerful enterotoxin is produced which causes severe ileitis and colitis and toxic shock. It should not be confused with pseudo-membranous colitis, which occurs in elderly patients after debilitating illness or operation. Infection with *Campylobacter* should be excluded by appropriate culture methods to identify the causative organism.

The onset is sudden, from two to seven days after antibiotic therapy. Colicky pain and nausea are rapidly followed by a state of collapse with rising temperature and pulse-rate and falling blood-pressure. Slight abdominal tenderness and distension are present, bowel sounds usually being normal. An offensive, blood-stained and watery green-yellow stool is passed. Rapid deterioration may lead to death in 48 hours. The severe fluid loss into the bowel leads to marked haemoconcentration.

Treatment with oral vancomycin and parenteral metronidazole should be instituted at an early stage. Fluid replacement with sodium chloride solution, plasma or dextran must be rapid to combat hypotension, and may require infusion of 10 to 20 litres in 24 hours.

Non-specific mesenteric lymphadenitis

The condition is a frequent cause of abdominal pain in children. Widespread enlargement of mesenteric lymph nodes is found, with slight reddening of the lower ileum or caecum. A moderate amount of clear intraperitoneal fluid is present. The histological appearance of the nodes is of non-specific inflammatory change; there is no evidence of tuberculosis. An adenovirus has now been cultured from the nodes and is the probable cause of the disease in the majority of cases.

The clinical presentation is characterised by repeated attacks of central abdominal pain of a dull aching nature with occasional bouts of colic. Vomiting is uncommon and the child is rarely acutely distressed, though a mild fever is present. Tonsillar and upper respiratory infections commonly exist. Abdominal tenderness is usually generalised, but may be localised in the right iliac fossa causing confusion with appendicitis. The site of tenderness may move medially on turning the patient on to the left side.

Operative treatment is not indicated, though appendicectomy is often performed because of suspicion of acute appendicitis. The prognosis is good, the condition subsiding after several months leaving no known after effects.

GRANULOMATOUS ENTERITIS (CROHN'S DISEASE)

Crohn's disease is a granulomatous condition, usually affecting the terminal ileum, but other segments of the intestinal tract, including oesophagus, colon (p. 205) and rectum, may be involved.

The *aetiology* is unknown, but because lymphatic obstruction is a prominent feature in the early stages it has been suggested that the condition may arise from blockage of lymph channels by ingested foreign particles or by altered products of fat metabolism. The histological appearance with giant-cell formation has led to the view that the lesion is tuberculous, but tubercle bacilli have never been isolated. Sarcoidosis has been implicated by some pathologists because of a similar histology; similar immunological phenomena can also be demonstrated in most patients, but the role of these in pathogenesis is obscure.

Pathology

The pathological changes can be divided into three main stages, although one progresses gradually to the other (Fig. 14.3).

1. An acute ileitis involves 15 to 30 cm of the terminal ileum. The bowel is swollen and hyperaemic, ulceration of the mucosa is a constant feature, the mesentery is thickened and the lymph nodes enlarged. This stage is often encountered at

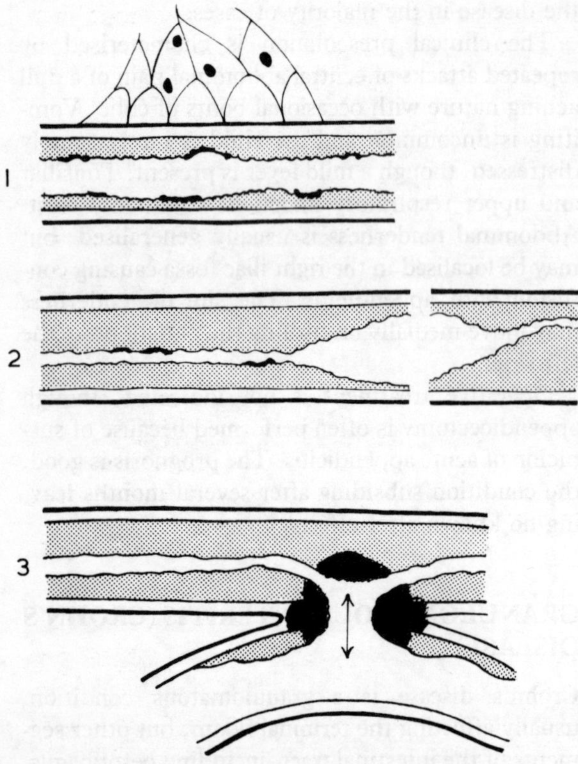

Fig. 14.3 Granulomatous enteritis. **Stage 1** Mucosal ulceration and submucosal inflammation. **Stage 2** Fibrosis and stenosis with involvement of areas higher in intestine. **Stage 3** Abscess and fistula formation.

operation for supposed acute appendicitis, and it is probable that 50 per cent of such cases subside spontaneously.

2. Marked fibrotic thickening and stenosis of the affected area is now evident. Similar areas may be present higher in the small intestine, whilst involvement of caecum, appendix and colon is not uncommon. The lumen is considerably narrowed by thickening of the submucosa, and in advanced cases it may become less than 5 mm in diameter, numerous irregular ulcers being present on the mucous surface.

3. Multiple abscess formation occurs in the later stages in the bowel and lymph nodes and is often followed by internal fistulae to adjacent intestine, bladder or rectum. Ill-advised appendicectomy may be followed by a fistula from the caecum extending through the wound to the skin.

The early histological appearance is of submucous lymphadenoid hyperplasia, lymphatic oedema being a marked feature. Eosinophilic and lymphocytic infiltration occurs; giant cells are common, but caseation does not take place.

Clinical features

The condition is more common in young adults. It presents with pain in the right lower quadrant of the abdomen accompanied by bouts of diarrhoea. In the early stage the attacks resemble acute appendicitis and laparotomy may be undertaken on a mistaken diagnosis. Fever, toxaemia and weight loss are present with the more advanced lesion and diarrhoea becomes troublesome. Features of a malabsorption syndrome may become evident from general mucosal abnormality or the formation of blind loops. Steatorrhoea and malabsorption of fat-soluble vitamins may occur in 60 per cent of patients and vitamin B_{12} deficiency may cause macrocytic anaemia. Persistent intestinal bleeding may lead to severe anaemia. Obstructive symptoms may be present leading to abdominal distension, but acute intestinal obstruction is rare. An inflammatory mass is often palpable in the right iliac fossa associated with tenderness and guarding. Fistulae may present on the abdominal wall or perineum or communicate with the bladder.

Barium small bowel enema examination may show an abnormality of mucosal pattern of the ileum in the early stages; in the presence of stenosis the barium outline of the bowel becomes narrowed, forming the classical 'string' sign of Kantor. Barium enema examination may be required to demonstrate the condition in certain cases and may also show lesions of the colon.

Treatment

The early stage discovered accidentally at laparotomy requires no treatment and excision of the affected bowel is not indicated as spontaneous resolution occurs frequently.

Conservative measures should be adopted in the first instance when the diagnosis has been made clinically. Bed rest, high protein low residue diet and vitamin supplements should be given until the lesion is quiescent, which may take several weeks or months. Excess fat should be avoided when steatorrhoea is present. Vitamin B_{12} or folic acid deficiency should be corrected. Anaemia is corrected by transfusion or iron therapy. Sulphasalazine is often beneficial and may be given over an extended period. Antibiotics are reserved for the treatment of secondary infection. Prednisolone (30 mg daily) may lead to dramatic improvement and maintenance dosage of 7.5 mg daily may help to prevent recurrence. Azathioprine as an immunosuppressive drug has been advocated but results are equivocal. The development of complications such as fistula, obstruction or perforation are indications for operative treatment.

Excision of the affected area is the procedure of choice. When there is a large inflammatory mass complicated by abscesses, exclusion by means of a by-pass operation may have to be undertaken. A vesico-intestinal fistula necessitates excision of affected bowel and closure of the bladder. The tendency for the lesion to recur higher in the ileum is notorious; it varies from 10 to 30 per cent, depending on the severity of the condition. Resection or anastomosis should therefore be well above the affected area. Repeated follow-up examination is necessary because of the tendency to recurrence and relapse after many years. Repeated operations may be inevitable in dealing with recurrent disease.

Tuberculosis

Tuberculosis of the intestinal tract, formerly a common condition, has now become rare in Great Britain. The lowered incidence follows the decline of tuberculosis generally and the almost complete elimination of bovine tubercle bacilli from milk.

It most commonly presents as a large granulomatous mass in the ileocaecal region and should be treated by chemotherapy. The only indication for surgery is to relieve obstruction by an ileotransverse colostomy, or to by-pass strictures of the small intestine.

Actinomycosis

Actinomycosis usually presents with abscess formation in appendicitis and leads to the formation of multiple fistulae through the appendicectomy wound. The diagnosis may be made on examination of the pus when the typical 'sulphur' granules are seen but an adequate biopsy should be taken if doubt persists. The response to antibiotic therapy is poor and a fatal outcome from widespread abscesses is common (p. 8).

Tumours

Tumours of the small intestine are rare and usually present with obstruction, although a benign growth may be present for several years without causing symptoms. No aetiological agents are known except in the case of multiple intestinal polyposis associated with melanin pigmentation of the lips, as described by Peutz and Jeghers, and inherited as a simple Mendelian dominant.

Adenomas and lipomas are the commonest benign lesions, but both occur less frequently than adenocarcinoma; the former are more usual in the ileum in contrast to carcinoma, which is found more often in the jejunum.

The benign tumour usually causes intestinal obstruction by intussusception, which may be preceded by mild attacks of colicky abdominal pain. Bleeding may occasionally be severe, but more commonly is slight though persistent, and results in hypochromic anaemia. The malignant lesion may be *adenocarcinoma* which is likely to cause obstruction by encircling the bowel wall. Mucosal ulceration is often followed by severe anaemia. *Lymphosarcoma* occurs as diffuse submucosal lesions which frequently reach large proportions. Wide resection of the affected loop and its mesentery is indicated for both malignant conditions. Radiotherapy can be employed post-operatively for lymphosarcoma or for the widespread inoperable lesion. The prognosis is poor, especially for adenocarcinoma, but cases of lymphosarcoma may survive for 10 to 15 years.

Carcinoid tumours

The majority of these tumours arise in the mucosa of the ileum, but they may also be found in the appendix, ovary, stomach and bronchus. The tumour varies in size from 1 to 10 mm and is of bright yellow colour. The histological appearance is of columnar cells showing frequent rosette formation and having a characteristic staining property with silver salts. The argentaffin cells synthesise small amounts of 5-hydroxytryptamine (5HT) which is deactivated in the liver. 5-hydroxyindolacetic acid (5HIAA) is excreted in the urine.

Ileal and colonic carcinoid metastasises to the liver where the secondary tumour produces larger amounts of 5HT, which pass directly to the systemic circulation and may cause manifestations of the carcinoid syndrome. Bronchial, pancreatic and gastric carcinoid tumours arise from the fore-gut; cell nest formation is less than in the ileal type and argentaffin staining not so marked. The concentration of 5HT is lower but the urine shows 5HIAA and 5-hydroxytryptophan. The hormone is passed directly to the systemic circulation from bronchial lesions and the carcinoid syndrome may result. Rectal tumours from the hind-gut are rare and are not associated with an altered metabolism of 5HT and the carcinoid syndrome.

Clinical features

Colicky abdominal pain and diarrhoea are the principal symptoms; weight loss may occur, and intestinal bleeding is rare. The lesion of the appendix produces symptoms and signs of appendicitis, the tumour being discovered accidentally at operation. Tumours of the ileum may present with obstruction.

The carcinoid syndrome which arises in ileal lesions with liver metastases and in bronchial tumours is characterised by the following features:

1. Flushing of the face, neck and chest which may be erythematous and can last from 2 to 10 minutes or be prolonged for 2 to 4 days in bronchial lesions. It is presumed to be due to bradykinin, the end result of the release of kallikrein, histamine and prostaglandins.
2. Intestinal hypermotility, which is evident by colicky pain and the passage of frequent soft watery stools due to an increased output of serotonin.
3. Heart disease, caused by deposits of fibrinous tissue on the internal elastic lamina, affecting the endocardium and pulmonary valve, and leading to pulmonary stenosis.
4. Asthmatic attacks.

The symptoms may be mild or become progressively severe and the course frequently extends over several years. The diagnosis is confirmed by estimation of increased levels of serum 5HT and urinary 5HIAA.

Treatment

Tumours of the appendix are adequately treated by appendicectomy. Tumours of the small intestine and colon are treated by wide resection of bowel and lymphatic drainage area. Resection of metastases in the liver may reduce the severity of attacks and retard the onset of pulmonary stenosis. The administration of an antagonist to 5HT such as methysergide or cyproheptadine will reduce flushing, bronchospasm and diarrhoea. Corticosteroids and phenothiazines also control flushing.

INTESTINAL OBSTRUCTION

Obstruction of the small or large intestine may be acute or chronic and result from a mechanical cause or from functional paralysis of the bowel wall. In this section, diseases of the large intestine will be included in so far as they are concerned with the production of intestinal obstruction as the same general principles of diagnosis and management are applicable.

Aetiology

Mechanical obstruction may be due either to blockage of the lumen by a foreign body or gall-stone, constriction of the bowel wall from a fibrous or neoplastic lesion, or by extrinsic pressure from fibrous bands or the neck of a hernial sac (Fig. 14.4). Paralytic ileus results from toxic damage to the nerve plexuses of the bowel wall occurring in peritonitis, or as a reflex mechanism following traction on the mesentery or fracture of the spine.

Pathology

Three forms of mechanical obstruction exist; (1) simple obstruction, (2) strangulation, (3) closed-loop obstruction.

Simple obstruction is followed by distension of the proximal intestine and collapse of the distal segment. Oedema and congestion of the bowel wall

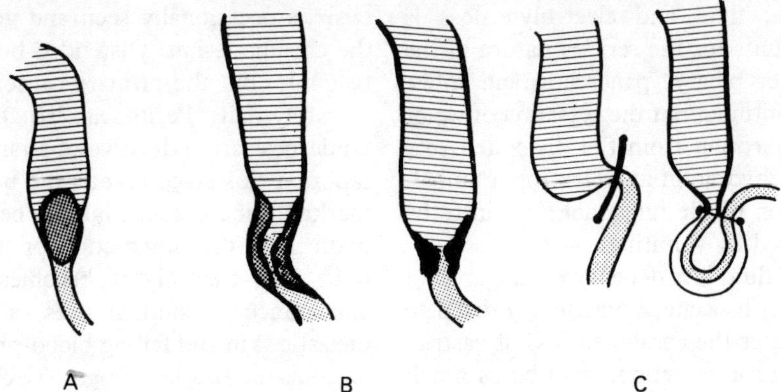

Fig. 14.4 The causes of intestinal obstruction. **A.** *Luminal* due to gall-stone or foreign body. **B.** *Mural* by inflammation or neoplasm. **C.** *Extramural* by fibrous band or hernial sac.

prevent absorption of fluid, electrolytes and digestive products. The distended bowel contains both food and the secretions of the intestinal tract, pancreas and liver, several litres of which may accumulate if the obstruction is low in the intestine. The fluid is light in colour at first, but becomes progressively more brown, due to the presence of altered blood which oozes from the congested mucosa. Gas derived from swallowed air and from bacterial fermentation slowly accumulates within the lumen. Small amounts of intraperitoneal free fluid form secondary to the congestion (Fig. 14.5A).

Strangulation usually commences with venous obstruction, but is followed by arterial occlusion resulting in rapid ischaemic changes in the bowel wall. The latter becomes oedematous and the colour changes from red to blue and later becomes a greenish-black. The development of gangrenous areas usually occurs first at the site of pressure from fibrous bands, neck of hernial sac, or on the antimesenteric border. It later spreads to involve whole segments of intestine and may be followed by perforation (Fig. 14.5B).

Closed-loop obstruction, which may follow adhesion or peritoneal bands, exhibits the changes of simple obstruction with the addition of a rapid rise of intraluminal tension in the affected segment. Congestion is followed by vascular thrombosis, which leads to the development of patchy gangrene of the mucosa, and the risk of perforation is considerable (Fig. 14.5C).

The systemic effects of intestinal obstruction are of

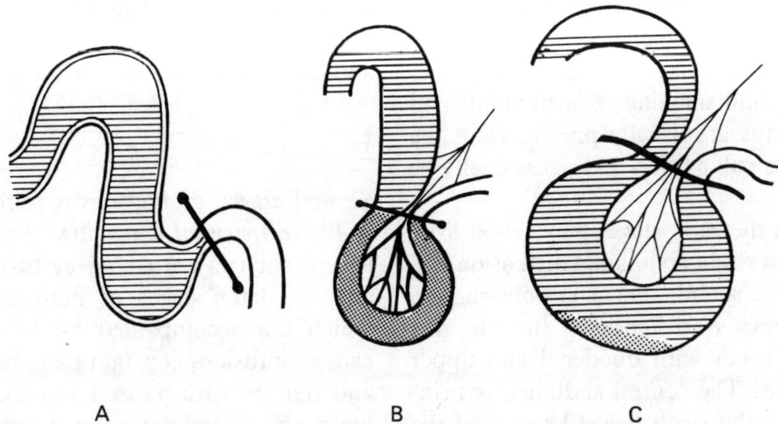

Fig. 14.5 The types of intestinal obstruction. **A**. Simple. **B**. Strangulation. **C**. Closed-loop. The dotted areas in **B** and **C** represent the development of gangrene of bowel wall.

great significance; fluid and electrolyte loss is marked and accounts for the serious nature of the condition. Gastric, biliary, pancreatic and intestinal secretions continue, but the cessation of water or electrolyte absorption from the distended segment results in dehydration and electrolyte imbalance. Regurgitation of the intestinal fluid into the stomach is followed by vomiting.

The severity of fluid loss depends on the level of obstruction. When it occurs immediately distal to the ampulla of Vater the combined loss of gastric, biliary and pancreatic secretions may be as much as 6 litres in 24 hours. Obstruction at a lower level results in a slower loss of fluid but when present for several days this also becomes serious. The loss of fluid is compensated at first by diminished excretion of urine with a low salt content. In later stages there is a reduction in blood volume and the development of intracellular dehydration. Sodium chloride deficiency and bicarbonate retention are the main changes in blood chemistry; potassium and magnesium loss become significant if obstruction persists for three or more days. Toxaemia resulting from bacterial growth and necrosis of tissues has been implicated as a cause of death in strangulation, but it probably plays only a minor role.

Clinical features

Pain is the common presenting symptom. It is colicky in nature and situated in the umbilical region with small intestinal obstruction, but below this with a colonic lesion. Vomiting occurs early with a high obstruction, but may be delayed or even absent in the large bowel type. The vomitus at first is colourless but soon becomes light brown, later dark brown and foul-smelling. Constipation and failure to pass flatus are usually present from the onset, although a small motion may occasionally be passed at first.

Examination in the early stages may reveal little abnormality except slight abdominal distension and an increase in bowel sounds. Persistent obstruction results in progressive distension, though this change does not occur with duodenal and upper jejunal obstruction. The central abdomen is principally involved in the small bowel lesion and the flanks with colonic obstruction, whilst volvulus of the colon produces gross distension. Visible peristalsis is occasionally seen and generally occurs in the chronic lesion. Distended bowel loops may be palpable, but the primary cause such as a tumour is rarely felt. Peritoneal irritation and rebound tenderness are indicative of strangulation. Auscultation at this stage reveals the bowel sounds to be markedly increased, high-pitched and tinkling in nature. As the obstruction progresses the loss of fluid and electrolytes becomes evident by the appearance of sunken eyes, a dry tongue, dry inelastic skin and falling blood-pressure, with onset of coma in the late stages. Great care should be taken in examination to exclude a femoral hernia and tumour of the rectum as causative lesions.

Investigations

Radiology is of value in establishing diagnosis and locating the level of obstruction. Plain films show the gaseous outlines of small intestine, generally lying in the central area, with fluid levels visible in the erect films. Colonic distension is identified by the outline of haustrations in a peripheral position (Fig. 14.6). Contrast radiography using 100 ml of radio-opaque fluid is at times used, but barium suspension should never be given by mouth because of the grave risk of aggravating an obstruction. A barium enema is occasionally necessary for the diagnosis of a colonic lesion.

Investigation of the serum electroytes alone does not give a clear indication of the state of dehydration and electrolyte imbalance, but is of value when taken in conjunction with the clinical picture. The haemoglobin and haematocrit levels are often raised, the serum chloride concentration lowered and the bicarbonate level elevated.

Diagnosis

Several *aspects of diagnosis* require consideration.

The differential diagnosis. Acute inflammatory lesions such as acute cholecystitis and appendicitis and the later stages of perforated peptic ulcer, which are accompanied by localised ileus, may cause confusion; constant pain, marked tenderness and rigidity with pyrexia and leucocytosis help to make the distinction. Acute pancreatitis may be confused with obstruction because of the profuse vomiting which is a prominent feature; it is

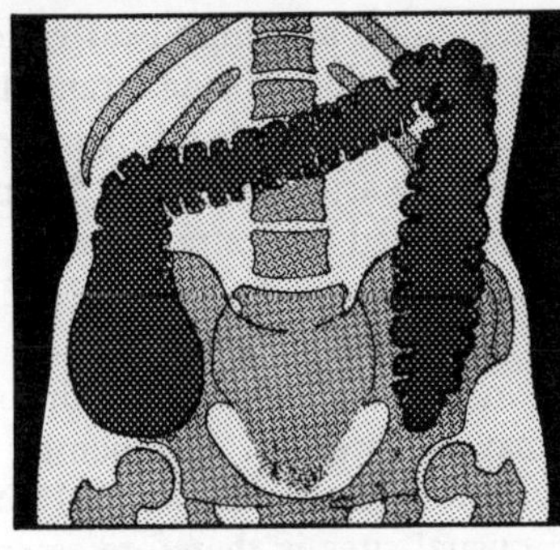

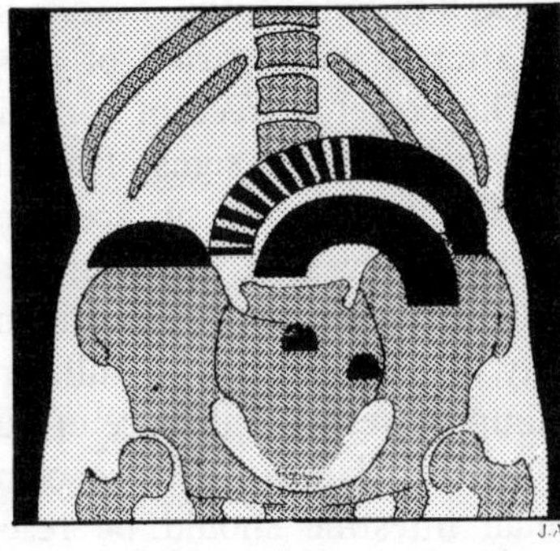

Fig. 14.6 The radiological appearances of intestinal obstruction. **A**. Large intestine. **B**. Small intestine.

excluded by the presence of tenderness, back pain, early peripheral vascular failure and a raised serum amylase level. Severe constipation, encountered more often in the elderly, is recognised by the impaction of hard faeces in the rectum and the response to enemas.

The level of obstruction may be diagnosed by the occurrence of early and profuse vomiting with little distension in high occlusion; lower ileal obstruction is accompanied by marked central distension, often with severe vomiting. The distension of colonic obstruction is seen in both flanks, the caecum often being markedly ballooned with gas; vomiting is slight or absent. Reference to the history and signs of the causative lesion frequently enables accurate localisation of the level of obstruction.

Differentiation of simple obstruction from strangulation is not easy in many cases. Strangulation usually has a rapid onset with severe colicky pain and, as a result of gangrenous change, is followed by local pain, tenderness and rigidity. It may also be accompanied by marked shock.

The nature of the obstructing lesion is often suggested by the history of the mode of onset. Intussusception presents in a young healthy child, whilst volvulus of the colon occurs in later life with the sudden development of gross distension. The history or scar of a previous operation may suggest adhesions or bands.

Cancer of the colon may be evident by a history of weeks or months of increasing constipation and bleeding culminating in an acute episode. Strangulated hernia is usually obvious, but the rare internal hernia may escape diagnosis. Special causes are considered further on page 184 *et seq*.

Treatment

Management of acute intestinal obstruction may be conservative or operative, in both instances correction of fluid and electrolyte imbalance being required as early as possible.

Preliminary management. Nasogastric aspiration should be employed to remove intestinal contents which regurgitate into the stomach. Long double lumen tubes are ideal for emptying the small intestine directly, but their passage is difficult and at times impossible.

The fluid and electrolyte loss occurring in the majority of cases of intestinal obstruction will require replacement. An approximate estimate of such loss may be obtained from a careful enquiry into the severity of vomiting, the amount of urine passed and a clinical appraisal of the degree of dehydration present.

The amount varies in individual cases, depending on the level of obstruction. During the initial 24 hours about 1 litre may be vomited, 1 litre may lie unabsorbed in the intestinal tract, 1 litre of urine may be passed and about 500 ml of insensible loss occur, the patient thus being deficient of 3.5 litres of fluid containing electrolytes. This loss becomes progressively more severe as vomiting increases, and after three days of complete obstruction the total deficit may be 12 litres. Complete replacement of this volume should not be undertaken immediately but spread over two or three days. Two litres of 0.9 per cent saline and 3 litres of 5 per cent glucose in water should be given every 24 hours, thereby counteracting the continued loss and slowly making good the deficit.

Severe salt depletion may present with collapse or even coma; replacement by 500 ml of 10 per cent sodium chloride then becomes necessary and results in dramatic improvement. Potassium deficiency arises after two to three days of vomiting or aspiration and may be prevented by the administration of 3 g of potassium chloride in each litre of saline. Fluid balance charts should be maintained at all times, and in determining progress estimation of serum electrolyte levels is helpful and should be performed daily (p. 35).

Conservative treatment is indicated in the early stage of colonic carcinomatous obstruction, which is often incomplete in nature, and which may later be treated by one-stage resection and anastomosis (p. 212). Simple obstruction of the small intestine from adhesions often responds to this therapy, and it is advisable in the recurrent case. The main disadvantage of conservative therapy is that strangulation may be overlooked, and cases of doubtful nature should therefore be treated by operation after preliminary management for 12 to 18 hours.

Operative treatment may either be directed to an obvious cause, such as a strangulated hernia, or a laparotomy may be necessary for the diagnosis and relief of obstruction, which may necessitate resection of bowel, colostomy or division of adhesions. It should be undertaken as soon as the patient can be prepared. Before induction of anaesthesia it is essential to pass a wide-bore stomach tube on all cases of obstruction to prevent sudden regurgitation of large amounts of fluid which may be aspirated and result in fatal asphyxia.

Post-operative care is outlined on page 39. It is important that suction and intravenous fluid replacement are not discontinued too soon; normal peristalsis with passage of flatus or stool should be awaited.

The common types of intestinal obstruction include the following.

Strangulated hernia

The external variety is the commonest cause of obstruction; internal hernia through a retroperitoneal fossa or a defect in the diaphragm is rare, and the exact diagnosis is seldom made before operation.

Inguinal hernia is the most common form, although the femoral and umbilical varieties have a sinister reputation for causing strangulation, the neck of the sac or a fascial band being responsible for constricting the arterial supply. A femoral hernia is often associated with strangulation of part of the bowel wall (Richter's hernia) (p. 142).

The principal complaint is of pain, both in the hernia and in the central part of the abdomen. Vomiting may be profuse. Frequently there has been no awareness of a hernia and careful examination of the usual sites is therefore essential in all cases of intestinal obstruction.

Surgical exploration of the hernia should be undertaken after a short period of pre-operative treatment. The bowel is freed of constriction and inspected for viability, the signs of which are persistence of a shiny peritoneal surface, a red-purple colour, which improves on warming with a moist pack, and slight but definite peristaltic movement. Non-viability is indicated by the dull, green-black surface of limp bowel with absence of pulsation in the mesentery and lack of surface oozing. Gangrenous small intestine should be resected, but large bowel is better managed by exteriorisation with the formation of a temporary colostomy. Gangrene, which is limited to the constricting rings caused by the neck of a hernial sac, can be oversewn.

Peritoneal bands and adhesions

These may follow previous intra-abdominal operations or infection, or they may be congenital, such as the attachment of a Meckel's diverticulum to the umbilicus. Adhesion of adjacent bowel loops leads to simple obstruction, whilst strangulation may follow torsion around a fibrous band. Laparotomy is indicated for most cases, with the exception of mild post-operative adhesions which often resolve with conservative measures.

INTUSSUSCEPTION

Invagination of one portion of the bowel into the adjacent distal segment is termed intussusception. It is the commonest cause of intestinal obstruction in babies.

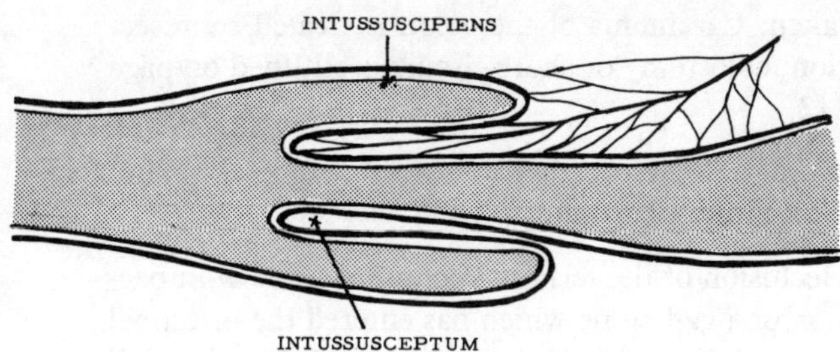

Fig. 14.7 Intussusception. The ileo-ileal variety is shown with the intussusceptum entering into the intussuscipiens.

Pathology

Enlargement of lymphoid patches in the ileum is a feature of the condition at this age. It has been assumed that infection must play a part, and an adenovirus has been isolated from the stool and mesenteric lymph nodes in a significant proportion of cases. Changes in diet at weaning may, by altering peristaltic activity, play a minor role in causation. In the older child and adult a tumour is the more usual cause.

Invagination of the intestinal wall is produced as a result of peristalsis acting on a mass of lymphoid tissue or tumour in the bowel wall. This process, called the intussusceptum, then acts as a foreign body and is carried further along the lumen of the distal bowel. The outer or ensheathing layer is termed the intussuscipiens (Fig, 14.7). The condition is isoperistaltic in the majority of cases. It usually commences in the lower part of the ileum forming the ileo-ileal variety, which generally passes into the colon to be termed ileo-colic. The less common ileo-caecal variety begins at the ileo-caecal valve where a prominent ring of lymphoid tissue forms the apex (Fig. 14.8).

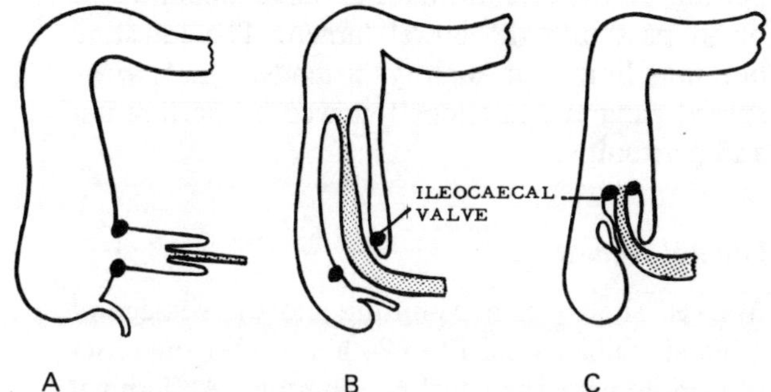

Fig. 14.8 Types of intussusception. **A.** Ileo-ileal. **B.** Ileo-colic. **C.** Ileo-caecal.

A mobile caecum or even a mesentery of the ascending colon is at times encountered permitting easier invagination of the distal colon. The intussusceptum is able to pass along the colon without hindrance until it is restrained by traction of the mesenteric vessels; occasionally it may extend as far as the anus. Primary colonic intussusception is uncommon and is usually only encountered in the adult in association with a tumour.

The invaginated bowel rapidly becomes oedematous, resulting in intestinal obstruction. Marked mesenteric lymphadenitis is a prominent feature. Interference with the arterial blood supply may then lead to gangrene of the intussusception with consequent peritonitis.

Clinical features

Healthy children from four to nine months of age are most commonly affected with a higher male incidence. The typical history commences with attacks of colicky abdominal pain manifest by crying and flexion of thighs and knees. Blood-stained stool and mucus are passed per rectum. Vomiting and abdominal distension develop with the progress of the intestinal obstruction. Physical examination reveals the presence of a sausage-shaped mass in the line of the colon, often noted first in the right hypochondrium, but later found in the left side of the abdomen. Rectal examination only rarely allows detection of the apex of the intussusception, but blood is frequently found on the examining finger. The late case exhibits marked abdominal distension, accompanied by severe shock and dehydration.

An accurate clinical diagnosis is possible in most cases, a barium enema being necessary only when doubt exists. Gastro-enteritis, intestinal obstruction due to volvulus, and the complications of a Meckel's diverticulum may cause confusion in diagnosis.

Treatment

Laparotomy and reduction of the intussusception by gentle manipulation of the bowel should be performed. On the rare occasions when irreducible or strangulated bowel is present it should be exteriorised and resected, leaving a temporary ileocolostomy for subsequent closure. Primary intraperitoneal anastomosis in such circumstances is more difficult and carries a higher mortality.

Volvulus

The small or large intestine may be affected. Involvement of the small bowel is usually associated with adhesion formation of the mesentery, which becomes narrowed at the base, allowing rotation of the bowel loop. Volvulus of the large intestine may affect a redundant pelvic colon or caecum (Fig. 16.6). Rapid gaseous distension of the bowel occurs, but gangrenous change is uncommon. Laparotomy is required for both varieties; reduction of the colonic volvulus may be aided by the passage of a rectal tube.

Tumour

Obstruction of the small intestine by tumour is uncommon although benign lesions such as lipoma or leiomyoma may block the lumen. The malignant cause is often a ring stricture and may be a carcinoma, lymphosarcoma or reticulum cell sarcoma. An episode of obstruction may be the first indication of disease, or it may be preceded by attacks of colicky pain, vomiting and unexplained anaemia.

Colonic carcinoma is a frequent cause of intestinal obstruction and the lesion is most often situated in the pelvic colon (p. 212). Distension of the small intestine arises when the ileocaecal valve becomes incompetent and allows back-pressure to be transmitted to the ileum. The clinical presentation is varied and the onset may be rapid with severe abdominal pain, vomiting and constipation, or there may be preceding vague pain, alternating constipation and diarrhoea and gradual distension. Plain-film radiography is often helpful in confirming and localising the lesion to either small or large intestine.

Treatment

Laparotomy is indicated in most instances and may be the only means of diagnosing a small intestine tumour. Resection of the growth and lymphatic field with end-to-end anastomosis is then undertaken. Carcinoma of the colon is treated by resection, colostomy or short-circuit as outlined on page 212.

Gall-stone obstruction

Occlusion of the terminal ileum may follow impaction of a gall-stone which has entered the intestinal lumen by ulceration through the gall-bladder wall into the duodenum. It is rare, but should be suspected in cases of intestinal obstruction with a previous history of cholecystitis (p. 246). The plain radiograph shows air in the biliary passages and on occasions a gall-stone in the lower abdomen.

MESENTERIC VASCULAR OCCLUSION

Pathology

Gangrene of long segments of intestine may result from thrombosis of the superior mesenteric artery secondary to atherosclerosis, or its occlusion by an embolus from heart or aorta. The inferior mesenteric artery is rarely affected. There is usually an associated thrombosis of the superior mesenteric vein; less commonly venous thrombosis may occur alone. The latter may be the result of retrograde thrombosis following splenectomy or portacaval anastomosis.

The majority of infarctions involve the ileum and only rarely does the occlusion affect the main trunk of the superior mesenteric artery, causing gangrenous change of the jejunum, ileum and the right half of the colon. At the onset the bowel becomes white, but venous stagnation quickly follows with a change of colour to bluish-red. A blood-stained peritoneal exudate forms and large amounts of blood pass into the bowel lumen. The intestine becomes limp and slightly distended, and widespread gangrene develops followed by perforation and peritonitis.

Clinical features

Marked shock, pain, vomiting and the passage of a blood-stained stool 12 to 24 hours after the onset of symptoms is the usual presentation. Abdominal distension and tenderness occur initially, rigidity developing later with the onset of peritoneal infection. A vague central mass of engorged intestine may become palpable and free peritoneal fluid may be detected. Bowel sounds are usually diminished, and rectal examination often reveals blood on the examining finger.

Treatment

Resuscitation by blood transfusion should be followed by laparotomy, when resection of long segments of small intestine and ascending colon may be necessary. The prognosis is poor and survival often accompanied by malnutrition, the severity of which depends on the amount of bowel resected. Embolectomy of the superior mesenteric artery is feasible but rarely successful, due to distal thrombosis subsequent on delay in diagnosis. A second laparotomy after 24 hours is occasionally necessary to deal with further gangrene which may have developed. In partial occlusion arterial reconstruction may be successful (p. 424).

PARALYTIC ILEUS

Functional paralysis of the intestine is a common and important cause of intestinal obstruction. It may follow an intraperitoneal or extraperitoneal lesion, the former being more common; peritonitis and operative manipulation are the principal factors. Spinal injury, chest infection and a retroperitoneal tumour occasionally induce ileus; gross meteorism is a feature of this form.

Post-operative paralytic ileus of mild degree follows the majority of abdominal operations, peristalsis normally recovering after 12 to 24 hours, but in certain instances paralysis persists for three to four days. Excessive handling of the small intestine, traction on the mesentery and dissection involving the sympathetic plexuses on the posterior abdominal wall are important aetiological factors.

Ileus secondary to peritonitis is probably due to toxic paralysis of the myenteric plexuses and results in patchy cessation of peristalsis. Bowel loops which are bathed in free pus or lie in an abcess cavity soon become distended, whilst other portions of the intestine not yet involved by infection retain their functional activity. In most cases of peritonitis there is an associated mechanical obstruction due to kinking of adherent intestine, but this rarely calls for surgical intervention.

The clinical onset of paralytic ileus is insidious. Painless abdominal distension is followed by vomiting, which in the later stages becomes profuse. No flatus or stool is passed per rectum. Dehydration and electrolyte imbalance are evident in the established condition. Diminished or absent bowel sounds help in the differentiation from mechanical obstruction. Radiological examination may be of value by demonstrating widespread and patchy distension of small and large intestine.

Treatment

Prevention is the foremost consideration, and regular abdominal examination with auscultation for bowel sounds should be undertaken in any condition liable to complication by ileus. If bowel sounds are absent and flatus is not passed, oral administration of fluids should be withheld and nasogastric suction and intravenous infusion commenced. Prompt treatment often prevents development of the well-established condition. Antibiotic treatment of peritoneal infection plays an important part in lessening toxaemia and thus limiting ileus. The administration of cholinergic drugs, such as prostigmine, is harmful. Similarly enemata and purgatives are better avoided in the early post-operative period. Treatment should be maintained until there is a return of bowels sounds. A trial administration of oral fluids is commenced and if retained and absorbed the nasogastric tube is removed. Recovery is accompanied by the passage of several foul-smelling loose stools.

Blind loop syndrome

Stasis in the lumen of the bowel as a result of obstruction, or from the development of large diverticula or the formation of redundant loops of small intestine may be followed by weight loss, diarrhoea and macrocytic anaemia. The condition is caused by alteration of bacterial flora in the jejunum resulting in either destruction or deficient absorption of vitamin B_{12}. Surgical treatment to correct the intestinal abnormality may be feasible. Antibiotic therapy and vitamin replacement may also be valuable forms of treatment.

APPENDIX

Anatomy

The appendix opens into the caecum about 2 cm below the ileo-caecal valve. Its termination corresponds with McBurney's surface marking on the skin, which is a point one-third of the distance from the lateral end of a line joining the anterior superior iliac spine to the umbilicus. The length of the appendix varies considerably, the average being 6 to 10 cm.

The position of the appendix shows considerable variation, which accounts for the variety of clinical presentations of disease. It is situated behind the caecum in 65 per cent of subjects, and in 30 per cent passes towards the pelvis or lies over the pelvic brim. It is uncommon for the appendix to be in relationship to the terminal ileum, but this position has serious significance because its proximity to the ileocolic vein may result in portal pylephlebitis. When directed medially perforation into the general peritoneal cavity is more probable.

The appendicular artery, a branch of the ileocolic artery, lies in the free border of the mesentery of the appendix which passes behind the terminal ileum. The collateral circulation is poor and early gangrene from vascular obstruction is common. The appendicular vein forms an important tributary of the portal system, a situation which may lead to severe portal pyaemia.

Lymphoid tissue is abundant and forms an almost continuous layer in the submucosa. The lymphatic drainage passes alongside the ileocolic artery to mesenteric nodes.

No useful function of the appendix is known in man. Absorption of water occurs from its lumen and accounts for the inspissation of retained faecal masses. Mucus is secreted by the lining cells and a mucocele may result from obstruction of the lumen.

Acute appendicitis

Acute inflammation of the appendix is common, accounting for the majority of abdominal emergency operations. Consideration of the history of the disease illustrates the great improvement which has occurred in recent years in the management of abdominal conditions. The annual death-rate for this seemingly simple condition was 3000 in 1938, but at the present time the figure is 180, the majority of these being in the age group 70–90 years. This marked improvement has resulted from earlier diagnosis and operation, better anaesthesia and improved methods of treatment of peritonitis with intestinal suction, fluid replacement and antibiotics.

Aetiology

Several explanations have been given to account for the varying incidence of this condition with age and race, but none adequately explains all the facts. The following points are important.

The disease occurs predominantly between the ages of 10 and 30 years when lymphoid tissue is abundant. It is rare below two years, and involution of the organ and its gradual replacement by fibrous tissue accounts for a low incidence in the aged.

The variation in racial incidence is probably related to diet. The frequency in the white races is attributed to the large proportion of meat consumed, while the lower incidence in other races may be related to a diet rich in cellulose, a substance which stimulates bowel activity and ensures emptying of the appendix. Stagnation of appendicular contents associated with constipation may have some bearing on the causation of acute inflammation. The hard faecolith, which in some instances becomes calcified, is an important cause of localised damage to the mucosa and may initiate acute inflammation. It also produces obstruction of the appendicular lumen, often associated with severe cases of appendicitis. Foreign bodies such as orange pips, lead shot and intestinal worms bear little relation to the causation of the disease. In most instances the organisms isolated from the appendix are *Esch. coli* and *Strept. faecalis*. An association of acute appendicitis and tonsillitis has been claimed, but definite confirmation is not readily obtained. No familial tendency has been shown.

Pathology

The severity of inflammation of the appendix varies considerably; it ranges from mild congestion of the

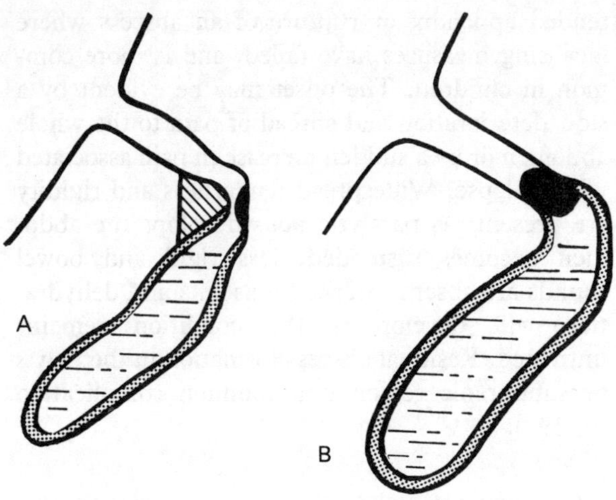

Fig. 14.9 The pathology of appendicitis. Inflammation of the appendix with distension by pus distal to obstruction due to **A.** Fibrosis; **B.** Faecolith.

mucosa to rapidly developing necrosis of the appendix wall. The degree of inflammation largely depends on the presence of obstruction of the appendicular lumen either by a faecolith or by scarring and adhesions from previous inflammation (Fig. 14.9).

The pathological changes can be classified as:

1. Catarrhal inflammation of the mucosa and submucous tissues. The appendix becomes slightly swollen and turgid, with increased vascularity. The mucosa is reddened and oedematous, and a mucous exudate is present in the lumen. Resolution occurs in many cases and may result in fibrosis of the appendix or a localised stricture which predisposes to the development of obstructive appendicitis on a subsequent occasion.

2. Obstructive appendicitis is the more usual type. The lumen may be blocked by fibrosis following previous inflammation or by a faecolith. The onset of inflammatory oedema causes a rapid rise in tension in the closed portion of the appendix resulting in venous occlusion, arterial thrombosis and localised gangrene of the appendicular wall which often lead to perforation. The significance of obstruction can be demonstrated by the contrast of marked inflammatory change distal to such obstruction with an almost normal appearance in the proximal part.

The appendix becomes adherent to adjacent viscera to a varying degree, depending on the rapidity of onset of the condition. Inflammatory adhesions are common and the omentum performs a well-recognised role in localising the inflammation by becoming adherent to the appendix, and in many cases enclosing it completely. The caecum and neighbouring abdominal wall often become inflamed and oedematous and adhere to each other.

Prior to perforation the lumen contains pus under tension. The pus and often the faecolith are discharged into the peritoneal cavity with the development either of a localised abscess or of generalised peritonitis, depending on the extent of the adhesions surrounding the appendix.

Clinical features

The illness usually commences with central abdominal pain accompanied by anorexia. The pain is of a dull aching nature, but in the obstructive case may be colicky. After several hours it becomes maximal in the right lower quadrant and is then constant and not colicky. The central abdominal pain is due to distension of the appendix and is referred via the tenth thoracic segment of the spinal cord. When the somatic peritoneum over the appendix becomes inflamed, pain is felt in the right iliac fossa. Nausea is a prominent symptom, occurring after the initial pain, and in most instances is followed by vomiting. The latter, commencing several hours after the onset of pain, is not generally profuse, but may be more marked in children. Constipation is more common than diarrhoea, the latter indicating an appendix lying in the pelvic position and causing irritation of the rectum. Frequency of micturition may similarly result from involvement of the bladder. A history of previous mild attacks of a similar nature is often forthcoming and lends support to the diagnosis.

Slight elevation of temperature is common; it rarely exceeds 38°C in uncomplicated cases, and if above 40°C a diagnosis of uncomplicated acute appendicitis is unlikely. The pulse-rate is usually raised. The appearance of a furred tongue and foul-smelling breath is helpful, particularly in children. The most important physical sign in establishing an early diagnosis is localised tenderness in the right iliac fossa. This should be elicited by careful palpation to determine its precise location; variation occurs, depending on the position of the appendix, but in the early stages the site of tenderness will be confined to a limited area near McBurney's point. Slight muscle guarding may be present at this stage, and as the disease progresses localised rigidity of the abdominal muscles becomes apparent. Generalised peritonitis is accompanied by diffuse tenderness, rigidity and distension of the abdomen.

Cutaneous hyperaesthesia is sometimes elicited in the right iliac fossa. Auscultation often reveals an absence of bowel sounds in the right iliac region; with the onset of paralytic ileus in the later stages of generalised peritonitis this becomes widespread. Rectal examination may demonstrate localised tenderness in the right side of the pelvis, providing valuable information in doubtful cases. At a later stage it may confirm the presence of a pelvic abscess.

Acute appendicitis is rare *under the age of two years*, and the difficulty of obtaining an accurate history under five years makes diagnosis less certain. Vomiting is a marked feature and may lead to confusion with gastro-enteritis or dietary indiscretion. A sore throat is a frequent accompaniment and may be associated with enlarged cervical lymph nodes. A temperature of 40°C is often found in babies with a corresponding tachycardia. Abdominal palpation to localise the site of tenderness and detect rigidity should be performed gently to avoid hurting the child.

In the *aged* the history is short and signs frequently minimal. Pain is not severe, and the onset of pelvic peritonitis is often confused with incomplete intestinal obstruction.

Complications

Peritonitis is the principal complication. It may be localised in the right iliac fossa or pelvis or may extend diffusely throughout the peritoneal cavity. *Local peritonitis* results from spread of infection through the appendicular wall or by perforation; in most cases further spread is prevented by localising adhesions of adjacent viscera and omentum. Peritonitis is not usually evident until the second or third day. The pain then becomes continuous, is aggravated by movement and there is an increase in the area of tenderness and rigidity. *Diffuse peritonitis* may follow sudden perforation of a distended appendix or rupture of an abscess where localising measures have failed, and is more common in children. The onset may be evident by a slow deterioration and spread of pain to the whole abdomen or by a sudden increase in pain associated with collapse. Widespread tenderness and rigidity are present; as paralytic ileus develops the abdomen becomes distended, less rigid and bowel sounds are absent. Marked toxaemia and dehydration will develop if the condition remains untreated. Residual abscess formation in the pelvis or subphrenic region is a common complication (p. 197).

Abscess formation

Localisation of infection with the development of an abscess is a common sequel of untreated acute appendicitis. Five to seven days after an attack of abdominal pain a characteristic tender mass is palpable in the right iliac fossa. The general condition at this stage is usually good, though a mild fever is common and a leucocytosis nearly always present. The abscess often lies behind or lateral to the caecum, but in rare instances may lie between coils of terminal ileum (Fig. 14.10).

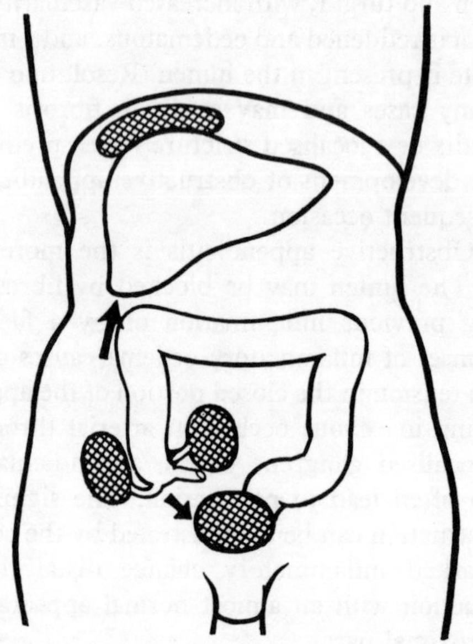

Fig. 14.10 The common sites of abscess formation following acute appendicitis

A pelvic abscess causes irritation of bladder and bowel and gives rise to frequent and painful micturition with diarrhoea and passage of mucus in the stool. Rectal examination is necessary to detect the abscess, as it becomes palpable in the abdomen only when very large. The pelvic abscess may rupture into the rectum or vagina with subsequent rapid improvement. The majority of abscesses subside spontaneously, the surrounding adhesions disappear almost completely, and at a subsequent laparotomy for appendicectomy little trace of the original infection remains.

Appendicitis is a cause of subphrenic abscess, which occurs by an intraperitoneal spread of infection lateral to the colon (p. 198). The more uncommon complications include portal pyaemia, intestinal obstruction, actinomycosis and faecal fistula following drainage of an abscess.

Investigations

Accessory investigations play little part in establishing the diagnosis, which should be made on careful evaluation of the clinical history and physical findings. Urine examination should be undertaken in every case though the presence of pus cells does not exclude a diagnosis of appendicitis. The white blood count is generally raised to 10 000 per cmm, but in the early case is of little help in establishing the diagnosis. In abscess formation there may be considerable leucocytosis. Serial counts may be helpful in assessing progress in these cases.

Differential diagnosis

The variety of presentation of acute appendicitis causes it to resemble several intra-abdominal and extra-abdominal conditions (Fig. 14.11). The majority are treated conservatively, whereas early operation is required for acute appendicitis. It should be emphasised that operation is preferable where any reasonable suspicion of appendicitis exists.

Pyelitis. This condition may present difficulty in diagnosis in young women and particular attention should be paid to a history of urinary symptoms accompanied by rigors, with pyrexia up to 42°C. Tenderness in the loin and over a wide area of the right side of the abdomen is often found. Urine

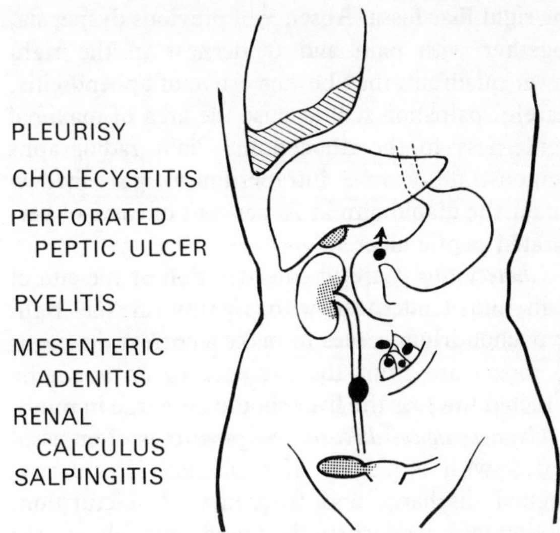

Fig. 14.11 The differential diagnosis of acute appendicitis

examination may reveal pus cells and motile organisms which should later be identified by culture.

Renal colic. This is characterised by intermittent colicky pain which may be severe and result in restlessness. Urine examination often shows red blood cells, few pus cells and no motile organisms. An immediate intravenous urogram may be necessary to confirm the diagnosis; it demonstrates poor concentration of the opaque medium in the affected kidney, and may indicate the site of impaction of a ureteric calculus.

Gastro-enteritis of specific or non-specific nature is commonly confused with appendicitis because the pain is situated in the epigastrium or umbilical region, but subsequent localisation in the right iliac fossa does not occur. Vomiting is an early feature and may initiate the illness. Diarrhoea is often profuse in enteritis, but may also occur with appendicitis. Tenderness is diffuse, the area of maximal intensity varying hourly.

Constipation is commonly associated with mild pain in the right iliac fossa, particularly in young girls. It results from distension of the caecum and appendix and can be excluded by the absence of vomiting and by the presence of a palpable caecum and descending colon. The pain is relieved by enemata.

Perforated peptic ulcer. A small anterior duodenal ulcer may on perforation spread gastric contents to the right iliac fossa. Absence of previous dyspepsia, together with pain and tenderness in the right lower quadrant, may be suggestive of appendicitis. Careful palpation will localise the area of maximal tenderness to the duodenum. Plain radiographs demonstrate a free intraperitoneal gas shadow under the diaphragm in 70 per cent of cases of perforated peptic ulcer.

Cholecystitis. Careful consideration of the site of pain and tenderness with rigidity in the right hypochondrium serves to make a correct diagnosis in most cases, but the presence of an appendix directed towards the liver should be borne in mind.

Gynaecological diseases. Salpingitis is often associated with a history of menstrual irregularity, vaginal discharge and frequency of micturition. Abdominal tenderness is found just above the pubis often near the midline, but right-sided salpingitis is difficult to distinguish from appendicitis. Vaginal examination reveals tenderness of the cervix, and an indurated mass may be palpable through the lateral fornix. A vaginal smear should be examined for pus cells and organisms, the Gram-negative intracellular diplococci of gonorrhoea being most often encountered.

Tubal pregnancy gives rise to lower abdominal pain with a history of menstrual irregularity. Signs of haemorrhage occur with rupture and may be followed by shoulder pain from diaphragmatic irritation. Vaginal examination reveals a swollen Fallopian tube.

Torsion of an ovarian cyst is accompanied by severe abdominal pain and repeated vomiting without nausea. A tender smooth swelling in the pelvis or lower abdomen may be detected soon after the onset and is unlikely to be confused with an appendix abscess.

Mesenteric adenitis. This presents considerable diagnostic difficulty in children. Tenderness is usually less definite than in appendicitis and nearer the midline where a vague mass may be palpable. Free fluid may occasionally be detected in the peritoneal cavity and may be demonstrated on a plain radiograph. Enlargement of cervical lymph nodes and tonsillar infection are often found.

Pneumonia poses a diagnostic problem in babies and young children. Pain from pleural inflammation may be referred to the abdomen, vomiting is uncommon, but gaseous abdominal distension with diminished bowel sounds is frequently encountered. The presence of an increased respiratory rate and physical signs of chest infection with lack of localised abdominal tenderness indicate the correct diagnosis, which must be confirmed by radiography. An exploratory operation should be avoided if there is a probability of pneumonia.

Diabetic abdominal pain. Colicky upper abdominal pain may occur in the ketotic diabetic subject. It is preceded by vomiting; tenderness is slight and muscular rigidity is usually absent. It is thought to be due to cramp of the accessory muscle of respiration associated with the low serum sodium and potassium levels found in ketosis. Treatment with insulin and saline infusion leads to relief of pain in three to four hours.

Treatment of acute appendicitis

Appendicectomy should be performed as soon as the diagnosis has been made. Conservative treatment is fraught with danger and should not be practised. In the early stages operation removes the source of infection and the risk of peritonitis due to rupture. Perforation with local or diffuse peritonitis does not preclude operation, in fact the continuing source of infection is better removed after a period of pre-operative preparation by gastric suction, parenteral fluids and antibiotics. At operation undertaken during the first two or three days a small abscess cavity may be found surrounding the appendix, but the latter should be removed if it is easily mobilised. The formation of an ill-defined inflammatory mass in the right iliac fossa is an indication for conservative management. Appendicectomy in such circumstances involves freeing protective adhesions and may result in damage to the friable caecum with production of a faecal fistula.

The development of a *localised abscess* indicates that the infection is being confined and *conservative* measures should then be employed in the initial stages. The diet is restricted to fluids. If vomiting is present, gastric suction and intravenous fluids should be prescribed. Resolution occurs in over 75 per cent of cases and is indicated by a falling temperature, diminished tenderness and decrease in size of the abscess. If fever persists or the abscess increases in size, incision and drainage are indicated, but no attempt should be made to remove the appendix. This can safely be carried out three months later when the inflammatory adhesions have almost completely resolved.

Appendicectomy

This operation is readily performed through a muscle-splitting incision in the right iliac fossa which gives direct access to the appendix. It has the further advantage that should peritoneal adhesions develop only the caecum is involved with less risk of subsequent intestinal obstruction.

Drainage of the peritoneal cavity is only required where a small collection of pus lies around the appendix. In generalised peritonitis it serves no useful purpose but peritoneal lavage with tetracycline in saline can be undertaken and antibiotic therapy with cephradine and metronidazole should be commenced. Post-operative infection of the wound is encountered with moderate frequency due to contamination by purulent exudate. Residual abscesses may occur after operation (p. 197). These are generally in the pelvis, but subphrenic abscess is also important.

CHRONIC APPENDICITIS

This term is probably a misnomer. A history of slight pain in the right iliac fossa accompanied by dyspepsia may be due to recurrent attacks of mild inflammation. The appendix is found to be fibrosed. The diagnosis is difficult; peptic ulcer, cholecystitis and pyelitis should be excluded by the clinical history and radiological investigation. The group of patients with recurrent pain and tenderness in the right iliac fossa often benefit from appendicectomy, but care should be taken to avoid indiscriminate removal of the normal appendix.

CARCINOID

Carcinoid of the appendix is the term used to describe a small yellow-coloured tumour which is seen in about 0.5 per cent of all appendices removed. The common site is near the tip. It is similar to argentaffin tumours of the small intestine and probably arises from Kulschitzky cells; the malignancy is low (p. 179). Functioning carcinoid syndrome is rare.

FURTHER READING

Cope, Sir Z. (1979). *Early Diagnosis of the Acute Abdomen*. 15th ed. Oxford: University Press.

Kirsner, J. B. and Shorter, R. G. (1980). *Inflammatory Bowel Disease*. 2nd ed. London: Kempton.

Kyle, J (1982). Surgery for Crohn's disease. Brit. J. Hosp. Med. 27, 482–487.

Shepherd, J. A. (1976). *Concise Surgery of the Acute Abdomen*. Edinburgh: Churchill Livingstone.

15

Peritoneum

Anatomy

The features of surgical importance relate to the peritoneal fossae and recesses as these are primarily concerned with the limitation of spread of infection. The greater omentum and the transverse mesocolon divide the peritoneal cavity into two major compartments and infection in one of these often remains confined there (Fig. 15.1).

The principal route for passage of infected material between the upper and lower abdominal compartments is the space on the lateral side of the ascending colon. The close relationship of the appendix to this space accounts for the not infrequent occurrence of subphrenic abscess following appendicitis. Similar recesses on each side of the pelvic colon direct infected fluid into the pelvis with the development of a pelvic abscess.

The lesser sac of peritoneum is readily infected from the pancreas and by perforation of ulcers on the posterior wall of the stomach. It communicates with the general peritoneal cavity through the epiploic foramen which rarely transmits infected fluid.

The *subdiaphragmatic area* may be divided into potential spaces which lie between the diaphragm, posterior abdominal wall, liver and adjacent viscera and above the transverse colon and its mesocolon. Four intraperitoneal and two extraperitoneal spaces

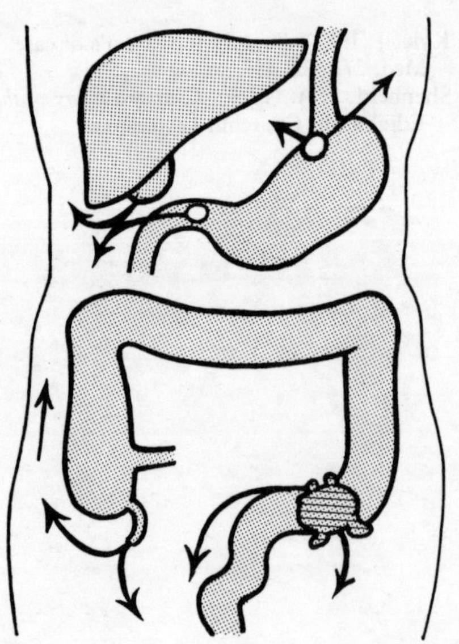

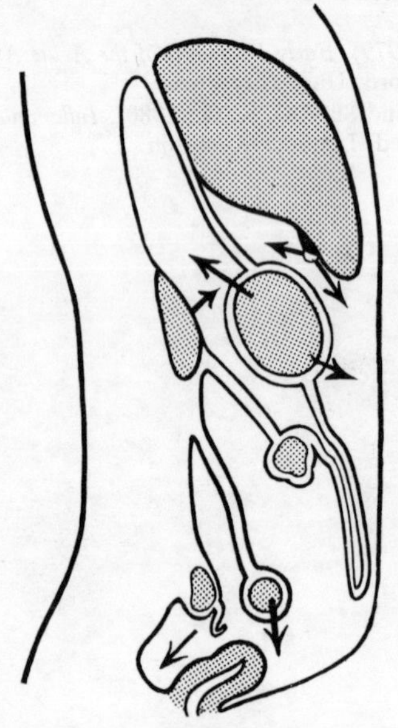

Lateral view

Fig. 15.1 The peritoneal recesses formed by viscera and omenta. The spread of infection is indicated by arrows.

are described. The latter, related to the bare area of the liver, are not surgically important. The two main subdivisions into suprahepatic and infrahepatic spaces are formed by the liver. Right and left areas are produced by the falciform ligament above the liver and ligamentum teres below the liver (Fig. 15.2,B). The right suprahepatic space is bounded posteriorly by the coronary ligament and extends over the dome of the liver. The right infrahepatic space lies between the liver and kidney (Fig. 15.2,A). The left suprahepatic space is not so clearly defined; it lies between diaphragm and left lobe of liver, fundus of stomach and spleen. The lesser sac of peritoneum constitutes the left infrahepatic space.

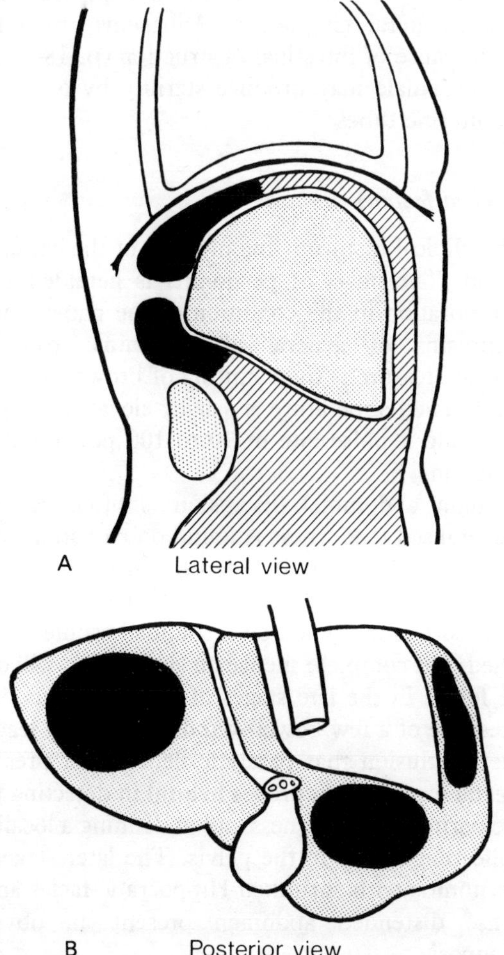

Fig. 15.2 Subphrenic abscess. **A**. Lateral view showing suprahepatic and infrahepatic abscess. **B**. Posterior view of liver showing position of right and left abscesses.

PERITONITIS

The commonest cause of acute infection of the peritoneal cavity is perforation of the intestinal tract, but it may also follow an operative procedure in the abdominal cavity or an induced abortion (Fig. 15.3). Acute peritonitis due to the pneumococcus occurring in young girls is now rarely seen.

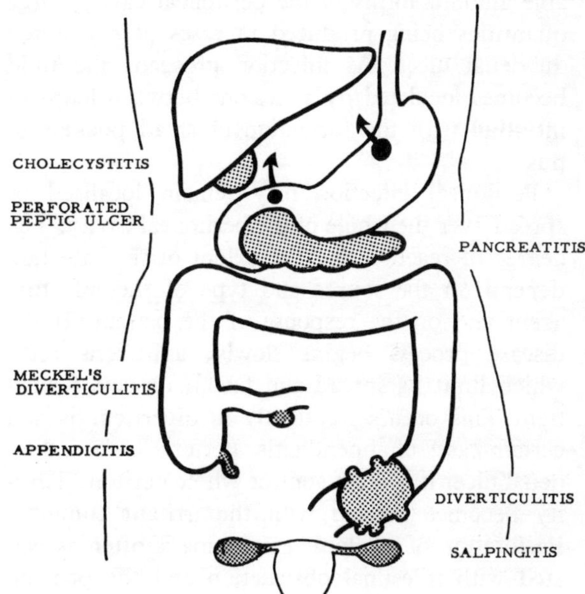

Fig. 15.3 The common causes of peritonitis

Perforated appendicitis ranks as the commonest single disease producing peritonitis. Perforated peptic ulcer and cholecystitis are prominent causes of upper abdominal peritonitis. Salpingitis, often gonorrhoeal in nature, is a frequent cause of pelvic infection in the young female. A haemoperitoneum, resulting from injury to viscera or rupture of an ectopic gestation, may become infected.

Peritonitis following operation is usually due to infection of a haematoma or the result of leakage at an anastomotic site in the intestinal tract. In the latter, particularly after gastric and colonic operations, it is often due to failure of operative technique, especially if the patient, is debilitated or inadequately prepared for surgery.

Pathology

The commonest organisms concerned in the production of peritonitis are *Esch. coli* and *Strept. faecalis*, often combined with *Bacteroides* sp. (p. 10), though many other pathogens have been incriminated. Actinomycosis is occasionally encountered following appendicular perforation.

The peritoneum becomes reddened in the initial stages and the surface sheen rapidly destroyed by an outpouring of fibrin. A serous exudate of variable amount forms in the peritoneal cavity, large quantities being produced in cases of perforated duodenal ulcer. As infection proceeds the fluid becomes loculated by adhesions between loops of intestine with the formation of small pockets of pus.

Peritoneal infection may remain localised or spread over the whole of the peritoneal cavity. The degree of reaction and the extent of the infection depend on the source and type of the infecting agent and on the response of the patient. If the disease process begins slowly, adhesions form which limit its spread and favour abscess formation. This occurs frequently in diverticulitis and certain cases of appendicitis. Perforation of a duodenal ulcer is sudden and the whole peritoneal cavity becomes flooded with the irritant contents. Perforation of a colonic carcinoma is often associated with intestinal obstruction and the pent-up fluid is poured into the peritoneal cavity, producing a particularly severe reaction. Biliary peritonitis from perforation of the gall-bladder produces a marked reaction with only slight localisation by adhesions. The response of the patient to infection is poor in the very young or aged and in cases of malignant disease or blood dyscrasia with inadequate leucocyte and antibody response. Continued administration of cortisone may limit antibody production and lessen resistance to infection.

Some degree of paralytic ileus is always present. If the infection is localised then only the loops of adjacent intestine become affected. Contamination of the whole peritoneal cavity causes a severe degree of ileus. This complication is one of the most serious aspects of peritonitis, and the excessive loss of body fluids into the bowel may account for the development of a shocked state. Toxaemia may be severe due to the large absorptive area of peritoneum in contact with infection.

If the peritonitis is allowed to progress untreated, the patient rapidly becomes dehydrated due to the passage of fluid and electrolytes into the paralysed bowel. The eyes become sunken, the mouth dry, and a state of circulatory collapse develops, which after it has been present for some hours will not respond to therapeutic measures and death ensues. This state is now uncommon because effective treatment is instituted at an earlier stage and the widespread use of antibiotics has helped considerably in combating the infection.

The late results of peritonitis are important. Adhesion formation is variable and after severe infection may be slight, whereas after abdominal operations it is often a marked feature. It is likely that ischaemia of omentum, peritoneum and bowel plays a considerable part in the development of adhesions which have been shown to provide valuable collateral circulation. Adhesions are a frequent cause of intestinal obstruction (p. 184), and in the female may produce sterility by occluding the uterine tubes.

Clinical features

The clinical history is mainly that of the causative lesion. The onset of peritonitis is heralded by a deterioration in the condition of the patient, who complains of generalised abdominal pain. A marked feature is the vomiting of brown intestinal fluid. The temperature is usually elevated to 38° to 40°C and a pulse-rate of 90 to 100 per minute is common.

Slight abdominal distension is often present. Generalised tenderness is found on palpation, with local or diffuse rigidity, depending on the extent of the infection. Rebound tenderness may be a marked feature. The bowel sounds become diminished, but complete silence on ausculation will only be found in the late stages of paralytic ileus. The presence of a few bowel sounds should not lead to the conclusion that paralytic ileus is not present. Rectal examination proves helpful in detecting pelvic peritoneal tenderness and in defining a localised collection of pus in the pelvis. The later stages of peritonitis with shrunken Hippocratic facies and a tense distended abdomen present an obvious diagnosis.

Ancillary investigations are seldom helpful, but an elevated white-cell count is to be expected and the serum electrolyte levels should be determined as they may be deranged by repeated vomiting. Plain radiographs of the abdomen may differentiate the distension from mechanical intestinal obstruction by showing patchy gaseous filling of small and large bowel without the presence of well-defined dilated loops. Free fluid between the coils is a marked feature. Perforation of the intestine may lead to accumulation of free intraperitoneal air.

Treatment

The principal requirements concern the *causative lesion*, the *bacterial infection* and the *paralytic ileus*. Removal of the source of infection is desirable and should be undertaken if the condition of the patient permits operation. If peritonitis has been present for 24 to 36 hours, pre-operative treatment with antibiotics, gastric suction and intravenous fluids should be given. Appendicectomy, cholecystectomy or closure of a perforated peptic ulcer may be readily performed, but other lesions, such as perforation in diverticulitis or carcinoma of the colon, may present a more difficult problem and drainage of the area of perforation or exteriorisation of a colonic loop may be preferred. Peritoneal lavage with saline or antibiotic solutions is useful in cases of severe contamination. Drainage of generalised peritonitis is not effective because of the loculation of infected fluid.

The principal organisms of infection are *Esch. coli* and *Strept. faecalis*, and a broad spectrum antibiotic is more likely to be effective. Cephradine or cefuroxime, gentamicin and metronidazole by intravenous or intramuscular route are widely used. Adequate dosage is essential both for initial treatment and in limiting the development of residual abscesses.

Paralytic ileus should be treated by withholding oral fluids and aspirating the stomach to withdraw the brown intestinal fluid which regurgitates into it. Fluid and electrolytes are given intravenously to replace this intestinal loss, which may be severe in some cases (p. 183). If the patient is shocked intravenous plasma expanders are beneficial. The administration of hydrocortisone is likely to benefit the few cases which have adrenal failure as a result of toxaemia (p. 26). Small doses of morphine are advocated by some surgeons; prostigmine or other cholinergic drugs are not now employed to stimulate peristalsis. Treatment should be continued until the gastric aspirate becomes clear and small in amount, the bowel sounds return to normal and the passage of flatus or faeces per rectum occurs. At this stage the patient often passes several foul-smelling fluid motions. The tendency to resume oral feeding too early should be resisted, fully developed paralytic ileus rarely recovering within 48 hours.

Residual abscess formation

The common sites for loculation of infected peritoneal fluid and the subsequent development of an abscess cavity are in the pelvis and in the subphrenic spaces (Fig. 15.4). A persistent fever and leucocytosis after an abdominal operation should arouse the suspicion of an abscess and ultrasound scanning is useful in confirmation.

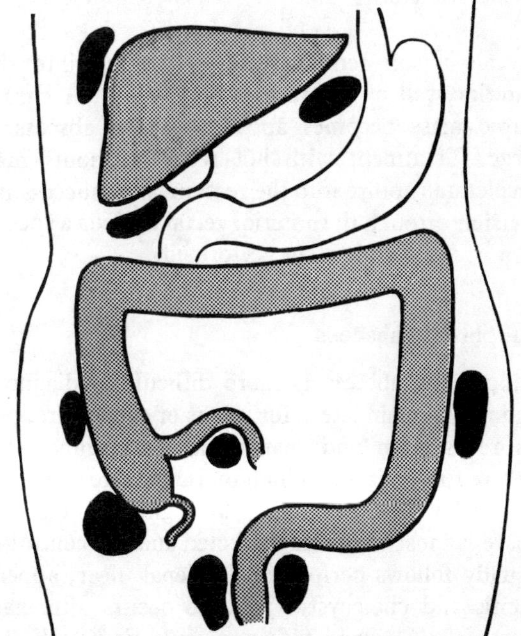

Fig. 15.4 The sites of residual abscess formation

Pelvic abscess

A pelvic abscess causes symptoms by irritation of neighbouring organs, diarrhoea and the passage of mucus per rectum after appendicitis being very suggestive of pelvic inflammation. Frequency of micturition with both red and white cells in the urine is a common finding. Rectal examination

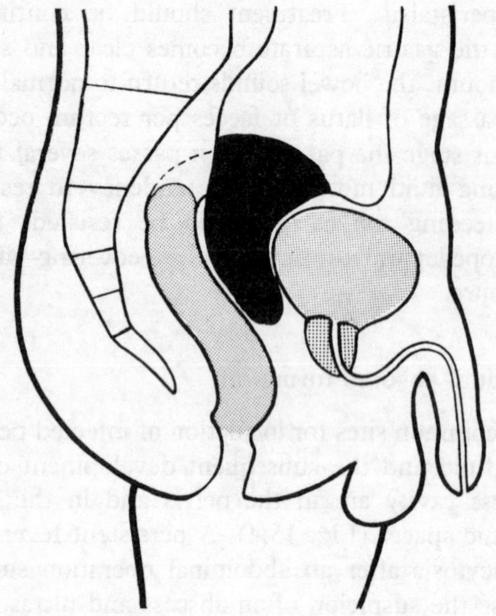

Fig. 15.5 Pelvic abscess, lying in close relationship with the bladder and rectum

reveals a soft tender swelling bulging into the anterior wall of the rectum (Fig. 15.5). A suprapubic mass becomes apparent if the abscess is large. Treatment with hot rectal washouts may accelerate rupture into the rectum. If unsuccessful, incision through the anterior rectal wall via a speculum is easily and safely performed.

Subphrenic abscess

Subphrenic abscess is more difficult to diagnose and may remain latent for weeks or even years, but its recognition and management are important. Severe toxaemia and a high mortality rate often follow delay in treatment. The right suprahepatic space is most commonly affected and the condition usually follows perforated duodenal ulcer, appendicitis and cholecystitis; it also occurs after gastrectomy. A mixed infection with *Esch. coli* and *Strept. faecalis* is usual.

Pain in the upper part of the abdomen is the most frequent symptom and may be referred to the shoulder. An intermittent fever is often present, and when occurring after intraperitoneal infection should arouse suspicion. Tenderness over the area of the abscess is an important localising sign. A small pleural effusion with associated basal crepitations is often to be found. Radiographic screening may show lack of diaphragmatic movement, whilst films may demonstrate an elevated diaphragm with a fluid level in the abscess cavity above the liver. Ultrasound scanning is generally helpful. The abscess should be drained, preferably by an extrapleural approach through the bed of the twelfth rib. If the lesion lies anteriorly or in the infrahepatic space it can be drained by an incision below the costal margin.

Tuberculous peritonitis

This condition is secondary to a focus elsewhere in the body, and coincident with the general decline of tuberculosis is not now commonly encountered. Infection usually reaches the peritoneum by direct spread from mesenteric lymph nodes, but may arise by blood stream spread from the lungs. It affects either sex and is commonest in the young adult.

Two main types of disease occur, the ascitic and the plastic, although adhesion formation and peritoneal exudation are common to both. The *ascitic type* is characterised by the production of large quantities of peritoneal exudate and the presence of tubercles on the peritoneal surface. The *plastic type* shows extensive adhesions, especially between loops of small intestine, which may lead to obstruction. The omentum is often rolled into a transverse mass in the epigastrium and caseation is common.

Clinical presentation is a gradual onset of abdominal discomfort and distension accompanied by generalised wasting; doughy masses may be palpable in the plastic variety. Laparotomy may be necessary in certain cases to establish the diagnosis and exclude malignant disease. Treatment is by anti-tuberculous drug therapy. Surgical relief of obstruction due to adhesions may be necessary at a later date.

Ascites

Peritoneal fluid may be present in excessive amounts from many causes. Serous fluid accumulates in tuberculous peritonitis, malignant disease and chronic nephritis. Congestive cardiac failure and cirrhosis of the liver produce large quantities of fluid. Examination reveals distension of the abdomen with shifting dullness on percussion of the flanks and a fluid thrill.

Paracentesis abdominis results in considerable relief of distension and embarrassed respiration and should be repeated as often as necessary. Intraperitoneal injections of radioactive gold suspension may prevent the accumulation of further fluid in malignant cases. Portacaval anastomosis for portal hypertension is only of occasional value in treating the associated ascites, medical measures using diuretics and spironolactone being more effective. Occasionally fluid may be transferred from the peritoneum to the venous system by means of a plastic tube incorporating a valve and joined to the jugular vein (Le Veen shunt).

Tumour

Primary peritoneal tumours are rare. Secondary deposits of carcinoma are common, the stomach and ovary being the main primary sites. Ovarian carcinoma often leads to ascites, which may be partially limited by removing the primary tumour and any large secondary deposits, including the greater omentum. Cytotoxic drugs such as cisplatin, cyclophosphamide or thiotepa can then be given systemically or intraperitoneally and may be of value as palliative therapy. Paracentesis should be performed as often as necessary to relieve any pressure symptoms due to malignant ascites.

Pseudomyxoma peritonei is an uncommon condition following rupture of a mucocele of the appendix or cystadenoma of the ovary. The peritoneal cavity is filled with gelatinous material, removal of which may be necessary to relieve distension; the causative lesion should also be removed.

FURTHER READING

Darrell, J. H. and Galland, R. B. (1980). Infection following abdominal operations. In *Recent Advances in Surgery*. 10. Ed. Taylor, S. Edinburgh: Churchill Livingstone.

Halliday, P. & Halliday, J. H. (1976). Subphrenic abscess: a study of 241 patients at the Royal Prince Edward Hospital, 1950–1973. Br. J. Surg., **63**, 352.

16

Colon

Physiology

The principal function of the colon is the absorption of the remaining water and electrolytes from the liquid chyme which is ejected through the ileocaecal valve. Approximately 600 ml of fluid enter the colon each day, and the majority is absorbed in the ascending colon, leaving only about 200 ml of water in the expelled faeces. Similarly absorption of electrolytes, of which sodium is particularly important, is mainly a function of the ascending colon. Potassium passes to the faeces by passive diffusion and by secretion in mucus, of importance in colitis and villous papillomas where the loss may be great. Ammonia is both produced and absorbed by the colon and is an important factor in portasystemic encephalopathy, following portacaval shunts in hepatic cirrhosis.

Considerable quantities of gas are found in the large intestine, mainly composed of nitrogen and arising from swallowed air. Diffusion from the bloodstream and bacterial decomposition of food, chiefly in the fluid conditions of the ascending colon, are further sources. The majority is expelled by the passage of flatus, but some is absorbed into the blood. In intestinal obstruction this mechanism is impeded and gross gaseous distension is a prominent feature.

Mucus is produced by the goblet cells in the colonic mucosa, and its function is to lubricate the passage of hard faeces, thereby protecting the mucosa from trauma. It is an alkaline secretion and aids in neutralising the irritating acids formed as a result of bacterial action.

The storage of faeces in the left half of the colon is the main function of this part of the large intestine. Mass peristalsis, initiated by the gastrocolic reflex which occurs after each meal, moves the contents into a more distant segment so that they finally collect in the pelvic colon. Such movements are controlled by the parasympathetic system, mainly the sacral component in the distal colon, and co-ordinated by the intrinsic nerves of the bowel wall. Further peristalsis forces the faeces into the rectum to produce an urge for defaecation.

MEGACOLON

This condition is one of dilatation of the colon without any clinically obvious organic cause. There are two main types, which at one time were confused; (*a*) Hirschsprung's disease or true megacolon, and (*b*) functional or acquired megacolon.

Hirschsprung's disease

Pathology

The abnormality in this congenital condition is present in the terminal and undilated portion of the large intestine, where an absence of ganglion cells interferes with normal peristalsis to produce subsequent obstruction. Usually only the rectum and sigmoid colon are affected, but the lesion may extend proximally to include the transverse colon. Gross hypertrophy of the whole of the muscular wall, followed by dilatation and secondary inflammatory changes in the mucosa, occurs proximal to the aganglionic segment. Bladder enlargement and urinary dysfunction may be associated in some cases.

Clinical features

Despite being the commonest congenital lesion of the colon the condition is rare and found in only 1 in 30 000 births. Other associated congenital abnormalities are unusual. There is a marked male preponderance of about 90 per cent, and although it is not hereditary it has been observed in several members of the same family.

Symptoms consist of constipation from birth or early infancy, becoming progressively more severe and obstinate. Diarrhoea may at times occur from fluid contents by-passing the obstructing faeces. Pain and vomiting are uncommon, but abdominal distension becomes pronounced after a few months. Interference with nutrition produces ill-health. Gross enlargement causes eversion of the lower ribs and dyspnoea, together with a tympanitic abdomen and protuberant umbilicus. Rectal examination is normal with no alteration in calibre and without the presence of loaded faecal material.

The diagnosis should be confirmed by a barium enema which demonstrates a variable length of apparently normal lower bowel and proximal dilatation. Oblique views are essential for adequate study of the area which may be obscured by a loaded colon. Transanal rectal wall biopsy is advisable and of value in differentiating the condition from acquired megacolon.

Treatment consists of removal of the aganglionic segment with end-to-end anastomosis. This generally involves resection of the rectosigmoid area with an anastomosis between the dilated colon and a short rectal stump. A combined abdominal and perineal approach is used. Preliminary transverse colostomy may be required where there is gross distension and debility, and this alone gives relief of symptoms. Operation is usually carried out at about the age of six months.

The results are good, although when conservative measures were employed, about 30 per cent did not survive more than two or three years.

Functional or acquired megacolon

This condition is not generally seen as early as Hirschsprung's disease, being found in children between two and four years of age. It is more common in boys, and is usually caused by a local lesion, such as an anal fissure, itself often the result of

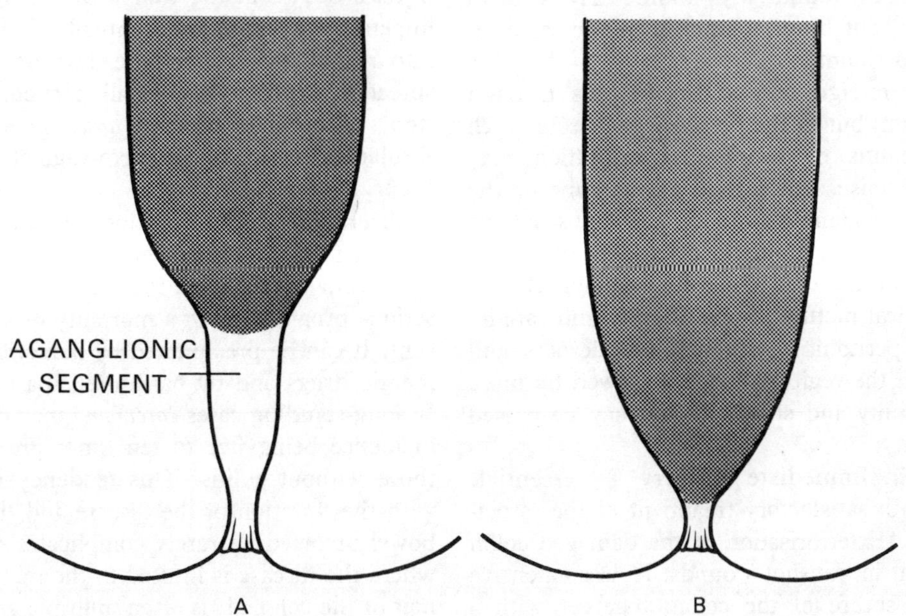

Fig. 16.1 Megacolon. **A.** Hirschsprung's. **B.** Functional.

faulty training in bowel habits. A vicious cycle may be induced with progressive constipation from fear of pain on defaecation. Increasing distension follows and faecal masses may be palpable in the abdomen. On rectal examination there is gross dilatation and hard and impacted faeces are easily felt, unlike Hirschsprung's disease, where the rectum is empty (Fig. 16.1). A barium enema confirms the dilatation and the absence of a distal portion of normal calibre.

Treatment involves evacuation of the bowel, either manually or by repeated enemata. Satisfactory training should be instituted subsequently, aperients and washouts being continued for several months until it is evident that the condition has been satisfactorily relieved.

Traumatic lesions

Injuries to the colon may be the result of an external force penetrating the anterior abdominal wall, or of an intraluminal force from an object either traversing the alimentary tract or introduced through the rectum. External colonic wounds are more frequent in war time, gunshot injuries being particularly serious from the extent of bowel devitalised. Incised wounds with a knife may occur in civilian life, but blunt trauma in motor car accidents is less common.

Ingested foreign bodies usually pass through normal colon, but in the presence of disease, such as diverticulitis or neoplasm, perforation may occur. The misuse of a rigid enema tube or the unsatisfactory manipulation of a colonoscope or sigmoidoscope may injure the colon. The damage is sometimes self-inflicted or may follow polypectomy.

The clinical picture is one of early and rapidly advancing peritonitis with pain, tenderness and guarding in the region injured, followed by more general rigidity and shock. Blood may be passed per rectum.

Treatment. Immediate surgery is essential, together with satisfactory treatment of the associated shock. Exteriorisation of the damaged colon is important in gunshot wounds. In less extensive lacerations suture of the colon, together with a temporary defunctioning colostomy, is adequate. Antibiotics should be prescribed.

ULCERATIVE COLITIS

Pathology

Various aetiological factors have been suggested in the causation of this disease—a specific organism or virus, an allergic phenomenon, an increase in the colonic enzymes which dissolve mucus—but none is entirely acceptable. A psychosomatic origin has been postulated, but although psychological factors may help to precipitate relapses there is no proof they are responsible for initiating the condition. It may be a disease of auto-immunity but evidence is lacking to establish this. It does appear to be more common in certain families. The condition begins in the rectum or rectosigmoid area and extends proximally to involve the whole or part of the large intestine. The terminal ileum is involved in 18 per cent of cases.

Early pathological changes are hyperaemia, congestion and oedema of the mucosa, which produce a reddened and granular appearance. Ulceration of the mucosa and submucosa may follow, which is initially patchy but may later become widespread. The intermediate areas of mucosa become congested and hypertrophied and give the appearance of pseudo-polypi. In chronic cases fibrosis occurs in the wall with narrowing of the lumen, the whole colon eventually being converted into a rigid and fibrotic tube. Infection rarely may spread through the bowel wall, particularly the rectum, to produce *perianal abscesses* and external fistulae. Occasionally a recto-vaginal fistula may occur.

Ulceration in some instances progresses to *perforation* and peritonitis. *Toxic dilatation* of the colon may occur in the acute fulminating type and is of serious prognosis with a mortality of about 25 per cent. It can be precipitated by narcotics, anticholinergic drugs and by barium enema examination. In long-standing cases *carcinoma* may develop, the incidence being five to ten times greater than in those without colitis. This tendency is increased with the duration of the disease and the extent of bowel involved. It rarely complicates distal colitis where the disease is limited to the rectum and left half of the colon. It is often multiple and scattered throughout the intestine, not being confined to the common site of the rectosigmoid. It appears to be preceded by epithelial dysplasia which, if severe, resembles carcinoma in situ. Metastases occur early and the prognosis is poor. In addition to the development of cancer, the following complications may occur: pyoderma gangrenosum and erythema nodosum, arthritis, sacro-iliitis, iritis, chronic anaemia and liver damage.

Clinical features

Males and females are equally affected, the greatest age incidence being in the third and fourth decades, although it may also occur in children. The onset is frequently abrupt and often related to a period of emotional strain, either occupational or domestic. The chief symptom is diarrhoea, often worse in the morning, and which may vary from five to twenty or more motions per day. This is usually followed by the passage of blood and slime, and may be accompained by abdominal colic. There are three main clinical types, but overlap is common.

1. Acute fulminating colitis
2. Severe chronic colitis
3. Mild chronic colitis

The acute fulminating type is accompanied by severe toxicity and carries a poor prognosis. Marked fluid and electrolyte loss and gross anaemia may contribute to death in a few days or weeks. Recovery may take place or the patient pass into the chronic state of ulcerative colitis.

In the severe chronic form the remissions may never be complete, and the frequent attacks produce gross incapacity, resulting in chronic invalidism.

In the mild chronic form the remissions may be complete and be of weeks or even years duration. The symptoms are seldom very severe and between attacks, and even during them, there is no disability.

On examination the general state of the patient varies with the clinical type, being apparently normal in the mild type and severely shocked in the fulminating form. Anorexia, nausea, vomiting, weight-loss, anaemia and fever may be present, tending to be more marked in the very young or the elderly. The abdomen is generally soft but the colon may be palpable and tender in the more severe case. There may be evidence of other complications, such as leg ulcers, painful joints and chronic debility.

Investigations

Haematological examination frequently shows an anaemia and raised E.S.R. whilst the blood chemistry is usually altered in the acute fulminating type to reveal fluid and electrolyte depletion. The stools vary from being semi-formed in the mild case to small volume ones with little faecal content but much blood and mucus in the seriously ill patient. Cultures are required to exclude specific dysenteries and *Campylobacter* and gonococci as well as the toxin of *Clostridium difficile* must be excluded. Sigmoidoscopy is essential. In the mild form the hyperaemic and friable mucosa bleeds easily when touched with the instrument but actual ulceration is seldom seen. Severe forms are recognised by oedema of the rectal valves, denuded and bleeding mucosa and mucopurulent discharge. In chronic cases polyps may be noted. A rectal biospy should be undertaken to confirm the diagnosis and differentiate it from Crohn's disease. Usually the inflammation is confined to the mucosa and does not extend into the submucosa. In long-standing cases colonoscopy and multiple biopsies can prove helpful in recognising pre-cancerous areas.

A plain radiograph is of value in diagnosing toxic dilatation. A barium enema is contraindicated in acute colitis and gentle bowel preparation advised in chronic disease but in the established case there is loss of mucosal pattern, lack of haustrations—which give a 'lead-pipe' appearance—and shortening of the colon with depression of flexures (Fig. 16.2).

Differential diagnosis

Although specific dysenteries must be excluded in addition to tuberculosis, the main lesions to be considered are Crohn's disease, large intestinal tumours and ischaemic colitis. The last named generally occurs in the elderly, often in the region of the splenic flexure and may either resolve completely or produce a stricture. The main confusion is with Crohn's disease of the large intestine but in the latter the onset is less sudden, a bloody stool is rare,

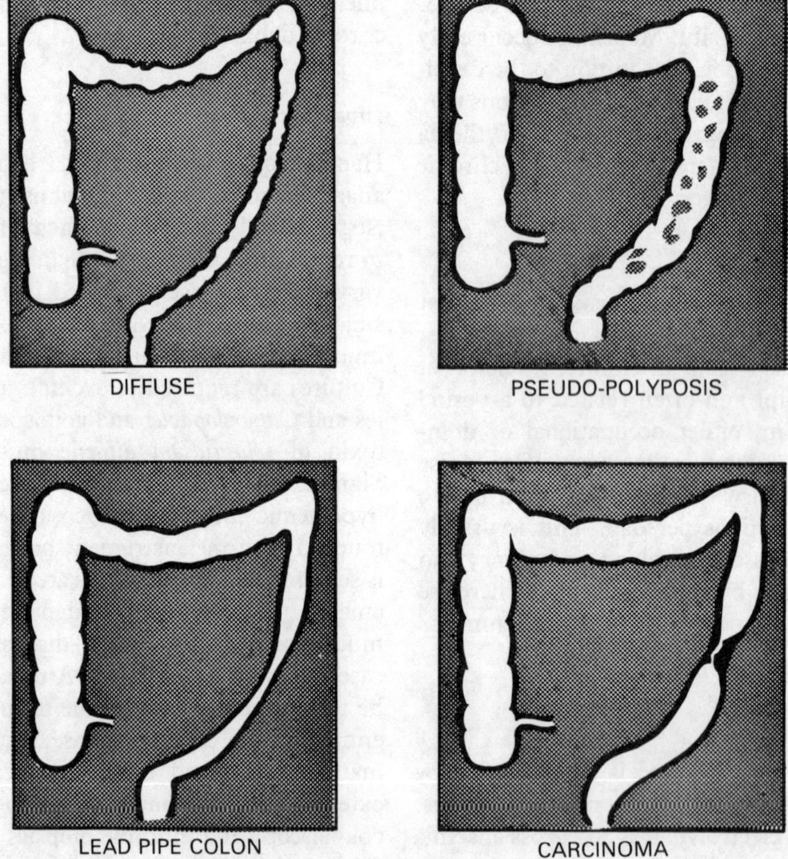

Fig. 16.2 Ulcerative colitis. The changes evident on radiological examination.

the anal region is more frequently involved than in ulcerative colitis, whilst radiologically strictures and internal fistulae are more likely in Crohn's disease.

Treatment

In the mild uncomplicated case a *medical regime* of rest, sedation and prolonged sulphasalazine therapy may suffice. In the more severe case bed rest, correction of anaemia and oral steroid therapy are required. Prednisolone applied topically in the form of a nightly rectal enema or suppository is also advisable. When symptoms disappear their frequency can be reduced but continued until the rectal mucosa is normal on sigmoidoscopy. Supportive sulphasalazine therapy should be continued indefinitely. In the *fulminating* form intravenous fluids, electrolytes and blood replacement are necessary, accompanied by adequate systemic steroids and metronidazole. Absence of good clinical response to medical management in five days is an indication for surgery.

Operative treatment is required for failure of an acute attack to respond to intensive medical management, toxic megacolon, severe bleeding and perforation. It is also indicated where chronic invalidism and intractable diarrhoea exist and will restore the patient to normal health. The grave hazard of cancerous change in long-standing cases, perhaps as high as 25 per cent where the disease has been present for ten or more years and affecting the whole colon, may be an additional indication for surgery.

The following surgical methods are available:

1 Panproctocolectomy
2 Total colectomy and ileo-rectal anastomosis

Panproctocolectomy is the procedure of choice in the majority of cases (Fig. 16.3A). In right-sided

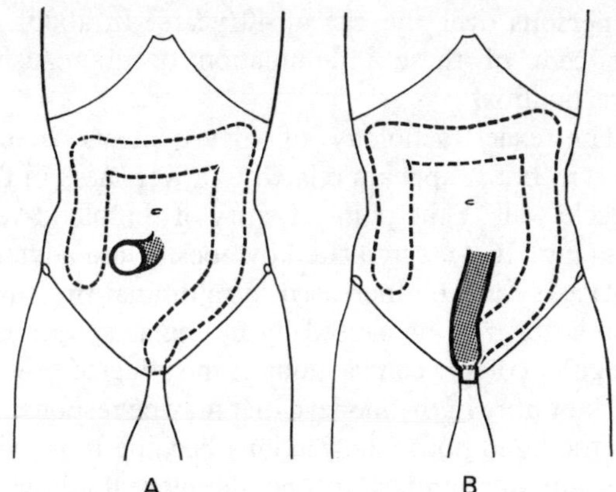

Fig. 16.3 The types of operation performed for ulcerative colitis. **A.** Panproctocolectomy with ileostomy. **B.** Resection of colon with ileorectal anastomosis.

or segmental colitis a more conservative resection can be performed. When the rectum is not extensively involved a low ileo-rectal anastomosis may be preferred, the patient being spared an ileostomy (Fig. 16.3, B). The bowels are usually opened four or five times a day and careful follow-up, including sigmoidoscopy, is essential to detect any subsequent neoplastic change in the rectal stump. If a diseased rectum is retained it may be the source of a later fulminating form or be responible for the persistence of the extra-bowel complications of the disease.

Although a permanent ileostomy is a disability, the availability of light plastic bags attached to slim flanges firmly adherent to the skin and which may be left in position for up to three weeks now permit a normal economic and social life. Some psychological readjustment in the first few weeks may be required, but trained stomatherapists can advise on any problems. Continent ileal reservoirs have been developed in recent years. Skill is required in their fashioning, but they may be constructed in the abdomen or in the pelvis following an ileo-rectal anastomosis. They can be emptied twice daily to the benefit of the patient.

GRANULOMATOUS COLITIS (CROHN'S DISEASE)

Pathology

The incidence of this condition affecting the large bowel has increased in recent years but the aetiology is unknown. The caecum or colon is involved in one-third of all cases of Crohn's disease whilst the large intestine alone is involved in about 10 per cent. The pathology is of discontinuous involvement of the bowel wall with three easily defined macroscopic types. There may be single or multiple strictures or ulceration of the mucosa with a characteristic 'cobble-stone' appearance of the latter. This is caused by fissures which surround islands of mucosa raised by oedema and inflammation. The bowel wall is thickened, small sarcoid granules may be seen on the serosa and the lymph nodes are usually enlarged (p. 177). Microscopically a sarcoid inflammatory reaction occurs in the bowel wall and often in the nodes. Fissuring is important and may extend through the wall. The picture may resemble non-caseating tuberculosis but there is a less florid reaction and the foci of epithelioid and giant cells are smaller and fewer in Crohn's disease.

Granulomatous colitis does not generally occur with ulcerative colitis, and less frequently affects the rectum and distal sigmoid colon alone. *Anal lesions* are usually not in direct continuity with the diseased bowel but appear to be separate, perhaps related to the lymphoid tissue around the anal glands. They occur in a quarter of the cases involving the terminal ileum, but in all those where the rectum is involved. They may be the first lesions encountered or there may be a latent period of months or years. At times they are the first indication of recurrence of the disease. Abscesses, fissures and fistulae may occur and ulceration can extend to involve the vulva, groins and natal cleft. There is an increased frequency of colonic carcinoma in long-standing Crohn's disease and it may also develop in excluded loops and fistulae.

Clinical features

Abdominal pain, diarrhoea and weight loss are common but rectal bleeding is less frequent than in ulcerative colitis. Tenderness and an abdominal mass due to pericolic thickening or infection, pyrexia and spontaneous external or internal fistulae may occur, the last not usually found in ulcerative colitis. In severe cases, toxic dilatation of the colon may take place. A past or present anal abnormality is common. Erythema nodosum, synovitis and iritis may be associated. Thickening and narrowing of the rectal wall may be found on digital examination. The mucosa is generally normal on sigmoidoscopy but when involved is less granular than in ulcerative colitis (p. 203), with patches of normal mucosa; biopsy should be performed. A double contrast barium enema demonstrating the 'cobblestone' changes of the mucosa and 'rose thorn' fissures is diagnostic. Strictures separated by normal areas also distinguish Crohn's disease from ulcerative colitis where a stricture is rare except after the development of carcinoma.

Treatment

Medical management with rest, sedation, high protein and calorie and low residue diet, codeine phosphate, sulphasalazine and steroids as in ulcerative colitis may effect an improvement. Immunosuppressive therapy has also been used but is not free of risk. Surgery is required when medical treatment fails or complications ensue. Localised lesions of the colon can be resected, but in extensive disease sub-total colectomy may be required. Recurrences may still take place and are often proximal to the anastomosis. Low anal fistulae should be laid open, but if high, and damage to the anal sphincters seems likely, simple drainage of the abscesses and curettage may suffice. The proximal disease must be treated. Total colectomy with excision of the rectum may be required in advanced cases.

DIVERTICULAR DISEASE

The colon is the most frequent site of diverticula in the alimentary tract and it is to inflammation of these colonic pouches that the term diverticulitis is generally applied.

Pathology

With the exception of the rare solitary diverticulum of the caecum, colonic diverticula are of the false or acquired type. They do not therefore contain all the coats of the bowel wall but are composed of prolapsed pouches of mucosa. The right half of the colon is seldom affected and the usual site is in the pelvic and descending portions. They are multiple in number and constitute the common condition of diverticulosis which is present in about 5 per cent of persons over the age of 40 years. In about 10 per cent of these inflammation occurs causing diverticulitis.

The exact aetiology of diverticulosis is not known, but it appears related to a weakness in the muscle wall at the point of entry of the blood-vessels (Fig. 16.4), aggravated by obesity and advancing years, and by increased intraluminal pressure. The latter may be caused by muscular spasm and irregular colonic contractions in the affected bowel. Lack of fibre in the modern diet may be responsible for the condition. Contractions become more vigorous in an attempt to propel the more fluid faeces with consequent rise in intraluminal pressure.

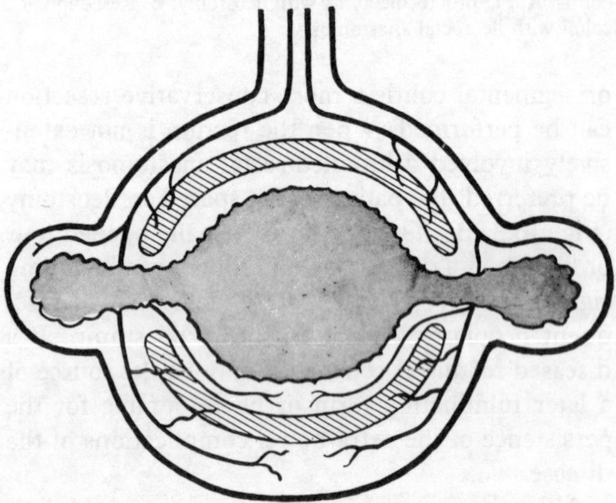

Fig. 16.4 Transverse section of the colon showing development of diverticula

The diverticula, most marked in the pelvic colon, are situated symmetrically in rows and frequently project into the appendices epiploicae. They commence as wide-mouthed pouches but become flask-shaped as faecal material enters and is not expelled, due to the absence of muscular contraction. The faeces become inspissated, the mucosa is injured and infection follows to produce diverticulitis. If the inflammation is acute there may be gangrene and peritonitis. Local abscesses may form, either intraperitoneally or as a pericolic collection of pus. These in turn may form a fistula, either internally into the bladder, vagina or small intestine, or externally. More frequently only minute perforation occurs with chronic changes of thickening of the

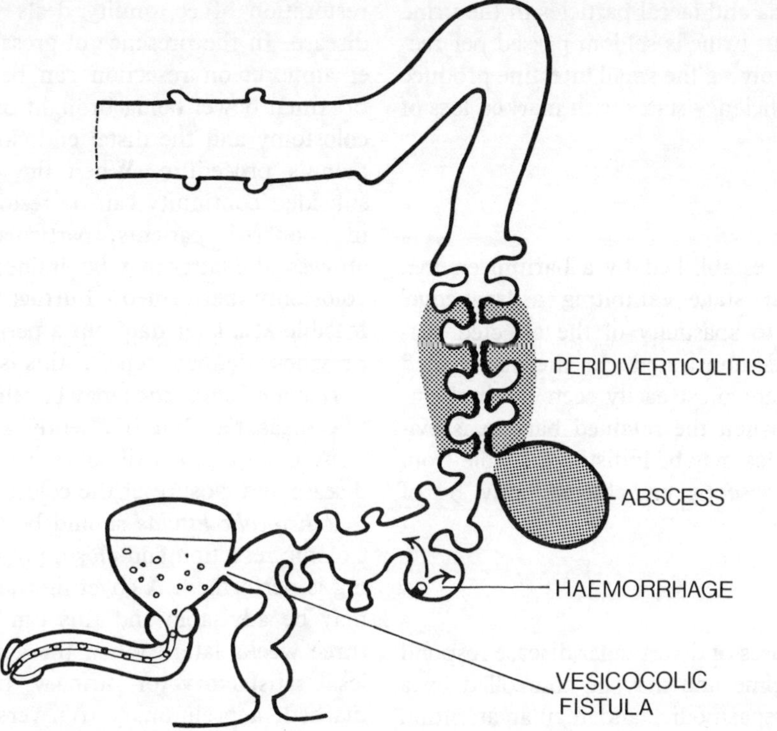

Fig. 16.5 The complications of diverticulosis of the colon

muscular coat due to hypertrophy of the longitudinal and circular muscle fibres, but the mucosa lining the lumen does not show gross ulceration. Localised inflammation in the pericolic tissues produces peridiverticulitis (Fig. 16.5). In long-standing cases deposits of fibro-fatty tissues are formed in the sub-serosa, the appendices epiploicae and in the mesocolon. These changes and the muscular hypertrophy result in a thickened, rigid and contracted segment predisposing to intestinal obstruction. This may be aggravated by contraction of the mesocolon with angulation and fixation to other structures. Malignant change does not occur in diverticulitis but can arise independently.

Clinical features

Middle-aged and elderly males, particularly the obese, are mainly affected. Diverticulosis is asymptomatic and not recognised clinically.

The main symptom of *acute* diverticulitis is sub-umbilical pain, later referable to the left iliac fossa, when the commonly involved pelvic colon is affected. Local tenderness and guarding occur and a mass is occasionally palpable. The temperature and pulse-rate are raised and signs of peritonitis may follow.

In *chronic* diverticulitis the symptoms are less definite, but the diagnosis is suggested by intermittent pain, generally of a dull nature but occasionally colicky, felt in the left iliac fossa. Dyspepsia, distension, constipation and at times recurrent diarrhoea may also be present. Bleeding occurs per rectum in about 20 per cent of cases generally in the elderly, but is only occasionally severe. Tenderness and a mass may be found in the left iliac fossa, and the clinical picture is easily confused with colonic cancer. Sigmoidoscopy should be performed to exclude distal malignant disease.

Obstructive symptoms are usually of large bowel variety due to stenosis but may be of small bowel type when the latter adheres to a diverticular area. The common fistula, the vesico-colic, is less likely in the female because of the interposition of the uterus, but is characterised by initial dysuria, frequency and haematuria. Resolution of the cystitis is usual and ascending renal infection is uncommon. Pneumaturia and faecal particles in the urine may be noted, but urine is seldom passed per rectum. Fistulae involving the small intestine produce diarrhoea and deficiency states with marked loss of weight.

Investigations

The diagnosis is established by a barium enema. A prediverticular stage exhibiting a 'saw-edge' appearance due to spasticity of the affected segments may be demonstrated. In the established case diverticula are most easily seen in the post-evacuation film when the retained barium is evident. Stenotic areas may be indistinguishable from cancer but colonoscopy and biopsy may be of value.

Treatment

Mild and early cases of diverticular disease respond to a medical regime and may be controlled by a bulky diet, anti-spasmodics and regular attention to the bowels. In acute diverticulitis conservative measures should also be adopted with bed rest and antibiotic therapy.

Indications for surgery

1. Failure of medical management
2. Presence of complications

Failure of response to a medical regime with repeated attacks of acute diverticulitis, progressive narrowing of the bowel and the inherent risk of complications is sufficient to warrant surgery which in recent years has become more safe. Resection of the diverticular area may be performed with restoration of continuity. This is generally completed in one operation after adequate bowel preparation but can be staged. In the latter, a transverse colostomy is first performed to defunction the distal bowel which is then washed out and the diverticular area resected three to six weeks later. The colostomy is closed two weeks afterwards.

Pericolic abscesses should be incised and drained.

Perforations require immediate laparotomy. If conditions are suitable immediate resection with restoration of continuity deals with the primary disease. In the presence of gross infection or oedematous colon resection can be undertaken, the proximal bowel being brought out as a temporary colostomy and the distal end closed as in a Hartmann's procedure. When the inflammation has subsided continuity can be restored. Occasionally in poor risk patients, particularly with a large abscess, the latter may be drained and a transverse colostomy performed. Further surgery may be feasible at a later date but a permanent colostomy provides adequate relief if this is not possible.

Intestinal obstruction may be relieved by conservative measures, but frequently a transverse colostomy is required with subsequent resection of the disease and closure of the colostomy.

Vesico-colic fistulae should be treated surgically. Colonic resection and closure of the bladder opening is performed. A covering transverse colostomy may be advisable and this can be closed two to three weeks later. When the general condition is less satisfactory or urinary tract infection is marked, a preliminary transverse colostomy may be advisable and the colonic resection performed six weeks later.

VOLVULUS

This condition involves a rotation, generally in an anticlockwise direction, of part of the large intestine around its mesenteric axis. The pelvic colon is the usual site and is frequently elongated and chronically distended. The caecum may also be involved, particularly when the ascending colon has an associated mesentery; less commonly the transverse colon is affected. A closed-loop obstruction ensues which may reach large dimensions. Continued twisting occludes the blood supply and gangrene, perforation and peritonitis follow.

Clinical features

The disease is more common in elderly men and associated with long-standing constipation. It is the most common cause of rapid gross distension of the abdomen. Following bouts of constipation there may be a sudden onset of lower abdominal colic, complete constipation and distension at first localised to the site of obstruction. In the pelvic colon the dilated loop may be seen through a thin abdominal wall, rising out of the pelvis, and accompanied by visible peristalsis. Tenderness over the loop or in the left iliac fossa may be noted. In later stages general distension with shock and peritonitis may follow. Radiography confirms the diagnosis, a plain film of the abdomen showing the distended loop. A barium enema may be required in less acute cases to determine the exact site involved.

Treatment

When the pelvic colon is affected, and in the absence of strangulation, a rectal tube may be carefully introduced through a sigmoidoscope to attempt deflation. If not easily successful immediate laparotomy is required with untwisting of the loop. Preliminary decompression of the bowel by puncture and suction or by manipulation of a rectal tube at the time of operation may be helpful. Volvulus of the caecum may be prevented from recurring by suturing it to the posterior abdominal wall. Strangulation or recurrent volvulus of the pelvic colon should be treated by resection or exteriorisation (Paul-Mikulicz) (Fig. 16.6).

BENIGN TUMOURS OF THE COLON

The majority are of epithelial origin, either adenomas or papillomas. Lipomas, leiomyomas, fibromas and angiomas occur only rarely. An endometrioma may involve the pelvic colon from without, and carcinoids have also been reported.

Epithelial tumours assume importance because of the undoubted risk of malignant change. They are frequently multiple and commonly involve the pelvic colon.

Adenoma is more common than papilloma and often occurs in children as a single polyp; malignancy does not supervene in childhood. It is composed of glandular epithelium, characterised by arising from a localised area of mucosa, and initially sessile, it later becomes pedunculated.

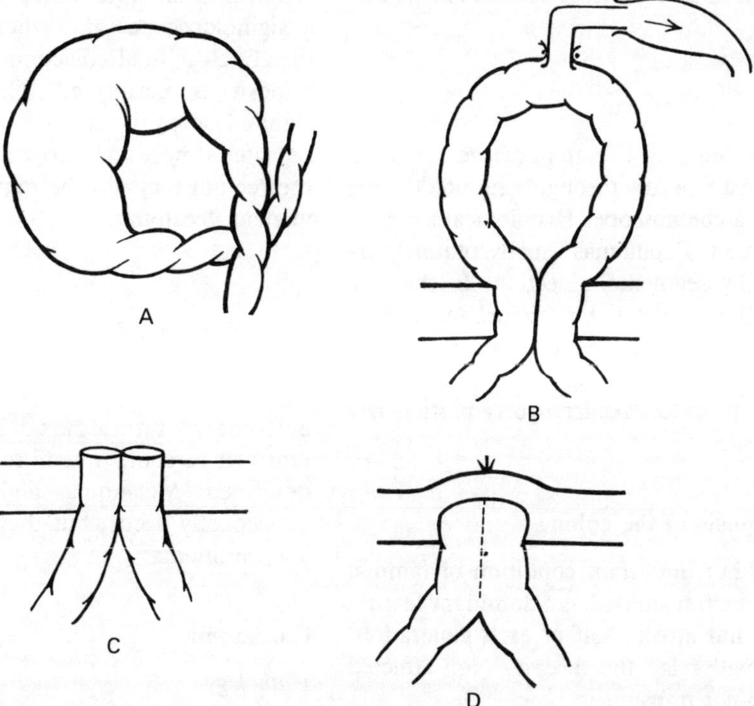

Fig. 16.6 Volvulus of the pelvic colon treated by Paul-Mikulicz type of resection. **A.** Volvulus. **B.** Loop of colon exteriorised and decompressed. **C.** Redundant loop excised. **D.** Closure of resulting colostomy.

Papilloma consists of proliferated epithelium arising from a wider area of bowel and bearing a connective tissue and vascular stalk. It may also be slightly pedunculated, but has a broad base and is more prone than an adenoma to undergo malignant change.

Clinical features

The chief symptom is rectal bleeding and if continuous may result in anaemia. It is more likely to be severe if an angioma is present, and if the bleeding is restricted to the time of the menses it is probably due to an endometrioma. A papilloma may produce diarrhoea or a discharge of mucus. A bulky tumour may intussuscept to give abdominal colic and obstruction. Frequently, benign tumours are asymptomatic and recognised on an incidental barium enema. The oral pigmentation of Peutz-Jeghers disease has been mentioned in small intestinal tumours (p. 179) where such neoplasms are more common, but it is occasionally found in association with colonic growths. The diagnosis is confirmed by a double contrast barium enema and colonoscopy.

Treatment

Adenomas of more than 1.0 cm in diameter should be removed by diathermy through a sigmoidoscope or more often a colonoscope. Histological examination is important. Papillomas usually require surgical excision by segmental resection. In the rare case of profound metabolic disturbance, preoperative fluid and electrolyte replacement is required. Careful follow-up by colonoscopy and radiology to detect recurrence is particularly important.

Familial polyposis of the colon

This is a rare but important condition of familial origin. It may be transmitted as a dominant feature by either sex and affects half of each generation, who in turn will relay the disease. Non-affected individuals do not transmit it.

Multiple polypi appear about the age of puberty diffusely scattered over all the mucosa of the colon and rectum and on section are shown to be adenomas. A period, which may last up to 10 years ensues, during which there are no symptoms despite the presence of polypi. Clinical recognition due to diarrhoea, followed later by blood and mucous discharge, is usual about the age of 21 years. In most cases cancer develops about the age of 25 years.

Familial polyposis may rarely be preceded by multiple exostoses or fibromas; this is helpful in determining those who are likely to be later affected by the disease. Sigmoidoscopy and a barium enema are essential investigations.

Treatment

Where feasible a comprehensive family tree should be compiled. This, combined with sigmoidoscopy of the children of affected members, is an important step in preventing the development of cancer. Sigmoidoscopy, initially required at about 13 years, should be repeated at 20 years and at five-yearly intervals until the age of 40 years.

In the established case the treatment is initial removal of all rectal polypi by diathermy through a sigmoidoscope, and when the rectum is completely clear total colectomy with ileo-rectal anastomosis is performed. Careful follow-up with sigmoidoscopy is essential and further diathermy repeated if necessary. In some instances excision of the rectum may also be required, incurring a permanent ileostomy.

MALIGNANT DISEASE OF THE COLON

Sarcoma

Sarcomas are rare, although lymphosarcoma, reticulum cell sarcoma and fibrosarcoma have all been described. Melanomas and malignant carcinoids occasionally occur, but the usual malignant lesion is a carcinoma.

Carcinoma

Pathology

Three known lesions are of aetiological importance—single colonic polyp, multiple polyposis and ulcerative colitis—but development may be independent of such conditions. The most common site, which is the pelvic colon, may be related to the stasis of carcinogenic substances or to the frequency of polypi. Next in order of frequency come the ascending colon, transverse colon, splenic flexure, caecum, hepatic flexure and descending colon. Macroscopically there are two main types, the proliferative and the annular, together with a less common ulcerative form with everted edges (Fig. 16.7).

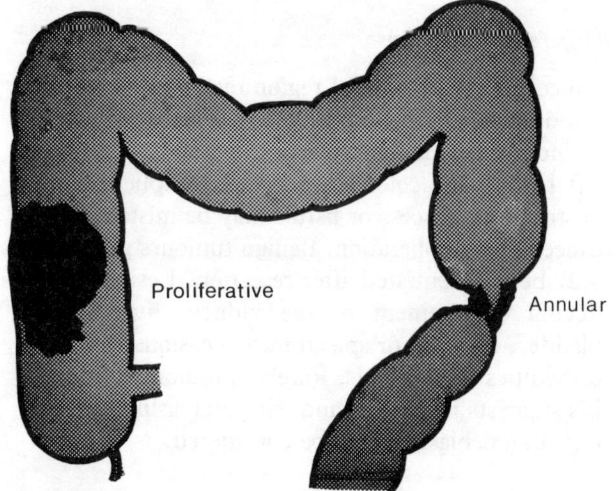

Fig. 16.7 The radiological appearance of carcinoma of the colon

The *proliferative* tumour is more often found in the right half of the colon, particularly in the caecal region, and is composed of a fungating cauliflower mass which projects into the lumen of the bowel. It is a slowly growing tumour which is less invasive than the annular type; due to its bulk mucosal necrosis is frequent and infection often supervenes. Mucoid degeneration may occur with disappearance of tumour cells and their replacement by mucoid material, the prognosis at this stage becoming worse.

The *annular* or scirrhous tumour is more common in the left half of the colon where it encircles the intestine, and by contraction resembles the tying of a string around the bowel. Ulceration is a late feature of this type. Microscopically the majority of colonic cancers are adenocarcinomas, but highly anaplastic tumours occasionally occur.

Spread takes place by direct invasion, by the lymphatics and by the bloodstream (Fig. 16.8).

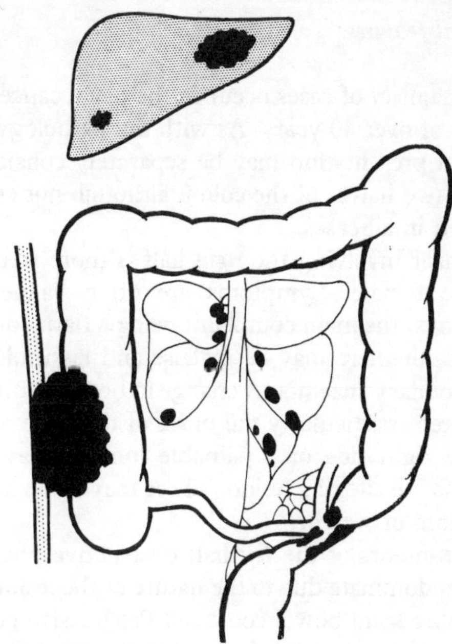

Fig. 16.8 Spread of carcinoma of the colon to the liver, abdominal wall, lymph nodes and small intestine with formation of a fistula

Local extension is both longitudinally and circumferentially in proliferative tumours in approximately equal amounts, but in annular growths it is almost entirely in a circumferential direction. The resulting stenosis produces hypertrophy and dilatation of the proximal bowel wall, whilst inspissated faeces collecting above the obstruction may cause pressure necrosis (stercoral ulceration). Intestinal obstruction and perforation follow earlier in the annular tumour than in the proliferative one which only obstructs the fluid faeces at a later stage.

Spread into the abdominal wall, bladder, ovary, small intestine or stomach may lead to the development of local infection, peritonitis or fistulae.

Lymphatic spread is most important and follows the vascular supply. The paracolic nodes at the point of division of the mesentery to surround the bowel are first affected, followed by spread to the intermediate group along the branches of the mesenteric vessels and thence to the central group surrounding the superior and inferior mesenteric trunks.

Bloodstream spread is via the portal vein to the liver, less commonly to the lungs and other sites.

Clinical features

The majority of cases occur in the usual cancer age group of over 40 years. As with the pathology, the clinical presentation may be separately considered in the two halves of the colon, although not clearly defined in all cases.

Cancer involving the *right* half is more frequent in the female. Symptoms are often vague and insidious, the main complaint being a flatulent dyspepsia, or there may be malaise and lassitude due to secondary anaemia. A change in bowel habit may be noted, particularly the onset of diarrhoea. Pain in the right side or a palpable tumour may later localise the site of a lesion. There may be an associated loss of weight.

In tumours of the *left* half obstructive phenomena predominate due to the nature of the lesion and the more solid bowel contents. Progressive constipation, the necessity of aperients for the first time and intermittent diarrhoea are typical symptoms, the last being due to inflammation and ulceration produced by faecal matter proximal to the obstruction. Attacks of abdominal colic, left iliac, or even right iliac pain due to caecal distension may follow. Recurring abdominal distension noted by a tightness of the clothes and audible borborygmi may be observed. The passage of blood on defaecation is a frequent complaint.

Initial symptoms may relate to a complication, particularly the distension, pain and constipation of an acute obstruction; vomiting does not occur unless the ileo-caecal valve becomes incompetent. Perforation of the tumour or of the bowel immediately proximal, from stercoral ulceration, may result in peritonitis.

On examination the tumour or a mass due to proximally impacted faeces may be felt in the abdomen. Hepatomegaly or ascites due to metastases may be noted in late cases, or peripheral distension or caecal tenderness from large bowel obstruction. There may be signs of peritonitis due to caecal rupture where the ileo-caecal valve continues to function, or superadded small intestinal obstruction if it becomes patent. Rectal examination may reveal a pelvic colon lesion which has prolapsed into the recto-vesical or recto-uterine pouch and is palpable through the rectal wall, or a more proximal tumour that has intussuscepted.

Sigmoidoscopy must always be employed and the faeces examined for the presence of occult blood. A barium enema may demonstrate an obstruction or the occasional occurrence of more than one primary growth.

Fibreoptic sigmoidoscopy is three times more likely to reveal a tumour than rigid sigmoidoscopy and should be employed in any doubtful cases, most lesions being in the left half of the colon.

Differential diagnosis

Cancer in the ileo-caecal region may easily be confused with an *appendix abscess, Crohn's disease*, actinomycosis or hyperplastic tuberculosis. In the left half of the colon *diverticulitis* complicated by obstruction, abscess or fistula may be mistaken for cancer even at operation. Benign tumours may also only be differentiated after resection. Lesions producing enlargement of the kidney, liver, gallbladder, stomach or spleen may occasionally cause difficulties in diagnosis. Rarely granulomatous colitis suggests neoplasia, and with increasing foreign travel amoebiasis has to be considered.

Treatment

The ideal solution is removal of the primary growth together with its associated lymphatic field and the restoration of alimentary continuity.

In *non-obstructed* cases pre-operative care should be directed to improvement of the general condition by blood transfusion where anaemia exists, and towards preparation of the bowel. It is not possible to sterilise the bowel of bacteria and operations should be carried out under antibiotic cover such as metronidazole to reduce infection. Mechanical cleansing of the bowel is more important in the left colon than in the right, and the removal of hard faeces is mandatory for successful anastomosis. Pre-operative starvation, oral magnesium sulphate, elemental diets and whole gut irrigation with saline or mannitol all have their advocates for this purpose.

The type of operation performed depends on the site and degree of invasion of vital structures (Fig.16.9). For growths in the caecum, ascending colon or hepatic flexure a right hemicolectomy should be carried out. Tumours of the transverse

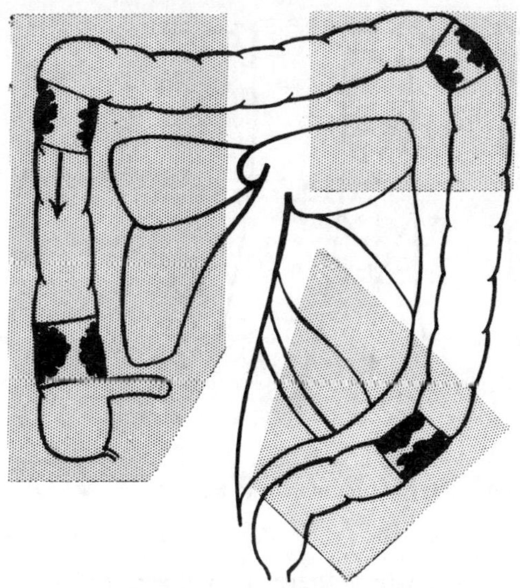

Fig. 16.9 The extent of resection of bowel and lymphatic field for carcinoma in various parts of the colon

colon should be excised, together with the whole of the transverse colon and a V-shaped portion of mesentery which includes the middle colic vessels. In cancers of the splenic flexure and descending colon the left colic vessels are ligated and the area supplied removed. In pelvic colon lesions the superior rectal and lower left colic branches should be ligated and the enclosed area of bowel resected. Tumours of the left half of the colon with extensive node involvement may require inferior mesenteric ligation and a left hemicolectomy.

Involvement of the abdominal wall does not preclude a cure, and if necessary resection of part of the parietes should be undertaken. Excision of solitary hepatic metastases or even partial hepatectomy may be a worthwhile procedure when the original growth can be removed. Removal of the primary tumour is the most satisfactory form of palliation and should generally be performed even in the presence of metastases.

Non-resectable tumours of the right half of the colon should be short-circuited by an ileotransverse colostomy; on the left half by a colocolostomy, or occasionally by a permanent colostomy. Resection may later be possible when any associated infection has subsided.

Obstructive lesions of the right colon can generally be treated by a hemicolectomy. Left-sided obstructed tumours can also be resected if the general condition is satisfactory, the proximal end being brought out as a colostomy and the distal end closed or sutured to the skin as a mucous fistula. Restoration of continuity can be later performed. Perforated tumours can often be dealt with similarly, but in the presence of a large abscess drainage and a transverse colostomy may be undertaken, resection being left until subsidence of infection. The prognosis in colonic cancer is related to the extent of spread. It is 80 per cent when confined to the bowel wall, but with lymphatic spread the 5-year survival figure falls to 30 per cent and it has not improved in the last 30 years.

Colostomy

In this procedure the colon is delivered to the surface and a definitive opening made into it in order to divert the faecal stream. It is most frequently performed in obstructive lesions, but may be required in the presence of intestinal perforation or fistula. The usual sites are in the transverse and pelvic colon. The former is generally to the right of the midline and called a transverse colostomy; the latter is placed in the left iliac fossa and known as a pelvic or left iliac colostomy. The colon in both regions possesses a mesentery permitting easier delivery of the bowel.

In either area two forms of colostomy may be fashioned: (1) terminal, (2) loop (Fig. 16.10).

A *terminal* or end colostomy is one in which the whole circumference of the bowel is divided and the faecal stream is therefore completely diverted. It is typically employed after abdomino-perineal excision of the rectum and is to be preferred in a transverse colostomy where distal resection is later proposed. Complete faecal exclusion diminishes infection and permits thorough cleaning of the affected region. The two loops of colon may be sutured together before division and designated a double-barrelled colostomy.

A *loop* colostomy is a more simple form of opening on the antimesenteric portion of a colonic segment. It is less satisfactory than the terminal colostomy as diversion is incomplete and faeces may pass into the distal loop, but it is quicker in performance and adequate when the general condition of the patient is poor.

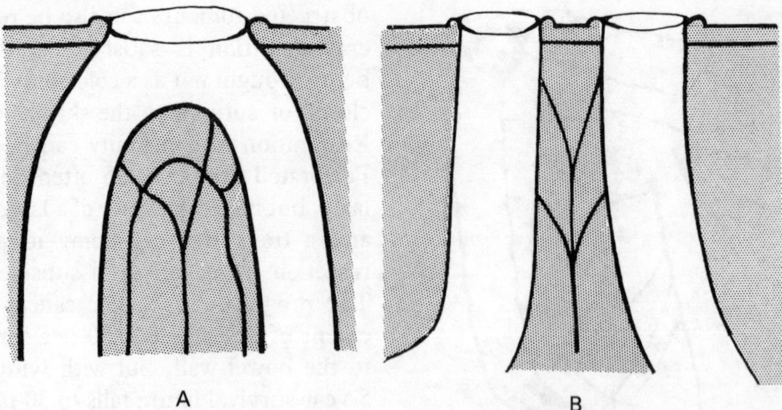

Fig. 16.10 Colostomy. **A.** Simple loop type. **B.** Double barrel defunctioning type of terminal colostomy.

A colostomy may be of a temporary or permanent nature. The former is usually placed in the transverse colon where it seldom interferes with later resection. When a permanent colostomy is required it should be placed as far distal as is compatible with the disease to permit the maximum amount of fluid absorption and render the disability more manageable.

Management

If a colostomy is to be a permanent feature, it is of help to effect an introduction to another patient who is successfully managing his own colostomy. The personal inconvenience may then be regarded in more correct perspective, and the pursuance of a normal life stressed with greater conviction. The stomatherapist can also give valuable advice.

In the first two to three weeks frequency of action and looseness of motion are common; the patient should be instructed that although control cannot be exerted the colostomy will later probably not act more often than twice in 24 hours. Restriction of fluid in the early post-operative days renders the motions less frequent. Personal experiment will indicate dietary articles of inconvenience, but roughage and fruit should be avoided in the first month or two. Where undue difficulty is experienced in bowel regulation Celevac is of value in obtaining a formed stool.

Daily colonic washouts with tap water are advocated by some but this procedure carries a small risk of bowel perforation and should only be undertaken where there is intelligent co-operation. No specific attention to the colostomy is the more usual routine. The opening should be covered with gauze and cellulose and supported by a light abdominal belt or girdle. Disposable adhesive plastic bags are a satisfactory alternative. Colostomy cups should not be worn as they produce herniation by suction.

The following complications of a colostomy may occur:

1. Stenosis
2. Herniation
3. Prolapse
4. Retraction
5. Small intestinal obstruction

Stenosis may be prevented by excision of an adequate circle of skin and skin-mucosal apposition when the colostomy is formed. If established it may require dilatation or refashioning. A hernia may occur around the colostomy and necessitate a belt or surgical repair. Prolapse of the colostomy may be mucosal or complete and follows on imperfections in technique. It is more frequent in a loop colostomy and the redundancy may require excision. Retraction, due to interference with the blood supply, may be serious if occurring in the first few days as peritonitis can follow intra-peritoneal recession. Urgent exploration may be necessary with formation of another colostomy. Small intestinal obstruction may occur if the paracolic gutter on the lateral side of the pelvic colostomy is not closed at the time of the initial operation.

FURTHER READING

Alexander-Williams, M. J. and Irving, M. (1982). *Intestinal Fistulas*. Bristol: Wright.

Brooke, B. N. and Wilkinson, A. (1980). *Inflammatory Disease of the Bowel*. London: Pitman.

De Cosse, J. J. (Ed.) (1981). *Large Bowel Cancer*. Edinburgh: Churchill Livingstone.

Ellis, H. (1982). *Intestinal Obstruction*. Hemel Hempstead: Prentice Hall.

Kyle, J. (1982). Surgery for Crohn's disease. *Brit. J. Hosp. Med.* 27, 482–487.

Thomson, J. P. S., Nicholls, R. J. and Williams, C. B. (Eds.) (1982). *Colorectal Disease. An Introduction for Surgeons and Physicians*. London: Heinemann.

17

Rectum and anus

Anatomy

The *rectum* extends from the pelvirectal junction at the middle of the third sacral vertebra to the upper end of the anal canal at the level of levator ani. It is approximately 15 cm long and possesses curves in both anteroposterior and lateral directions. The former follows the line of the sacrum, the latter is initially to the right then to the left and, finally, assumes a midline position. The peritoneum which almost completely surrounds the upper part then sweeps laterally covering only the anterior portion, and in the lower one-third the rectum has no peritoneal coat. In the male the peritoneum is reflected anteriorly on to the bladder at the rectovesical pouch, which is about 7 cm from the anus. In the female it forms the pouch of Douglas where it is reflected on to the uterus at a slightly lower level.

Within the lumen are three valves composed of the circular muscle lined by mucosa. The main one, which is always well-marked, is at the level of the peritoneal reflection on the right side, and distal to it the rectum balloons out to form the ampulla. The remaining two valves lie above and below the main one on the opposite wall and are of smaller size. The function of the valves is to support the faeces.

The *anal canal* is understood by surgeons to extend from the anorectal ring, where the large intestine passes through the levator ani, to the anal margin. It measures approximately 4 cm in length and is related anteriorly to the membranous urethra and the bulb of the penis in the male, and to the lower part of the vagina in the female.

The pectinate line, denoted by small anal valves, represents the region of the proctodeal membrane, and the differing mucosa above and below it is important. Above it consists of lax mucosa with folds which are immediately above the valves and known as columns of Morgagni. At first columnar the cells become cuboidal in shape just proximal to the pectinate line. Below the latter the mucosa becomes firmly adherent to the deeper structures. It is initially transitional but assumes a modified squamous appearance, finally becoming true skin at the anal margin.

The muscular arrangement is surgically important (Fig. 17.1). The longitudinal muscle of the colon and rectum is continued distally to the inferior border of the internal sphincter, where it breaks up into strands which pass outward through the lower part of the perianal region. The circular muscle of the rectum thickens at the anorectal ring and continues distally as the *internal sphincter*, completely surrounding the anal canal before terminating just above the level of the anus. It is an involuntary muscle. The *external sphincter* may be regarded as an outer cylinder of muscle surrounding the inner cylinder of the internal sphincter. The lower part lies below and lateral to the lower end of the internal sphincter and is attached to the skin of the perianal region. More proximally the posterior fibres are attached to the coccyx forming the anococcygeal raphe. The deeper portion of the external sphincter is annular with no posterior attachment but fuses at the upper end with levator ani. The **anorectal ring** is formed at this point, being comprised of the levator ani, the deeper portion of the external sphincter and the circular and longitudinal coats of the rectum. It may be recognised by palpation and may be seen on proctoscopy. Division will result in incontinence.

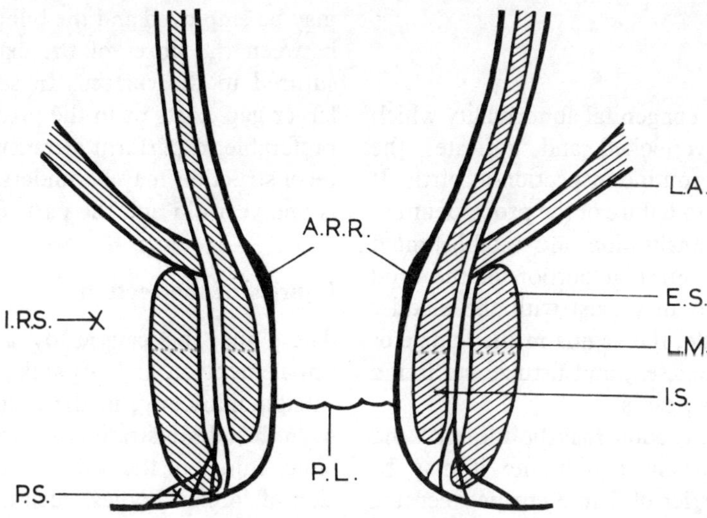

Fig. 17.1 Anatomy of anorectal musculature. I.R.S., ischiorectal space. P.S., perianal space, A.R.R., anorectal ring. P.L., pectinate line. L.A., levator ani. E.S., external sphincter. L.M., longitudinal muscle. I.S., internal sphincter.

The arterial supply to the rectum is chiefly through the superior rectal artery, which is the main continuation of the inferior mesenteric artery. At the beginning of the rectum it divides into a right and left branch, and the former in turn divides into an anterior and posterior division. These three main branches terminate at the columns of Morgagni at 3, 7 and 11 o'clock with the patient in the lithotomy position. This is surgically important as the venous drainage follows the arterial supply and explains the characteristic position of the main venous cushions in haemorrhoids. The middle rectal artery, a branch of the anterior division of the internal iliac artery, reaches the rectum in the lateral ligament and supplies the area locally. The inferior rectal artery, a branch of the internal pudendal artery, is distributed to the anal canal.

The middle and inferior rectal veins drain into the internal iliac veins, whilst the superior rectal vein continues as the inferior mesenteric vein which is a tributary of the splenic vein and hence the portal system. A communication thus exists between portal and systemic systems at the lower end of the rectum.

The lymphatic drainage follows the line of venous return, the main pathway accompanying the superior rectal vein. The route includes the pararectal, the superior rectal and inferior mesenteric nodes. Some lymphatics accompany the middle rectal vessels and below the level of the pectinate line drainage is to the inguinal lymph nodes.

The nerve supply of the rectum and anal canal above the level of the pectinate line is by sympathetic and parasympathetic nerve fibres. The sympathetic supply is partly by branches of the inferior mesenteric plexus and partly by the presacral nerves from the preaortic plexus commencing in the second, third and fourth lumbar sympathetic ganglia. The parasympathetic supply comes from the second, third and fourth sacral nerves. Sympathetic function is to inhibit the rectal wall and stimulate the internal sphincter. The parasympathetic nerves stimulate the wall and inhibit the sphincter. Distal to the pectinate line the anal canal is supplied by the inferior haemorrhoidal nerve which also supplies part of the external sphincter.

Anal glands, usually between four and eight in number, are present in the anal canal as blind outgrowths from the anal crypts. They are found in the submucosa, the internal sphincter, and may reach as far as the longitudinal muscle. Outward and downward extension occurs but they are not seen above the level of the anal valves. They are important in providing a route of infection from the anal canal to the submucous and inter-sphincteric spaces.

Imperforate anus

Pathology

This is an important congenital abnormality which may initially be overlooked and indicates the necessity for careful routine inspection at birth. It is believed to be due to failure of the proctodeum to undergo complete canalisation and establishment of contact with the terminal portion of the hind gut. Communications may exist with the bladder or urethra in the male, the vagina in the female or the perineum in either sex, and fistulae are found in more than half the cases.

The extent of obstruction may be minimal and due only to a persistent membrane; it may be moderate with a barrier of 2 to 3 cm between the termination of the rectum and the exterior; it may be severe with a long gap to the surface. The external sphincter develops separately from mesoderm and is unaffected by the anomaly.

Clinical features

Although the diagnosis should be obvious at birth, occasionally it is delayed for several days until the absence of meconium or signs of obstruction are noted. Where a fistula exists meconium may be observed in the urine or escaping from the vagina. The appearance of dimpling of the skin in the mid-line indicates the presence of an external sphincter. When the gap is minimal, bulging may be seen in the anal area when the child cries or strains.

Investigations

Radiographs are of value after 18 to 24 hours. Swallowed gas has by this period reached the terminal bowel, and if a marker is applied to the buttocks in the region of the anal sphincter and the child placed in a head-down position an accurate estimate of the extent of the gap may be determined.

Treatment

Where only a thin membrane is present incision is adequate. Daily dilatations should be continued for three months, the mother's gloved index finger being a satisfactory means. In moderate cases, with a gap of not more than 2 cm, a perineal approach may be employed and the blind loop brought down between the fibres of the external sphincter and sutured to the surface. In severe cases, where a larger gap exists or in the presence of fistulae, it is preferable to perform a transverse colostomy, and reconstruction may be undertaken when the child is one year old and the parts of larger size.

Injuries of the rectum

These may be caused by a gunshot wound or impalement on a sharp spike. Technical mistakes in sigmoidoscopy, in the excision of rectal polypi or in the administration of enemata may be responsible. Injury to the wall may also follow the ingestion of foreign bodies, such as meat bones, which frequently form an abscess. Occasionally it may occur after the self-introduction of foreign bodies for the relief of pruritus ani or for self-gratification. Severe perineal tears associated with parturition may injure the rectum. Whatever the cause, but particularly with penetrating injuries, associated damage to the bladder, peritoneal cavity or lumbosacral plexus may take place.

Clinically shock, peritonitis and rarely a pneumoperitoneum, which may be confirmed radiologically, will be encountered in upper rectal injuries. Damage to the lower portion may be relatively symptomless unless it is complicated by associated injury to the bladder or nerve plexus. Perirectal inflammation is an important sequel with wide-spread cellulitis.

Treatment should be immediate and any foreign body, particularly an introduced portion of clothes, must be removed. Laparotomy should be performed for intraperitoneal injuries and the perforation sutured. Extraperitoneal tears should be drained adequately. A colostomy should be performed if there is injury to the internal sphincter and incontinence. Wounds of the bladder require suture and transurethral catheter drainage.

Proctitis

Pathology

Inflammation of the rectum not infrequently forms part of a proctocolitis, for example, ulcerative colitis or dysentery. The condition then assumes greater importance due to its extent. When localised the cause may lie in injury or infection, such as gonorrhoea, tuberculosis, lymphogranuloma inguinale, bilharzia, syphilis, or thread worms in children. Extensive or inadequately guarded irradiation and allergy are other causes.

In the acute form the mucosa is hyperaemic and oedematous and there may be associated ulceration. The condition may persist and become chronic with a thickened mucosa and contracted rectal wall.

Clinical features

Tenesmus is the chief symptom and there is frequently some bleeding on defaecation. Mucous discharge is common with perianal excoriation and pruritus. Rectal examination is often painful in the acute stage, and the characteristic inflammatory changes are easily recognised on proctoscopy. Sigmoidoscopy is essential to exclude any proximal disease, and the possibility of carcinoma has to be considered. A rectal swab for bacteriological examination should be taken and biopsy performed of any ulceration.

Treatment

Any known cause must first be removed, and if the infection is part of a more general inflammatory state treatment must be directed to the major lesion. Specific infections require treatment of their cause with the correction of any secondary anaemia. Liquid paraffin softens the motions and reduces trauma to the affected area.

Stricture of the rectum and anus

Pathology

The most common cause of severe stricture is a venereal infection, lymphogranuloma inguinale. It is caused by a filter-passing virus which particularly affects the lymphatics and implicates women more often than men. The latter are infected by direct contact. A perirectal lymphangitis develops with secondary rectal stenosis at a distance of 2 to 8 cm from the anus. Other causes include a congenital form due to persistence of the proctodeal membrane with narrowing in the anal canal, trauma from penetrating injuries or stenosis following haemorrhoidectomy. A number are also due to pelvic irradiation, particularly for carcinoma of the cervix. Specific infections, such as syphilis, tuberculosis, dysentery or gonorrhoea, seldom account for the condition, but Crohn's disease or ulcerative colitis may occasionally cause a benign stricture, and carcinoma of the rectum or anus may produce a malignant one.

Clinical features

Progressive constipation is the main complaint, although there may also be symptoms of bleeding and discharge from the underlying cause. Pipestem stools may be produced and later faecal impaction and intestinal obstruction. Stercoral ulceration can lead to perforation, peritonitis and fistula formation. Digital examination reveals the presence of a stricture and biopsy determines the exact nature.

Treatment

Gentle dilatation with graded Hegar's dilators performed twice weekly until a satisfactory passage is obtained, and then at infrequent intervals, suffices in most cases. Internal proctotomy followed by dilatation may be employed for post-operative benign strictures in the lower third of the rectum, whilst a colostomy may be required for high strictures or those not responding to dilatation. Malignant lesions are considered separately (p. 228).

Prolapse of the rectum

Pathology

Two types exist: partial, when only the mucosa is prolapsed, and complete, when all coats of the rectal wall are involved. *Partial* prolapse is common and usually encountered in young children and in the elderly. In childhood malnutrition and faulty bowel habits with straining at stool for prolonged periods are frequent precursors. In old age loss of sphincter control, urinary obstruction due to stricture or prostatism, chronic bronchitis or haemorrhoids may be responsible.

Complete prolapse is rare and generally found in adult females. It may be caused by pelvic injury at parturition, although it occurs in patients who have never borne children, who are thin and show other evidence of visceroptosis. It also occurs in the excessively stout. The condition is in effect a 'sliding hernia' involving first the anterior and later the posterior rectal wall.

Clinical features

The main symptoms are bleeding, mucous discharge and a reducible swelling which at first appears only on defaecation but which later persists. In complete prolapse the complaint is of a large swelling which appears on coughing or straining, later even on standing, which dilates the anus and produces faecal incontinence.

At examination the prolapse may be demonstrated by asking the patient to strain in the left lateral position. The full extent should be determined and palpation indicates the type. In complete prolapse small intestine may be noted anteriorly in the peritoneal pouch. Sphincteric tone is poor. Ulceration, thrombosis, irreducibility and gangrene may follow. Severely prolapsed haemorrhoids or intussusception may cause confusion, but the latter is distinguished by the finding of a space between the descending bowel and the rectal wall.

Treatment

Conservative management suffices for minor degrees, with attention to bowel habit. Children should be trained to defaecate without undue delay, and at first may be required to perform this function lying on their side with the buttocks supported. The prolapse should always be reduced and maintained by pad and bandage or strapping across the buttocks. In adults any underlying cause should be removed and faradism and sphincter exercises commenced where necessary.

Operative treatment in children consists of linear cauterisation of the rectal mucosa to produce underlying adhesions in the minor case. In the *partial* type in adults, where the extent of the prolapse is not more than 5 cm a Thiersch operation should be performed. This consists of introducing an encircling ligature of wire in the perianal region after the prolapse has been reduced, which narrows the anus to the diameter of one finger. When this fails a haemorrhoidectomy type of operation will often suffice. Surgical treatment of the *complete* prolapse is carried out through the abdomen. The most satisfactory procedure is the insertion of a polyvinyl alcohol (Ivalon) sponge prosthesis. This is placed so as to encircle the posterior four-fifths of the rectum, after returning the prolapse within the peritoneal cavity. The sponge is anchored to the sacrum and retains the rectum in position by its capacity to produce considerable fibrosis. An alternative but more serious procedure is to perform an anterior resection of the redundant rectum. Recurrence can occasionally take place after either method.

HAEMORRHOIDS

The term *internal* haemorrhoids refers to a plexus of veins of the superior rectal system situated just above the mucocutaneous junction. The anal submucosa is thickened into three cushions, each composed of a plexus of veins supported on a smooth muscle elastic tissue stroma.

Pathology

The anatomical disposition of the main tributaries of the superior rectal vein into left, right anterior and right posterior divisions results in the formation of the three primary haemorrhoids at 3, 7 and 11 o'clock when examination is performed in the lithotomy position. Intermediate cushions, generally four in number, may occur and are known as secondary haemorrhoids.

The cause is obscure but hard stools and straining may cause the cushions to swell with venous suffusion and downward displacement. There is often a hereditary factor and there may be an association with a lack of fibre in the Western diet. Obesity and pregnancy or other intra-abdominal tumour may also be factors.

Clinical features

The principal and often sole symptom is bleeding. This initially occurs only with defaecation and may

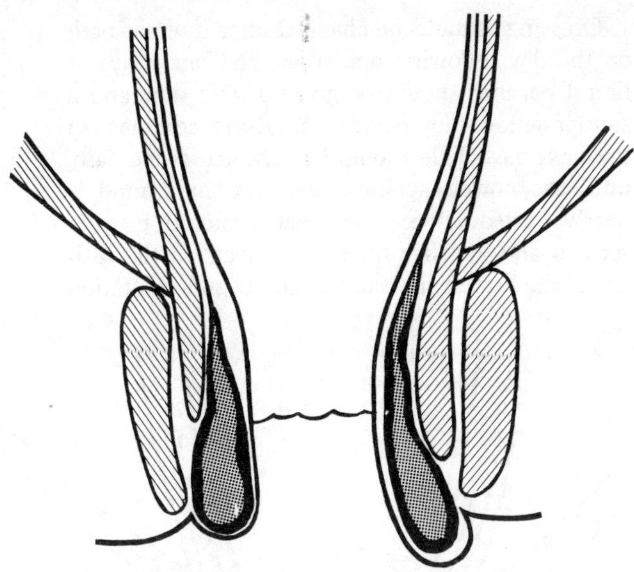

Fig. 17.2 Prolapsing haemorrhoids

be slight, staining the pan or noted on the toilet paper, but later may be noted independently of bowel action and be excessive. It is always bright red blood. Swelling or prolapse may follow, serving to classify haemorrhoids into three degrees:

First degree haemorrhoids produce bleeding but no prolapse.

Second degree haemorrhoids prolapse with defaecation but return spontaneously (Fig. 17.2).

Third degree haemorrhoids prolapse on defaecation or other form of straining but do not return spontaneously.

It is to be stressed that pain is not a symptom of simple haemorrhoids and only occurs in the presence of complications. Haemorrhoids cannot be felt unless they have undergone thrombosis. Inspection, to include the act of straining on the part of the patient, should be followed by proctoscopy to determine their extent and site. Sigmoidoscopy is essential to exclude a neoplasm.

Complications

Irreducibility may follow prolapse as a result of spasm of the anal sphincter; the affected haemorrhoid becomes painful and oedematous and thus further prevents reduction. *Thrombosis* in the vein may ensue and *strangulation* follows interference with the arterial blood supply. *Infection, gangrene* and *ulceration* are additional complications. More seriously, infection may spread to produce *pylephlebitis* and *portal pyaemia*. Fibrosis may occur in a thrombotic pile to produce a fibrous *polyp*, which in turn may tear the anal mucosa and cause a *fissure*. Persistent blood loss from internal haemorrhoids may be responsible for a severe degree of *secondary anaemia*, the primary cause occasionally being overlooked. Lastly, chronic irritation due to a prolapsed third degree haemorrhoid may produce metaplasia and *carcinomatous change*.

Treatment

Conservative measures include adequate attention to the bowel habit by means of exercise, high fibre diet and aperients, together with reduction in obesity. These may be sufficient in mild cases to prevent further symptoms and should be adopted where the increased congestion is of a temporary nature, such as occurs with a pregnant uterus.

Injection therapy is beneficial in first degree haemorrhoids. It may also be used in uncomplicated second degree ones, but is only palliative. For economical reasons it may be considered satisfactory, and with repeated injections many years of relief can be obtained. This form of treatment must not be employed for third degree haemorrhoids.

The solution used is 5 per cent phenol in arachis oil, and the aim is to produce a perivascular fibrosis around the base of the pile in the submucosa, thereby obliterating the lumen of the vessel and drawing up the haemorrhoid (Fig. 17.3). The injection is given through a proctoscope with the patient in the left lateral or knee-elbow position. Usually a total of about 10 ml is employed (Fig. 17.4), the mucosa being stretched by the solution until the superficial minute blood-vessels become visible—the striation sign. Further injections three to four weeks later may be necessary if symptoms persist.

Operation is required for third degree haemorrhoids and is the treatment of choice in the majority of second degree piles.

Pre-operative preparation includes an aperient 48 hours and an enema 24 hours before operation. Haemorrhoidectomy should be performed by excision and ligature of each primary pile, the base

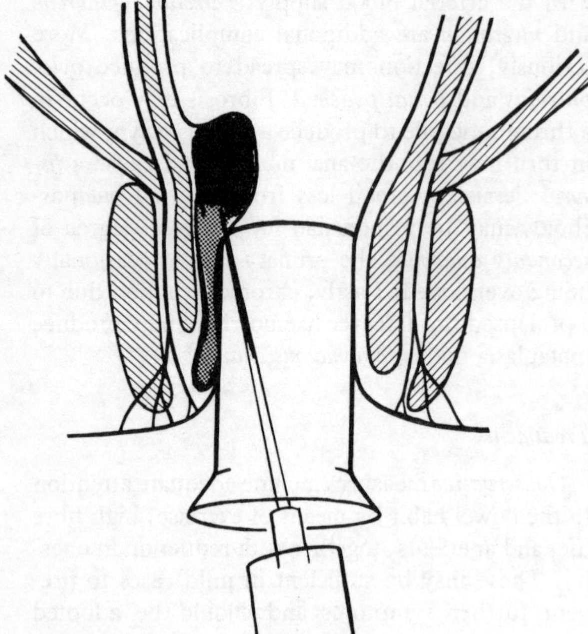

Fig. 17.3 Injection of haemorrhoid

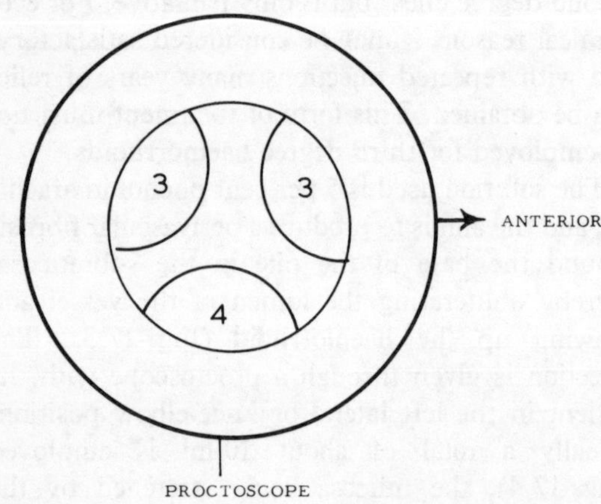

Fig. 17.4 A method of recording haemorrhoid injections.

being transfixed (Fig. 17.5). It is of importance to leave a bridge of skin and rectal mucosa intact between each raw area or stenosis will follow (Fig. 17.6). Secondary haemorrhoids may be removed at this operation only if this principle is not violated, otherwise they should be treated later by injection or further surgery when the wound has healed.

Dressings should be changed after a warm bath on the day following operation. Half an ounce of liquid paraffin should be given at this time and a similar amount of paraffin emulsion commenced the next day. This should be repeated twice daily until the bowels act normally and the wound is nearly healed. Twice daily baths should be prescribed and an olive oil enema given on the fifth day if the bowels have not acted. Digital dilatation

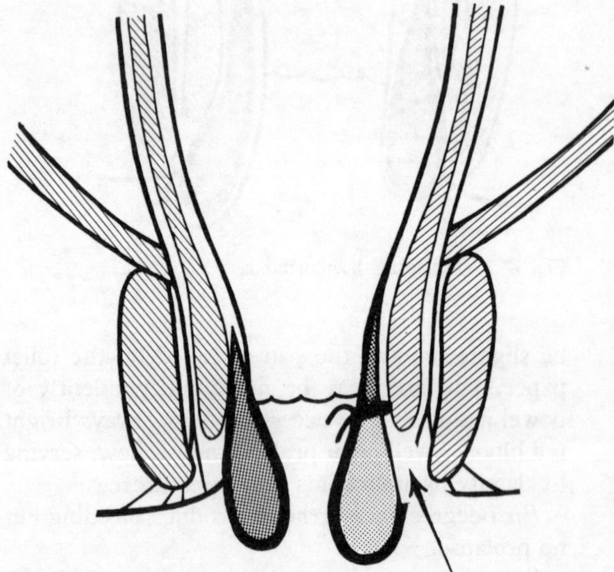

Fig. 17.5 Haemorrhoidectomy. Excision and ligature at base of haemorrhoid.

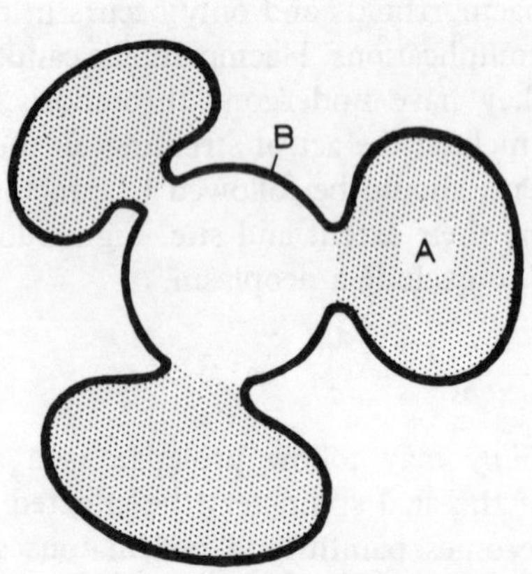

Fig. 17.6 Haemorrhoidectomy. A. Raw area at site of removal. B. Skin and mucosal bridge.

of the anal canal should be performed from the sixth day until the wounds have healed.

Complications include stricture, retention of urine, reactionary haemorrhage due to the slipping of a ligature and secondary haemorrhage six to ten days post-operatively. Control of the latter is most conveniently obtained by inserting a Foley catheter into the rectum, inflating the balloon and applying traction.

Alternative surgical procedures include rubber band ligation of the haemorrhoids, which has limited use; cryosurgery, which may produce copious prolonged mucous discharge; and eight-finger dilatation of the anus and lower rectum under general anaesthesia, followed by the passage of anal dilators for several weeks.

External haemorrhoids are only of importance in the condition of *perianal haematoma*. Excessive strain at work, play or stool, frequently occurring in young adult males, may result in rupture of an inferior rectal vein with the production of a tense, localised and tender swelling at the anal margin. If untreated, resolution generally occurs, but infection and a perianal abscess may supervene.

Patients who attend within four days of onset of the lesion should have the clot evacuated under local anaesthesia with immediate symptomatic relief. After this period pain is less marked and local compresses of lotio plumbi are adequate.

ANORECTAL ABSCESS

A thorough appreciation of the anatomy of the anorectal region is essential for the understanding and management of these abscesses. They assume particular importance because of the liability to proceed to fistulae-in-ano with the attendant discomfort and inconvenience. A suitable classification relates them to their anatomical site (Fig. 17.7).

1. Perianal
2. Submucous and intersphincteric
3. Ischiorectal
4. Pelvirectal

Perianal abscess

This, the commonest form, is a superficial condition in the region of the anus arising as a result of infection in a hair follicle or anal gland, a sebaceous or sweat gland or in a perianal haematoma. It may follow a chronic anal fissure or result from downward extension of a submucous or intersphincteric abscess. Rupture may occur on to the perianal skin or into the anal canal with the formation of a sinus, or the track may be complete to produce a fistula.

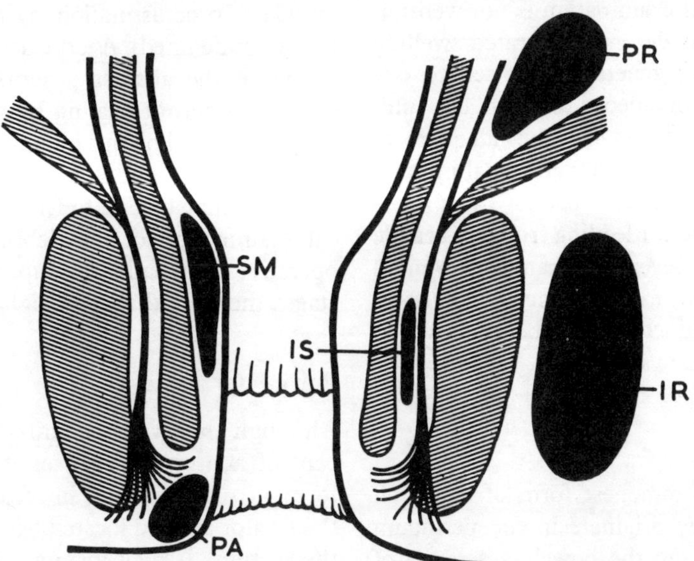

Fig. 17.7 Anorectal abscess; S.M. = submucous; P.A. = perianal; P.R. = pelvirectal; I.R. = ischiorectal; I.S. = intersphincteric.

Clinical features

All anorectal abscesses are more common in men than in women. The perianal variety causes pain and throbbing with signs of superficial abscess formation adjacent to the anal margin. There may be an associated anal fissure. General disturbance is usually slight. Early and adequate drainage is important, the wound being allowed to granulate from its depth. Loose packing, never a tight one, may aid this and frequent baths are essential.

Submucous and intersphincteric abscesses

The submucous abscess is a less common form which arises in the lower rectum or upper anal canal deep to the mucous membrane. It may follow infection in a haemorrhoid or anal gland, be the result of the misplacement of an injection for such a condition, or be associated with a foreign body. Rupture may take place into the bowel. The intersphincteric abscess may be caused by anal glandular infection and be responsible for other anorectal abscesses.

Clinical features

Pain is experienced within the rectum and becomes more severe with defaecation. Rupture brings considerable relief. Rectal examination is not well tolerated but reveals a tender and indurated swelling within the anal canal, generally localised to one lateral wall. Where spontaneous drainage has commenced hot rectal washouts may be adequate to clear up residual infection. A longitudinal incision to include the most dependent part of the abscess is more usually required. Bleeding from the friable mucosal edges may be severe, but can be prevented by using diathermy to make the incision. Dissection between the sphincters may be required to drain an intersphincteric abscess.

Ischiorectal abscess

This is the second commonest form of anorectal abscess. Infection may originate in the perineum but usually follows from the bowel as a result of injury from a foreign body or in association with haemorrhoids. It may rarely be blood borne. The usual agent is the *Esch. coli*, although gas gangrene organisms are occasionally responsible. Inflammation spreads rapidly in the lax areolar tissue of the ischiorectal fossa with its impoverished blood supply, and extension behind the anus may occur to involve the other ischiorectal fossa. Eventual rupture into the bowel below the anorectal ring, less commonly at the skin of the perineum, may result. Occasionally the levator ani is penetrated with the formation of a pelvirectal abscess.

Clinical features

This is usually a condition of some severity with pronounced constitutional effects of malaise, pyrexia and tachycardia. Locally there is considerable pain in one or both ischiorectal fossae. There may also be pain on defaecation. There is frequently an indurated and tender swelling of the affected side with oedema of the overlying skin. In obese patients such signs are not always obvious and gentle bimanual palpation with the finger in the rectum will enable them to be detected more easily. Softening and fluctuation are late manifestations and if a fistula is to be prevented treatment must be initiated before these signs are noted. Crepitus is indicative of gas gangrene infection and toxaemia may be pronounced.

Treatment consists of early wide incision and drainage; procrastination by antibiotic therapy is to be condemned. A cruciate incision to the full extent of the abscess is employed and the flaps excised to permit healing by granulation from the deepest parts. The pus obtained should be cultured for organisms, and as a small proportion of such abscesses may be due to Crohn's disease, histological examination of the debris is advisable. Postoperative daily baths are important and in the early stages the wound may be lightly packed.

Pelvirectal abscess

Although this type accounts for only about 5 per cent of anorectal abscesses it is the most serious form, arising as it does in the cellular tissues above the levator ani and located between this muscle and the rectum. It may form as an extension from an ischiorectal abscess, but more commonly follows disease within the pelvis. The cellular tissue is continuous with that of the pelvic mesocolon, within the broad ligament and around the base of the bladder, and disease in any of these regions may be responsible. Thus diverticulitis, appendix abscess, ulcerative colitis, Crohn's disease, endometriosis, prostatic and bladder infections and the inflammation around a carcinoma may all be a cause. Occasionally it may be due to a tuberculous abscess from osteomyelitis of the vertebrae or pelvic bones. Spread may also occur from within the rectal lumen. When established, extension may take place upwards to involve the peritoneal cavity, downwards to penetrate the levator ani and subsequent rupture in the perineum, or pus may enter the bowel above the anorectal ring to produce a sinus or fistula. Due to inadequate drainage, even following treatment, and with persistent intra-abdominal pathology recurrent abscesses are frequent.

Clinical features

The picture may resemble a large ischiorectal abscess with marked constitutional disturbance and a tender high mass on rectal or vaginal examination. When the levator ani is perforated the signs are those of an ischiorectal abscess. The previous history is important in determining an underlying cause. Treatment is by incision and adequate drainage through the corresponding ischiorectal fossa. The opening in the levator ani should be sought and either stretched or incised laterally to permit the insertion of a wide drainage tube after satisfactory evacuation of the pus. Similar bacteriological and histological investigations and after-treatment, as mentioned under ischiorectal abscess, should be performed.

FISTULA-IN-ANO

This condition is almost always the result of an anorectal abscess which ruptures both into the bowel and on to the surface of the skin. The term also includes sinuses which form when the abscess bursts only into bowel or on to the skin. A convenient classification relates them to the anorectal musculature.

1. Subcutaneous
2. Submucous and intermuscular
3. Anal:
   - Low
   - High
4. Anorectal

Subcutaneous fistula (Fig. 17.8A)

This type is the end result of a perianal abscess and lies subcutaneously in the perianal region superficial to the sphincters. It may be complete or incomplete. In common with anorectal abscess and other anal fistulae, it is more often seen in the adult male.

Similar symptoms obtain for all complete fistulae of a persistent faecal discharge on to the surface of the skin around the anus. In a subcutaneous fistula the opening is near the anal margin. Palpation reveals induration in long-standing cases. A probe passed through the fistula is encountered superficially at the lower end of the anal canal.

Treatment consists of opening up the fistulous track by an incision carried down on an indwelling probe. The wound is then enlarged in an outward direction, the overlying skin edges excised and a wide but shallow area allowed to granulate.

Submucous and intermuscular fistulae (Fig. 17.8B & C)

These follow rupture of a submucous or intersphincteric abscess. There may be an opening at the anal margin or it may lie within the anal canal. The submucous fistula lies in the submucosa; the intermuscular one between the circular and longitudinal muscle. Induration may be noted on rectal examination. Treatment is to lay open the fistula by a longitudinal incision as for a submucous abscess.

Anal fistula (Fig. 17.9A)

Two forms are recognised—the low and the high. The former, which is the commonest type of fistula-in-ano, is usually due to rupture of a perianal abscess, but may follow anal gland infection. The track enters the anal canal at the level of the pectinate line or near it and usually traverses the lower part of the internal sphincter. The high variety

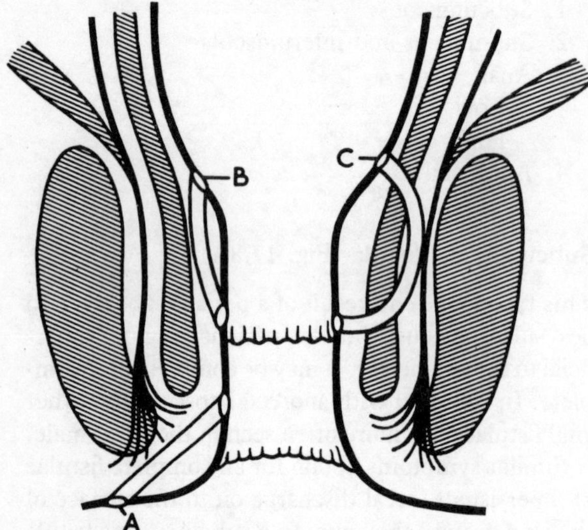

Fig. 17.8 Fistula-in-ano. **A.** Subcutaneous. **B.** Submucous. **C.** Intermuscular.

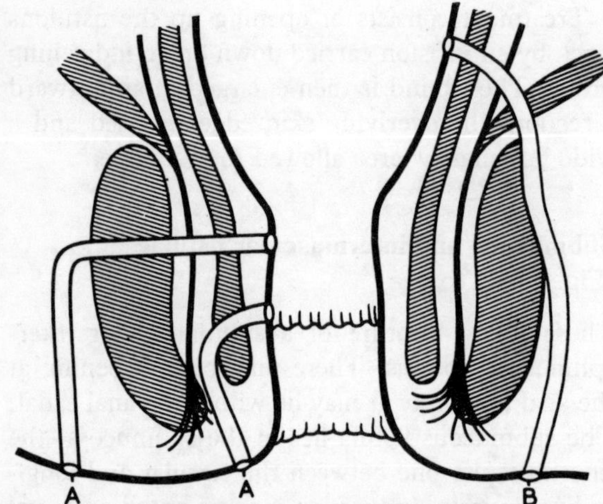

Fig. 17.9 Fistula-in-ano. **A.** Anal. **B.** Anorectal.

results from rupture of an ischiorectal or intersphincteric abscess. The track enters the anal canal at a higher level than in the low variety, but always enters it below the anorectal ring.

The diagnosis is made from the previous history of an abscess, a persistent faecal discharge and the finding of a fistulous opening which is outside the anal margin. In those with an external opening lying anterior to a line drawn transversely through the anus, the internal opening is on a corresponding radius towards the anus. Where the external opening lies posterior to this line the internal opening, due to the presence of the anococcygeal raphe, is in the midline.

Treatment involves laying open the track and obtaining adequate drainage. Division of the superficial portion of the sphincters is essential. In a high fistula an extensive wound may result, but secondary tracks must be opened up and drained. The relationship of the internal opening to the anorectal ring is of paramount importance and it must be constantly remembered that division of this will result in incontinence. Where it may be in danger a two-stage operation is preferable. At the first stage the superficial part of the sphincters is divided and a silk ligature applied to the deeper part of the fistula. Two weeks later, when scar tissue has formed, traction on the ends of the ligature will indicate the exact relationship to the anorectal ring, which may be both palpated and seen on proctoscopy, and the remaining track laid open without danger. Histological examination of the wall of the fistula should be performed as a small proportion are due to Crohn's disease (p. 205).

Anorectal fistula (Fig. 17.9B)

This serious and complicated fistula results from rupture of a pelvirectal abscess. The main track extends above the levator ani and there may not be an opening into the rectum above the anorectal ring. Subsidiary openings into the anal canal may be found, whilst the external opening is often placed at a considerable distance from the anus. Care must be taken in probing this type of fistula not to penetrate the rectal wall above the anorectal ring when no previous opening exists. The ramifications may be determined by the introduction of a radio-opaque dye. In all chronic fistulae, particularly where induration is a feature, the possibility of malignant change must be considered.

Treatment is difficult and often requires several operations. The principle of establishing adequate drainage must be maintained and excision of the skin of the ischiorectal fossa and meticulous pursuance of all tracks is indicated. Side openings into the anal canal should be laid open, but never the anorectal ring, even when a superior opening exists. With patience and care healing may be obtained. Underlying abdominal pathology should be removed. The wound is allowed to granulate, digital palpation being performed regularly to prevent pocketing and to relax the sphincter.

Pilonidal sinus

Pathology

The cause of this condition is not known. Previously it was assumed that all cases were of congenital origin, due to a developmental abnormality in the sacrococcygeal region. This is probably correct in some instances, but recently it has been suggested that in the majority it is an acquired lesion. An excess of thick, dark hair in the region, associated with trauma, such as a hard seat—it was known as Jeep disease in the Second World War—may cause penetration of the skin or sweat glands with subsequent cyst formation. The latter lies in the subcutaneous tissues where it is subject to trauma; infection and sinuses frequently follow. The histological picture reveals a lining of squamous epithelium containing hairs and epithelial debris.

Clinical features

Symptoms usually occur between the ages of 20 and 30 years and dark-haired men are more often affected. The history is generally one of inflammation in the sacrococcygeal area progressing to an abscess with later discharge, at times blood-stained, and subsequent sinus formation. Repeated infection is common with multiple secondary sinuses which lie in a lateral position. The condition may simulate a fistula-in-ano, but a probe passed into the most anterior sinus is found to proceed in a backward direction towards the sacrum and not anteriorly towards the rectum. There may also be a tuft of hair projecting from one of the openings.

Treatment of the acute abscess is by incision and drainage, together with the removal of any associated hair. For the more common chronic lesion an elliptical incision to include all the ramifications of the sinus should be followed by complete excision. Primary closure may be obtained. Recurrence is not infrequent following direct suture and a Z-plasty procedure of rotating the flaps enhances the chances of success and subsequent prevention. An alternative is to allow the wound to granulate.

ANAL FISSURE

Pathology

This condition consists of a tear in the epithelium at the lower end of the anal canal. In the majority of cases it occurs posteriorly in the midline at the point of decussation of the superficial fibres of the external sphincter where lack of support adds to the liability of injury. The fissure is usually produced by the passage of hard faeces and consequent overstretching of the mucosa in a patient accustomed by habitual purgation to small and liquid stools. Occasionally a fibrous polyp or ingested foreign body may be responsible.

Chronicity often occurs. The margins become indurated, the fissure deepens and fibrosis and contracture take place in the underlying internal sphincter. A characteristic ‘sentinel tag’ forms at the lower end of the fissure, composed of indurated and oedematous skin. Infection frequently follows on its deeper aspect.

Clinical features

Pain in the perianal region, initiated by defaecation and persisting for several hours afterwards, is characteristic. It is frequently severe and results in the patient being afraid to open the bowels. Further constipation aggravates the condition. There may be associated slight bleeding noted at defaecation and pruritus ani is common. With infection there may be a purulent discharge.

Inspection with satisfactory retraction and illumination furnishes the diagnosis. The epithelial split is easily seen and the sentinel pile observed in chronic cases. Rectal palpation reveals chronicity but may be too painful in the acute case. When the condition has subsided full rectal examination must be undertaken to exclude any underlying cause of the symptoms.

Treatment

Acute minor lesions may respond to bowel regulation, local hygiene and pain relief from the application of an analgesic ointment, such as Xylocaine, immediately after defaecation. More refractory cases often benefit from the daily insertion of a blunt dilator. The instrument should be well lubricated with a similar analgesic ointment and passed night and morning for three weeks, being retained for two or three minutes at a time. Anal sphincter stretching, using local or general anaesthesia, to the extent of four fingers and maintained for several minutes is commonly employed. Transient faecal incontinence in the elderly and prolapse of associated large haemorrhoids are possible complications.

Chronic lesions where fibrosis prevents stretching should be treated by sphincterotomy in which the lower half of the internal sphincter is divided, an incision being made through the base of the fissure to expose the muscle which is then divided (Fig. 17.10). In order to obtain satisfactory drainage the incision is carried on to the skin for about three centimetres. Any associated pathology, including a 'sentinel tag' should be excised at the same time. The wound becomes painless in five or six days and healing is complete in about three weeks. The daily use of a dilator post-operatively from the fifth day is essential until the wound has healed. An alternative procedure is a lateral sphincterotomy.

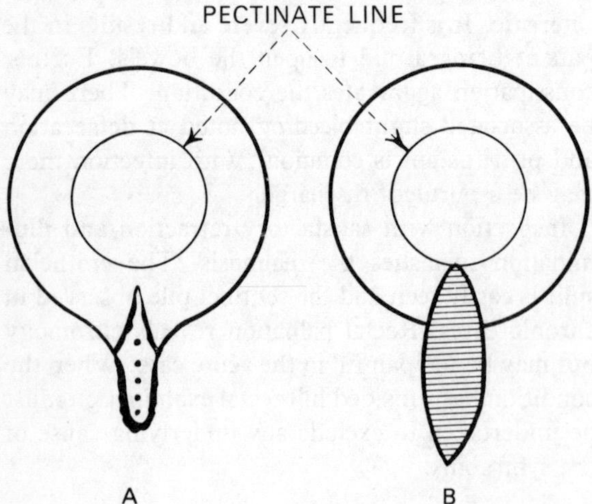

Fig. 17.10 Anal fissure. **A**. The fissure does not reach the pectinate line. **B**. Sphincterotomy incision reaches pectinate line and divides the internal sphincter.

BENIGN TUMOURS

These are essentially similar to those described in the chapter on Colon (p. 209), but a *villous papilloma* is more often present in the rectum than in the colon and is particularly important because of the higher risk of malignant change. Rarely the tumour may produce profuse mucous diarrhoea with gross fluid and electrolyte loss, particularly potassium depletion. Two to three litres per day may be passed per anum, causing lassitude, oliguria, acidotic respiration and even sudden collapse. Careful biopsy to exclude neoplasia is required and the tumour should be removed. Small low lesions may be severed with diathermy or excised, but often an anterior resection is required (p. 230). When profound metabolic disturbance is present prior management by intravenous therapy is essential.

A *papilloma of the anus* or an anal wart may occur. It is infective in origin and due to a virus. The warts are frequently multiple and progress rapidly at the anal margin, even extending into the anal canal, due to the moisture of the region. They may be associated with an anal discharge, cause pruritus and produce bleeding. Biopsy may be required to determine the exact pathology and exclude venereal infection. They may be treated medically by means of podophyllin or by surgical excision or diathermy should this fail.

CARCINOMA OF THE RECTUM

This is a condition of considerable importance and accounts for more than 10 per cent of all cancers. It is the most common site of carcinomas which involve the large bowel. The lesion may arise *de novo* or similar aetiological factors to that of colonic cancer, that is familial polyposis, ulcerative colitis and pre-existing polypi, may be responsible.

Pathology

The tumour arises at one of three sites: (1) the upper end or rectosigmoid region, (2) the midrectum or ampulla and (3) the lower end.

Growths of the upper third of the rectum are the most common and constitute 70 per cent of rectal carcinomas. They are usually annular tumours and similar in structure to those of the left half of the colon. Lesions of the middle third are generally proliferative growths with a cauliflower appearance. Diminution of the blood supply due to their bulk results in superficial necrosis and at times ulceration. They account for 25 per cent of rectal cancers. Tumours of the lower third are the least common, about 5 per cent, and usually present as a malignant ulcer with raised everted edges (Fig. 17.11). Histologically most tumours are adenocarcinomas, although some anaplastic forms occur. Spread occurs locally, by lymphatics and by the blood stream.

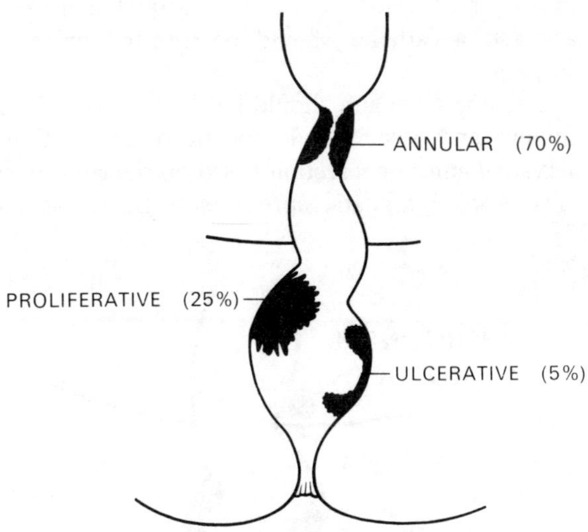

Fig. 17.11 Sites of carcinoma of the rectum

Local spread in the wall of the rectum is initially more marked in a circumferential than in a longitudinal direction and a period of two years is considered to be an average time for complete encirclement of the bowel. Penetration through mucosa, submucosa and muscle wall occurs and is of greater importance than the size of the tumour. Extrarectal structures become involved later with posterior spread to the sacrum and sacral plexus, laterally into the pararectal tissues and anteriorly to invade bladder, prostate and seminal vesicles in the male or uterus and vagina in the female. High growths extend to the peritoneum and numerous seedling deposits may occur. Low tumours may directly invade the anal canal and even the perianal skin.

Lymphatic spread occurs when the muscle wall has been penetrated and in almost all cases is in an upward direction. The pararectal glands are initially involved, followed by spread to the glands accompanying the superior rectal vessels and eventually those surrounding the inferior mesenteric artery. Distal lymphatic spread downwards or laterally only takes place when normal drainage is blocked by tumour. It does not occur in more than 1 per cent and the inguinal nodes then become involved.

Blood stream spread is usually a late feature, except in the rare instances where emboli enter a vein in penetrating the bowel wall. The main pathway is to the liver via the portal system, but systemic spread to the lungs and elsewhere may occur. Occasionally the hepatic metastasis appears to be a solitary one.

Dukes' classification of pathological groups based on resected operation speciments has proved valuable in assessing prognosis (Fig. 17.12). In Group A spread is limited to the rectal wall; in Group B it has extended to the extrarectal tissues but without lymph node involvement; in Group C there are regional node metastases.

Clinical features

The majority affected are over the age of 40 years, but the condition is not infrequently encountered in younger patients. Men suffer twice as frequently as women. A previous history of ulcerative colitis or polyposis coli may be obtained in some instances.

It is convenient to divide the symptoms into those produced by tumours in the three different sites. Rectosigmoid growths present a similar clinical picture to those of the left half of the colon with increasing constipation or alternating constipation and diarrhoea. Intermittent abdominal fulness, audible borborygmi or pain in the right iliac fossa from caecal distension may occur from stenosis and obstruction. Ampullary tumours are frequently large before they are recognised clinically by tenes-

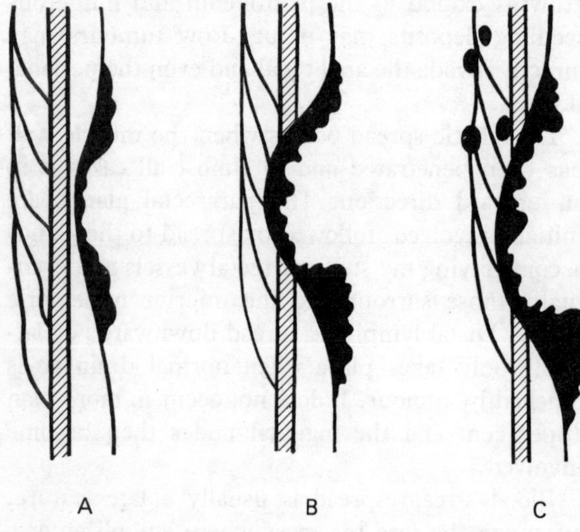

Fig. 17.12 Dukes' classification of carcinoma of the rectum. **A**. Confined to rectal wall. **B**. Extension to extrarectal tissues. **C**. Metastasis to lymph nodes.

mus, bleeding and mucous discharge, often described as diarrhoea. Low growths cause bleeding, tenesmus and perianal pain. General symptoms of loss of weight, anorexia and cachexia are late manifestations of the disease, as are dysuria, sciatica, fistula, jaundice and swelling of the lower limbs.

Abdominal examination is often negative, but there may be signs of intestinal obstruction, hepatomegaly or other masses and ascites.

In the majority of cases the tumour is palpable on rectal examination (Fig. 17.13). There may be evidence of haemorrhoids from venous obstruction. The site and size of the tumour, together with its fixity, should be noted. A high rectal growth may prolapse and become easily palpable and any secondary tumour in the rectovesical pouch or pouch of Douglas should be detected.

Sigmoidoscopy is essential to inspect the growth, to determine the distance of the lower edge from the anal margin and to obtain a biopsy, which must be performed in all cases. A barium enema is only of value in demonstrating obstruction at the pelvirectal junction or in showing associated colonic pathology. It should not be relied upon for the diagnosis of rectal cancer. If bladder involvement is suspected cystoscopy should be carried out.

Treatment

The majority of rectal tumours do not respond to radiotherapy and surgery is to be preferred.

Fixity of the tumour on rectal examination, particularly anteriorly in the male, where there is no additional barrier such as the uterus in the female, may be a contraindication to radical surgery, but abdominal exploration should be advised as infection may be the cause of immobility. Ascites, jaundice and widespread metastases are also contraindications to radical surgery.

Pre-operative preparation should include correction of any anaemia, breathing exercises, and bowel preparation by colonic and rectal washouts and antibiotics in a similar regime to that employed for colonic cancer (p. 212). The male urethra may be in danger where dissection of the growth is necessary and a catheter should be inserted prior to surgery.

The operative aim should be the removal of the tumour and associated lymphatic drainage. Conservative anterior resection based on the constancy of upward lymphatic spread is being employed

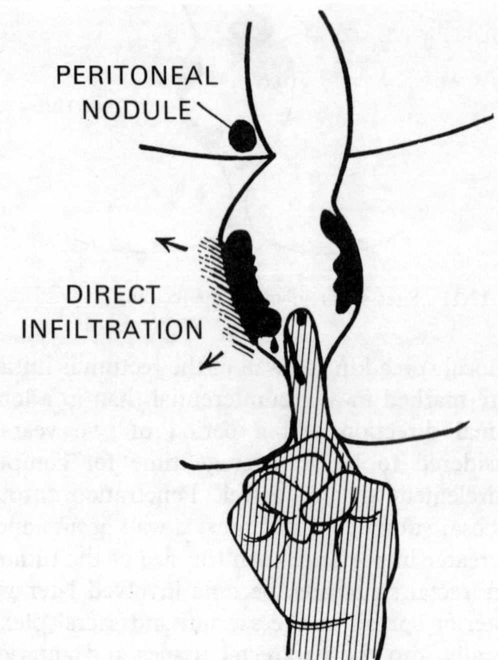

Fig. 17.13 The features of carcinoma found on rectal examination

more frequently at the present time. The availability and use of the stapling gun has enabled lower anastomoses to be performed with retention of the anal sphincter. Tumours whose lower edge is approximately 6 cm from the anus can be treated in this manner. A temporary transverse colostomy may be needed to allow healing of the anastomosis. For lower growths the method of choice is a synchronous-combined abdominoperineal excision of the rectum performed by two surgeons working simultaneously. This involves a permanent left iliac colostomy.

The end results of untreated rectal carcinomas are often so pitiable with protracted and progressive pain and fistulae that palliative resection of the primary tumour should be undertaken wherever possible, despite the presence of obvious intra-abdominal spread. Colostomy alone is unsatisfactory and should be withheld, except in the presence of obstruction or when it may markedly reduce infection. It may be performed in conjunction with radiotherapy to the primary growth to diminish the risk of obstruction.

Other procedures include Hartmann's operation in which the tumour is removed from above and a colostomy established, but the anal canal is not disturbed. The absence of a perineal wound speeds convalescence and it has a limited place in the elderly. Diathermy excision may be used for growths which lie below the peritoneal reflection and which cannot be removed by other means. It may palliate the excessive mucous discharge, which is often troublesome. A pelvic clearance operation to include the removal of bladder and prostate or uterus and adnexae, together with the rectum, when these structures are implicated is occasionally a worthwhile procedure. It poses additional problems with ureteric transplantation into proximal colon and a 'wet colostomy,' or into a reconstructed ileal bladder, which gravely restrict its indications.

Prognosis

Rectal carcinoma carries a reasonably good outlook. Young patients withstand operation better than the elderly, who are more prone to develop pulmonary and urinary complications, but the rate of tumour growth is probably more rapid. The outlook is better in females as the wider pelvis facilitates a more satisfactory dissection and the uterus provides a barrier to bladder involvement.

Operability is often as high as 70 to 80 per cent, and of those subjected to surgery the mortality is about 5 per cent. Dukes has shown that in Group A cases there is an 80 per cent five-year survival rate; in Group B a 60 per cent five-year survival rate, and in Group C a 30 per cent five-year survival rate.

Other rare malignant conditions include sarcoma of the rectum, generally a lymphosarcoma, and malignant melanoma which usually arises in the anorectal region. Surgery should be employed where feasible, or radiotherapy used as a palliative measure for lymphosarcoma, but the prognosis is poor.

CARCINOMA OF THE ANUS

Two types of tumour are encountered. The first and more common is an adenocarcinoma, which is an extension of a rectal growth. The second, which accounts for about 3 per cent of cancers of the rectum and anus, is a squamous-cell carcinoma. It may be of low malignancy, with keratinisation and cell nests, or of high malignancy without either of these features. It may originate at the anal margin where growth is slower, or in the anal canal. The former is more common in men, the latter in women. Tumours of the anus are generally of low malignancy. Spread is both local and to the inguinal lymph nodes.

Bleeding and pain on defaecation are the principal symptoms. The lesion is recognised as a warty-looking mass at the anal margin or within the canal with characteristic induration. A biopsy is essential to confirm the diagnosis and small growths may be excised locally or treated with interstitial irradiation. Larger tumours or those involving the anal canal require an abdomino-perineal excision. The inguinal regions must be kept under observation and a block dissection performed if palpable nodes persist after the subsidence of any infection.

FURTHER READING

Goldberg, S. M., Gordon, P. H. and Nivatvongs, S. (1980). *Essentials of Anorectal Surgery*. New York: Lippincott.
Goligher, J. C. (1980). *Surgery of the Anus, Rectum and Colon*. 4th ed. London: Bailliere Tyndall.
Keighley, M. R. B. (1982). Prevention and treatment of infection in colorectal surgery. World J. Surg. 6, 312–320.
Thomson, H. (1981). Haemorrhoids: A contemporary appraisal. In *Surgical Review*. 2. Eds. Lumley, J. S. P. and Craven, J. L. Tunbridge Wells: Pitman Medical.

18

Liver and biliary tract

THE LIVER

Physiology

The liver plays an important role in body metabolism and its cells appear capable of many functions.

1. *Bile secretion*. The daily output of bile in a normal adult is 1000 ml, the main constituents being bile pigments, bile acids, cholesterol, mucin, inorganic salts and water. Bile pigment or unconjugated bilirubin is formed by the breakdown of haemoglobin in the reticulo-endothelial system, particularly the spleen, and carried to the liver where it is conjugated with glucuronic acid and excreted. Bilirubin is a tetra-pyrrole formed from haemoglobin after removal of the iron atom and the protein part of the molecule. Bilirubin cannot pass the glomerular membrane into the urine unless it has passed through the liver cells and become conjugated. In obstructive jaundice this water soluble conjugated bilirubin is present in the blood giving a 'direct' van den Bergh reaction, and also in the urine. In haemolytic jaundice, the unconjugated bilirubin, being insoluble in water, cannot reach the urine (acholuric jaundice) but gives an 'indirect' reaction in the serum. In hepatocellular jaundice, both conjugated and unconjugated forms may be present in the serum giving a 'biphasic' van den Bergh reaction.

In the small bowel bilirubin is converted to stercobilinogen, some of which is absorbed and then either excreted in the bile again or excreted through the kidneys as urobilin (0 to 4 mg per day). The colour of the stool is due to the contained stercobilin (up to 300 mg per day) and hence the importance of daily inspection of the stools of the jaundiced patient.

2. *Formation and destruction of red blood cells*.
3. *Production of immune bodies*.
4. *Storage and metabolism of carbohydrates*.
5. *Metabolism of cholesterol*.
6. *Metabolism of lipids*.
7. *Metabolism of proteins*. Albumin and the proteins fibrinogen and prothrombin concerned in blood coagulation are made in the liver, but the immunoglobulins are mainly synthesised elsewhere in the body.
8. *Control of ammonia catabolism*. The ammonia produced by bacterial breakdown of proteins in the alimentary tract is carried to the liver and also to the kidneys, where it is metabolised to urea. Failure of this mechanism may lead to 'ammonia intoxication'.
9. *Detoxication of drugs and hormones*.

Liver function tests are performed: (*a*) to differentiate the type of jaundice, (*b*) to aid in the diagnosis of liver-cell damage and (*c*) to determine the prognosis. Many tests are described, since no single one is satisfactory. The following are commonly used in surgical practice.

1. *Serum bilirubin*. Normal values are 5–16 μmol per litre. Jaundice becomes appparent above 35 μmol per litre.

2. *Serum proteins*. Normal serum albumin is 49 g per litre, and globulin 28 g per litre. Normal individuals produce 10 to 16 g albumin daily, but this is markedly reduced in severe liver disease, producing a fall in serum albumin; many patients with liver disease also have an increased plasma volume, which reduces the serum protein concen-

tration. Serum globulin levels increase in chronic liver disease, due to the activity of the reticulo-endothelial system, globulin being mainly formed by the plasma cells. But since the serum albumin and globulin reflect different functions, the albumin-globulin ratio is meaningless.

3. *Flocculation tests*. These depend upon empirical alterations in the serum proteins. Thymol turbidity is the most reliable of these, the normal value being 0 to 4 units. It becomes raised about the third week of virus hepatitis and may remain positive for many months. It is usually normal in obstructive jaundice. Other flocculation tests are the zinc sulphate test and colloidal gold test which become positive about the second week of virus hepatitis, but remain normal in cholestasis.

4. *Serum alkaline phosphatase*. The normal value is 3 to 13 King-Armstrong units. In obstructive jaundice levels are usually over 30 K-A units, but smaller rises are seen in hepatitis. Raised levels are found in bone diseases, particularly Paget's disease, bony metastases and hyperparathyroidism.

5. *Serum transaminases*. Aspartate aminotransferase (formerly known as serum glutamic oxaloacetic transaminase, SGOT) is present in heart, liver and other tissues; the normal serum level is 5 to 17 international units per litre but varies with the method of determination used. Raised levels indicate liver cell destruction, but normal or low values may occur even in disease of fatal severity. High levels are also seen in myocardial infarction, but rarely cause confusion. Alanine aminotransferase (formerly known as serum glutamic pyruvic transaminase, SGPT) is more specific for liver damage, but disappears from blood after sampling so that it is less useful. Normal serum level, again depending on the method of determination used, is 4 to 13 international units per litre.

6. *Bromsulphthalein test*. A 5 per cent solution of bromsulphthalein is given by slow intravenous injection in a dose of 5 mg per kg body weight. After 45 minutes a venous sample is taken and the amount of bromsulphthalein retained is measured photometrically. Normal is up to 3 per cent retention. It is a useful test for liver cell damage in the absence of jaundice.

7. *Prothrombin level*. Since prothrombin is synthesised in the liver, it is deficient in liver cell disease. A decrease is also seen in obstructive jaundice, due to lack of absorption of the fat-soluble vitamin K from the intestine, but this can be corrected by giving vitamin K_1 intramuscularly.

Liver scanning methods

Liver isotope scanning. Radioactive colloidal gold (^{198}Au) or technetium (^{99m}Tc) are taken up by the Kupffer cells and can be scanned for gamma rays. 'Cold areas' produced by tumours, cysts or abscesses may be seen and the scan also gives an indication of the overall shape and size of the liver.

Ultrasound scanning. Grey-scale ultrasound scans are an excellent method of demonstrating cysts, abscesses and dilated bile ducts in the liver. They can sometimes show tumours and metastases, unless obscured by nearby intestinal gaseous distension. The method is very useful in demonstrating stones in the gall bladder and bile ducts.

Computerised tomography (CT) scanning. Results are similar to ultrasound, although slightly better in demonstrating tumours, but less accurate for showing stones in the biliary tract, since these are usually too small to visualise.

Invasive methods

Needle biopsy of the liver. A special needle which removes a small fragment of liver tissue is inserted under local anaesthesia in the 8th, 9th or 10th intercostal space in the right mid-axillary line. The biopsy is removed whilst the breath is held in expiration. Intraperitoneal haemorrhage may occasionally follow, and in patients with biliary obstruction there is the additional danger of intraperitoneal leakage of bile.

Selective coeliac axis arteriography. The tip of an arterial catheter passed via the femoral artery is directed into the coeliac axis or hepatic artery. Radiographs show variations in blood supply and can delineate the extent of hepatic tumours.

Traumatic lesions

Pathology

The liver may be injured by direct or indirect violence; the former may be associated with a blow or crushing force to the lower chest or abdomen, or from gunshot or stab wounds. Indirect violence may result from sudden deceleration, produced by a fall from a height or a head-on collision between vehicles. In the presence of disease, such as glandular fever or malaria, even minor trauma may rupture the liver. Damage to other intra-peritoneal organs or the lungs may also be sustained. The extent varies from contusion of liver substance to complete rupture or separation of a portion of a lobe, the right lobe being principally affected. There are often lacerations on the anterior or superior surface and a subcapsular haematoma may form. Profuse bleeding and leakage of bile may be serious consequences.

Clinical features

A history of closed injury to the lower chest or upper abdomen may be obtained, or the presence of an open wound in the area may suggest the diagnosis. Pain, initially in the right upper quadrant, tends later to be more general and may be referred to the right shoulder or scapular region. Tenderness and guarding in the right hypochondrium is usual and the amount of shock is variable, increasing with the degree of internal haemorrhage. When considerable quantities of blood have escaped free fluid may be detected and an increased but fixed dullness found on the right side. In late stages abdominal distension and ileus occur. The clinical picture may be overshadowed by that of associated lesions.

Treatment

Many liver injuries do not require surgery and provided that blood transfusion can control shock, conservative treatment by bed rest and analgesics is sufficient. If bleeding is not controlled or there is evidence of spreading peritonitis from an associated lesion, laparotomy is required. Loose or pulped liver should be removed and lacerations sutured. Careful exploration to detect other injuries must be performed and the peritoneal cavity drained to prevent the accumulation of bile and blood. Secondary haemorrhage, liver abscess and a biliary fistula are the commonest post-operative complications. Following operation antibiotics should be administered if there is severe liver necrosis, a retained foreign body or associated bowel damage.

The risk of delayed rupture of a subcapsular haematoma warrants observation of suspected cases of liver damage in hospital for 10 to 14 days.

INFECTIONS OF THE LIVER

Virus hepatitis

This condition is the most common cause of jaundice in adults. At least two viruses have been isolated. (1) Hepatitis A virus (HAV), responsible for *infective hepatitis*, is the more common, being excreted in the faeces and may be carried by flies. It has an incubation period of 15 to 50 days and a mortality of 1 to 2 per 1000. (2) Hepatitis B virus (HBV) causing *serum hepatitis*; this is transmitted only by injection, after which the incubation period is 50 to 160 days. The usual source is a blood or plasma transfusion, but infection may follow any injection with a contaminated hypodermic needle or close physical contact. An infected blood donor is capable of transmitting the disease for many years and HBV infection carries a much higher mortality than HAV. Potent sources are massive transfusions, such as those used in heart-lung bypass, renal dialysis, pooled human plasma and blood products such as human fibrinogen or antihaemophilic globulin. A variety of laboratory tests are used in the detection of HB antigen (HB Ag) and HB antibody (HB Ab), the elimination of HB Ag carriers being particularly important in the selection of blood donors. Australia antigen can be identified by electron microscopy or immunological tests and is specific for serum hepatitis. The test is valuable in identifying symptomless carriers as well as in determining the aetiology of some forms of cirrhosis and chronic liver disease.

Clinical features

Nausea, anorexia, malaise and mild abdominal pain precede the onset of jaundice by several days. The liver enlarges towards the end of this stage, after which the jaundice appears rapidly. The liver is usually palpable and often the spleen. The jaundice disappears slowly after about 10 days, but may last longer in older patients. In protracted cases liver biopsy or laparotomy may be necessary to exclude extrahepatic biliary obstruction.

Features of obstructive jaundice may develop in some cases of virus hepatitis making the differential diagnosis difficult. This may be due to 'bile thrombi' blocking the minute biliary ducts. A hepatitis-like clinical picture is occasionally seen after halothane (Fluothane) anaesthesia, being a hepato-cellular jaundice due to idiosyncrasy to the drug. More than one halothane anaesthetic is usually responsible, the first being followed by undiagnosed fever and a transient rise in serum bilirubin. The second anaesthetic is followed immediately or within two weeks by jaundice, which may be fatal.

Treatment

Pooled non-specific immunoglobulin effectively prevents infective hepatitis in personnel exposed to the virus. Protection against serum hepatitis needs specific high-titre Australia antigen immunoglobulin, but is useful in medical workers who have been at risk in renal dialysis or cardiac by-pass units.

Acute pyogenic infections

Pathology

Most liver abscesses formerly arose from portal system infection, often secondary to appendicitis in young people. This is now rare, due to earlier diagnosis and the use of antibiotics. Severe pyogenic infections are now usually secondary to obstruction of the biliary tract by stones or stricture. However there are still four main routes along which infection reaches the liver.

1. *Portal vein*. Portal pyaemia may result from suppuration in the pelvis or gastro-intestinal tract, where conditions such as appendicitis, diverticulitis and occasionally strangulated haemorrhoids are responsible. The mechanism is either through septic emboli or pylephlebitis, a septic thrombophlebitis of the portal vein. Actinomycosis may reach the liver by the portal vein from the ileocaecal region. In the newborn, umbilical sepsis may reach the liver along the umbilical vein.

2. *Cholangitis*. Infection in the obstructed bile ducts above a gallstone, stricture or cancer is now the commonest cause of liver abscess. In the Far East ascaris or liver flukes (*Clonorchis sinensis*) in the bile ducts often lead to suppuration. Cholangitic abscesses are often multiple.

3. *Hepatic artery*. Pyaemic liver abscesses may complicate staphylococcal osteomyelitis or pneumonia.

4. *Direct spread*. Penetrating liver wounds, secondary infection of an amoebic abscess or spread from a subphrenic abscess are rare causes of liver infection.

The liver may be enlarged by multiple small abscesses or a single, thick-walled abscess. Multiplicity is usual in portal pyaemia, septicaemia or suppurative cholangitis. The portal vein may contain pus and blood clot and the abscesses are mainly in the right lobe, in relation to the portal tracts. Microscopy shows a heavy parenchymal infiltration with polymorphonuclear leucocytes around the abscesses. When the infection is due to a cholangitis, the foci are in the smaller bile duct radicles. In pyaemia and septicaemia metastatic abscesses may be found in the lungs, kidneys or brain. Most liver abscesses are due to Gram-negative bacilli, such as *Esch. coli* or *Proteus vulgaris*, but *Staph. pyogenes* and *Strept. faecalis* are also common; *Salmonella typhi* and *Brucella* are sometimes found.

Clinical features

There are general signs of severe, deep-seated infection with swinging temperature, rigors, profuse sweating and tachycardia. Hypotension and shock may occur in Gram-negative bacteraemia. Tenderness and enlargement of the liver, jaundice and ascites are characteristic. The mortality of pyogenic liver abscess is high.

Investigations

Repeated blood cultures are essential; they are more likely to be positive when taken during or immediately after a rigor. There is leucocytosis and anaemia and the serum bilirubin may be raised. X-rays reveal a high, immobile right diaphragm and fluid-levels may be present if the organisms are producing gas. An ultrasound scan may demonstrate the lesion whilst an isotope scan of the liver may reveal a 'cold' area and selective coeliac arteriography is often useful (p. 234).

Treatment

Antibiotics should be used in severe intra-abdominal infections and may prevent development of liver abscess. Established liver infection requires identification of the responsible organism and for this purpose liver biopsy may be needed. The appropriate antibiotic can then be given. Cholangitic abscesses may require relief of the associated biliary obstruction by T-tube drainage of the common bile duct. Single, large liver abscesses are drained by a low intercostal incision, although aspiration sometimes suffices.

Amoebic abscess

Pathology

Entamoeba histolytica, the organism responsible for amoebic dysentery, reaches the liver by the portal vein from the submucosa of the colon. Multiple hepatic foci produced by liquefactive necrosis are common and cause no symptoms unless they coalesce to form a large abscess, which is usually single. The postero-superior part of the right lobe is the commonest site.

The pus is usually sterile and is composed of broken-down liver cells, rather than leucocytes. *Entamoeba histolytica* can usually be found in the wall of the abscess, but secondary infection with pyogenic organisms may occur. An untreated amoebic abscess may rupture through the diaphragm causing an empyema or lung abscess and the patient may cough up pus; rarely it may rupture into the peritoneal cavity.

Clinical features

The condition is usually encountered in males between 20 and 40 years who have lived in the tropics. About one quarter give a history of amoebic dysentery, sometimes many years previously. The onset is usually gradual, with increasing ill-health the cause of which is difficult to diagnose. Fever is variable, but there may be severe sweating or rigors. The patient looks ill, with a peculiar sallow complexion. There is dull pain in the liver area, sometimes referred to the back, but if perihepatitis is present pain may be sharp and referred to the tip of the right shoulder. Local tenderness over the liver may be severe and the enlarged viscus is usually palpable. There may even be bulging of the intercostal spaces or a palpable swelling in the epigastrium. Percussion over the lower right chest may cause pain and a pleural effusion or pulmonary consolidation is sometimes found.

Investigations

There is a moderate leucocytosis (12000 to 16000 per cmm) with 70 to 80 per cent polymorphs, but in long standing cases the white cell count may be normal. A mild anaemia may be present. Fresh, warm stools should be examined on several occasions for the presence of cysts and amoebae. Sigmoidoscopy may show ulcers if colitis is active and scrapings from the base should be examined for amoebae. A haemagglutination test for *Ent. histolytica* is specific in hepatic amoebiasis. Radiographs and screening of the chest may demonstrate pulmonary signs and limitation of movement of an elevated diaphragm. Ultrasound scanning may demonstrate the cyst which may be confirmed by isotope scanning. A dramatic response to metronidazole 400 mg three times daily for five days suggests a correct diagnosis.

Treatment

Metronidazole 400 mg three times daily for five to ten days may be used. Alternatively, emetine hydrochloride 60 mg subcutaneously daily for ten days is given, but toxic side effects are common. Emetine should be continued with chloroquine 1.0 g daily for two days, followed by 0.5 g daily for three weeks. When a liver abscess can be localised it should be aspirated as an adjunct to drug treatment and secondary infection treated with the appropriate antibiotics.

Actinomycosis of the liver

The liver is involved by portal vein or direct spread from a lesion in the ileocaecal region. The infection tracks in the substance of the liver, producing a honeycomb of communicating abscesses and marked surrounding fibrosis. Sinuses may communicate with the abdominal wall and adjacent viscera. The patient becomes ill and anaemic, with a large, tender liver and multiple sinuses on the overlying skin. Characteristic 'sulphur granules' may be seen in the pus, the diagnosis depending upon staining and culture of actinomyces. Massive doses of penicillin should be continued for six weeks or more.

Hydatid disease of the liver

Pathology

Hydatid disease is due to infestation by the dog tapeworm, *Taenia echinococcus*. Man, sheep and cattle are intermediate hosts and are infected by the cyst or larval stage and the disease is commonest in Australia, New Zealand, Wales and Cyprus. The dog is infected by eating the viscera of sheep or horse liver and it then harbours the tapeworm in the intestine, the terminal segment containing about 500 ova. Man is infected by handling the dog, or by eating contaminated vegetables; the ova are liberated from their chitinous envelope by digestion in the intestine, from where they migrate into the portal vein and are carried to the liver. Consequently 70 per cent of eventual cysts are hepatic, but a few ova pass through the liver and are spread by the systemic circulation. Pulmonary hydatid cysts arise in 20 per cent and about 10 per cent occur in spleen, brain or bone.

The cyst is composed of three layers (Fig. 18.1).

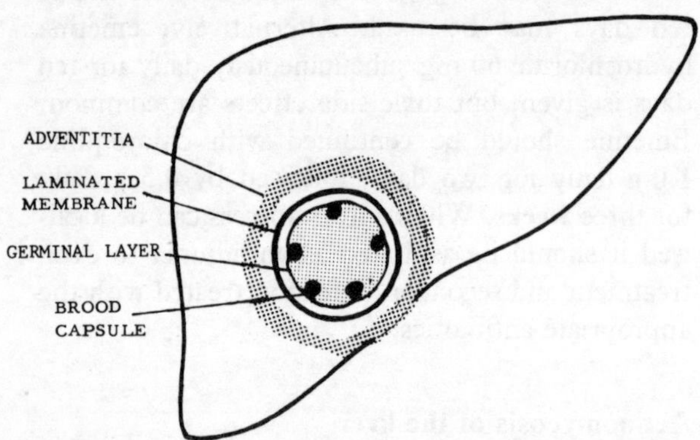

Fig. 18.1 Hydatid cyst in liver

The *adventitia* is derived from the host and consists of fibrous tissue which may calcify. The *laminated layer* is intermediate and can be stripped away from the adventitia. The inner *germinal layer* is derived from the parasite and consists of a single layer of nucleated cells, which produce a number of *brood capsules*, projecting into the cavity of the cyst. The scolices develop in these capsules and are eventually extruded into the main cyst so that daughter cysts are common. The clear fluid within the hydatid cyst therefore contains sand-like scolices, brood capsules, and daughter cysts, all of which are capable of forming secondary cysts. The fluid contains a foreign protein which sensitises the host.

Complications of hydatid cyst are: (1) *Rupture* into the peritoneal cavity, biliary ducts, intestine or lung which may result in dissemination. (2) *Secondary infection*, especially following rupture into the bile ducts, to produce a pyogenic liver abscess. (3) *Hydatid allergy* may lead to recurrent urticaria or severe anaphylaxis.

Clinical features

The cyst may be symptomless or cause pain over the liver. A swelling extending below the costal margin may be apparent but fluctuation is rare. Urticaria or skin rashes may result from sensitisation and jaundice may occur from obstruction of the bile duct in the porta hepatis. Physical signs may be absent when the cyst is in the upper part of the liver, but irregular enlargement of the lower edge due to multiple cysts is fairly common.

Investigations

Eosinophilia of more than 6 per cent occurs in the majority of cases. A positive haemagglutination test is more reliable than the older Casoni intradermal test, but remains negative in 20 to 30 per cent of patients with living cysts and a higher proportion of patients in which the cysts are dead. Radiography may reveal calcification in cysts and elevation or alteration of the right diaphragm outline and barium studies may reveal displacement of stomach or colon. Ultrasound liver scanning usually shows one or more cystic cavities, containing typical multiple acoustic shadows due to the daughter cysts. Hepatic isotope scanning may show a 'cold area'.

Treatment

Mebendazole 2 g daily for three to six months has been used, but its efficacy remains uncertain. Therefore the cysts should be removed surgically. Aspiration of the contents, after carefully towelling off the area to prevent spillage, should be followed by installation of 2 per cent formalin or hypertonic saline to destroy the parasites. The cyst is then dissected away from its adventitial layer and removed. Occasionally a partial hepatectomy or hepatic lobectomy may be necessary. The cysts sometimes communicate with the bile ducts and post-operative bile leakage may occur from the wound drain.

TUMOURS OF THE LIVER

Benign tumours include simple adenoma and haemangioma and are rare. Malignant tumours of the liver are common and include both primary and secondary neoplasms.

Primary neoplasms

Primary carcinoma of the liver may arise in a previously normal organ but the majority occur in patients with cirrhosis. About 15 per cent of patients dying with cirrhosis in Great Britain have complicating liver carcinoma, but the incidence varies with the aetiology of the cirrhosis, being highest in multinodular hyperplasia complicating virus hepatitis, in which a multicentric growth may occur; the lowest incidence occurs in alcoholic cirrhosis. It often complicates haemochromatosis and sometimes parasitic infections such as schistosomiasis and clonorchiasis. The incidence of primary liver carcinoma has a wide geographical variation, being highest in East African Bantus and in Oriental races, where it may be related to ingestion of aflatoxin, a carcinogen produced by a mould found in stored grain. It is usually encountered before the age of 40 in Negroes and between 40 and 60 years in white races and is four to six times more common in men. There are two histological types: (1) *malignant hepatoma*, arising from the liver cells and associated with portal cirrhosis in about 85 per cent of cases, occasionally with haemochromatosis; (2) *malignant cholangioma*, originating in the intrahepatic bile ducts and rarely associated with cirrhosis and then usually the biliary variety.

Clinical features

Symptoms are mainly general, with rapid wasting, low fever and anorexia; sudden deterioration may occur in a known cirrhotic subject. Upper right abdominal pain may be present with a palpable mass due to liver enlargement. Jaundice is not invariable, but ascites is found in half the patients. Radiography may show distortion of the diaphragm and selective coeliac arteriography may outline the tumour, which may also be identified in a liver isotope scan. A raised level of serum alpha fetoprotein is often present but this can also occur in serum hepatitis.

Treatment

Partial hepatectomy is occasionally practicable, particularly for localised tumours and in childhood. The procedure is less hazardous when the left lobe is affected. Cytotoxic drug therapy or embolisation of the hepatic artery using Gelfoam introduced by selective coeliac axis catheterisation may induce necrosis of the tumour which may be palliative, but the average life expectancy from the onset of symptoms is less than one year. Liver transplantation has been employed in specially selected cases.

Secondary neoplasms

The liver becomes involved in about one-third of all cancers, irrespective of whether the primary growth is drained by systemic or portal veins. The sinusoidal hepatic circulation appears to provide a favourable site for the growth of malignant cells.

Metastatic deposits may reach the liver by the following routes:

1. *Portal vein*. Malignant emboli arise in the gastro-intestinal tract.

2. *Hepatic artery*. Carcinoma of the bronchus and breast, melanomas and adrenal tumours disseminate by this route; the malignant cells probably reach the systemic circulation from the primary growth by lymphatic spread via the thoracic duct.

3. *Lymphatic*. There may be retrograde lymphatic permeation, along the portal tracts from the hilum of the liver, from tumours of stomach or bowel, or spread along the falciform ligament from the breast.

4. *Direct spread* from carcinoma of the stomach or gall-bladder may occur.

The metastases vary from one or two microsopic nodules to enormous deposits. They form white, well-demarcated areas in which necrosis may occur, producing an umbilicated appearance in superficial lesions. Perihepatitis may complicate these and cause pain. Deposits in the porta hepatis can cause obstructive jaundice and the portal vein or inferior vena cava may be obstructed by pressure or thrombosis.

Clinical features

Most liver metastases are first detected at operation for the primary abdominal condition. Others present with an enlarged liver and deterioration of general health with fever, and pain accompanied by obstructive jaundice or ascites. The liver may feel hard and irregular with palpable nodules or be considerably enlarged to below the umbilicus.

Liver function tests may remain normal even in the presence of large metastases but there may be a rise in serum bilirubin, alkaline phosphatase or transaminase levels. Needle biopsy may be used to provide material for histological examination and avoid the need for laparotomy. Isotope scanning and selective coeliac arteriography may also be useful in determining the site of the metastases in the liver.

Treatment

Resection of an apparently solitary liver metastasis is occasionally feasible but rarely curative. Pain should be relieved by analgesics and the pruritis of deep jaundice by antihistamines or methyl testosterone. Regression of liver metastases may be obtained by hepatic artery embolisation or palliation achieved with cytotoxic drugs.

Homotransplantation of the liver

The donor liver is taken from the cadaver of a patient with the same blood group and close histocompatibility with the recipient. Serious difficulties may arise from interference with the normal blood clotting mechanism and with rejection. The latter may be modified by prolonged immunosuppressant treatment with prednisolone, azathioprine (Imuran) and antilymphocytic serum. Survival over a period of months has been recorded but further basic research is needed to enable transplantation to be of widespread clinical use.

JAUNDICE

Pathology

Jaundice is a yellow pigmentation of the tissues by bile pigment, associated with an increase in serum bilirubin. A variety of causes can be responsible, either alone or in combination; it is convenient to consider these under the following headings:

1. Haemolytic jaundice

Normal destruction of worn-out red cells by the reticulo-endothelial system releases about 6 g of haemoglobin a day. In haemolytic conditions as much as 45 g of haemoglobin may be released and the liver responds by greatly increased excretion of bile pigment, with only a slight rise in serum bilirubin to 30 to 50 μmol per litre, due to incomplete excretion. Clinical jaundice is not usually evident. The excreted bile pigment is converted in the colon to stercobilinogen, small amounts of which are reabsorbed and excreted in the urine as urobilinogen, some being oxidised to urobilin. Urobilinogen and urobilin are normally absent from the urine but are present in haemolytic jaundice. Bilirubin is not present in the urine, because it is in the unconjugated form which is not excreted by the glomeruli. Haemolytic jaundice is associated with dark urine, due to urobilin, but contains no bilirubin—the so-called *acholuric jaundice*.

2. Hepato-cellular jaundice

Acute liver cell failure is a common cause of jaundice, the depth of which parallels the extent of the damage. In chronic liver cell failure, such as occurs in cirrhosis, jaundice is usually absent. The most frequent cause of hepato-cellular jaundice is virus hepatitis, but it is also noted in hepatic artery occlusion, cirrhosis of the liver, yellow fever, damage by hepato-toxic drugs such as carbon tetrachloride and phosphorus, and occasionally after repeated halothane anaesthesia. The mechanism for the jaundice is complicated, being a combination of failure in the transport of bilirubin from the serum to its site of conjugation in the liver cell, impaired excretion into bile canaliculi and regurgitation of excreted bile from the canaliculi into the liver cells. In addition to this gross interference all along the route of bilirubin excretion, there is often increased haemolysis and cholestasis.

The earliest clinical abnormality is the presence of both bilirubin and urobilinogen in the urine and this occurs before jaundice is apparent. Urobilinogen disappears when jaundice is well established because the liver cells become incapable of excreting any pigment into the bile. Urobilin reappears in the urine during recovery of the liver cells and provides a useful indication of this stage. In hepato-cellular jaundice both conjugated and unconjugated bilirubin are present in the serum, as revealed by the van den Bergh reaction. The level is variable but is usually between 85 and 350 μmol per litre.

3. *Cholestatic jaundice*

Failure of bile to reach the duodenum is known as cholestasis. This may be due to (*a*) *extra-hepatic cholestasis* (with mechanical obstruction of the bile ducts) due to gall-stones, tumours of the bile duct, pancreas and ampullary region, bile duct atresia and stricture, choledochus cyst and parasites such as *Clonorchis sinensis* (a fluke) and the round worm, *Ascaris lumbricoides*; (*b*) *intrahepatic cholestasis* (without mechanical obstruction) seen in chlorpromazine jaundice or as a complication of acute virus hepatitis. Longstanding cholestasis, due to any cause, produces the pathological picture of biliary cirrhosis, in which there is fibrosis in the portal tracts, proliferation of bile duct cells and accumulation of bile pigment in the lobules; portal hypertension eventually occurs.

The liver enlarges and the biliary tree becomes widely dilated and the contained bile colourless and viscous, due to mucus secretion of glands in the wall of the ducts (white bile). Ascending cholangitis results from secondary infection. Bile is normally secreted at a pressure of 150 to 250 mm of water, but production ceases when the pressure rises to about 350 mm. The bile regurgitates into the liver cells and is reabsorbed by the sinusoids; it also enters the blood stream by rupture of distended bile canaliculi and by absorption through lymphatics. A gradual increase in conjugated serum bilirubin occurs during the first three weeks of obstruction; this being dialysable, is excreted by the glomeruli and can be detected in the urine, which becomes dark and frothy. At the same time bile salts accumulate in the blood and may cause severe pruritus. If bile does not reach the duodenum the stools become pale.

In intrahepatic cholestasis the lesion lies within the liver cell and appears to be a disorder of function rather than structure and the actual mechanism is largely unknown. There is often no hepatomegaly, the bile ducts are not dilated and cholangitis is absent. The pathological lesion may lie anywhere between the liver cells and the smaller bile ducts. Cholestatic jaundice develops in 1 to 2 per cent of patients taking phenothiazine derivatives such as chlorpromazine, usually after about a week. It is also occasionally seen during pregnancy and in association with contraceptive pills. Other causes of intrahepatic cholestasis are primary biliary cirrhosis and a form of congenital biliary atresia affecting the small branches of the ducts within the liver.

CAUSES OF JAUNDICE

1. Haemolytic jaundice

Excessive bilirubin production

Congenital and acquired haemolytic diseases

2. Hepato-cellular jaundice

Infections

Virus hepatitis
Yellow fever
Weil's disease (Leptospirosis)
Infective mononucleosis
Pylephlebitis and suppurative infections

Metabolic

Cirrhosis of the liver, portal and post-necrotic

Toxins

Phosphorus
Carbon tetrachloride
Amanita phalloides (toadstool)
Senecio alkaloids

Drugs

Halothane (Fluothane)
Hydrazine mono-amine oxidase inhibitors
Alcoholic hepatitis.

3. Cholestatic jaundice

a) Extrahepatic obstruction

Congenital:
Atresia of bile ducts
Choledochus cyst
Traumatic:
Bile stricture
Neoplastic:
Tumours of bile ducts, pancreas and ampullary region
Metabolic and infective:
Gall-stones
Parasitic:
Ascaris lumbricoides and *Clonorchis sinensis*.

b) Intrahepatic cholestasis

Intrahepatic bile duct atresia
Primary biliary cirrhosis
Virus hepatitis (also hepato-cellular)
Recurrent jaundice of pregnancy
Contraceptive pills and phenothiazines (chlorpromazine).

Clinical features

The onset of jaundice is most rapid in hepato-cellular jaundice and slowest in cholestatic jaundice; both tend to produce a more intense colour than haemolytic jaundice because conjugated bilirubin is soluble in body fluids. Prolonged obstructive jaundice may produce a greenish tinge to the skin, due to oxidation of bilirubin to biliverdin. After the serum bilirubin has fallen to normal during recovery from any form of jaundice, the patient may remain yellow for several days as a result of staining of the tissues, particularly the skin and ocular sclera which have a high elastic content.

Investigations

Examination of the blood reveals a leucocytosis in obstructive jaundice with cholangitis, and in malignant disease. A low total white cell count (1500 to 3000 per cm) with a relative lymphocytosis is seen in virus hepatitis. In haemolytic jaundice examination of blood reveals spherocytosis and immature cells (normoblasts and reticulocytes) and erythrocyte fragility is increased. Coombs' test is positive in idiopathic haemolytic anaemia, but negative in congenital haemolytic anaemia.

Bilirubin is present in the urine during the first few days of virus hepatitis and drug jaundice. A negative bilirubin test with an excess of urinary urobilinogen is found in haemolytic jaundice. In obstructive jaundice due to malignant disease, bile does not reach the alimentary tract and urobilinogen is usually absent from the urine, which contains bile pigment and bile salts. Biliary obstruction also produces pale stools in which bilirubin is absent. The stools should be tested for occult blood, present in ampullary or duodenal carcinoma. The serum bilirubin is raised above 35 μmol per litre in clinical jaundice; the level being proportional to its severity. High levels (250 to 350 μmol per litre are seen in malignant obstruction and occasionally in virus hepatitis. In jaundice due to gall-stones, obstruction is often incomplete and the serum bilirubin variable and less high. The serum alkaline phosphatase is raised above 30 K-A units in most cases of biliary obstruction. The serum proteins should be estimated; in hepato-cellular jaundice there is a low serum albumin and raised γ-globulin, whereas in cholestatic jaundice the albumin is normal but the α_2-and β-globulins are raised. Serum aspartate aminotransferase is raised in hepatitis, as an indication of liver cell damage.

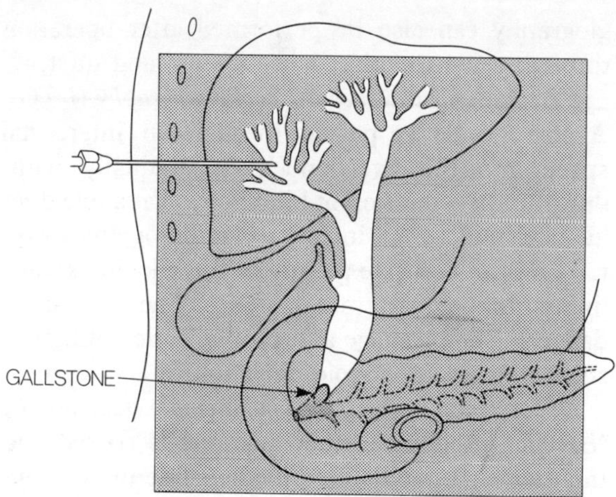

Fig. 18.2 Percutaneous transhepatic cholangiogram outlines distended biliary ducts due to impacted gallstone

A plain radiograph of the abdomen may indicate liver and spleen size and reveal 10 per cent of gall-stones. A barium meal may show an ampullary or duodenal carcinoma and often reveals expansion of the duodenal loop in pancreatic carcinoma. Cholecystography is not helpful when the serum bilirubin level is above 35 μmol per litre, since insufficient medium is secreted. Ultrasound scanning of the liver usually shows dilated intrahepatic ducts in patients with mechanical obstruction by tumour, stone or stricture. Percutaneous cholangiography (Fig. 18.2) may give additional information on the precise level of obstruction and the probable cause. If the bile ducts are not dilated, a surgical cause for the jaundice is unlikely and needle biopsy of the liver may be more helpful in providing the diagnosis. These procedures carry a small risk of bleeding or bile leakage in jaundiced patients. ERCP (p. 244) is useful in selected cases. Laparoscopy with inspection of the liver and direct biopsy may be helpful.

Differential diagnosis

The common clinical causes of jaundice are acute virus hepatitis, carcinoma of the head of the pancreas and ampullary region, cholestatic drug jaundice and choledocholithiasis. Less frequent causes are carcinoma of the hepatic ducts, hepatic metastases, bile duct strictures, primary biliary cirrhosis, Weil's disease and haemolytic jaundice. Most cases can be distinguished by careful history-taking and examination, supported by the urine, faeces and serum biochemical tests. In *virus hepatitis* there is rapid development of jaundice after prodromal symptoms of anorexia and fever and the liver becomes enlarged and tender. In *pancreatic carcinoma* there is weight loss and progressive jaundice, with eventual evidence of complete biliary obstruction. Pain is a common accompaniment. In *cholestatic drug jaundice* there is the history of drug therapy and the jaundice develops rapidly. *Gallstone obstruction of the common bile duct* may produce the triad of intermittent jaundice, fever and abdominal pain, but any of these features may be absent.

Treatment

The principal problem in management concerns the necessity for and correct timing of surgical intervention to relieve extrahepatic biliary obstruction. Jaundice is rarely a surgical emergency and it can be wise to delay exploration for two to three weeks, whilst tests are repeated to exclude virus hepatitis and drug jaundice. An unnecessary general anaesthetic in a patient with hepato-cellular jaundice may precipitate catastrophic liver failure. Operation is indicated when biliary obstruction is clearly present, after correction of anaemia and restoration of a normal prothrombin level by parenteral vitamin K_1 administration. Many cases of malignant obstruction show advanced and inoperable disease at operation, but an attempt should be made to relieve the jaundice and the distressing itching which accompanies it, by means of a palliative short-circuit. Where biliary obstruction is severe, the serum bilirubin may be reduced prior to operation by inserting a fine catheter through the liver into a dilated bile duct and leaving it in place until the patient is ready for operation. In some patients the radiologist can pass a plastic catheter through the biliary stricture, and in this way malignant strictures can be permanently intubated as an alternative palliative procedure to surgery in carcinoma of the main bile ducts and head of pancreas. Care must be taken so that a curative lesion such as a gallstone or early ampullary carcinoma is not overlooked.

GALL-BLADDER AND BILE DUCTS

Physiology

One litre of bile is secreted each day by the liver at a pressure of up to 250 mm of water. This pressure is maintained by the tone in the sphincter of Oddi, diverting some bile up the cystic duct into the gall-bladder where bile salts, bilirubin and cholesterol are concentrated tenfold by absorption of water and electrolytes. Bile passes into the duodenum as soon as the gall-bladder is full, as well as during periodical relaxations of the sphincter of Oddi. Gall-bladder contraction with simultaneous relaxation of the sphincter of Oddi occurs at intervals through fasting, and also when fatty substances pass into the duodenum after a meal, due to release of the hormone cholecystokinin. The sphincter is also influenced by parasympathetic action, and by duodenal peristaltic waves traversing the ampullary region. The sphincter of Oddi is contracted by morphine, so that pethidine is a more suitable analgesic for biliary colic.

Bile secretion ceases when the ductal pressure rises above 350 mm of water as a result of obstruction and eventually the bile in the duct is replaced by a watery fluid containing mucus (white bile) secreted by mucous glands in the wall of the main bile ducts. This indicates prolonged and complete biliary obstruction, usually with poor hepatocellular function.

Radiological investigation of the biliary system is an important method of assessing pathological changes. *Cholecystography* depends upon the absorption from the gut and concentration in the bile of iodine-containing phenolphthalein derivatives. Pheniodol or Telepaque taken by mouth may be revealed in the gall-bladder by radiography after 12 hours. The normal organ contracts to about half size after a fatty meal. Cholecystography is seldom practicable when the serum bilirubin is above 35μmol per litre. *Cholangiography* may be undertaken by the intravenous injection of Biligrafin (iodipamide), which demonstrates the bile ducts and is particularly useful when the gall-bladder has been previously removed. *Operative cholangiography* entails the injection of radio-opaque medium into the exposed ducts at operation, and cholangiography can also be performed after operation through a T-tube placed in the common duct.

Percutaneous transhepatic cholangiography (PTC). A fine needle is passed through an intercostal space into the liver and then gradually withdrawn until aspiration of bile shows that a bile duct has been punctured. Injection of radio-opaque material gives an accurate picture of the bile ducts, outlining tumours, stricture or stones. There is a small danger of bile leakage and prophylactic antibiotics should be given to avoid cholangitis.

Endoscopic retrograde cholangiopancreatography (ERCP). A flexible duodenoscope is passed and the duodenal papilla identified. A fine plastic cannula can then be introduced into either the common bile duct or the main pancreatic duct and these structures filled with radio-opaque fluid. This method allows identification of stones and tumours in both the biliary tract and the pancreas. It is also possible to enlarge the opening of these ducts into the duodenum by division of the sphincter with diathermy (endoscopic sphincterotomy). This method can be used for removing stones from the common bile duct. There is a risk of bleeding and of cholangitis after this procedure and it is usual to give a prophylactic broad spectrum antibiotic.

Congenital anomalies

The liver and biliary tree develop as a diverticulum from the primitive fore-gut and although the ducts are originally patent they become filled at one stage by solid epithelium, recanalisation taking place later. Some of the developmental anomalies of the type seen in biliary atresia are due to failure of this process. The gall-bladder may be absent, double, rudimentary or intrahepatic; rarely it has a mesentery and may undergo torsion.

Congenital atresia of the bile ducts

There are a number of variants of this uncommon condition, in which obstructive jaundice appears during the first week of life and becomes progressively more severe. The site of the obstruction may be in the minute intrahepatic bile ducts or the extrahepatic channels. The prognosis is poor, but children may live for several years without any bile reaching the duodenum. The only chance of cure is by operation, although correction is only possible in about 16 per cent of cases by anastomosis of a suitable duct to the duodenum or jejunum.

Choledochus cyst

In this congenital lesion there is dilatation of part of the common duct, usually the supraduodenal part, accompanied by intermittent obstructive jaundice due to obstruction of the distal common duct. It is commonest in girls under 10, who usually present with intermittent pain in the right subcostal region, together with episodes of jaundice, fever, and a palpable, cystic swelling below the liver. Anastomosis of the cyst to the duodenum or jejunum relieves the symptoms.

GALL-STONES

Cholesterol is held in solution in the bile by the detergent action of the bile salts, which form macro-molecular aggregates called *micelles*. Many factors upset this equilibrium causing the solids of the bile to come out of solution. The colloids in the bile are also important, since precipitation of protein or mucus provides nuclei for the accretion of layers of cholesterol or bile pigment. The precise aetiology of gall-stones is not understood, but a number of factors are important and frequently interact.

Factors concerned in the production of gall-stones include biliary stasis, changes in the constituents of the bile, infection and epithelial changes in the gall-bladder.

1. *Biliary stasis*. The normal gall-bladder never empties completely and the small residue of concentrated bile remains separate from the new bile entering from the liver. When stasis is more marked, cholesterol and bile pigment tend to precipitate in this residue, particularly near the interface between the old and the new bile. Occasionally a cholecystogram reveals a horizontal line of gall-stones 'floating' between these different layers of bile.

Temporary obstruction of the cystic duct, usually due to impaction of a stone, causes the secretion of mucus by the gall-bladder wall; the rise in pressure impedes the blood supply to the mucosa and the contained bile causes chemical inflammation and further mucosal damage. During this process concentric deposits of cholesterol, bilirubin and calcium are laid around a central nucleus of purulent debris or previous cholesterol stone. The process is often repeated with further episodes of obstruction.

2. *Changes in constituents in the bile*. Patients with congenital haemolytic jaundice or any form of chronic haemolysis frequently develop bile pigment stones, due to greatly increased excretion of this substance. It is less certain that changes in dietary cholesterol produce stones and there is no increased incidence in conditions like myxoedema and diabetes, in spite of the raised serum cholesterol. Bile is normally supersaturated with cholesterol, so that it is a common constituent of gall-stones. A low bile salt concentration leads to precipitation of cholesterol and may occur on diets rich in sucrose and in patients on the contraceptive pill.

3. *Infection* reduces the concentration of bile salts and may cause precipitation of solids, whilst clumps of bacteria provide a nucleus for the accretion of other substances from the bile. However, most gall-stones develop in sterile bile, and in acute cholecystitis the bile is usually sterile at the onset.

4. *Epithelial changes in the gall-bladder*. Hypertrophy of the naturally occurring crypts in the gall-bladder wall may occur, resulting in *adenomyomatosis of the gall-bladder*. This condition is commonest in women between 20 and 40. Tiny stones often develop in these crypts and later make their way into the lumen of the gall-bladder where they enlarge. *Cholesterosis* of the gall-bladder ('strawberry') is due to deposition of cholesterol in macrophages in the submucosal layer. These deposits may become pedunculated and ultimately give rise to cholesterol stones.

Types of gall-stones

Three main types are encountered: (1) mixed, (2) cholesterol and (3) pigment. Others such as calcium carbonate stones are rare.

Mixed stone is the common form, accounting for

about 80 per cent of biliary calculi. The brownish stones are usually multiple, smooth and facetted from contact with each other. Mainly composed of cholesterol, bile pigments and calcium salts laid down in concentric layers, there may also be some protein matrix. There may be sufficient calcium to make them radio-opaque.

Cholesterol stone is frequently single and light in weight. It consists of coarse whitish crystals which radiate from the centre. The calculus is not radio-opaque and is usually found in the absence of infection.

Pigment stones are small, crumbly and dark brown or black. They contain bile pigment with a variable amount of calcium and protein matrix. They are seldom radio-opaque.

Investigations

As a result of their low calcium content only about 10 per cent of gall-stones are radio-opaque, compared with about 90 per cent of urinary calculi. Calcification of the gall-bladder wall is occasionally revealed in a plain radiograph. Cholecystography can demonstrate gall-stones not evident on the plain film and also failure to opacify the gall-bladder outline indicates obstruction of the cystic duct by stone.

Complications of gall-stones

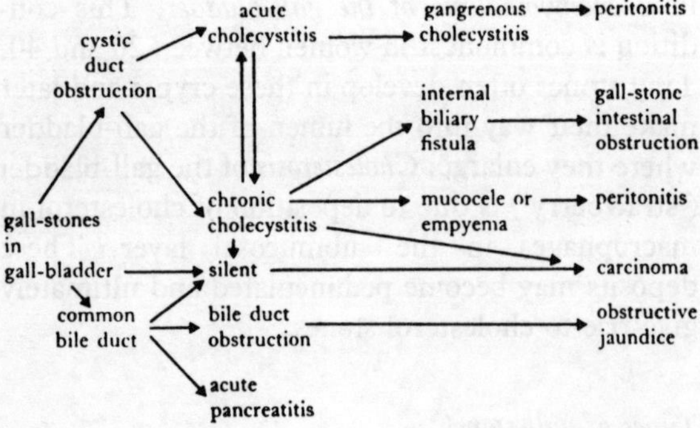

Disease of the gall-bladder is rare unless gall-stones are present. Symptoms usually begin when stones pass into the cystic duct causing biliary colic. Impaction produces obstruction, the resulting inflammatory changes constituting acute or eventually chronic cholecystitis. Sometimes stones pass through into the common bile duct where they again may produce obstruction, usually leading to jaundice. Stones are frequently silent whilst lying in the gall-bladder, and they may also be symptomless in the common duct.

Acute cholecystitis may progress to gangrene and perforation of the gall-bladder, leading to peritonitis; but more often the stone moves relieving the obstruction and the inflammation subsides. It may proceed to chronic cholecystitis or this may arise independently. A stone impacted in Hartmann's pouch may ulcerate through into the duodenum or transverse colon. Intestinal obstruction may then develop from impaction of this stone in the bowel, usually the terminal ileum. Persistent obstruction of the gall-bladder results in its distension with mucus or pus, producing a mucocele or empyema of the gall-bladder. Carcinoma of the gall-bladder is an occasional complication of long-standing gall-stones. Acute pancreatitis may follow the passage of a stone down the common bile duct, the oedema obstructing the adjacent pancreatic duct or the stone actually impacting at the ampulla of Vater.

Acute cholecystitis

Pathology

In 95 per cent of cases, the inflammation is the result of obstruction of the cystic duct by a gall-stone. In the remainder there is a primary bacterial infection of the gall-bladder wall, such as occurs in typhoid and paratyphoid fever, or occasionally during septicaemia from other organisms.

Impaction of a stone in the cystic duct or neck of the gall-bladder produces distension of the viscus by retained secretion and mucus, impairment of blood supply and increased permeability of the gall-bladder wall. The retained bile and especially the bile salts cause chemical inflammation of the mucosa, but the extent to which bacterial infection participates is uncertain. Bile is usually sterile during the first 24 hours, but intestinal organisms can often be cultured subsequently. The gall-bladder appears distended and its serosa oedematous. It contains turbid fluid which may become purulent and the mucosa appears red and inflamed, with patchy greenish necrosis. The obstructing stone is usually palpable in the region of its neck and the cystic lymph nodes are enlarged. In most attacks, the inflammation is localised by the adjacent transverse colon and omentum and the process subsides after a few days. Infarction of the gall-bladder wall occasionally occurs, causing gangrene of the gall-bladder followed by perforation and diffuse peritonitis.

Clinical features

Females are affected three times more commonly than males and are usually over 40 years, but no age group is exempt. A previous history of similar attacks is common, but in the elderly an acute onset is frequently the first indication of gall-bladder disease. The chief symptom is pain, often starting during the early part of the night, and situated in the right upper abdomen or epigastrium. It is usually a continuous, severe ache with exacerbations. Intermittent colicky pain is uncommon. The pain may be referred to the right infrascapular region and sometimes to the tip of the right shoulder but usually localises in the right upper abdomen below the ribs, being aggravated by abdominal movement and deep breathing. Nausea, vomiting and flatulence are usual and constipation is often present. Fever up to 40 °C may develop. The important physical signs are tenderness, guarding and rigidity in the right hypochondrium. Localisation of the tenderness to the ninth costal cartilage anteriorly with a sudden catch of the breath during inspiration is important confirmation. Occasionally there is a palpable, tender mass in the right hypochondrium. Jaundice is rare in uncomplicated cholecystitis.

Investigations

A plain radiograph of the abdomen may give positive evidence of radio-opaque gall-stones, but about 90 per cent are non-opaque. Ultrasound scanning usually confirms a distended gall-bladder containing stones. The leucocyte count may be raised. The serum amylase is normal or slightly raised.

Differential diagnosis

Confusion occurs with conditions both above and below the diaphragm. Myocardial infarction, pleurisy, pulmonary embolism and pneumonia must be considered. The abdominal conditions of perforated duodenal ulcer, acute pancreatitis and acute appendicitis require elimination. In appendicitis, vomiting is usually infrequent and pyrexia slight, whilst the site of tenderness is lower. Pancreatitis may be difficult to differentiate, but severe central abdominal and left infrascapular pain, marked tachycardia and central abdominal tenderness with a marked rise in serum amylase are all typical of acute pancreatitis.

Treatment

Most cases resolve on a conservative regime. General measures include bed rest, intravenous fluids and relief of pain with pethidine. Severe cases need antibiotics, ampicillin being satisfactory. Deterioration of the patient's condition during conservative treatment may indicate the onset of gangrene of the gall-bladder wall and it is wise to explore the abdomen and perform cholecystectomy. This operation is technically feasible during the first three days of acute cholecystitis, provided the surgeon is experienced. In elderly, frail patients drainage of the gall-bladder (cholecystostomy) is sometimes advocated as a simpler procedure than emergency cholecystectomy. If operation is not undertaken for the acute attack cholecystectomy should be performed about two months later when the inflammation has subsided, because recurrent attacks are common.

Chronic cholecystitis

Pathology

Chronic cholecystitis seldom occurs in the absence of gall-stones. It may follow repeated attacks of acute cholecystitis or develop insidiously. The gall-bladder may be enlarged or shrunken and fibrotic. The thickened wall appears white and may even calcify. The contained bile is turbid or purulent and there may be one or many gall-stones. The mucosa is ulcerated and scarred with areas of granulation tissue. When the organ is distended with mucus or pus, the terms *mucocele* and *empyema of the gall-bladder* are often used, but the turbid pus of empyema is often sterile on culture.

Adenomyomatosis is a condition in which there is hypertrophy of mucus-secreting glandular tissue in the gall-bladder wall giving it a spongy appearance, particularly in the fundus, and in the body, where an hour-glass stricture may develop. Small calculi frequently arise in these glandular crypts, from which they may eventually migrate into the lumen. Some lymphocytic infiltration accompanies these changes, but bacterial infection is uncommon. The condition is commonest in women between 20 and 40 years.

Cholesterosis (*'strawberry' gall-bladder*) is due to accumulation of yellow lipid material including cholesterol esters in the submucosal layer. It occurs when the concentration of cholesterol in the bile is raised, the gall-bladder wall absorbing the lipid and storing it in foamy macrophage cells. The deposits may become pedunculated and give rise to cholesterol stones.

Clinical features

Commonly there are repeated attacks of acute cholecystitis which vary in severity from a transient attack of right subcostal pain to an episode lasting several days. In other cases symptoms are ill-defined, with a feeling of abdominal distension. nausea and right subcostal discomfort, usually with referral to the back of the right chest. Right subcostal tenderness is usually present but clinical signs are sometimes absent.

Investigations

Cholecystography is reliable, revealing radiolucent gall-stones or indicating failure of the organ to opacify, but the latter may also be due to failure of the patient to ingest the test material, failure in absorption due to diarrhoea or vomiting, or failure of the liver excretion. Ultrasound scanning usually shows a thick-walled gall-bladder containing stones.

Differential diagnosis

Chronic cholecystitis may be confused with peptic ulceration, hiatus hernia, carcinoma of the stomach, renal calculi or pyelitis, recurrent appendicitis and functional dyspepsia. Anginal pain or myocardial infarction may be difficult to distinguish even with the help of an electrocardiograph. Chronic pancreatitis may accompany gall-stones, but is particularly suggested by backache, steatorrhoea and diabetes, whilst the serum amylase may be raised and pancreatic calcification may be visible on a plain radiograph.

The presence of gall-stones or a non-functioning gall-bladder on cholecystography is highly suggestive but care must be taken to exclude the above diseases because chronic cholecystitis often co-exists.

Treatment

Cholecystectomy is the procedure of choice. Medical measures can only be palliative and the incidence of complications is high. Particular care is necessary to avoid damage to the common bile duct and hepatic artery. Unsuspected stones may occur in the common bile duct, *operative cholangiography* being commonly employed to detect them. 'Silent' gall-stones may be left until such a time as they begin to cause symptoms, which does not always happen; the chance of such a patient developing cancer of the gall-bladder is insufficient to justify routine cholecystectomy in the absence of symptoms.

Typhoid cholecystitis

The biliary tract is infected in about 0.2 per cent of typhoid patients, although circulating typhoid bacilli are regularly excreted in the bile. Acute typhoid cholecystitis occurs as a rare complication during the second week and should be treated by cholecystectomy. Chronic typhoid cholecystitis presents a health hazard because a symptomless carrier state is produced in which the organisms are continuously excreted in the faeces. A previous history of typhoid fever can always be obtained. Cholecystectomy should be advised, but may fail to cure the carrier state when there is an associated infection of the bile ducts. Ampicillin or co-trimoxazole should be given following the operation.

Common duct stones (Choledocholithiasis)

Pathology

Most stones found in the common or hepatic ducts have originated in the gall-bladder; this includes calculi presenting after cholecystectomy, these having been overlooked during the original operation. Occasionally a stone may develop above a common duct stricture and in the Far East they arise in ducts infested with liver fluke or round worm. Any number of stones may occur, usually of mixed composition, but pigment stones are present in haemolytic anaemia. Biliary stasis is usually present, either from the obstruction of the stone or associated pathology, so that the bile becomes opaque and brown (biliary mud) and bacterial infection is common. The stones usually lie free in the lumen of the duct but may impact in the ampulla of Vater or at other levels. Intermittent obstruction is usual from temporary impaction of the stone often complicated by infection. Complete obstruction occasionally occurs and the common duct becomes filled with 'white bile', although this more often follows malignant obstruction.

Accompanying infection produces thickening of the wall of the dilated common duct, and ulceration and desquamation of its epithelium. This inflammation may spread up into intra-hepatic bile ducts and produce multiple cholangitic abscesses. The cut surface of the liver shows irregular cavities containing bile-stained pus, communicating with the ducts. *Esch. coli* is the commonest infecting organism. In long-standing cases liver function becomes impaired by a combination of obstruction and infection, and biliary cirrhosis may develop. Common duct stones are occasionally silent or they may present for the first time as fulminating acute pancreatitis, due to sudden obstruction at the ampulla of Vater.

Clinical features

The majority of patients develop intermittent attacks of pain, fever and jaundice, but any or all of these features may be absent. The pain usually is continuous and severe and situated in the right upper quadrant, radiating through to the right infrascapular region. Associated vomiting is common. The fever is characteristically intermittent and accompanied by sweating, rigors and considerable malaise. It may reach 40°C in acute cholangitis and the blood culture may be positive during the episodes. Occasionally marked prostration with hypotension is due to Gram-negative septicaemia and renal failure may follow.

The jaundice is usually mild and obstructive (cholestatic) in type, with dark urine, pale stools and pruritus, but bile duct obstruction is seldom complete and some pigment usually reaches the stools. Frequently there are no abnormal physical signs apart from mild jaundice and epigastric or hepatic tenderness. The gall-bladder is usually impalpable, being shrunken from chronic cholecystitis and *Courvoisier's law* may be applied. This states that in obstructive jaundice a palpable distended gall-bladder is not the result of gall-stones. However, rarely an enlarged gall-bladder can be felt and in long-standing cases, the liver may be enlarged.

Investigations

The urine contains bilirubin and sometimes bile salts. The serum bilirubin is raised to about 50 to 150 μmol per litre and the alkaline phosphatase elevated, but the remaining liver function tests are usually normal, unless severe hepatic damage is present. If a stone obstructs the main pancreatic duct, a sharp rise in serum amylase occurs. A plain radiograph may indicate radio-opaque stones in the gall-bladder and, more medially, along the common duct. Ultrasound scanning may show the stones within a dilated common duct and can be used in the presence of jaundice. Endoscopic retrograde cholangiography can also be done but carries a slight risk of causing ascending cholangitis. With the subsidence of jaundice a cholecystogram will provide evidence of gall-bladder disease and an intravenous cholangiogram usually demonstrates a dilated common duct and may show the contained stones. During a fever, blood culture may identify the organism and allow determination of sensitivities for appropriate antibiotic therapy. Aspiration liver biopsy is seldom advisable due to the risk of bile leakage.

Differential diagnosis

In the presence of obstructive jaundice distinction between calculous and malignant disease may be difficult. Fluctuation in the intensity of the jaundice, intermittent fever and the presence of pain suggest a stone, whilst painless increasing jaundice and a palpable gall-bladder are more indicative of neoplasm (Fig. 18.3). Acute virus hepatitis may also be difficult to exclude in the first two weeks of jaundice, but anorexia, liver tenderness and impairment of liver function may point to this diagnosis.

Treatment

Small stones may pass into the duodenum, but surgical removal is generally necessary. Antibiotics such as tetracycline, ampicillin or gentamicin may improve the associated cholangitis, but the infection will recur unless the stones are removed. Pre-operative vitamin K_1 and the correction of anaemia, fluid and electrolyte imbalance are advisable. The common duct is opened and all calculi removed, usually through an incision in its supraduodenal part, but an impacted stone at the ampulla may require opening of the duodenum and division of the sphincter of Oddi. Operative cholangiography is valuable in confirming that all stones have been removed (Fig. 18.4). Alternatively operative choledochoscopy can be employed. The chronically diseased gall-bladder should also be removed. Postoperative drainage of the common bile duct by a T-tube is advisable and this should be removed about the tenth to twelfth post-operative day, preferably after a further cholangiogram via the tube to exclude any residual stones. If these are found they may be flushed into the duodenum, removed

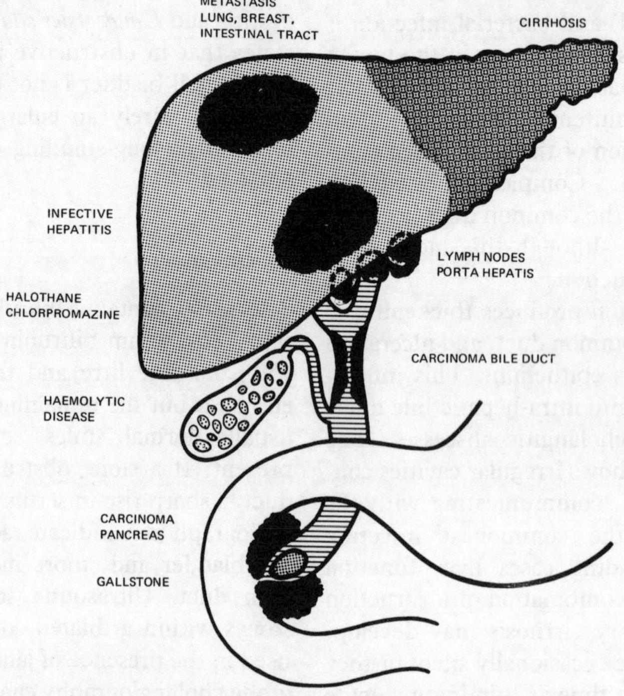

Fig. 18.3 The common causes of jaundice

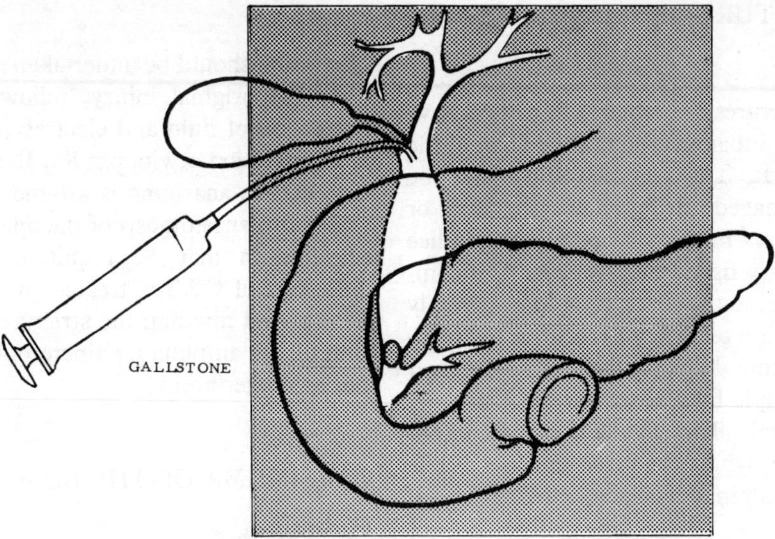

Fig 18.4 Operative cholangiogram

by the radiologist using a basket appliance passed along the T-tube track six weeks after operation or by an endoscopist using a similar method through the duodenal sphincter. Further surgery is now seldom needed for residual biliary stones.

Post-cholecystectomy syndrome

Symptoms which persist or return after cholecystectomy are due to the following causes. (1) Wrong initial diagnosis, for instance when symptoms are due to an underlying hiatus hernia, chronic pancreatitis or gastric ulcer; (2) presence of residual calculi in the common or hepatic ducts; (3) traumatic stricture of the main bile ducts or inflammatory stricture at the sphincter of Oddi; and (4) a cystic duct stump or neuroma. Diagnosis is greatly helped by intravenous cholangiography or ERCP (p. 244), which reveals or excludes any abnormality of the common or hepatic bile ducts. If any biliary abnormality is discovered, endoscopic sphincterotomy or surgery is usually advised to improve the drainage of the common duct.

CARCINOMA OF THE GALL-BLADDER

Pathology

Carcinoma of the gall-bladder is an uncommon tumour, usually complicating long-standing gall-stones. It is an adenocarcinoma in 90 per cent of cases, but squamous metaplasia may occur. The lesion may occur anywhere in the organ and usually infiltrates widely into the liver, duodenum, colon and stomach. Lymphatic spread occurs to nodes around the common bile duct and pylorus. Blood-stream spread is less common.

Clinical features

Females are affected more often than males in the ratio of four to one. There may be a long history of calculous disease, with a recent alteration in symptoms. The pain may become constant, with progressive jaundice, weight loss and the presence of a palpable mass. Occasionally the tumour is an unsuspected finding in the course of cholecystectomy for gall-stones.

Treatment

Cholecystectomy together with excision of locally invaded structures offers the only chance of survival. This may necessitate excision of the right lobe of the liver, but the growth is usually advanced by the time it is discovered. The best results are obtained when the diagnosis is made histologically in a gall-bladder removed for stones.

BENIGN STRICTURE OF THE BILE DUCTS

Pathology

Most benign strictures are either due to operative trauma or chronic inflammation in the region of the sphincter of Oddi. The common duct may be inadvertently damaged during cholecystectomy or partial gastrectomy. Following operation jaundice occurs and a biliary fistula may appear. The common duct proximal to the stricture becomes grossly dilated and there is a tendency to recurrent cholangitis, with the eventual development of severe liver damage and multiple liver abscesses or biliary cirrhosis. An external biliary fistula may be complicated by infection, whilst the persistent loss of bile salts leads to vitamin deficiency, particularly of vitamin K.

A benign stricture of the sphincter of Oddi may occur in women between 50 and 70 and is probably inflammatory in origin. The dilated common duct usually contains stones or biliary mud.

Clinical features

Complete obstruction of the bile duct is indicated by rapid onset of progressive jaundice, which may cease with the establishment of a biliary fistula. The persistence of biliary leakage for more than a week after gall-bladder surgery suggests that organic obstruction may be present. Intermittent pain and fever are usual. Injection of radio-opaque material along the fistula may demonstrate an obstruction with dilated proximal duct and intrahepatic tributaries.

Stricture of the sphincter of Oddi causes recurrent fever and jaundice, often with pain. Radiological investigation of the biliary tract may be carried out as outlined on p. 244.

Treatment

Operation should be undertaken as soon as possible after the original injury, following pre-operative correction of fluid and electrolyte balance and the administration of vitamin K_1. Excision of the stricture and re-anastomosis around a T-tube is preferable but anastomosis of the dilated duct to a loop of jejunum may be required. Stricture of the sphincter of Oddi is treated by opening the duodenum and dividing the stricture with reconstruction of the ampulla (sphincteroplasty) or endoscopic sphincterotomy.

CARCINOMA OF THE BILE DUCTS

Pathology

The most frequent site is the right or left hepatic duct, but the tumour may arise in any of the extrahepatic bile ducts. Histologically the growth is a columnar-cell adenocarcinoma which grows slowly, producing obstructive jaundice except when only one hepatic duct is affected. Spread is both local and to adjacent lymph nodes. Proximal dilatation of the duct system occurs and death is due to liver failure. Radical excision of bile ducts may be feasible in selected cases; palliative intubation by means of PTC or ERCP (p. 244) may be helpful in relieving jaundice and pruritus.

FURTHER READING

Cotton, P. (1980). Non-operative removal of bile duct stones by duodenoscopic sphincterotomy. Brit. J. Surg. 67, 1–5.

Sherlock, S. (1981). *Diseases of the Liver and Biliary System*. 6th ed. London: Blackwell.

Smith, R. Lord, and Sherlock, S. Dame. (1981) *Surgery of the Gall Bladder and Bile Ducts*. London: Butterworth.

19

Spleen. Portal hypertension

THE SPLEEN

Congenital disorders

The spleen is seldom absent. *Accessory spleens* occur in 10 to 20 per cent of the population. These splenunculi are often situated along the splenic vessels, at the hilum of the spleen, rarely in the mesentery or greater omentum. It is important to remove accessory spleens at the time of splenectomy for acholuric jaundice. Splenomegaly may be caused by a *solitary dermoid cyst* or occasionally be part of a *polycystic disease*.

Infective splenomegaly

Many infectious disorders produce splenic enlargement. *Bacterial* causes include typhoid, paratyphoid, typhus, anthrax, tuberculosis, Weil's disease, syphilis and septicaemia. More marked splenomegaly is seen in the *protozoal* diseases, malaria, kala-azar and Egyptian splenomegaly. Of the *parasitic* infestations, hydatid cyst is a rare cause of an enlarged spleen.

TRAUMA

The spleen is the commonest intraperitoneal organ to be ruptured, most cases following direct trauma in road and industrial accidents due to a crushing injury. Indirect trauma by falling from a height may be responsible, whilst penetrating stab and gunshot wounds may also involve the spleen. There may be associated rib fractures and occasionally damage to the left kidney. The diseased spleen not infrequently ruptures from minimal injury in malaria, leukaemia and infectious mononucleosis; spontaneous rupture has also been recorded.

Hilar avulsion and fragmentation of the spleen result in profuse haemorrhage and are generally associated with severe trauma. In some instances the splenic capsule exercises restraint on the underlying bleeding with the formation of a subcapsular haematoma. This usually ruptures, but occasionally there is conversion to a blood cyst or organisation of the haematoma. Minimal bleeding with an associated capsular tear may cause a perisplenic haematoma (Fig. 19.1). The anatomical position of the spleen tends to localise such an effusion, particularly when bleeding is slow. The diaphragm may be raised, the colon depressed and the stomach displaced, the whole collection becoming walled off

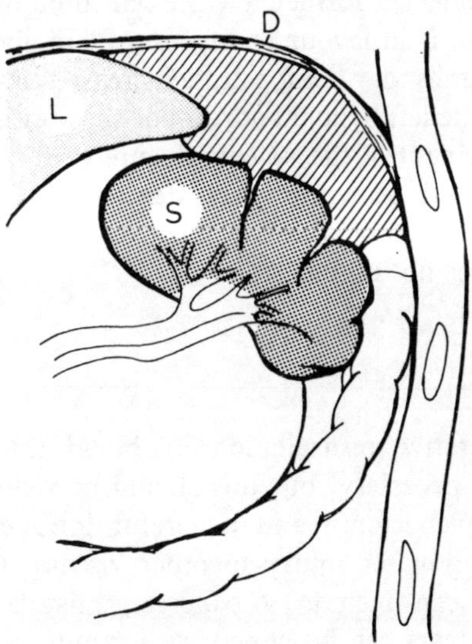

Fig. 19.1 Rupture of spleen leading to formation of perisplenic haematoma between diaphragm (D) and liver (L)

by adhesions between alimentary tract and abdominal wall. Intraperitoneal rupture may later occur.

Clinical features

The picture is dependent on the amount and rapidity of blood loss, but commonly the initial shock caused by traumatic rupture passes and leaves abdominal pain, which is made worse on breathing and may be referred to the left shoulder. General examination will reveal variable features of internal haemorrhage and shock. Pallor is constant, but the development of tachycardia or fall in blood-pressure may be delayed. The abdomen moves well on quiet respiration, but pain is usually worsened by deep respiration. Rigidity and tenderness in the left hypochondrium are constant but may never be marked. Dullness may be detected in both flanks, and may be shifting on both sides or fixed on the left. Rectal examination may detect a fullness with some tenderness in the rectovesical pouch.

'Delayed rupture', due to the sudden bursting of a subcapsular haematoma, may take place, usually between the third and ninth day. It is often precipitated by minor trauma and presents a picture of severe blood loss.

The diagnosis of complete rupture is seldom difficult, but in doubtful cases where a perisplenic haematoma has formed a white cell count of 15 000 per cmm is in favour of rupture. Plain abdominal radiographs may demonstrate increased tissue density in the left hypochondrium or show evidence of displacement of the splenic flexure or diaphragm. Ultrasound scanning may demonstrate a perisplenic haematoma or a torn spleen, but a negative scan does not exclude injury.

Treatment

Pre-operative resuscitation by blood transfusion may be necessary, but this should be followed by early splenectomy and a careful intraperitoneal examination for injury to other viscera. Complications can include a pancreatic fistula. Small splenic tears can be closed with catgut sutures to avoid the need for splenectomy; this is particularly applicable in children as splenectomy diminishes the resistance to infection in this age group.

HAEMOLYTIC ANAEMIA

This group of blood disorders is encountered in both congenital and acquired forms and is due to destruction of the red blood corpuscles either by the cells of the reticulo-endothelial system or in the circulating blood.

Congenital haemolytic anaemia

Pathology

This is a familial condition in which there is an increased fragility of the red cells. It is transmitted by either parent as a Mendelian dominant and may be inherited by either sex. The underlying cause is believed to be an enzymatic abnormality in the red cells. The characteristic feature is the abnormal shape of the red corpuscles which tend to be biconvex and smaller than normal (microspherocytosis). There is also an increased fragility, the life span being reduced to less than 14 days as compared with the normal 120 days. As a result of such destruction immature red cells (reticulocytes) are seen in abundance. There is splenomegaly and perisplenitis. Increased haemolysis gives rise to hyperbilirubinaemia and the formation of pigment gall-stones. Hepatomegaly is occasionally encountered and pigment deposition may produce biliary cirrhosis.

Clinical features

Both sexes are equally affected. Symptoms usually commence in the first decade, but are generally mild. Anaemia and jaundice vary in degree and the spleen becomes palpable. Patients with a mild form of the disease may continue without ill-health for many years into middle age. In others haemolytic crises occur which can prove rapidly fatal. In such acute episodes there is abdominal pain, fever, nausea and vomiting, together with severe anaemia, deepening jaundice and splenomegaly. Biliary colic and obstructive jaundice are not common despite the finding of gall-stones in 60 to 70 per cent of patients. Rarely chronic leg ulcers are encountered.

Investigations

Examination of the blood reveals a moderate normochromic anaemia, but in a crisis the red-cell count may fall to 1 000 000 per cmm. The reticulocyte count is raised to 5 to 20 per cent, although this may also fall in a crisis, becoming raised afterwards to 50 per cent. The *fragility test* is pathognomonic. The red cells are unduly fragile in hypotonic saline solution. Normally haemolysis commences at 0.45 per cent and is complete at 0.3 per cent; in congenital haemolytic anaemia these figures are 0.75 to 0.4 per cent. The serum bilirubin is raised above 20 μmol per litre with an indirect van den Bergh reaction, Coombs' serological test for immune globulin is negative. A plain radiograph or cholecystogram may demonstrate gall-stones.

Treatment

Splenectomy is indicated during a remission. Gallstones when present should be treated by cholecystectomy. Blood transfusion should be avoided unless severe anaemia is present since gross haemolytic transfusion reactions are common. Following splenectomy the osmotic fragility of the red blood cells is not cured and haemolysis occurs to a lesser degree, but the anaemia is improved and leg ulcers heal.

Other haemolytic anaemias are acquired and may be caused by a variety of factors. These may be grouped as follows: (*a*) Infective: streptococci, staphylococci, *Cl. welchii*, malaria. (*b*) Toxic: lead, arsenic, sulphonamides. (*c*) Haemolysins: haemolytic disease of the newborn (erythroblastosis foetalis), incompatible blood transfusion and auto-immune haemolytic anaemia.

Auto-immune haemolytic anaemia occurs more commonly in females and in the third decade of life. It is due to the circulation of auto-agglutinins and autohaemolysins, which damage the red cells. Splenomegaly occurs, but there is no family history. Coombs' test is usually positive. Steroids are often effective in those cases which do not remit. Splenectomy has little place, but may be tried if all else fails.

Purpura

The appearance of areas of haemorrhage in skin or mucous membrane is a manifestation of this disease. It is important surgically as it may produce gastro-intestinal and uterine bleeding, intussusception and signs suggestive of acute intestinal obstruction.

The cause is a deficiency of blood platelets and two types are recognised: (1) primary (idiopathic) thrombocytopenic purpura, and (2) secondary (symptomatic) purpura. The latter may be due to infections such as tuberculosis, drugs such as arsenicals, benzene, gold salts, sulphonamides and chloramphenicol, excessive radio-therapy, leukaemia and secondary malignant disease of bone. In these cases the thrombocytopenia is secondary to bone marrow dysfunction.

Idiopathic thrombocytopenic purpura

This condition mainly afflicts children and young adults. The cause of deficient platelets is unknown, although it may be an antigen-antibody reaction. Ecchymoses, gastro-intestinal and urogenital bleeding are common, but haemarthroses are rare. Remissions and relapses are frequently seen and the disease runs a chronic course. There may be few physical signs apart from subcutaneous bruising and occasionally a palpable spleen, but inflation of a sphygmomanometer cuff sufficient to obstruct the venous return in a limb generally produces obvious petechiae.

Examination of the blood may show a hypochromic microcytic anaemia and a bleeding time prolonged above 15 minutes. The coagulation time is normal, but poor retraction of the clot and a low platelet count (40 000 per cmm or below) are usually present.

Treatment

Spontaneous recovery is seen, particularly in children. A conservative approach should be adopted initially in all cases, and includes blood transfusion and steroid therapy. Splenectomy is required when there is failure of response or relapse on medical treatment and in severe cases. Prolonged bleeding time and increased capillary fragility are dramatically improved. The platelet count rises to a maximum in 48 hours and may precipitate spontaneous thromboses. This thrombocyte response is not permanent, but symptomatically 80 per cent of patients are improved.

Neoplasms

Primary tumours of the spleen are rare and include angioma and fibrosarcoma. Involvement in Hodgkin's disease, lymphatic and myeloid leukaemia is common, but the presence of secondary malignant deposits in the spleen is rare.

Indications for splenectomy

Congenital: Cystic spleen, torsion.

Traumatic: Rupture of the spleen.

Neoplastic: Primary fibrosarcoma, reticulosarcoma.

Blood disease: Congenital haemolytic anaemia, acquired haemolytic anaemia, thrombocytopenic purpura.

Splenectomy may be combined with mapping of the intra-abdominal lymph nodes to determine the extent of Hodgkin's disease. It is performed in total or subtotal gastrectomy for carcinoma of the stomach. The discomfort caused by a large spleen in leukaemia, kala-azar, Hodgkin's disease and malaria may also necessitate removal. In these and other conditions, portal hypertension for example, evidence of hypersplenism is a further indication.

The physiological effects of splenectomy include a leucocytosis, increased platelet count and increased coagulability of the blood within the first two months, together with a mild anaemia and erythropenia. After several months a relative lymphocytosis or eosinophilia occurs. The bone marrow in young people becomes more proliferative and red marrow replaces yellow. Splenunculi when present hypertrophy.

PORTAL HYPERTENSION

The normal portal venous pressure is between 75 and 150 mm of water, and portal hypertension is said to occur when it exceeds 160 mm.

Physiology

The portal venous pressure, being higher than that in the hepatic vein, normally directs the flow of blood through the hepatic sinusoids into tributaries of the hepatic vein. Arterial blood from branches of the hepatic artery enters these sinusoids, whilst other hepatic arterioles supply the structures in the portal tracts. In cirrhosis of the liver this vascular arrangement becomes altered and much of the blood no longer perfuses the liver cells but instead passes from the portal radicles into hepatic venules through sinusoids that short-circuit the regenerative liver lobules. The latter also compress the hepatic venules and some of the portal venous blood is diverted into portasystemic collaterals. As a result of these intra- and extrahepatic shunts, perfusion of the liver cells with portal blood is greatly reduced. The liver lobules continue to be supplied by hepatic artery blood, which passes into the sinusoids, so that part of the rise in portal pressure is the result of this arterialisation. It is the bizarre anatomy of the regenerative liver lobules, rather than the accompanying fibrosis, which is responsible for portal hypertension in cirrhosis of the liver.

The portal venous pressure may be determined by direct manometry, using a saline-filled vertical tube connected to a needle which may be introduced by percutaneous splenic puncture, or placed in a mesenteric vein during surgery. Percutaneous splenic puncture also allows the performance of portal venography after the rapid injection of 40 ml of 70 per cent radio-opaque dye (diodone). The hepatic vein pressure may be determined by retrograde passage of a cardiac catheter through the right side of the heart and inferior vena cava into a hepatic vein under radiological control. The normal wedged hepatic vein pressure is about 5 to 6 mm Hg but may be raised to 25 mm Hg with the presence of cirrhosis. The normal portal pressure is about 8 mm Hg rising to between 20 and 35 mm Hg in portal hypertension.

PATHOLOGY

Aetiology

Portal hypertension may be more precisely classified according to its anatomical localisation.

1. Extrahepatic portal hypertension

This is seen particularly in children as a result of umbilical sepsis spreading along the umbilical vein and left branch of the portal vein (umbilical thrombophlebitis following exchange transfusion or other neo-natal infection). In later childhood portal pylephlebitis following appendicitis may be responsible. In adults the portal vein may thrombose in blood diseases such as polycythaemia, or as a result of compression by malignant deposits in the porta hepatis. Cavernous transformation of the portal vein is probably the result of enlargement of venae comitantes and recanalisation following thrombosis.

2. Intrahepatic portal hypertension

(*a*) *Pre-sinusoidal*, where the responsible lesion is in the portal tracts, as may occur in schistosomiasis or rarely when the portal tracts are infiltrated by sarcoid or reticulosis.

(*b*) *Post-sinusoidal* portal hypertension occurs in cirrhosis. It may be the result of alcoholic cirrhosis, but in Great Britain it is more often due to previous virus hepatitis or an unknown cause (chronic hepatitis). Another variety is noted in veno-occlusive disease, a disorder seen in Jamaica after drinking medicines made from Bush teas and in other regions after plant toxins; obliteration of minute hepatic venules occurs, producing back-pressure in the portal system.

The collateral circulation (Fig. 19.2)

Most of the diverted blood finds its way into the azygos and hemiazygos systems and through the left renal vein into the inferior vena cave (porta-systemic collaterals). Porta-portal collaterals may occur in some cases of extrahepatic portal vein obstruction, the flow re-entering the portal vein in the porta hepatis beyond the block.

In portal hypertension as much as 90 per cent of the portal flow is directed through portasystemic communications which mainly occur at the following sites:

1. *Gastro-oesophageal*, between the oesophageal branches of the left gastric vein and the intrathoracic systemic veins. Oesophageal varices develop in the submucous layer of oesophagus and cardia and may result in severe haemorrhage.

2. *Anorectal*, between the superior rectal tributary of the inferior mesenteric vein and inferior rectal veins.

3. *Periumbilical*, along relics of the umbilical veins in the falciform ligament to superficial veins of the anterior abdominal wall.

4. *Retroperitoneal* in the bare area of the liver, the lieno-renal ligament and the omentum.

The spleen

Particularly in children the spleen is enlarged, due to back-pressure, and its sinusoids are dilated; there is leucopenia, thrombocytopenia and anaemia (secondary hypersplenism). The hypersplenism persists after relief of the portal hypertension, unless the spleen is also removed.

Ascites

The development of ascites in hepatic cirrhosis usually indicates a poor prognosis. Portal hypertension (1) raises the capillary filtration gradient in the abdominal viscera, but the ascites is also due to (2) sodium retention associated with hyperaldosteronism, (3) low serum albumin, and (4) increased production of hepatic lymph.

Liver cell failure

Impairment of liver function in portal hypertension occurs partly from the original causative disease and partly from failure of normal perfusion of the regenerated liver cells within the lobules. The appearance of jaundice in cirrhosis usually indicates severe hepato-cellular damage. Liver cell failure often complicates a severe haemorrhage from oesophageal varices, major surgery or even paracentesis of ascitic fluid.

Hepatic encephalopathy

Products of intestinal metabolism which pass into the systemic circulation may produce severe cerebral disturbance or coma (portasystemic encephalopathy), particularly if liver cell function is poor or the degree of shunting severe. Ammonia is one

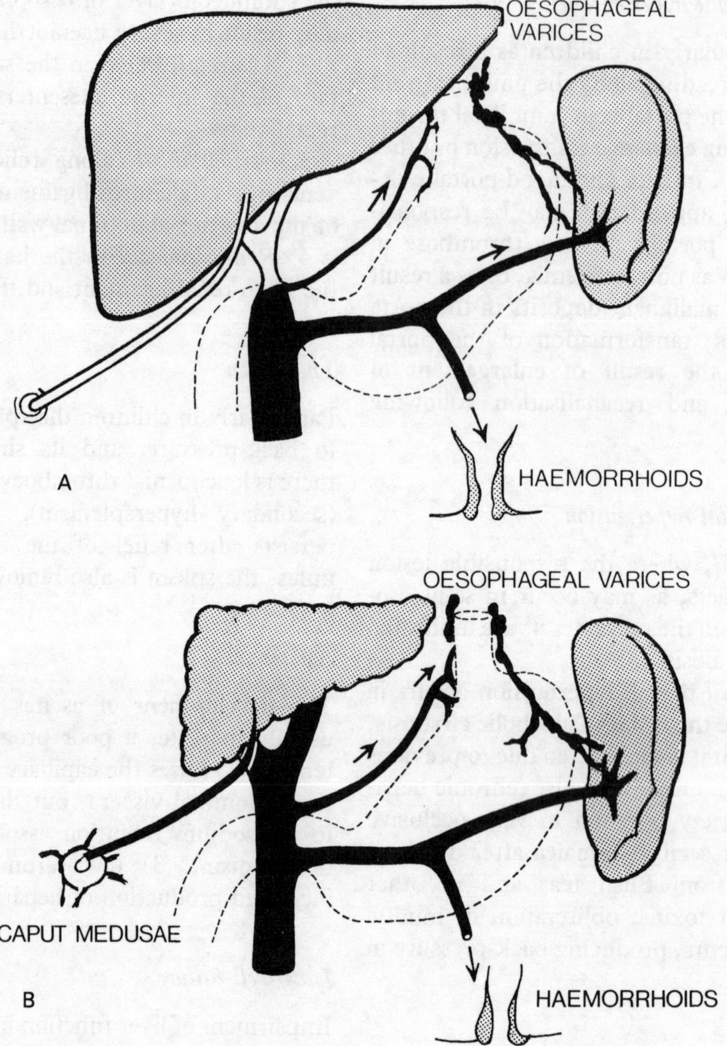

Fig. 19.2 Collateral circulation in portal hypertension. **A.** Extrahepatic obstruction. **B.** Intrahepatic obstruction.

of the responsible agents, but tryptophan and other metabolites are also important. The efficacy of broad-spectrum antibiotics in the relief of hepatic encephalopathy suggests that at least some of the toxins are produced by intestinal bacteria.

Clinical features

A history of alcoholism or previous virus hepatitis may be obtained. Neonatal sepsis may precede the appearance of an extrahepatic portal block in childhood. A sudden, profuse haematemesis may be the first symptom and precipitate liver failure or even hepatic coma. Anorexia and morning vomiting are common in cirrhosis. A sallow appearance with facial and truncal telangiectasia may be noted. Dilated veins radiating from the umbilicus are a feature as well as palmar erythema. Splenomegaly is usually marked and in advanced cirrhosis jaundice and ascites are present.

Investigations

A full blood count shows anaemia, leucopenia and thrombocytopenia, indicative of hypersplenism. Liver function tests may be abnormal and a serum albumin below 30 g per litre indicates severe impairment. The chest radiograph may show enlargement of the azygos veins. A barium swallow and meal demonstrates oesophageal and gastric varices and helps to exclude other causes of gastro-intestinal bleeding. Oesophagoscopy is the principal method of demonstrating such varices. Selective angioportography entails catheterisation of the superior mesenteric and coeliac axis arteries, shows opacification of the portal venous system during the late phase of the injection and is the best way of confirming the portal obstruction and planning its surgical relief. Direct confirmation of the portal hypertension can be obtained by measuring the intra-splenic pressure, the portal venous pressure at operation or the wedged hepatic venous pressure by cardiac catheterisation.

Differential diagnosis

Other causes of haematemesis such as peptic ulcer, oesophagitis, carcinoma of the oesophagus and stomach require exclusion. The bleeding of oesophageal varices is characteristically profuse and the blood wells up the oesophagus without effort. Causes of splenomegaly and hypersplenism, such as haemolytic anaemia, leukaemia and reticulosis must be differentiated. Causes of ascites such as constrictive pericarditis, mesothelioma and abdominal carcinomatosis must be considered. Portasystemic encephalopathy must be distinguished from delirium tremens and acute alcoholism.

Treatment

Severe haemorrhage requires immediate blood replacement, but this alone is insufficent. Vasopressin (Pitressin) 20 units should be given by intravenous infusion over 10 minutes and may control profuse oesophageal bleeding by lowering portal pressure, which it achieves by causing intense splanchnic vasoconstriction. The injections may be repeated every four hours, but they cause unpleasant side effects and become less effective with repetition. Neomycin 6 g daily should be administered to diminish the intestinal bacterial content and the risk of encephalopathy, whilst blood in the bowel should be removed by enemata. If hepatic coma appears imminent 20 per cent dextrose should be given into a large vein through a cannula. Intravenous vitamin K_1 should always be given to control the bleeding tendency of prothrombin deficiency.

If bleeding continues, compression of oesophageal and gastric veins is required, best obtained by using a triple-lumen rubber tube, bearing two inflatable balloons and a channel for gastric aspiration. The distal balloon compresses the subcardiac gastric veins and the proximal ballon those at the lower end of the oesophagus. The tube is kept under slight traction (Fig. 19.3). Twenty-four hours after inflation the balloons are released and if further bleeding occurs immediate treatment is indicated.

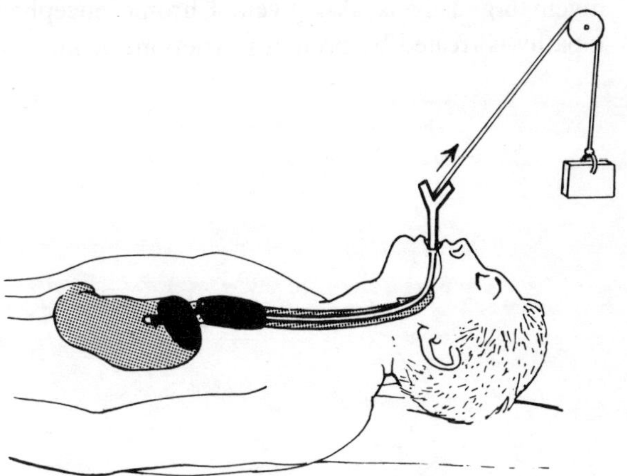

Fig. 19.3 Sengstaken triple-lumen tube for arrest of haemorrhage from oesophageal varices

Failure to control haemorrhage by tamponade necessitates an emergency procedure. A number of methods are available. Sclerosants may be injected into or around the bleeding varices through a fibreoptic oesophagoscope and this may be repeated if further bleeding occurs. Oesophageal transection using the stapling gun introduced through a gastrotomy can also be helpful in an emergency situation. Ligation of the lower oesophageal and upper gastric veins may be performed at the same time and these measures may be permanently effective. Another alternative is the embolisation of the bleeding vessels via a catheter passed through the liver into the portal and left gastric veins. Although a more major procedure, in the absence of ascites, jaundice or hepatic coma, an emergency portal decompression by a shunt operation may be undertaken with either a portacaval, mesocaval or splenorenal anastomosis. These operations may also be employed after initial control of haemorrhage by one of the other methods. The principal complication of portacaval shunting is the development in 20 per cent of severe encephalopathy, together with some acceleration of the underlying liver disease when cirrhosis is present. The encephalopathy which follows portasystemic shunting operations is due to ammonia and intestinal toxins by-passing the liver directly to the brain. To prevent this, anaemia should be corrected before operation and protein intake reduced for a week afterwards. Oral neomycin 6 g daily is also given. Chronic encephalopathy is treated by protein restriction, neomycin and lactulose and occasionally by ileorectal anastomosis to exclude bacterial breakdown within the colon. When ascites is present paracentesis should be avoided as it leads to further protein depletion. A low sodium diet is prescribed (less than 20 mmol daily) supplemented by diuretics (frusemide 40 to 80 mg daily and spironolactone 100 to 200 mg daily).

FURTHER READING

Johnston, G. W. (1981). Bleeding oesophageal varices: management of shunt rejects. Ann. R. Coll. Surg. Engl. 63, 3–8.

MacDougall, B. R. D., Westaby, D. and Williams, R. (1982). *Variceal Bleeding*. London: Pitman.

Sherlock, S. (1981). *Diseases of the Liver and Biliary System*. 6th ed. London: Blackwell.

20

Pancreas

Physiology

Pancreatic juice is a watery, alkaline fluid produced by the acini in response to both nervous and chemical stimuli. The hormonal response is produced by secretin and pancreozymin, released by the passage of acid chyme into the duodenum. The total volume is 1200 to 2000 ml a day. The three main enzymes—lipase, amylase and trypsin— are responsible for splitting fats, starches and proteoses respectively. Their continued loss, as in a fistula, leads to rapid depletion of sodium and base in addition to skin excoriation. Lack of pancreatic juice in the intestine leads to malabsorption of fat and protein. Pancreatic function tests are seldom satisfactory and have been largely replaced by scanning and endoscopic pancreatographic methods. Diabetes mellitus due to impaired insulin production is seen in pancreatitis and carcinoma. Hyperinsulinism occurs in some islet cell tumours.

Congenital anomalies

Annular pancreas. The second part of the duodenum is encircled by pancreatic tissue.The disorder is explained by incomplete migration of the ventral anlage with subsequent fusion. It may be symptom-free or present in adult life as duodenal obstruction, for which duodeno-jejunostomy is the best treatment.

Heterotopic pancreatic tissue is seen most commonly in the stomach, duodenum and jejunum, and occasionally in association with Meckel's diverticulum. Any pathological change occurring in normal pancreas may also take place in heterotopic pancreatic tissue, which is also liable to ulcerate and give rise to severe gastro-intestinal bleeding.

Fibrocystic disease of the pancreas is part of the hereditary abnormality of mucus secretion (mucoviscidosis). The disorder principally affects the lungs and pancreas, the viscid mucus producing obstruction of these organs with recurrent respiratory infection and pancreatic fibrosis. The pancreatic lesions are present before birth, and 10 per cent of cases present with meconium intestinal obstruction or peritonitis. In infants and older children bronchiectasis and steatorrhoea lead to chronic poor health and weight loss. Cirrhosis of the liver with portal hypertension is a further complication. In addition there is an abnormality of sweat secretion; the detection of a high salt content helps to confirm the diagnosis.

Traumatic lesions

Severe injury to the pancreas may be associated with other visceral injuries, such as ruptured spleen or intestine, when the diagnosis is often only made at laparotomy. The organ may also be transected by closed violence, probably by compression across the front of the vertebral bodies. With milder trauma a pseudo-pancreatic cyst (p. 264) may slowly develop and present at a later date. The pancreas can also be damaged during abdominal surgery, particularly operations for duodenal ulcer, splenectomy and removal of the left adrenal gland. A pancreatic fistula may result (p. 265).

ACUTE PANCREATITIS

Aetiology

Acute pancreatitis can be initiated in several different ways. It is probable that obstruction to the pancreatic duct with or without reflux of bile is responsible in the majority of instances. The following theories are postulated.

1. *Obstruction in the ampullary region* due to spasm, oedema or fibrosis of the sphincter of Oddi. In a small number of cases an impacted gall-stone may be encountered. Often there is co-existent cholecystitis, and reflux of infected bile into the pancreatic duct may be responsible. The commonest cause is probably a small gall-stone passing down the common duct and obstructing the pancreatic duct which lies nearby.

2. *Obstruction to the pancreatic duct* by intraduct stones, round worms (ascaris),tumours, small duct epithelial metaplasia and surgical ligation can cause pancreatitis, probably initiated by sudden secretory stimulation of the organ.

3. *Alcohol* can cause pancreatitis, perhaps by inducing a viscid secretion which obstructs the smaller ducts. In susceptible individuals the intake of alcohol need not be excessive.

4. *Regurgitation of duodenal contents* may account for some cases of pancreatitis following partial gastrectomy due to incompetence of the valvular mechanism at the sphincter of Oddi and abnormal pressures in an obstructed afferent loop.

5. *Atherosclerosis* and pancreatitis often co-exist and localised infarcts may activate the pancreatic juice.

6. *Blood-borne and lymphatic infection* from neighbouring sites or secondary to virus infection, such as mumps.

7. *Miscellaneous factors* include heavy meals, hyperparathyroidism and familial hyperlipidaemia, all of which appear to induce secretion and activation of the pancreatic ferments. Trauma to the pancreas during partial gastrectomy or other abdominal operations may also be responsible.

Pathology

Autodigestion of the gland occurs with liberation of enzymes into and around the pancreas, the pathological features varying with the stage and severity of the attack. In mild cases slight oedema occurs with subsequent resolution, whilst in severe cases diffuse necrosis is followed within a few hours by a fatal termination. In moderate cases oedema and necrosis are usual, the latter being patchy and followed by autodigestion of the gland by activated enzymes. Haemorrhage resulting from digestion of the blood-vessel walls may be noted in the pancreas, in the retroperitoneal tissues or as a blood-stained effusion into the peritoneal cavity, occasionally into the pleural cavity particularly on the left side. Collections in the subphrenic regions or the lesser sac forming a pseudopancreatic cyst may develop later and be followed by infection. Recovery may be accompanied by complete resolution and there is rarely any permanent impairment of pancreatic function.

Fat necrosis is a characteristic feature and is due to the action of the liberated lipase on the fat converting it into fatty acids and glycerol, the former combining with calcium to form insoluble soaps. Small white areas occur within the gland, on the surface of the mesentery or are scattered throughout the peritoneal cavity. The haemorrhage of severe pancreatic necrosis is mainly the result of digestion of blood vessels by activated trypsin. A high level of all three pancreatic enzymes occurs in the blood during the early stages of pancreatitis but the serum amylase is most readily estimated.

Clinical features

Sex distribution is equal and the majority of patients are over the age of 40 years. The severity of symptoms varies with the type of attack, the prognosis being grave in the fulminating form. A history of previous mild episodes is common. The onset is usually heralded by severe pain, which is generally continuous. It is situated in the epigastrium or left hypochondrium, and characteristically radiates to the back or lower chest. The pain may last for several days with a poor response to analgesics. Nausea and vomiting are early and persistent features. Rarely haematemesis may occur from gastro-intestinal congestion. Pronounced shock and prostration are characteristic of the severe case and may be accompanied by pallor, sweating and cyanosis, the last caused by extreme circulatory failure. Moderate pyrexia and marked tachycardia occur. Tenderness and rigidity, not initially severe, later become more pronounced and widespread and may be followed by abdominal distension and the presence of free fluid. Slight jaundice may become apparent after 24 hours. Bruising and induration of the peri-umbilical region or flank may develop about the third day.

Complications include hypovolaemic shock, severe electrolyte disturbance, paralytic ileus or renal failure. Residual abscess is uncommon but may occur in the subphrenic region, whilst accumulation of pancreatic fluid and necrotic debris in the lesser sac leads to a pseudocyst. Diabetes may occur in the severe or recurrent attack and occasionally tetany results from acute hypocalcaemia.

Investigations

The serum amylase is raised above 1500 international units per litre and usually reaches a figure greatly in excess of this if estimated within 48 hours, but a high level may sometimes be obtained in perforated peptic ulcer or in cholecystitis. The urinary amylase is also raised, but a 24-hour sample is required and the investigation is less satisfactory. Occasionally the blood sugar is raised and glycosuria may occur. The serum calcium may be lowered. A plain radiograph of the abdomen may show gaseous distension and fluid levels in the small intestine, the presence of associated gall-stones or pancreatic calculi, the absence of free intraperitoneal gas seen in many cases of perforation, or narrowing of the gas shadow of the transverse colon directly over the pancreas due to surrounding oedema. Ultrasound scanning may show an enlarged pancreas and demonstrate stones in the biliary tract.

Differential diagnosis

This includes perforated peptic ulcer, acute small intestinal obstruction, mesenteric thrombosis, leaking and dissecting aortic aneurysm, ruptured oesophagus, acute cholecystitis and cardiac infarction. Pain in the back, local tenderness over the left hypochondrium, surgical shock out of proportion to the physical signs, together with the high serum amylase are important features in the correct diagnosis but the latter may only be made at laparotomy.

Treatment

Management is conservative in the established case. Control of pain is essential and since morphine causes spasm of the sphincter of Oddi pethidine is to be preferred. Gastric suction is started and an anti-cholinergic given to diminish pancreatic secretion. In severe cases the blood volume may be greatly depleted and intravenous fluids and electrolytes are required. Blood transfusion may be needed to correct anaemia. The intravenous administration of aprotonin (Trasylol) has been advocated but is not universally accepted. It is a protease inhibitor which acts on the pancreatic cells. Antibiotics should be given prophylactically to counteract infection, and cortisone administered if there is suspected adrenal failure. The occurrence of diabetes may necessitate treatment with diet and insulin, whilst tetany may require injections of 10 per cent calcium gluconate.

Operative treatment is required when the diagnosis is uncertain. In the absence of biliary tract disease the abdomen should be closed without drainage. When gall-stones are present cholecystectomy should be performed and a careful search made for an impacted stone at the ampulla. Surgical treatment is also required for the complications of pseudopancreatic cyst, fistula or subphrenic abscess.

CHRONIC PANCREATITIS

Aetiology

This is a comprehensive term used to describe a number of different diseases. (1) Chronic relapsing pancreatitis; (2) recurrent acute pancreatitis; (3) primary pancreatic lithiasis; (4) the lesions due to ductal obstruction. Chronic alcoholism may be important in the first two of these.

Pathology

Chronic pancreatitis resembles hepatic cirrhosis in being the end stage of a number of disorders, all of which eventually result in destruction of the acini and replacement fibrosis. When obstruction is present the ducts become dilated and form irregular cyst-like cavities containing glairy or milky fluid. Calcification is common and the deposits are confined to within the ducts. Microscopy reveals widespread replacement fibrosis, the islets of Langerhans usually remaining. Pancreatic necrosis is seen in recurrent acute pancreatitis but not in the other varieties, since enzyme production is impaired.

Clinical features

Pain is common and is usually felt in the upper abdomen radiating to the back. It may be severe and persistent and lead to alcohol or drug addiction. Weight loss, steatorrhoea and diabetes may occur but in some instances pain may be absent. Obstructive jaundice is occasionally encountered and leads to confusion with carcinoma of the head of the pancreas. Slow progression of the disease is usual, leading to malnutrition, cachexia, bronchopneumonia and death.

Investigations

Examination of the faeces may reveal an increase in undigested muscle fibres. The serum amylase may be raised in an acute exacerbation. Glycosuria and a typical diabetic type of glucose tolerance curve may be found. Duodenal intubation is not a reliable method of assessing pancreatic function. Radiography may show calcified opacities in the region of the pancreas or the presence of gall-stones in a plain film. Enlargement of the head of the pancreas may be demonstrated by widening of the duodenal loop on barium examination. Endoscopic retrograde cholangiopancreatography may demonstrate duct abnormalities. Pancreatography during surgery may elucidate the cause of an intrapancreatic obstruction.

Treatment

The dietary management of deficiency states is of value in the initial stages. Small frequent meals should be advised, and if there is marked steatorrhoea the fat intake reduced to about 45 g a day. High protein and carbohydrate foods should be given together with extra fat-soluble vitamins A and D. Pancreatin tablets should be taken with meals to substitute for the loss of enzymes. Diabetes is treated by insulin or diet.

Surgical treatment is advisable in persistent and progressive cases. Where gall-stones or biliary duct pathology exist, cholecystectomy and exploration of the common bile duct should be undertaken. Division of the sphincter of Oddi by the transduodenal route (sphincteroplasty) is often performed with the object of removing any obstructive element at the ampulla and reducing the opportunity for bile to enter the pancreatic duct. Endoscopic sphincterotomy is now more often used. When the disease is advanced, excision of the tail of the pancreas and implantation of the remaining duct into the jejunum is to be preferred. Transplantation of the common bile duct into the duodenum or jejunum is an alternative to sphincteroplasty. The more radical measure of pancreaticoduodenectomy is only rarely required.

Pancreatic cysts

Pathology

Pancreatic cysts may be classified into true or false varieties, the latter being known as pseudocysts and comprising the majority of lesions. **True** cysts include (*a*) *congenital* cysts which are generally multiple and may be associated with polycystic disease elsewhere; (*b*) *retention* cysts which are small and related to intermittent or partial obstruction of the pancreatic duct, and (c) *cystadenomas*, multiloculated tumours composed of spaces lined by high epithelium and containing projecting papillary processes. True cysts occur most commonly in the body and head of the pancreas. **Pseudocysts** arise as a result of pancreatitis or injury to the organ. A collection of necrotic tissue, blood and pancreatic juice forms in the lesser sac. Some pseudocysts communicate with the pancreatic ducts, when the cavity may then contain large amounts of pancreatic enzymes. External drainage of such a cyst may produce a fistula. Unlike the true variety, false cysts do not possess an epithelial lining, being surrounded by a wall of fibrous tissue.

Clinical features

Some cysts are asymptomatic, others give rise to epigastric pain or discomfort, nausea, vomiting and abdominal swelling which is usually felt more to the left of the midline. Infection and rupture of the cyst occur rarely. Confusion may arise with a mesenteric or ovarian cyst or a splenic, hepatic or renal swelling. Retroperitoneal tumours or cysts may be difficult to differentiate. A plain radiograph may show a rounded upper abdominal soft tissue mass and barium studies demonstrate indentation of surrounding viscera. Ultrasound scanning is useful in detecting pancreatic and pseudopancreatic cysts. It can be repeated at regular intervals to note any change in size of a cyst or to determine the thickness of the wall of a pseudocyst.

Treatment

Drainage should be undertaken in large cysts when the wall is sufficiently thick, which may be some weeks after the onset. It is preferably performed internally by anastomosis of the cyst wall to the posterior wall of the stomach. Resection of pancreatic tissue is necessary in malignant cysts.

Pancreatic fistula

External discharge of pancreatic juice is liable to persist as a result of the high pressure generated during pancreatic secretion and the resistance produced by the sphincter of Oddi. There are two principal results: (1) diversion of electrolytes and in particular sodium and base, produced by the loss of up to two litres of alkaline secretion; (2) severe excoriation of the skin surrounding the opening by the activated pancreatic ferments. Diagnosis depends upon the identification of pancreatic ferments in the secretion, and the track can be demonstrated by the injection of radio-opaque material. Treatment includes urgent parenteral replacement of fluid and electrolytes and protection of the skin surrounding the fistula from further digestion by the use of a barrier cream of aluminium paint. If the discharge does not cease within a few weeks implantation of the fistula into the intestinal tract may be required.

NEOPLASMS OF THE PANCREAS

Tumours of the pancreas arise either from ampullary and duct epithelium or from the islet tissue.

Carcinoma of the pancreas and peri-ampullary region

Carcinoma involving the head of the pancreas, ampullary region, distal common bile duct and some tumours of the duodenum present a number of similar diagnostic and therapeutic problems.

Pathology

There are no known aetiological factors, but a benign papilloma of the duodenal papilla, pancreatic and bile ducts may become malignant. Pancreatitis does not predispose to the formation of carcinoma. About 80 per cent of all pancreatic carcinomas are found in the head and ampullary region.

Peri-ampullary tumours arise in the ampulla, duodenal papilla or terminal bile or pancreatic ducts. They form either a papillomatous growth or a flat ulcerating tumour producing early obstruction at the lower end of the common bile duct (Fig. 20.1, B). Duodenal ulceration may occur or the lesion may bulge into the lumen from the ampulla.

Carcinoma of the gland itself arises from the epithelium of the smaller ducts or acini. It is a spheroidal cell type and generally scirrhous, but occasionally is an encephaloid tumour. Mucoid, cystic and haemorrhagic changes may take place and pancreatic duct obstruction is common. The majority arise in the head of the pancreas and present a hard irregular and nodular surface (Fig. 20.1,A).

Spread takes place locally, by the lymphatics and by the blood stream, the effects varying with the type and situation of the tumour. Local spread in lesions of the head involves the common bile duct and duodenum, with dilatation of the biliary tract including the gall-bladder, uniform enlargement of the liver and the secretion of white bile in long-standing cases. Peri-ampullary growths produce noticeable effects at an early stage, but are slow to disseminate. In tumours of the body local spread is often more marked. In later stages ascites follows portal vein thrombosis or secondary peritoneal deposits. Lymphatic spread takes place to adjacent nodes, and blood stream metastasis is mainly to the liver, but may involve bones and lungs.

Clinical features

Men are affected twice as commonly as women, and the disease is chiefly of the middle and older

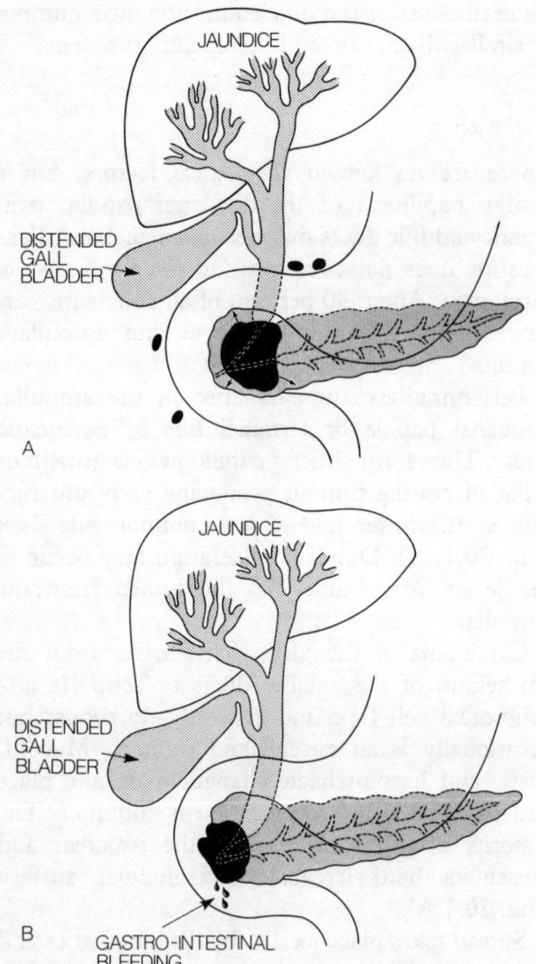

Fig. 20.1 Carcinoma of the pancreas. **A.** Tumour of the head of pancreas. **B.** Peri-ampullary tumour.

age groups. Jaundice, at times accompanied by pain, occurs in 90 per cent of tumours of the head, particularly peri-ampullary growths, but is late or absent in lesions of the body and tail. Jaundice is usually deep and progressive, but may fluctuate in peri-ampullary growths when obstruction is incomplete. Epigastric pain is an important feature in lesions of the body and may radiate through to the back. Vague dyspepsia, anorexia and weight loss may precede the onset of jaundice and diarrhoea may occur.

Examination may reveal a palpable gall-bladder, jaundice and some hepatomegaly; occasionally ascites or an abdominal mass due to pancreatic tumour may be found. Anaemia is common in peri-ampullary growths. Migratory thrombophlebitis, particularly in the lower limbs, may rarely be the only positive finding.

Investigations

Liver function tests and the presence of bile in the urine may help to confirm an obstructive jaundice. Occult blood may be found in the faeces in ampullary growths and steatorrhoea may occur. Barium meal examination may show widening of the duodenal loop or bulging of the pancreas into the duodenum above or below the ampulla. CT scanning may reveal the tumour. Occasionally selective coeliac angiography and endoscopic cholangiopancreatography (p. 244) are useful. In jaundiced patients, where ultrasound liver scanning confirms that the biliary ducts are dilated, a percutaneous transhepatic cholangiogram will accurately show the level and type of obstruction, which is usually near the lower end of the common duct (p. 244).

Differential diagnosis

Obstructive jaundice from common duct stone, chronic pancreatitis and metastatic liver carcinoma must be excluded. Lesions producing abdominal and back pain such as penetrating peptic ulcer, osteoarthritis of the spine, renal lesions and aortic aneurysm, together with anaemia from gastro-intestinal bleeding, require differentiation.

Treatment

Pre-operative intramuscular injections of vitamin K_1 should be given for several days to correct the low prothrombin level and consequent tendency to bleed. In the absence of spread, tumours of the head and peri-ampullary region should be treated by radical pancreaticoduodenal resection. Unfortunately this operation is only rarely possible and the likelihood of early recurrence usually makes it inadvisable in growths of the neck and body. In most cases relief of jaundice is readily obtained by palliative cholecystojejunostomy, with the addition of gastro-jejunostomy if duodenal obstruction appears imminent.

NEOPLASMS OF THE ISLET TISSUE

Islet-cell tumours are usually adenomas and only rarely malignant; they are generally 1 to 2 cm in diameter, but may reach a large size on occasions. The adenoma is purple in colour and encapsulated, a high proportion being found in the body and tail of the pancreas. Carcinomas spread to the regional lymph nodes and to the liver, but may be slow growing and hormonally active. A variety of hormonally active tumours are produced by the various specialised cells of the islets. In order of frequency these are (1) insulinoma; (2) gastrinoma; (3) rare tumours, such as vipoma (vasoactive intestinal peptide) and glucagonoma.

Clinical features

Insulinoma. This is a tumour of β cells. Irregular attacks of hypoglycaemia occur with increasing severity and frequency. In the earlier stages vague symptoms of lassitude and abdominal discomfort occur, particularly during fasting. Attacks of intense hunger follow with sweating, trembling, and fainting. More damaging neurological symptoms and signs, namely inco-ordinated movements, dysarthria, diplopia, hallucinations and convulsions, may take place, whilst emotional instability and confusion may result in admission to a mental hospital. Obesity is common since eating relieves symptoms. Intellectual impairment is a late complication. The components of Whipple's triad are diagnostic. (1) Attacks of nervous or gastro-intestinal disturbance during fasting or exercise. (2) Hypoglycaemia with a blood glucose level below 2 mmol per litre. (3) Rapid relief after giving glucose.

The glucose tolerance test may be of value if continued to six hours when it may show a flat hypoglycaemic curve. A 12 to 36-hour fast generally reproduces the symptoms and blood should be taken for simultaneous glucose and insulin assay. An inappropriately high insulin level for the blood glucose level is diagnostic of hyper-insulinism. Electroencephalography during a hypoglycaemic attack shows characteristic changes. Localisation of the insulinoma prior to surgery is important and can be done by a combination of selective arteriography and portal vein sampling. A plastic catheter passed through the liver into the portal, splenic and superior mesenteric veins enables serial blood samples to be taken at a number of sites. These samples are then processed by radio-immunoassay; a peak level indicates the suspected site of the tumour.

Gastrinoma (Fulminating peptic ulcer or Zollinger-Ellison syndrome). In this rare syndrome gastric hypersecretion is due to a gastrin-like substance produced by a pancreatic tumour that is usually malignant. Associated tumours may also occur in other endocrine glands, particularly the parathyroid and pituitary glands, giving rise to the condition of multiple endocrine adenomatosis (MEA I) syndrome. Severe peptic ulceration develops and tends to recur rapidly after conventional medical or surgical therapy, frequently in an atypical site such as the jejunum. Gastric hypersecretion occurs to the extent of 2 or 3 litres of gastric juice during an overnight aspiration and fasting serum gastrin levels on radio-immunoassay are markedly raised.

Vipoma. (Pancreatic cholera syndrome.) This very rare syndrome consists of extreme watery diarrhoea of cholera-like intensity due to the production of a vaso-active intestinal peptide by the pancreatic islets. The abnormal peptide can be identified by radio-immunoassay.

Treatment

Removal of the tumour requires accurate pre-operative localisation, particularly in insulinoma which is the commonest condition, although the tumour may be small (about 1 cm). Removal of an insulinoma or a vipoma usually cures the disorder, but in gastrinoma (Z-E syndrome) total gastrectomy is often necessary in order to prevent the gastric hypersecretion and the consequent severe peptic ulceration. Streptozotocin may be helpful in malignant insulinoma and cimetidine in malignant gastrinoma. The slow progress of the malignant endocrine tumours may allow survival for many years with satisfactory control of their symptoms.

FURTHER READING

Deveney, C. W., Deveney, K. S. and Way, L. W. (1978). The Zollinger-Ellison syndrome—23 years later. Ann. Surg. 188, 384–393.

Smith R. (1978). Cancer of the pancreas. J. Roy. Coll. Surg. Edin. 23, 133–50.

21

Adrenal glands

Physiology

The function of the glands is to produce hormones from both cortex and medulla. The former is essential for the preservation of life. Adrenocortical hormones may be divided into three main groups:

1. Glucocorticoids.
2. Sex hormones:
   - Oestrogens.
   - Androgens.
3. Aldosterone.

The glucocorticoids and sex hormones, but not aldosterone, are under the control of the pituitary through the adrenocorticotrophic hormone, ACTH. The main glucocorticoids are hydrocortisone (cortisol) and cortisone, known also as 17-oxogenic steroids from their chemical structure, and are concerned with organic metabolism. The sex hormones influence the secondary sexual characteristics and comprise both oestrogens and androgens. The latter are measured chemically as the non-phenolic 17-oxosteroids. Aldosterone is a powerful salt-retaining hormone concerned with the maintenance of electrolyte balance. The medullary hormones consist of adrenaline and noradrenaline; the former increases cardiac output, the latter peripheral resistance through vaso-constriction, both effectively raising the blood-pressure.

LESIONS OF THE CORTEX

Pathology

This may take one of the following forms:

1. Hyperplasia.
2. Adenoma.
3. Carcinoma.

Hyperplasia is almost always bilateral; adenoma and primary carcinoma are generally unilateral. Small pea-like adenomatous projections from the surface of the gland are not uncommonly found at necropsy and are of no clinical significance. Macroscopically large adenomas and carcinoma may resemble each other, and are usually round with a lobulated surface. Often soft in consistency the cut surface shows areas of necrosis and haemorrhage intersected by bands of fibrous tissue. In hyperplasia the histological changes usually affect the zona fasciculata with proliferation, but in some cases of Cushing's syndrome the glands appear microscopically normal. The cells are well-differentiated in adenomas and resemble normal adrenal architecture except where necrosis and haemorrhage have altered the picture, but the capsule is well-defined. A number of carcinomas exhibit a similar appearance, but anaplasia with numerous mitotic figures and capsular invasion is more common. Spread occurs by invasion of neighbouring adjacent structures, particularly the kidney and renal vein, by lymphatics to the adjacent nodes, and by bloodstream to lung and liver.

Clinical features

These may be most conveniently related to the type of hormone produced and be classified as follows. A small proportion of adenomas and carcinomas are hormonally non-productive.

1. Cushing's syndrome—excess glucocorticoids.
2. Adrenogenital syndrome—excess sex hormones.
3. Conn's syndrome—excess aldosterone.
4. Non-hormonal syndrome.

Cushing's syndrome

This condition was first described by Harvey Cushing, who found it associated with a basophil adenoma although it may occur with other types of pituitary adenoma. The clinical picture is characteristic and may differ little in hyperplasia, adenoma or carcinoma. A similar state may also be apparent following steroid administration and the syndrome may also be observed in association with non-endocrine tumours such as carcinoma of the lung, thymoma, pancreatic carcinoma and bronchial adenoma as well as ovarian tumours (*ectopic ACTH syndrome*).

Young adults are most frequently affected, and women five times more commonly than men. Obesity is prominent but of specific distribution. The moon-shaped face, the 'buffalo hump' of cervicodorsal fat and adiposity of the trunk are usually present, the normal limbs in contrast being apparently thin. Endocrine changes are also responsible for the well-marked striae of abdomen, upper thighs and shoulder regions. There is an increased tendency towards bruising and a plethoric appearance. Hypertension, causing severe headaches or disturbance of vision and leading to cardiac failure or uraemia, is common. Osteoporosis, particularly of the vertebrae, with backache and vertebral compression or pathological fracture is frequent. Amenorrhoea and impotence, an insulin-resistant diabetes, and emotional disturbances and psychoses may all occur. In children there may be retarded growth. Increased skin pigmentation may be seen in the ectopic ACTH syndrome where melanotropins may be secreted.

Adrenogenital syndrome

Overproduction of the sex hormones is generally restricted to the androgens with resulting virilism; oestrogenic excess with feminism is very rare.

Virilism

The clinical effects are dependent on the age of the patient at the time of hormonal production.

Female pseudo-hermaphroditism may be produced by adrenal hyperplasia before birth. In childhood, when most cases are due to a tumour, the main features in girls are an early appearance of pubic and facial hair with enlargement of the clitoris, associated with increased growth and at times hypertension. In boys the secondary sexual characteristics are noted early and the external genitalia and prostate may be of adult size. Increased muscular development with pubic, axillary and facial hair is responsible for the 'pocket Hercules' appearance. Acne, hypertension and hoarseness may complete the picture.

In the adult the change mainly affects the premenopausal female as virilism, is very rare after the climacteric, and produces little demonstrable change in the male. Hirsutism with male distribution is early, together with premature baldness. Increased muscular development, with a masculine appearance and deepening of the voice and acne may all follow. Amenorrhoea and loss of libido may occur, with enlargement of the clitoris and diminution in breast size.

Feminism

The most prominent feature is gynaecomastia, with breast tenderness. Testicular atrophy, loss of libido, diminished penile size, thinning of the beard and a female hair distribution may all occur.

Mixed syndrome

Not infrequently a combination of Cushing's syndrome and the adrenogenital syndrome is present and the two may be regarded as opposite extremes of a broad hormonal range.

Conn's syndrome

This uncommon condition of primary aldosteronism is usually due to adenoma. They are generally single and small in size. It should be suspected if hypertension and hypokalaemia are present provided other causes for the latter, such as diuretics, are excluded. Clinically there may be severe recurrent muscular weakness and transient paralysis, tetany, paraesthesia, polyuria and polydipsia. Hypertension without oedema is found. Arrhythmia, cardiac failure or cerebral thrombosis may ensue.

Non-hormonal syndrome

Although pain and a palpable swelling in loin or

abdomen may be noted in hormonal tumours, it is the main presentation of non-hormonal lesions. In carcinoma, haematuria may occur with invasion of the kidney, or symptoms from metastases may be the primary feature.

Investigations

(1) *Laboratory* examinations are important. Plasma cortisol (normal range 280 to 700 nmol/1) and urinary cortisol levels are increased in Cushing's syndrome and there is a loss of the diurnal variation, normally high in the morning and low at night, in the early stages of the disease. Urinary 17-oxosteroids (normal range 35 to 85μmol/24 hr) are raised in virilising lesions. Cortisol suppression by dexamethasone, 2.0 mg six-hourly for two to three days produces a fall in 17-oxogenic and 17-oxosteroids in hyperplasia, but no alteration in carcinoma. Adenomas give equivocal results. The *plasma ACTH* level is high when the cause of Cushing's syndrome lies in the pituitary gland or in ectopic ACTH secretion, this differentiating those of primary adrenal origin. The *metyrapone* test is also valuable in determining a primary pituitary or adrenal cause of hyperadrenocorticism. In an autonomous adrenal tumour where ACTH is suppressed there will be no increase in 17-oxogenic steroids in response to metyrapone. In Conn's syndrome the plasma and urinary aldosterone levels are high and the renin level low. Stimulation with intravenous frusemide does not increase the level of aldosterone, and failure to reduce the level after three days of intramuscular deoxycorticosterone acetate (DOCA) indicates an autonomous cause, probably an adenoma. (2) *Radiological* investigations include radiography of the abdomen, which may show calcification in a tumour, and in some instances intravenous urography may reveal kidney displacement, but the best method of localisation is by CT scanning. Ultrasound may also be of value and adrenal angiography may occasionally be required. Where hormonal changes are present radiography of the hands may reveal early ossification in the adrenogenital syndrome. A radiograph of the spine may show osteoporosis in Cushing's syndrome.

Differential diagnosis

Non-hormonal tumours require to be differentiated from the more common renal swellings—hypernephroma, Wilms' tumour or benign cysts—and from other adrenal neoplasms. Ovarian tumours must be excluded by pelvic examination, and rarely the interstitial tumour of the testis must be considered.

Treatment

Total adrenalectomy should be performed in adrenal hyperplasia. The abdominal route is usually preferred, although the posterior approach may be advantageous in obese or poor risk patients. Steroid cover before, during and after surgery is essential and total adrenal replacement therapy must be maintained indefinitely. When an extra-adrenal tumour is present its removal may cause regression of adrenal hyperplasia, but it is often malignant with a poor prognosis. Adenomas and carcinoma should be removed by unilateral adrenalectomy or combined with nephrectomy when the kidney is involved. Contralateral adrenal atrophy may exist and post-operative steroid maintenance is essential. When surgery is unsuitable due to widespread metastases, chemotherapy using o,p'DDD may be helpful, particularly in those exhibiting Cushing's syndrome.

The *post-adrenalectomy syndrome* may develop after surgery. It is recognised by skin pigmentation and an enlarging pituitary fossa demonstrated by radiography. The latter may press on the optic chiasma with constriction of the visual fields. Pituitary tumour development is responsible although not usually capable of recognition prior to operation. It can be confirmed by a rapidly rising ACTH level. Treatment is by pituitary irradiation using implants of yttrium 90 (p. 323).

LESIONS OF THE MEDULLA

The only surgically important conditions are the benign tumours, ganglioneuroma and phaeochromocytoma, and the malignant neuroblastoma.

Ganglioneuroma

This is an encapsulated, often lobulated tumour, generally of small size. Histologically there are numerous well-differentiated nerve cells with bundles of non-medullated fibres accompanied by Schwann cells. Malignant change to a neuroblastoma may occur. Clinically the ganglioneuroma remains unrecognised until it becomes palpable. If it undergoes malignant change the clinical picture is that of neuroblastoma. An intravenous or retrograde pyelogram may reveal kidney displacement. Treatment is by removal.

Phaeochromocytoma

Pathology

Macroscopically this is spherical or oval in shape, well-encapsulated and often with large and dilated veins coursing over the surface. The cut area presents a reddish-brown appearance with haemorrhage and necrosis and at times calcification. Rarely malignant change may supervene, and occasionally they occur bilaterally and may even be multiple. They may be found anywhere along the sympathetic chain, aorta and inferior vena cava between the diaphragm and bladder, and at times even in the thorax. Histologically the tumour consists of polygonal cells arranged in cords staining dark brown in colour with chromic acid.

Clinical features

Phaeochromocytomas occur almost exclusively in adults, generally between 40 and 50 years, and women are twice as frequently affected as men. It may form part of multiple endocrine adenomatosis (MEA II) and be associated with a parathyroid adenoma or medullary thyroid carcinoma. There is an increased incidence in neurofibromatosis. The characteristic picture is one of paroxysmal attacks of hypertension, lasting several minutes or hours, at gradually decreasing intervals. Between attacks the blood-pressure is usually normal, but it may be raised and careful differentiation from benign and malignant hypertension is then required. Straining, changes of posture, local pressure or emotion may produce an attack. Symptoms include headache, palpitations, nausea, sweating, pain in the abdomen, chest or back, and coldness, blanching and tingling in hands or feet. Cardiac and renal failure, myocardial infarction and cerebral thrombosis may follow. Cushing's syndrome, hyperthyroidism and Conn's syndrome require differentiation.

Investigations

Measurement of the urinary catecholamines—noradrenaline and adrenaline—or their major urinary metabolites—hydroxymethoxymandelic acid (HMMA) and the metanephrines is the most satisfactory method of diagnosis. An increase is characteristic and less likely to produce false positives or negatives than pharmacological tests but certain substances such as tetracycline, bananas and vitamins interfere with the test and must be avoided. Phentolamine is the most commonly used pharmacological test, 5 mg being given intravenously and the blood-pressure measured every half minute for 10 minutes. A fall greater than 25 to 35 mm Hg denotes a positive result but the test requires maximum caution. The radiological investigations are similar to those for an adrenocortical tumour but should be delayed until medical control of the hypertension has been obtained. Then angiography may localise a growth and measurement of noradrenaline and adrenaline in the inferior vena cava may differentiate adrenal and extra-adrenal lesions. The former which are the more usual mainly secrete adrenaline, the latter noradrenaline.

Treatment

Removal of the tumour is required and is followed by a return to normal blood-pressure unless structural changes have occurred. The pre-operative and operative use of α- and β-blocking agents which inhibit the action of noradrenaline and adrenaline is important and should be used before angiography or venous sampling is undertaken. Phenoxybenzamine and propranolol should be given for at least three days before operation to control hypertension and tachycardia. Phentolamine may be required for a hypertensive crisis during the handling of the tumour and noradrenaline and angiotensin are occasionally necessary to combat the hypotension which can follow its removal.

Neuroblastoma

Pathology

Considerable variation in size exists, and many tumours resemble an embryoma, but are more nodular. Soft and vascular with a greyish-red cut surface there is a tendency to necrosis and haemorrhage, and occasionally calcification. Microscopically it is composed of small round or polyhedral cells in a scanty stroma. Some attempt at differentiation is seen in the less rapidly growing lesions where 'rosette formation', due to grouping, is apparent. Further differentiation produces recognisable nerve cells and the picture of a ganglioneuroblastoma. Spread is both by the bloodstream and lymphatics, with a special predilection for the skeletal system. In consequence many cases of suspected Ewing's tumour of bone are now known to have been due to a small occult primary neuroblastoma.

Clinical features

Eighty per cent of cases occur before the age of five years, and Wilms' tumour (p. 287) is the only malignant lesion more frequently found in childhood. There is an equal sex ratio. The primary growth may be recognised as a painless abdominal or loin swelling, but often the first indication is due to metastases. There may be pallor, anorexia and loss of weight, with recurrent pyrexia from tissue necrosis. Pathological fracture or pain and swelling of peripheral bones may occur. Skull metastases may cause unilateral exophthalmos and hepatomegaly is frequent.

Investigations

A blood count may reveal an anaemia. Radiography may show calcification of the primary tumour or skeletal or pulmonary metastases, and intravenous urography indicates kidney displacement. CT scanning is of value in outlining the lesion. Aspiration biopsy of a palpable tumour should be performed.

Treatment

A combination of surgical removal and radiotherapy is to be preferred. A combination of cyclophosphamide and vincristine is useful in chemotherapy.

FURTHER READING

Harrison, T. S., Gann, D. S., Edis, A. J. & Egdahl, R. H. (1975). *Surgical Disorders of the Adrenal Gland*. New York: Grune and Stratton.

Scott, H. W. Jr., Dean, R. H., Oates, J. A., Robertson, D., Rhamy, R. K. and Page, D. L. (1981). Surgical management of phaeochromocytoma. Am. Surg. 47, 8–13.

22

Kidney and ureter

ACUTE RENAL FAILURE

Acute renal failure is a common medical emergency characterised by anuria (failure of the formation of urine) or oliguria. Anuria must be clearly distinguished from retention of urine in which urine is not voided from the bladder and from uraemia, which is the clinical state arising from renal failure. In order to understand the mechanism of anuria, it must be remembered that plasma is first filtered from the glomerular capillaries, that enormous quantities of water and some electrolytes are then absorbed during passage of the filtrate down the renal tubules, and that the greatly altered filtrate known as urine then passes into the renal pelvis. Anuria may result from a disturbance of any of these stages and may therefore be due to **prerenal, renal** or **postrenal** (obstructive) causes. Examples of *prerenal* factors include peripheral and central circulatory failure and hypovolaemia, due to haemorrhage, dehydration, loss of plasma, septicaemia, intravascular haemolysis and drug overdose, which result in an insufficient glomerular blood flow. Dissecting aneurysm of the aorta is another cause since the renal arteries become blocked by stripping of their coats. *Renal* causes include acute tubular necrosis due to widespread tubular damage by chemicals or drugs, mismatched blood transfusions, septic abortion, acute blood loss, postoperative infections and extensive burns. The tubular epithelium is capable of regeneration, but it may take up to three weeks for this to occur. The diagnosis of the renal cause may be obvious from the history but frequently it is necessary to resort to renal biopsy by a special needle, or open technique, if a bleeding tendency is likely. *Postrenal* (obstructive) type is suggested by a history of complete anuria, the causes including bilateral ureteric or lower urinary tract obstruction from any cause, including stones, and occasionally from precipitation of sulphonamides in the collecting tubules.

Treatment of anuria

Prerenal anuria

The two most common surgical causes of anuria are hypotension and dehydration, the correction of which are urgent requirements. The small quantities of urine passed are of high specific gravity, since the kidneys concentrate normally and the urinary urea content may be normal or increased (250 to 500 mmol per day). These findings are important distinctions from renal anuria due to tubular damage. In the majority of cases intravenous fluid therapy is necessary and this must be given sufficiently rapidly to increase blood volume and restore glomerular filtration.

Renal anuria

Intrinsic (renal) failurc is likely to be present when the sodium concentration of the urine is below 10 mmol per litre, the urea concentration above 333 mmol per litre and there are no casts in the urine. A common error is delay in considering dialysis; some indications for employing this are as follows:

(*a*) Poor or deteriorating clinical state, infection, overhydration, cardiac problems, hypercatabolic states and bleeding tendency.
(*b*) Blood urea over 50 mmol per litre.
(*c*) Serum potassium above 7 mmol per litre.
(*d*) Total serum bicarbonate below 15 mmol per litre.

The rapidity of biochemical changes is more relevant than absolute values.

Conservative measures employed, where dialysis is being considered, are:

1. Restriction of fluid intake to 400 ml per day, with increments for measured gastro-intestinal and urinary losses and also for raised temperature and respiration rate.

2. Correction of acidosis by infusion of sodium bicarbonate or lactate.

3. As *hyperkalaemia* is a common cause of death by cardiac arrhythmia, important prophylactic measures include adequate removal of devitalised tissue and pus, treatment of infection and provision of adequate calories to prevent protein catabolism. Cation exchange resins, such as Resonium-A, given orally or rectally may be effective, particularly pending dialysis. Other short-lived emergency remedies include intravenous hypertonic glucose (100 ml of 50 per cent dextrose covered by 10 units of soluble insulin), sodium bicarbonate (300 ml of 1.4 per cent solution) and calcium gluconate (10 ml of 10 per cent solution), when electrocardiographic changes are present.

4. Adequate calorie intake, particularly if nausea or vomiting occur, may require an intravenous route. The use of carbohydrates as the only source of calories is undesirable, more so when nutrition has to be continued for longer than a few days, and a protein hydrolysate should be used. An adequate calorie supply to uraemic patients minimises protein breakdown. If oral feeding is feasible there will be sufficient carbohydrate and fat to provide 1000 calories per day, although severe fluid restriction limits the form in which this is taken. During the anuric period drugs such as morphine, digitalis, streptomycin and gentamicin that are normally eliminated by the kidney should be used with great caution.

Dialysis

The management of acute renal failure has been improved in latter years due in part to the introduction of dialysis. Those undergoing this therapy may be allowed a more liberal diet and fluid intake. The two methods used are haemodialysis and peritoneal dialysis.

Haemodialysis. This is achieved by means of the **artificial kidney,** which is an apparatus in which the blood is passed through tubes of semipermeable material lying in a bath of fluid of such osmotic constitution that unwanted electrolytes pass from the blood to the surrounding fluid. In this way it is possible to remove excess potassium and urea and adjust acid-base equilibrium, leaving the other blood constituents unchanged. Haemodialysis can also be used when there has been circulatory overloading due to over-transfusion or water intoxication, in order to extract the excess of water from the patient's blood. The modern machine consists of sterilised coils of cellophane tubing which are connected to radial artery and cephalic vein; a pump ensures adequate flow. Coagulation of blood in the coil is prevented by the use of heparin. Careful control of the constituents of the bath surrounding the coils is essential to permit safe extraction of plasma electrolytes. Rapid dialysis may be achieved by large-capacity machines. The dialysis proceeds for about six hours on each occasion. Where the method is necessary for the correction of over-hydration or pulmonary oedema, 'ultrafiltration' can be used whereby positive pressure is applied to the blood in the pump allowing extremely rapid removal of water or sodium from the patient's blood. The main indications for haemodialysis are a persistent rise in serum potassium levels above 7 mmol per litre or serious hyperkalaemic changes seen in the electrocardiograph, a blood urea over 50 mmol per litre, or a bicarbonate below 15 mmol per litre. Dialysis may need to be repeated several times at intervals of a few days. Where chronic renal failure exists intermittent treatment extending over many months may be employed. The loop of plastic tubing is inserted into a forearm artery and vein and retained permanently as an artificial arteriovenous fistula (Scribner shunt). This is connected to the apparatus on attendance at the dialysis unit.

Peritoneal dialysis. This method is now frequently used, being relatively simple and not requiring a specialised unit. It should be used with caution in the presence of peritonitis or following recent abdominal surgery. It is to be preferred if there is a danger of haemorrhage or in patients with shock or severe cardiovascular disease. A plastic cannula is inserted into the peritoneal cavity using local anaesthesia. Two litres of a pre-warmed solution similar to the electrolyte content of normal serum are introduced, allowed to remain within the peritoneum for about half an hour and then removed. The process is repeated several times over twelve hours, thereby correcting the majority of electrolyte constituents in the blood. When urea production is unduly rapid the method may fail to eliminate all the urea. Protein loss may be significant and there is some risk of peritoneal infection. It is less efficient than haemodialysis.

Diuretic phase. The onset of diuresis is encouraging but treatment should be continued until the blood urea is falling progressively. Electrolyte and water replacement may be necessary and when protein restriction is no longer required a diet of high nutritional value should be given to correct the incurred malnutrition.

Postrenal anuria is caused by obstruction to the urinary flow such as fibrosis, tumours or calculi in the ureter and invariably requires urgent surgical treatment. It is virtually the only acute renal failure causing complete anuria and diagnostic cystoscopy and retrograde pyelography are mandatory to elucidate the cause and relieve it where appropriate by passing bilateral ureteric catheters. This may induce adequate drainage, but nephrostomy is at times required.

CONGENITAL ABNORMALITIES OF THE KIDNEY

One organ may be absent, hypoplastic or be in an ectopic situation, usually in the pelvis or iliac fossa.

Horse-shoe kidney is the most common of several different types of congenital fusion of the two kidneys (Fig. 22.1). The isthmus is generally inferior being crossed by the inferior mesenteric artery which effectively prevents further ascent of the fused kidney. The pelves and ureters also pass down in front of the isthmus. The abnormality can therefore be recognised in a urogram since the renal pelvis on each side lies almost directly in front of its own calyces which appear to be directed medially. Hydronephrosis may develop as a complication, either due to pelvi-ureteric causes or to obstruction by the isthmus. Stone formation and infection occur because of stagnation of urine.

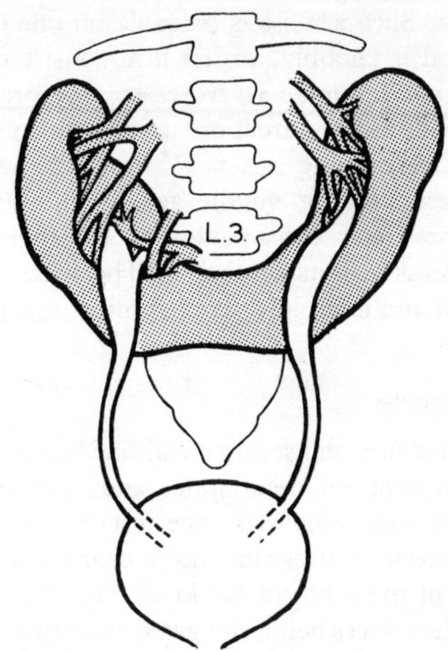

Fig. 22.1 Congenital fused kidneys (Horse-shoe). The pelvis and ureter lie anterior to the kidney substance.

Congenital polycystic kidneys

The cause of this disease, which is often familial, is unknown, although it has been suggested that it is due to a failure of the mesonephric tubules to join the metanephros. The infantile form is due to a recessive gene and is always bilateral. It is often accompanied by cyst formation in the liver, lungs or pancreas. Adult polycystic disease is due to a dominant factor and although the cysts are formed early in life they enlarge slowly and do not usually give rise to symptoms until the third decade. The kidneys contain large numbers of cysts, many of which bulge beneath the capsule, through which pale yellow fluid can be seen or thick yellow or haemorrhagic fluid as a result of infection or haemorrhage into the cysts. The cysts enlarge gradually, with eventual atrophy of the remaining renal substance. Many of the adult patients die from renal failure or hypertension.

Clinical features

(1) *Due to the enlarged kidneys*. There may be aching pain in the loins and the physical signs of a renal

swelling. Such a mass is palpable on one or both sides and is knobbly, with a firm consistency. (2) *Due to renal failure*. Severe cases may present in childhood with retardation of growth and bone changes resembling rickets. More often the symptoms begin during middle age, with headaches, drowsiness and constipation or diarrhoea. The blood-pressure is usually raised. The urine contains albumin and has a low, fixed specific gravity.

Investigations

The blood urea and serum creatinine become raised as renal function deteriorates and tests of renal function (creatinine clearance test) are abnormal. An intravenous urogram shows characteristic distortion of the pelvis of the kidney by the multiple cysts, the calyces being elongated and often dilated. Aortography may be necessary to confirm the diagnosis and exclude tumour, and ultrasound or isotope scan provide confirmatory evidence.

Treatment

Eventual renal failure may be delayed and pain relieved by Rovsing's operation, which consists of exposure of the kidney and puncture of as many cysts as possible. Haemodialysis may be required temporarily to correct temporary acute renal failure; intermittent dialysis is used in selected cases of renal failure awaiting renal transplatation. Treatment is mainly for the control of hypertension and infection to which the cysts are prone. Surgical decompression of one or more cysts may be required because of haemorrhage, infection or obstruction of the ureter by a cyst, but this does not improve renal function. Rarely nephrectomy is required for severe symptoms or bleeding.

Solitary cysts

These are fairly common, being either congenital or occurring as the result of tubular obstruction. They are usually serous but may be haemorrhagic and are of variable size.

Clinical features

If the cyst is large enough it may be recognised as a symptomless renal swelling. Occasionally loin pain from haemorrhage or infection may direct attention to the lesion. Intravenous urography shows a rounded filling defect of the calyces which may be confirmed by ultrasound. Renal arteriography demonstrates the same area to be devoid of vessels, but final diagnosis usually rests on percutaneous puncture and injection of radioactive contrast or on surgical exploration. In simple cysts deroofing is sufficient treatment but excision may be required.

Congenital abnormalities of the ureter

Congenital abnormalities of the ureter include duplication, ureterocele, megaureter, retro-caval ureter, and ectopic ureter.

Duplication of the ureter is frequently seen in excretory urograms and is due to the formation of two ureteric buds on one side. The commonest type is a double renal pelvis, with the two ureters joining in their upper two-thirds, but they sometimes open separately into the bladder or have an ectopic opening lower down. In such duplex ureters, the upper ureter opens below the other into the bladder. Double ureter seldom causes any symptoms and treatment is usually unnecessary.

Ureterocele. This is a curious abnormality, apparently the result of a congenital stenosis of the lower end of the ureter, which balloons into the bladder with each peristaltic wave; it occasionally causes back pressure upon the ureter and kidney and consequent pain in the iliac fossa or loin.

An **ectopic ureteric orifice** is an occasional cause of incontinence in children. The abnormality is commoner in girls, the orifice opening into the lower urethra, vestibule or vagina. Since the other ureter may open normally into the bladder the child may pass urine naturally in addition to being wet.

INJURIES OF THE KIDNEY AND URETER

Rupture of the kidney

This injury is not common as the kidney is encased in a dense layer of fascia and fat formed from extraperitoneal connective tissue, which maintains its general position on the psoas and quadratus lumborum alongside the vertebral column, to some extent protected by the lower thoracic cage. Open injuries are rare but are seen with penetrating wounds of the abdomen and back. The majority of injuries follow direct violence such as a blow on the loin or the crushing trauma seen in football injuries or road traffic accidents. It may also occur in intra-abdominal injuries. The kidney is compressed between the twelfth rib and the sides of the vertebral bodies. Minor contusion of the parenchyma and sub-capsular haematoma occur most commonly but cortical lacerations of differing severity from a complete calycocortical tear or amputation of the lower pole occur, which latter is usually lethal. Haematuria may be obvious and is due to a calyceal tear but internal bleeding into the perinephric space is clinically more important.

Clinical features

After the initial injury there is dull pain in the loin, which may become severe if clots are passing down the ureter. Occasionally with the patient supine there may be pain in the shoulder, indicating that blood has penetrated the peritoneal cavity and reached the under-surface of the diaphragm. The flank may appear full and is extremely tender; there is reflex rigidity in the loin and iliac fossa. The urine is blood-stained.

Treatment

Irrespective of the severity of the haematuria or haematoma in the loin, a conservative regime should be adopted. Morphine is administered for sedation and careful observation maintained for signs of continued or reactionary bleeding, such as increased pallor, sweating or a fall in blood-pressure. The haemoglobin level and blood group are determined, and the appearance of each specimen of urine passed is noted. An intravenous urogram should be performed as soon as possible, mainly to determine the function of the opposite kidney in case nephrectomy becomes necessary, but it may be valuable, as may angiography, in assessing the possibility of conservative renal surgery. Blood transfusion may be required. In most cases haemorrhage gradually ceases without recourse to surgery and the damaged kidney recovers its function. Severe, continued bleeding suggests that large vessels are torn and indicates the need for urgent nephrectomy. Surgery is also necessary if damage to other abdominal viscera is suspected. Late complications, such as perinephric infection, require surgical drainage. Pre-existing hydronephrosis made apparent by minor trauma may need definitive surgery.

Injuries of the ureter

The ureter may be accidentally ligated or divided during operations upon the uterus, rectum or sigmoid colon. This may result in the gradual development of hydronephrosis in the obstructed kidney or the appearance of a urinary fistula. Anastomosis of a divided ureter should be attempted in the upper two-thirds but in the lower third it is more satisfactory to re-implant the ureter into the bladder. In extreme cases with urinary fistula formation nephrectomy may be required.

HYDRONEPHROSIS

Hydronephrosis is a persistent dilatation of the renal pelvis, which also tends to involve the calyces, and to a greater or lesser extent causes atrophy of the renal parenchyma. When it occurs without organic obstruction, the term *primary* or *idiopathic* hydronephrosis is used to distinguish it from hydronephrosis *secondary* to obstruction in the ureter or bladder. Both primary and secondary hydronephrosis may be unilateral or bilateral.

Pathology

Primary or *idiopathic hydronephrosis* is the most common type seen in young people (Fig. 22.2). The majority of cases are probably due to intrinsic abnormalities leading to failure of transmission of peristaltic waves from the renal pelvis to the ureter. Pelvi-ureteric adhesions binding the upper ureter to the pelvis are frequently seen and in a few cases may be the primary cause of the obstruction. Rarely is vesico-ureteric reflux of urine a contributory factor in pelvi-ureteric hydronephrosis.

It was previously thought that hydronephrosis was often due to obstruction of the pelvi-ureteric

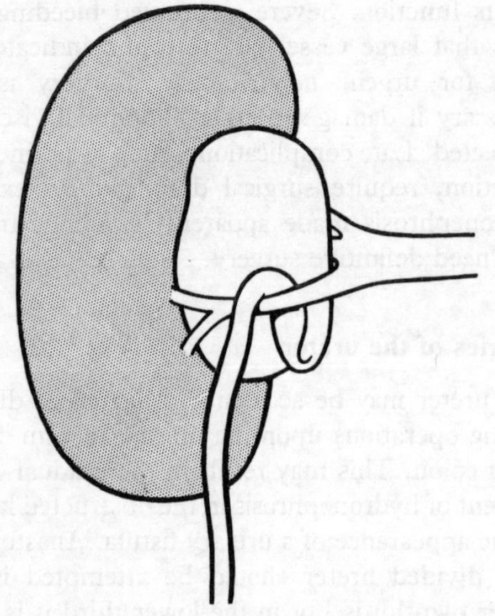

Fig. 22.2 Primary hydronephrosis. The dilatation of the pelvis ends at the pelviureteric junction and is not caused by the aberrant artery.

region by vessels directed to the lower part of the hilum or aberrant vessels going to the lower pole of the kidney. This explanation is rarely satisfactory, since the dilatation nearly always ends at the pelvi-ureteric junction rather than at the site of an aberrant or infrapolar artery. Such vessels are common and when hydronephrosis is present they may kink the upper end of the ureter and cause periods of obstruction to an already dilated pelvis. Rarely are vessels the sole cause of hydronephrosis.

Secondary hydronephrosis. The unilateral form is usually due to obstruction of the ureter. Bilateral hydronephrosis is due to a lesion in the bladder, bladder neck or the urethra. Common causes of ureteric obstruction include ureteric calculus, stricture, or neoplasm and pressure from without by pelvic tumours such as fibroids. Bilateral hydronephrosis may be caused by a vesical calculus or neoplasm, prostatic hypertrophy, bladder-neck obstruction, carcinoma of the prostate or a urethral stricture. It also occurs during pregnancy, possibly due to relaxation of smooth muscle in the wall of the ureter.

Clinical features

Pain or discomfort may be noted in the loin, flank or iliac fossa due to distension of the renal pelvis. Occasionally there may be intermittent attacks of severe pain, accompanied by oliguria, which are due to transient complete obstruction of the hydronephrosis. Symptoms may be due to the complications of hydronephrosis, such as urinary infection, stone formation, hypertension or renal failure. In some instances hydronephrosis produces no symptoms. Frequently there are no physical signs, but if the hydronephrosis is large it may be palpable bimanually in the loin as a smooth or cystic swelling moving on respiration, with a band of resonance anteriorly.

Investigations

Urine examination may not demonstrate any abnormality, or pus cells and organisms will indicate infection. Intravenous urography is diagnostic, provided that renal function is adequate to concentrate the dye, and shows dilatation of the pelvis and calyces with delay in emptying down the ureter. Doubtful cases may be proven by giving a water-load during radiology. Panendoscopy and cystoscopy are necessary in bilateral hydronephrosis to determine whether the cause lies in the bladder. Retrograde pyelography may be required to outline the pelvis if the excretory urogram is unsatisfactory, but should be followed immediately by definitive surgery. A radio-active isotope renogram is helpful in diagnosis and a typical obstructive pattern may disappear a few months after effective surgery.

Complications

1. *Infection* is common, producing pain and tenderness in the loin, with increased urinary frequency and fever. Pyonephrosis is a more severe degree of this complication, in which the renal pelvis becomes a bag of pus and is due to infection with pyogenic organisms.

2. *Calculus formation* may occur in a primary hydronephrosis from urinary stasis or infection.

3. *Renal failure and hypertension*. Progressive renal failure with uraemia and hypertension is the end result of severe bilateral hydronephrosis. The raised intrapelvic pressure produces gradual atrophy of the renal parenchyma which becomes reduced to a thin shell. Further destruction may occur from infection.

The pyelonephritis which complicates a unilateral hydronephrosis sometimes leads to high blood-pressure, caused by the production of angiotensin. In younger patients removal of the diseased kidney may be followed by return of the blood-pressure to normal, but it usually fails to do so owing to the development of arterial disease in the opposite kidney as a result of the hypertension.

Treatment

Nephrectomy should be performed only when the affected kidney is severely damaged and the remaining organ healthy. In other cases *pyeloplasty* should be undertaken; this involves a plastic repair of the enlarged renal pelvis, with the object of improving drainage at the pelvi-ureteric junction (Fig. 22.3). In secondary hydronephrosis the underlying disease generally requires more urgent treatment than the hydronephrosis which it causes. Infection in a hydronephrosis is usually controlled by antibiotics in the initial stages, but relapse is frequent. Nephrectomy is usually necessary for recurrent infection and failed pyeloplasty.

Renal artery obstruction

Fibromuscular hyperplasia is an important, although uncommon, cause of obstruction to the renal artery in early life. Similarly, stenosis due to atheroma generally affects a localised area near the origin of the renal artery in adults. Both are important though rare causes of hypertension, which may be treated surgically before there is any appreciable degree of renal failure. The condition should be suspected in a hypertensive patient if a bruit is audible over the renal artery. Intravenous urography may show shrinkage of the cortex of the kidney on the affected side, but the concentration of the dye is sometimes increased, giving a denser pyelogram than the normal side. The diagnosis can be confirmed by renal angiography. Treatment is by direct arterial surgery to restore the blood flow.

URINARY CALCULUS

Pathology

The usual sites of stone formation in the urinary tract are the kidney, bladder and prostate. The stones may be called primary when they develop in a normal urinary tract and secondary when they follow infection or stasis. Many cases of urolithiasis are due to reduced fluid intake, particularly in hot climates or working conditions.

Primary stones may be due to a metabolic abnormality, and in particular an increased urinary excretion of calcium. This occurs in hyperparathyroidism, during prolonged immobilisation of patients with fractures or spinal disease, in Paget's disease of bone, renal tubular acidosis, idiopathic hypercalcuria, vitamin D overdosage and neoplastic disease. Uric acid stone formation occurs in gout, polycythaemia and leukaemia, usually due to crystallisation from dehydration or reduction in urinary *p*H. Some cases are due to hyperuricaemia. A rare abnormality is cystinuria, transmitted by a recessive gene. Occasionally primary oxalate stones are due to a metabolic defect causing hyperoxaluria.

Secondary stones develop when the urine is

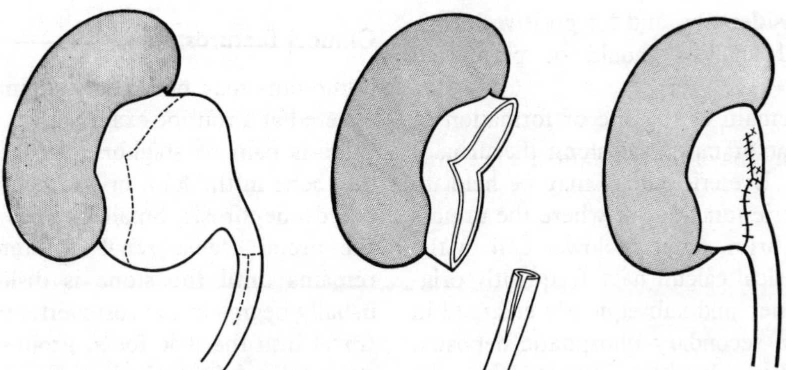

Fig. 22.3 Pyeloplasty for hydronephrosis

infected, due to the presence of proteinaceous debris, which acts as a nucleus for subsequent crystallisation. Calculus formation is most common in a strongly alkaline urine, the alkalinity being caused by the presence of urea-splitting bacteria such as *Staph. aureus* or *B. proteus*. This type of stone is usually composed of ammonium magnesium phosphate ('triple phosphate'). Urinary stasis is another principal cause of stone formation, accounting for the appearance of calculi in a hydronephrosis or hydroureter and of vesical calculi in prostatic obstruction.

Types

About 60 per cent of urinary calculi contain calcium oxalate; a further 30 per cent are composed of phosphates and the remaining 10 per cent include urates, uric acid, cystine and calcium carbonate. *Calcium oxalate* forms hard, whitish stones, which may become darkened by continual staining with blood. They arise usually in an acid urine and are radio-opaque. Curious spiky stones, variously called 'mulberry', 'hedgehog', 'jackstone' or 'sea-urchin' calculi, are forms of oxalate calculus. *Phosphatic* calculi are white and crumbly and occur in an alkaline urine. They may adjust their shape according to their position, such as the 'staghorn calculus' of the renal pelvis. These large calculi are composed of triple phosphates and are generally radio-opaque. *Uric acid* and *urate* stones are more common in the bladder than in the kidney; they are yellowish or occasionally purple and are not radio-opaque. *Cystine* stones, the result of a familial metabolic error, resemble hard candle-wax and are radio-opaque. The colour and shape of urinary stones varies considerably, and for positive identification chemical analysis should be performed after removal.

Calculi may remain at the site of formation in kidney or bladder or may pass along the urinary tract (Fig. 22.4). Ureteric calculi may be held up at the pelvi-ureteric junction, or where the ureters cross the pelvic brim, or at its lower end in the bladder wall. Vesical calculi have frequently originated in the kidney and subsequently enlarged in the bladder from secondary phosphatic deposits. Occasionally calculi become impacted in the urethra, usually behind a stricture. Urinary stones may cause the following complications:

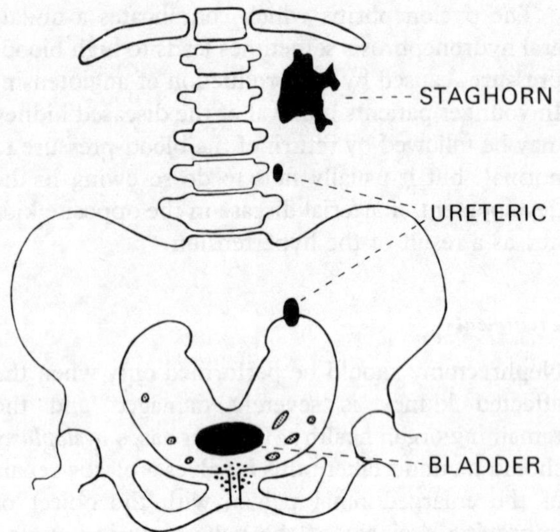

Fig. 22.4 Urinary calculi. The common sites at which calculi are demonstrated radiologically. Phleboliths in the pelvis and prostatic calculi are common associated findings.

1. *Infection*. Obstruction may lead to cystitis, pyelonephritis, pyonephrosis or perinephric abscess.
2. *Secondary hydronephrosis* is generally due to intermittent obstruction.
3. *Calculous anuria* may be caused by obstruction of one ureter the other kidney having been diseased or previously removed, or from the presence of bilateral stones.
4. *Neoplasia*. A squamous-cell carcinoma of the renal pelvis may develop in areas of epithelial metaplasia, caused by the presence of long-standing calculi.

Clinical features

Symptoms may be absent, albuminuria being discovered at a routine examination, but more usually there is pain. A staghorn calculus may produce a dull ache in the loin, or backache may result from a hydronephrosis. Smaller stones, which impact in the ureter, cause renal or ureteric colic which remains until the stone is dislodged. The pain usually begins in the costovertebral angle, but may travel into the iliac fossa, groin or genitalia. Ureteric colic frequently lasts for several hours and may be accompanied by shock. Haematuria is common and at times profuse whilst frequency may occur if the calculus is close to the ureteric orifice.

A vesical calculus occurs more commonly in men than in women and in the latter the majority are caused by an introduced foreign body. A bladder stone causes frequency of micturition and pain in the lower abdomen and genitalia. The pain may be worsened by jolting, although in stone formation secondary to prostatic hyperplasia there may be no symptoms, since the calculus lies in the sump of stagnant urine behind the elevated trigone. At times the pain is referred to the external meatus and usually occurs at the end of micturition when the stone sinks to the floor of the bladder. Infection is often present and aggravates the pain during micturition.

Physical examination may reveal lumbar or iliac tenderness or a palpable hydronephrosis. A large vesical calculus may be felt on rectal or vaginal examination and occasionally urethral calculi are palpable.

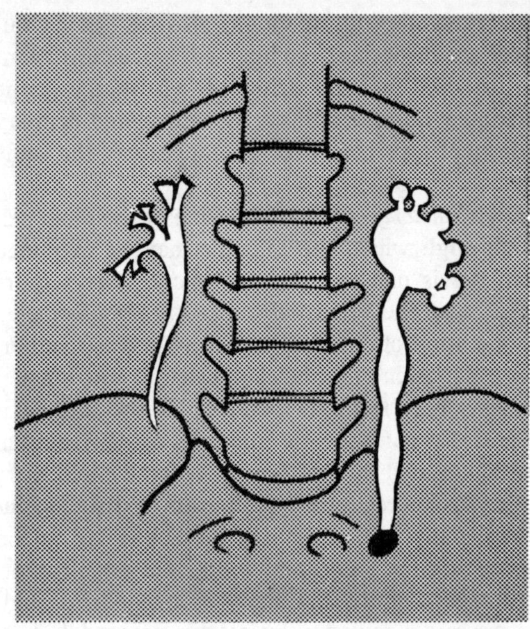

Fig. 22.5 Intravenous urogram demonstrating hydronephrosis and hydroureter due to a calculus held up at the level of the pelvic brim

Investigations

The urine may contain albumin and microscopy reveal red blood cells or pus. Most urinary stones are radio-opaque due to a high calcium content, and radiography of the abdomen may show the calculus in the line of the urinary tract. A lateral view helps to locate a calculus in the renal area. Intravenous urography should be performed, if necessary during an attack of ureteric colic. The presence of some small opaque and non-opaque stones can at times only be diagnosed in this way. Radiographs show the degree of function on the diseased side and whether obstruction is present (Fig. 22.5). During an attack of ureteric colic a nephrographic outline may be obtained on films delayed for several hours and it is important to do an after-micturition film to show up the lower end where a stone frequently lodges. If the kidney fails to excrete sufficient dye then a retrograde ureterogram may be necessary and is best performed with an 'acorn' bulb ureteric catheter. Vesical calculi are confirmed by cystoscopy.

Many urinary stones are caused by metabolic abnormalities and the serum calcium and uric acid levels should be determined. If uric acid calculi are present the urinary uric acid and urinary *p*H require to be measured. Further investigations of hypercalcuria may need to be performed, and when a stone is obtained it should be analysed chemically. In about 5 per cent of patients with a calculus the serum calcium is raised and this may be the only indication that a parathyroid tumour is present.

Treatment

It is not necessary to remove all urinary calculi, but progressive renal impairment through obstruction and pyelonephritis may be avoided by removal of calculi which are too large to pass normally.

Renal calculus

Surgical treatment is indicated if the radiographic shadow is symptomatic and more than 1 cm in diameter, as natural elimination is then unlikely. Moulding of the calculus to the shape of calyx or pelvis often indicates that it has been present for some time. Operation should also be carried out where the urine has been infected, since permanent sterility will not be achieved whilst the stone remains within the kidney. An underlying primary hydronephrosis may need pyeloplasty at the same time.

Pyelolithotomy entails an incision of the renal pelvis through which the calculus may be extracted from pelvis or calyx. Larger calculi may require incision of the renal substance (*nephrolithotomy*), an operation often complicated by severe haemorrhage. Division of a branched calculus into smaller portions may facilitate removal. If the kidney is extensively damaged by infection or obstruction, partial or total *nephrectomy* is generally necessary but the use of regional hypothermia or drug inosine allows temporary clamping of the renal blood supply without significant functional impairment, permitting unhurried surgery in a bloodless field. Per-operative radiography of the exposed kidney provides verification that a kidney is free of calculi after operation.

Ureteric calculus

Severe ureteric colic usually indicates movement of the stone which is likely to pass during the existing attack or within the next few weeks. Treatment should at first be conservative by analgesics, such as pethidine, or morphine with atropine, followed by the ingestion of large quantities of fluids. Full investigation of the urinary tracts should be undertaken when the acute attack has subsided. In the absence of infection or significant obstruction between attacks of colic a stone can be treated conservatively for an indefinite period. Stones over 5 mm diameter are less likely to pass spontaneously and if the diameter of the calculus is more than 1 cm eventual removal is probable. Progressive dilatation of the renal pelvis, impairment of renal function and infection are indications for early operation. The presence of a ureteric calculus in cases of bilateral stone or unilateral kidney requires urgent surgery.

The stone may be dislodged by the passage of a ureteric catheter, or special basket extractors can be used to catch and withdraw it. These should be used with caution as damage to the ureteric wall may occur. It is preferable to perform these manoeuvres under radiographic control using an image-intensifier. Enlargement of the ureteric orifices by diathermy incision may be necessary for stones impacted in the lower end of the ureter. Open *ureterolithotomy* is performed if these measures fail or complications are present, the ureter being approached by an extraperitoneal exposure.

The management of bilateral renal stones is difficult, but small stones which are not causing symptoms may be left untreated. Any patient who has had urinary calculi should be advised to increase their fluid intake to prevent the formation of a concentrated urine at any time during a 24-hour period, as this considerably lessens the risk of recurrent stone formation.

A vesical calculus may be crushed with a special instrument (lithotrite) and the contents evacuated in the operation of *litholapaxy*, or the stone be removed by a suprapubic operation (*lithotomy*). A urethral calculus should be removed directly or displaced into the bladder and treated as a vesical calculus.

INFECTIONS OF THE KIDNEY

Acute pyelonephritis (acute pyelitis)

Pathology

Acute bacterial infection of the parenchyma of the kidney may occur in a previously healthy patient or as a complication of operations or disease of the urinary tract. Although infection may start in the pelvis (pyelitis), there is invariably spread up the collecting tubules and pyelonephritis is a more accurate term. Multiple small abscess may occur in the cortex, some of which are visible under the capsule of the kidney.

The principal routes of infection are through the bloodstream and by reflux along the ureters. The infection is usually bilateral, and if unilateral an underlying abnormality such as a stone or congenital defect should be suspected.

Clinical features

Pain in one or both loins is typical and is usually accompanied by vomiting; painful and frequent micturition is a common but not invariable complaint. There is a fever of 38° to 40°C, often with rigors. Examination usually reveals renal tenderness. The commonest organism is *Esch. coli*, which occurs in an acid urine, but the urine becomes strongly alkaline in staphylococcal and *B. proteus* infections. Investigations show a leucocytosis, and microscopy of the urine demonstrates numerous leucocytes and organisms, often visibly motile; there may be many red blood cells. The Gram film confirms the presence of bacteria and culture reveals the responsible organism; the sensitivity of this to the more common antibiotics should be determined.

Differential diagnosis

Acute pyelonephritis is a common cause of sudden fever in children. It is also important to exclude it where the complaint is of pain in the loin or iliac fossa and the suspected diagnosis appendicitis, diverticulitis or renal colic.

Treatment

In the initial 24 to 48 hours, during which time the bacterial sensitivities are being completed, preliminary treatment with septrin or ampicillin should be commenced. When repeated rigors are present and bacteraemia suspected, blood cultures should be taken. If the blood urea and creatinine levels are within normal limits gentamicin should be given. The fluid intake should be moderately high. If the patient is vomiting intravenous fluids are essential because dehydration and electrolyte imbalance rapidly develop. If improvement occurs the above regime should be continued for five to seven days, but if there is no change after 48 hours the appropriate antibiotic should be administered. When urinary infections fail to respond to these measures, the cause is usually a persistent pathological abnormality in the urinary tract, and full investigation should be undertaken to determine its nature, which is usually obstructive.

Chronic pyelonephritis

Pathology

Chronic or recurrent infection of the kidney produces widespread cortical scarring, with consequent irregular shrinkage of the organ. This may lead to renal failure or hypertension, often in young adult life. The presence of structural damage in the parenchyma makes recurrence of the infection likely. The route of infection is probably similar to that of acute pyelonephritis.

Clinical features

In infancy anorexia, loss of weight or failure to thrive are the main symptoms. In older children fever or abdominal pain may occur. Urinary symptoms may be absent, although there is sometimes increased nocturnal frequency or enuresis. In adults there may be thirst and polyuria, or evidence of hypertension and renal failure. Apart from the occasional presence of fever, renal tenderness is absent and there are no abnormal physical signs. The diagnosis depends upon the finding of leucocytes and organisms in the urine and their subsequent culture, the bacteriology being similar to that of acute pyelonephritis. Intravenous urography is essential and may show enlargement of the calyces and thinning of the cortical substance of the kidney. In many patients showing these changes, reflux of urine from the bladder into the ureter can be demonstrated during voiding on a micturating cysto-urethrogram. Whether this is a cause or an effect of the pyelonephritis remains uncertain.

Differential diagnosis

Progressive renal failure in a patient with small contracted kidneys may be due to chronic glomerulonephritis or renal arteriolosclerosis. Chronic pyelonephritis is distinguished by the isolation of the causative organism and the presence of pyuria. Pyelonephritis may co-exist with a congenital malformation such as hydronephrosis or megaureter, which will be revealed in the intravenous urogram.

Treatment

The severe sequelae of pyelonephritis make it important to treat every urinary infection promptly and efficiently. In chronic pyelonephritis the relapse rate is between 10 and 20 per cent, regardless of the particular antibiotic used. It is therefore necessary to follow these patients carefully and reexamine the urine after a period of three months. In cases with renal impairment drugs such as nitrofurantoin should be used with caution but relapse may be treated after two weeks of high dose therapy with long-term chemotherapy using drugs such as hexamine mandelate (Mandelamine) or low-dose sulphonamides, co-trimoxazole, nitrofurantoin or nalidixic acid provided that the responsible organism is sensitive. When used for long-term therapy, toxic side-effects may develop. In using any drug, treatment should be guided by repeated bacteriological studies and sensitivity tests, the drug being withdrawn to determine the possibility of long-term remission. When vesico-ureteric reflux on micturition exists, transplantation of the ureter may be necessary, but in minor degrees of reflux, providing there is no appreciable upper renal tract abnormality, a conservative policy can be adopted by preventing infection. If recurrent urinary tract infection occurs despite adequate therapy or there are increased upper renal tract changes or urethral outflow obstruction then surgery is necessary, the ureters being re-implanted into the bladder (uretero-neo-cystostomy).

Suppuration in the kidney

An abscess may develop in the renal pelvis (*pyonephrosis*), renal parenchyma (*pyaemic abscess* or *carbuncle of the kidney*), or around the kidney (*perinephric abscess*). The infection is usually due to *Staph. aureus* or to the coliform bacillus.

Pathology

Pyonephrosis is a complication of ureteric obstruction, usually due to a stone. The pelvis of the kidney becomes filled with pus and may be lined by granulation tissue.

Pyaemic abscess is a blood-borne staphylococcal infection; there may be a recent history of boils or osteomyelitis. The abscess usually causes widespread destruction of the substance of the kidney.

Perinephric abscess is usually a complication of one of the two preceding conditions, as a result of spread of infection through the renal capsule. Occasionally it may originate in a tuberculous pyelonephritis. This should be excluded in cases in which initial culture of the pus proves sterile.

Clinical features

The diagnosis may prove difficult despite general malaise. There is often little pain and urinary symptoms are uncommon. Remittent fever to 40° to 41°C is usual and there may be rigors. Deep tenderness is felt in the loin, and often slight bulging of the flank results from oedema, but obvious swelling is rare.

The urine may or may not contain pus and organisms. A plain radiograph may show enlargement of the soft tissue outline of the kidney or loss of the lateral outline of the psoas muscle, due to local oedema. Renal stones may be apparent. An intravenous urogram is sometimes helpful in indicating an obstructive cause.

Treatment

Surgical drainage is nearly always necessary. The kidney should be exposed in the loin, care being taken not to open the peritoneum. Suppuration within the kidney usually requires nephrectomy, but this may be better carried out at a later operation in two or three weeks time when the acute inflammation has subsided as conservative renal surgery including calculi removal may be an effective procedure. Renal carbuncle, if diagnosed with certainty, can be treated by antibiotics. Nephrectomy may be necessary when the kidney is totally destroyed or there is no response to antibiotics.

RENAL TUBERCULOSIS

Pathology

The earliest lesions in the kidney are multiple tuberculous foci in the cortex, near the glomeruli, the result of haematogenous spread from a primary focus usually in the chest but occasionally in the lymph nodes of the neck, mediastinum or abdomen. These lesions usually heal without further progression, but continue to harbour live tubercle bacilli and re-activate later should there be a fall in the general resistance of the patient. When renal lesions develop the primary infection has usually healed. Enlargement of one or more cortical foci takes place either in one kidney or on both sides ulcerating into the collecting system and also pro-

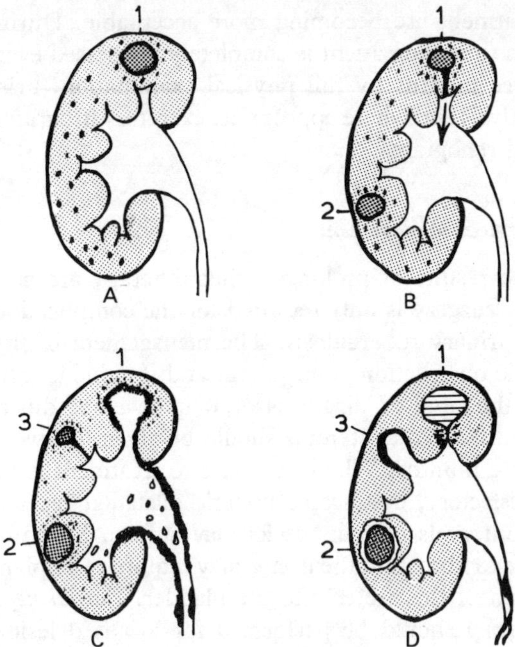

Fig. 22.6 Pathology of renal tuberculosis
A. Multiple blood-borne foci with activity in single focus in upper pole (1). **B.** Fistula develops into upper calyx. Activity commences in focus (2). **C.** Ulcero-cavernous stage. Focus (1) has formed a cavity in the pyramid and lesions (2) and (3) enlarge. Tuberculous follicles appear in the pelvis and ureter. **D.** After treatment with chemotherapy. Cavity (1) becomes closed. Focus (2) calcifies and focus (3) remains open. Strictures develop in the ureter.

ducing tuberculous bacteriuria. These coalesce and may spread throughout the kidney (*tuberculous pyelonephritis*) with areas of caseation and even calcification before any symptoms occur. The onset of symptoms coincides with spread of the disease towards the renal papillae, the formation of medullary lesions and rupture of a caseous focus into one of the calyces, causing infection of the renal pelvis and the production of an apparently sterile pyuria. This conversion of the lesion from a 'closed' to an 'open' infection exposes the patient to the danger of tubercle bacilli spreading down the lymphatics of the ureter, or being washed into the bladder with the urine. In this way the bladder, and in the male the prostate, seminal vesicles or epididymis are often infected. The opposite kidney may also become involved either through reflux or by re-activation of previously silent foci. In advanced urinary tuberculosis both kidneys are nearly always diseased.

Established renal tuberculosis is sometimes called the *ulcero-cavernous lesion*. Multiple caseous lesions are present in the parenchyma, some of which communicate with a partially ulcerated pelvis, diffusely infiltrated with tuberculous foci. The three narrowest areas of the urinary tract at which stricture formation takes place are the uretero-vesical junction, the pelvi-ureteric junction, and the necks of the calyces. If the effects of this fibrosis are severe, total destruction of the kidney takes place with the occurrence of an '*autonephrectomy*'.

The earlier stages of renal tuberculosis sometimes heal without treatment, and this also occurs after obstruction of a calyx or at the pelvi-ureteric junction. Advanced urinary tuberculosis rarely heals without treatment and complications include *tuberculous pyonephrosis, tuberculous perinephric abscess* or *renal failure* from extensive pyelonephritis. Severe lesions may be induced to heal with chemotherapy, often leaving sequelae such as strictures of the ureter and contraction of the bladder.

Clinical features

Urinary tuberculosis occurs mainly between 15 and 40 years and in old age. It is slightly commoner in men. The early lesions are symptomless, but there may later be frequency, haematuria and pain. Frequency of micturition, particularly at night, is often the first and only symptom of renal tuberculosis and in advanced disease may be very distressing. Painless haematuria is common, a few patients also having aching pain in the loin, ureteric colic due to passage of clots or debris, or strangury. General symptoms such as loss of weight, evening pyrexia or lassitude may predominate. Following arrest of the disease most patients are cured of their symptoms, but during the healing process a few treated by chemotherapy develop symptoms due to fibrosis in the ureters or bladder; thus loin pain may follow hydronephrosis or severe frequency may be the result of a small and fibrotic bladder.

Examination may show the general condition to be good and local abnormal signs may be absent, but there may be a palpable kidney or seminal vesicle and thickening in the spermatic cord, vas or epididymis. Epididymo-orchitis may be acute and present with a painful large hydrocele. When the overlying skin becomes involved and adherent, sinus formation takes place posteriorly. Rarely a cold abscess presents in the loin.

Investigations

Examination of the urine is essential and the finding of sterile acid pyuria is characteristic. Three successive early-morning urine specimens should be examined for the presence of tubercle bacilli by staining the centrifuged deposit by the Ziehl-Neelsen method. Acid-alcohol-fast bacilli can usually be discovered, but a culture must be made on Loewenstein-Jensen medium. Sensitivity tests should be carried out on any cultures that are found to be positive. Rarely is guinea-pig inoculation necessary. Confusion may occur with the smegma bacillus or rarely with schistosomiasis or abacterial pyuria.

Intravenous urography is important in determining the extent of the disease and the response to treatment. The position of calcified areas in the kidney is shown and there is often irregularity and distortion of the clayces, due to ulceration. Later the pelvis and ureter become irregular or dilated. The chest should be radiographed, but active pulmonary tuberculosis is rarely found. Cystoscopy is not essential but when performed may show oedema of a ureteric orifice or scattered shallow ulcers of the bladder. Retrograde pyelo-ureterography is only required when high-dose intravenous urography has failed to delineate abnormalities in the kidney and drainage system such as strictures. Isotope renography is helpful in monitoring the progress of the disease under treatment, particularly the demonstration of ureteric obstruction before and after treatment.

Treatment

General measures together with chemotherapy are of prime importance. During the first 12 weeks, or until drug sensitivity reports are available, three of the following drugs should be given in combination—streptomycin, pyrazinamide, isoniazid, ethambutol and rifampicin. Pyrazinamide is helpful in the acute phase combined with isoniazid and rifampicin. Combinations of two drugs are necessary for at least one year after the disease appears to be quiescent. Using rifampicin shorter courses of treatment are becoming more acceptable. During this time the patient is completely reassessed every three months by full physical examination, urine analysis and where appropriate excretory urography and renograms.

Surgical management

The results of prolonged chemotherapy are good and surgery is only required for the complications of urinary tuberculosis. The management of ureteric obstruction is important and if demonstrated at the time of diagnosis or if it develops during treatment, oral steroids should be given for two to three months. Where response to treatment is not satisfactory, cystoscopic ureteric dilatation repeated at intervals of four weeks may suffice. Strictures due to fibrosis in the ureter may require re-implantation of the ureter into the bladder. *Partial nephrectomy* should be performed for localised lesions which fail to heal with chemotherapy and continue to flood the urine with tubercle bacilli. Alternatively caseous foci may be curetted and the renal capsule partially resutured (cavernostomy). *Uretero-nephrectomy* is preferable if one kidney is severely destroyed and unlikely to recover and the other is almost normal. The kidney and all of the ureter are removed through separate incisions, as the stump of a diseased ureter might be a continued reservoir of infection.

Contraction of the bladder may in some cases require diversion of urinary flow on to the anterior abdominal wall by means of an ileal conduit. Both ureters are implanted into a short length of isolated ileum, one end of which is closed, whilst the other is brought out to drain into an ileostomy appliance. The continuity of the ileum is restored by anastomosis (Fig. 22.8). An alternative is caecocystoplasty, in which the isolated caecum is anastomosed to the lower portion of the bladder. In females it may be necessary to reduce the urethral outflow resistance by urethrotomy, using an urethrotome.

TUMOURS OF THE KIDNEY AND URETER

Primary tumours involve the renal parenchyma, the pelvis and the ureter (Fig. 22.7). Secondary

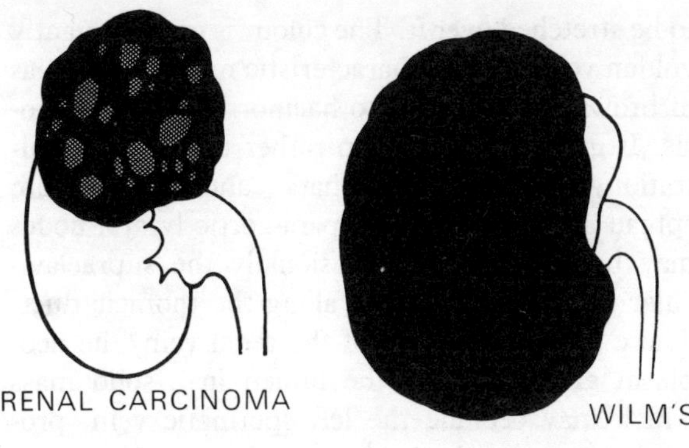

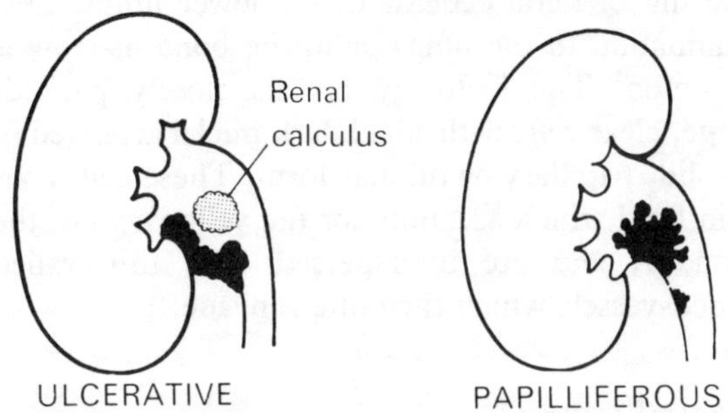

Fig. 22.7 Tumours of renal parenchyma and pelvis

deposits are less common; they arise chiefly from carcinoma of the lung and in the reticuloses.

A. Tumours of the parenchyma

Benign

Angioma, fibroma, adenoma

Malignant

Embryoma or sarcoma (Wilms' tumour)
Renal carcinoma ('hypernephroma')

B. Tumours of the renal pelvis and ureter

Benign

Papilloma

Malignant

Papillary carcinoma
Squamous-cell carcinoma

TUMOURS OF THE PARENCHYMA

Benign tumours of the parenchyma have little clinical significance, although an angioma is a rare cause of painless haematuria.

Nephroblastoma (embryoma) of the kidney (Wilms' tumour)

This is the commonest intra-abdominal malignant tumour of childhood and usually occurs before the age of four years. The peak incidence is at the age of three years. It may be associated with congenital abnormalities and genetic factors may be involved.

The tumour has a pinkish or greyish appearance, expanding the substance of the kidney from which it becomes sharply delineated by a pseudocapsule of connective tissue; the remaining substance may be seen at one or other pole. Most of the tumours grow rapidly producing areas of haemorrhage and necrosis, sometimes with cyst formation.

This histology shows a mixed appearance, with primitive renal tubules and primitive striated muscle fibres, lying in an undifferentiated and mesenchymal stroma. Cartilage, osteoid and adipose tissues are sometimes found. The tumour arises from neoplastic change in a malformation of the kidney, which accounts for the variegated structure. Metastasis occurs by the retroperitoneal lymphatics or by the bloodstream, to involve the lungs, liver, bones and superficial tissues.

Clinical features

The usual presentation is a large, solid, lobulated swelling discovered in the flank of a small, pale infant. It tends to protrude forward rather than into the loin and may be too large to move on respiration. Abdominal pain is rarely severe and microscopic haematuria occurs in about one-third of patients. Anaemia and weight loss are usually found when metastasis has taken place.

The differential diagnosis includes hydronephrosis, multicystic kidney, splenic enlargement, adrenal neuroblastoma, so that an intravenous urogram should always be performed. Radiography of the chest is mandatory to exclude pulmonary metastases. A staging of the disease is based on clinical examination, investigation and careful surgical and pathological documentation. The most popular form used is that by the National Wilms' Tumour Study Group as follows:

Stage I: The tumour is confined to the kidney and is completely resected.
Stage II: The tumour extends beyond the kidney but is completely resected.
Stage III: There is residual tumour confined to the abdomen.
Stage IV: Haematogenous metastases are present.
Stage V: Bilateral tumour.

Radical nephrectomy should be undertaken without delay after correction of anaemia, and a complete lymph node dissection from the diaphragm to the aortic bifurcation performed. A course of radiotherapy should be started as soon as the wound has healed. Chemotherapy may produce a cure together with surgery and radiotherapy, but it has an important role in palliation, the two most effective drugs being actinomycin D and vincristine.

Courses may be repeated at intervals of three months up to 15 months from the time of diagnosis. Gastro-intestinal and haematological side effects dictate modifications in treatment. Surgical excision of metastatic disease limited to a resectable anatomical segment of an organ should be performed. With a radical approach to treatment 80 per cent of all children can be cured, a higher success rate being achieved in infants treated during the first year of life.

Renal carcinoma (adenocarcinoma)

Pathology

The theory of Grawitz, that the lesion arose from ectopic adrenal tissue, was based upon the yellow colour of the tumour and its histological similarity to normal adrenal tissue. This is no longer believed, and since the term hypernephroma is unsatisfactory it is more accurate to refer to the neoplasm as a renal carcinoma.

The tumour can arise anywhere in the kidney substance but is generally at one or other pole, frequently the upper. It appears encapsulated, has sharp margins and the remains of the kidney seem to be stretched over it. The colour is predominantly golden yellow, with characteristic mosaic-like areas of brown and red, due to haemorrhage and necrosis. It grows by expansion rather than direct infiltration, but both lymphatic and bloodstream spread are common. The para-aortic lymph nodes may be involved, or occasionally the supraclavicular group, from spread along the thoracic duct. There may be invasion of the renal vein, the neoplasm growing along the lumen in a solid mass which may occlude the left spermatic vein, producing a varicocele, or along the inferior vena cava, causing bilateral oedema of the lower limbs. Dissemination to the lungs or to the bone marrow is common. The histology reveals closely packed, large, clear cells with small dark nuclei arranged in a solid, papillary or tubular form. These cells contain lipid which accounts for the yellowness of the tumour, and are interspersed with thin-walled blood-vessels which they often invade.

Clinical features

Renal carcinoma is commonest from 40 to 60 years. The usual presentation is haematuria, pain or abdominal swelling. There may be general symptoms such as loss of weight, pyrexia or anaemia, or attention may first be drawn to some metastasis such as a pathological fracture, pulmonary deposit with cough or haemoptysis, or obstruction of the inferior vena cava.

The tumour is not always palpable, but may constitute a typical renal swelling. In the presence of haematuria immediate cystoscopy should be undertaken to determine from which side the bleeding occurs. In the absence of frank haemorrhage, microscopic examination of the urine should be performed and may show an increase in red blood cells.

Radiography of the abdomen may show enlargement of the renal outline. An intravenous urogram may reveal distortion or obliteration of one or more of the renal calyces, which often become drawn out by the expansion of the tumour, producing a spidery appearance. Rarely is retrograde pyelography necessary but aortography or selective renal arteriography may show tumour circulation in a space-occupying lesion. Ultrasound scanning will distinguish a solid from a cystic lesion. Lymphography and inferior vena cavography may be used in order to stage the tumour more accurately (T.N.M. classification). A radiograph of the chest may show large, discrete 'cannon-ball' deposits, although smaller secondaries are more common.

Treatment

The diseased kidney should be removed, either through a curved loin incision, which may have to be extended into the chest if the tumour is very large or through an abdominal approach. Ligation of the renal pedicle is advisable as an initial step to prevent dissemination through handling of the tumour. Post-operative radiotherapy is advisable when the tumour has been incompletely removed but there is no evidence to show that pre- or post-operative radiotherapy improves the prognosis in all cases. Pre-operative embolisation, performed at the time of selective renal angiography, is helpful in reducing the vascularity of the tumour and may facilitate removal.

TUMOURS OF THE RENAL PELVIS AND URETER

Pathology

Papillary tumours arise from the transitional epithelium lining the renal pelvis and ureter and are often multiple. All tumours of low-grade potential (papilloma and papillary carcinoma) should probably be regarded as low-grade papillary carcinoma, the incidence being mainly seen between 30 and 50 years, whilst the maximum incidence of invasive carcinomas is between 40 and 60 years.

The multiplicity of these transitional-cell tumours is probably due to a wide field of epithelium becoming increasingly unstable over the course of many years so that several tumours eventually arise at about the same time. The epithelium may be susceptible to various carcinogens or abnormal metabolites. Another explanation is that they are liable to seed by direct implantation through cells passing down the ureter in the urinary stream. It is probable that both methods occur. Macroscopically they are nodular proliferative growths which closely resemble their counterparts in the bladder. The papillary tumours are composed of a central core of connective tissue, surrounded by a mass of fronds covered by transitional epithelium. The carcinomatous variety tends to appear more sessile, with thicker epithelium, contains more mitoses and has a liability to local infiltration at the base.

Squamous-cell carcinoma of the renal pelvis is usually a complication of long-standing renal calculi, which cause squamous metaplasia in the epithelium and eventual malignant transformation. These tumours form flat, ulcerated, sloughing lesions which usually infiltrate widely into the surrounding tissues.

Clinical features

The majority present with painless haematuria, which may at times be profuse and be accompanied by the passage of clots. Ureteric colic with radiation of pain from loin to groin or genitalia may result. Backache and swelling in the loin due to hydronephrosis from the obstructive effect of a tumour are occasional symptoms. Physical examination is generally unhelpful, and the diagnosis must be made on cystoscopy when blood may be seen spurting from the ureter, or by intravenous urography which may show the appearance of a translucent filling defect in the renal pelvis, or dilatation and irregularity of the ureter. Retograde ureteropyelography may be necessary to localise tumours or confirm the multi-focal nature of the disease. A radioactive isotope renogram may show an obstructive pattern.

Treatment

The kidney and ureter should both be removed because of the multi-focal nature of the disease and the marked tendency to recurrence. The operation (*nephro-ureterectomy*) is performed through a posterior loin incision and a separate lower abdominal wound to remove the lower end of the ureter together with full thickness of bladder tissue.

TRANSPLANTATION OF THE URETERS

Diversion of the normal outflow of urine through the bladder may be required in congenital defects such as exstrophy of the bladder and spastic paraplegia, in advanced tuberculosis of the bladder and for certain vesical tumours. Three methods are available.

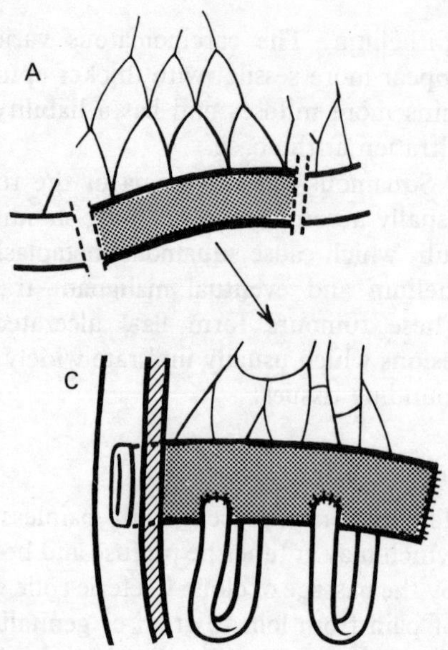

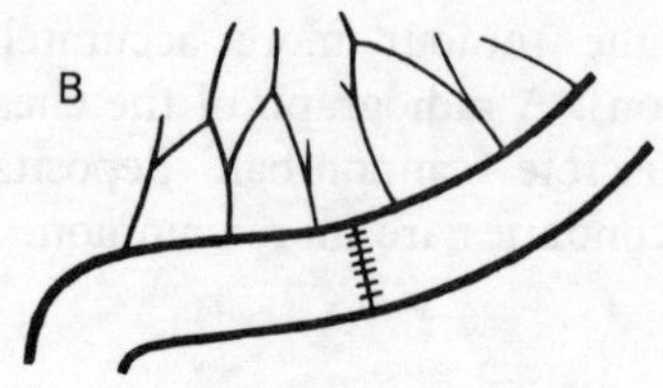

Fig. 22.8 Uretero-ileostomy. **A.** The length of ileum is isolated. **B.** Intestinal continuity is restored. **C.** The ureters are implanted into the ileum which leads through the abdominal wall.

Uretero-sigmoidostomy involves implantation of both ureters into the sigmoid colon where urine collects before being voided per rectum.

Uretero-ileostomy necessitates construction of an *ileal conduit*; this is a short loop of ileum removed from continuity with the bowel and closed at one end. Urine collects therein and passes into an ileostomy appliance attached to the abdominal wall (Fig. 22.8).

Cutaneous ureterostomy may be performed in the iliac fossa as a loop procedure in children to deflate obstructed ureters or as a cutaneous end ureterostomy to relieve obstruction in the younger age group.

The method using sigmoid colon is preferred in some countries where a uretero-ileal conduit with the necessary appliance is not acceptable, and in patients who refuse to wear the appliance, and may be preferred in elderly patients, or in palliative procedures because of easier post-operative management. It has several disadvantages, in particular a liability to urinary infection and metabolic disturbances resulting from absorption of urinary electrolytes by the colonic mucosa. These factors may together lead to a condition of *hyperchloraemic acidosis* which the already damaged kidneys are unable to correct without vigorous medical treatment. Hyperchloraemic acidosis is characterised by marked muscular weakness and vomiting. The patient appears ill, with a rapid pulse and hypotension. The serum chloride and urea are elevated, due to reabsorption in the colon, and the bicarbonate is low. Treatment requires continuous drainage of the sigmoid colon by rectal tube, antibiotic therapy and intravenous administration of sodium lactate. It may be possible to prevent further attacks by encouraging the patient to void frequently and administering alkalis regularly. A lax anal sphincter particularly in the elderly may pose a problem of incontinence of urine. Some of these problems may be overcome by forming a 'bladder' from a rectal stump and bringing out an end sigmoid colostomy in the left iliac fossa.

Uretero-ileostomy requires an ileostomy appliance, but is free from the complications of the previous method. It is therefore preferable in young patients and in those who already have renal damage.

In children with *spina bifida* problems needing a urinary conduit, it is often easier to isolate a loop of redundant sigmoid colon, transplant the ureters into the sigmoid conduit and restore bowel continuity.

FURTHER READING

Blandy, J. P. (Ed.) (1976). *Urology*. Oxford: Blackwell.
Newsam, J. E. (1982). Genito-urinary surgery. In *Essential Surgical Practice*. Eds. Cuschieri, A., Giles, G. R and Moossa, A. R. Bristol: Wright.

23

Bladder and urethra

BLADDER

Physiology

The function of the bladder and urethra may be assessed to some extent by symptomatology, clinical examination, static radiography and endoscopy but its functional evaluation is far better served by urodynamic measurement. The clinical use of the detrusor pressure during filling of the bladder through a small intra-urethral catheter, its response to coughing, change of posture and during voiding can be coupled with the flow rate measurement.

Synchronous evaluation can be performed radiologically by ciné cystourethrography. The urethral pressure profile is a graphical record of pressure within the urethra at successive points along its length. For the maintenance of continence the intra-urethral pressure must be greater than intra-vesical pressure. A knowledge of the urethral closure pressure is useful in testing patients with sphincter weakness and in assessing the level of obstruction in those patients with neurogenic disturbances. Several sphincteric mechanisms exist, including the so-called internal sphincter at the normal bladder neck. The normal opening of the bladder neck is related to detrusor and trigonal function. Other important mechanisms for the maintenance of urinary continence are the total intrinsic urethral resistance mechanism and the extrinsic 'striated muscle' sphincter. Most of these investigations require sophisticated apparatus coupling catheters to pressure transducers, but quite simple estimation of the urinary flow rate may be achieved. Normal flow rate is between 20 and 25 ml per second with a detrusor pressure of approximately 50 cm of water.

Neurogenic disturbances of micturition

The spinal reflex centre controlling the act of micturition lies in the second, third and fourth sacral segments, at the level of the twelfth thoracic and first lumbar vertebrae. Both motor and sensory arcs pass in the pelvic splanchnic nerves to the detrusor muscle and urethral sphincters. Neurogenic disturbance of micturition may follow congenital lesions *spina bifida* and *sacral agenesis* and acquired lesions *traumatic paraplegia*, *spinal tumour*, *disseminated sclerosis*, and *tabes dorsalis*. Overflow incontinence, urinary infection and bilateral hydronephrosis, with or without stone formation, are frequent complications.

The level and type of cord damage influences the outcome. In traumatic paraplegia, the bladder is at first paralysed and atonic for several weeks (**spinal shock**). If the lesion is above twelfth thoracic level, the spinal reflex centre, being below this, may then resume activity, producing an **automatic bladder.** This enables a male patient to remain dry, wearing a urinal and initiating reflex emptying of the bladder by some sensory stimulus such as stroking the thighs. When the cord lesion involves the sacral segments, as occurs in cauda equina damage, the reflex centre is unable to function and an **autonomous bladder** results. Although there is a large residual urine, passive emptying can sometimes be produced by exerting pressure directly over the bladder.

During the stage of spinal shock catheterisation is necessary and a fine plastic catheter and aseptic technique eliminates infection. Patients with automatic and autonomous bladders can often manage well after training and practice. Permanent catheter drainage is undesirable. A male patient is better off with a reflex or expressible bladder, but if this cannot be managed, continuous incontinence is acceptable into a penile incontinence appliance and bag. Perurethral resection of the bladder neck or division of the external urethral sphincter may be necessary to reduce the outflow resistance in a chronically distended bladder. In females intermittent self-catheterisation on a twice-daily basis is a useful technique in dealing with chronically distended bladders. Diversion of urine to an ileostomy bag (uretero-ileostomy) is indicated in progressive hydronephrosis with renal failure, severe vesicoureteric reflux, intractable pyelonephritis and continuous incontinence in women.

Congenital exstrophy of the bladder

This is a congenital abnormality in which the anterior wall of the bladder fails to close. In the complete form the total mucous membrane is exposed, in the lower part of which the two ureteric orifices continually leak urine. The child is persistently wet and smells of ammoniacal urine. In addition the pubic symphysis is usually widely separated, causing an ungainly, waddling gait. Epispadias is also present and there may be inguinal herniae. As in most severe congenital defects, other organs such as the heart and kidneys may be abnormal, and an imperforate anus may be present. Treatment should be carried out at about four years of age. The ureters are implanted into the sigmoid colon or an isolated ileal loop (ileal conduit); the mucosa of the bladder is then removed and the ventral hernia closed.

Traumatic rupture of the bladder

Rupture of the bladder occurs from direct violence or as a complication of fracture of the pelvis. The rent may be intraperitoneal or extraperitoneal; the latter is more common. Combined rupture of the bladder and urethra occurs in 20 per cent of patients sustaining urological damage with fracture of the pelvis. Extravasated urine from an injured bladder or urethra is relatively harmless for 24 hours, if the urine is not infected, thus providing ample time for resuscitation and treatment of other major injuries, according to their priority.

Intraperitoneal rupture occurs when the bladder is full. It may occur after trauma and is a rare complication of cystoscopy or instrumentation. The tear is in the fundus of the bladder, from which urine escapes into the general peritoneal cavity, resulting in signs of diffuse peritonitis. Treatment entails immediate repair, via the peritoneal cavity, leaving an indwelling urethral catheter.

Extraperitoneal rupture is an occasional complication of fractures of the pelvis and results in extravasation into the prevesical space. There is failure to pass urine and a tender swelling is produced above the pubis which may later extend up the anterior abdominal wall; the pulse rate rises more rapidly than in intraperitoneal rupture.

The bladder should be explored and in view of the frequency with which injury is associated with a ruptured urethra, suprapubic catheter drainage is advisable for three weeks. This should be followed by a urethrogram and panendoscopy to confirm that the urethra is normal, thus allowing urine to be passed spontaneously after spigotting the suprapubic tube.

Diverticula of the bladder

Pathology

The majority are of the 'pulsion' variety, as the result of obstruction at the neck of the bladder. Rarely a congenital form related to the urethra or a 'traction' variety secondary to pelvic cellulitis may occur. The commonest type occurs in idiopathic bladder-neck obstruction, but it may complicate senile enlargement of the prostate, or other causes of urethral outflow obstruction such as stricture or urethral valves.

The diverticulum when large is often single and the opening usually found lateral to the ureteric orifice. It is presumed that there is an associated weakness of the bladder wall at this site in those cases where a diverticulum develops. The lesion is composed of a pouch of mucous membrane surrounded by fibrous tissue but without a muscle coat; it is therefore unable to empty by its own contraction. Perivesical fat often adheres to the outer wall. Gradual increase in size may obstruct the lower end of the ureter and the diverticulum may reach similar dimensions to that of the bladder, particularly during micturition. Disturbance of the vesico-ureteric mechanism allows reflux of urine on micturition to occur in some cases. Complications include (*a*) infection, (*b*) stone formation, (*c*) carcinoma and (*d*) hydronephrosis.

Clinical features

Most diverticula occur in males between 50 and 70 years of age. Unless complicated they are symptomless and are generally recognised during the investigation of intractable cystitis or bladder-neck obstruction. Rarely the phenomenon of 'double micturition' may take place. This is due to distension of the pouch during urination as the result of contraction of the bladder. When the latter relaxes urine escapes from the diverticulum and may be voided. Frequency, haematuria, backache or pyrexia may occur as a result of a complication.

Investigations

Examination of the urine may show pus cells and organisms and a radiograph may demonstrate calculi in the diverticulum, although these are uncommon. An intravenous urogram may reveal hydronephrosis and the bladder films show that the organ fails to empty completely. The diverticula are often visible in these cystograms, but catheter cystography is necessary when renal excretion of the medium is poor (Fig. 23.1). Cystoscopy reveals the orifice of a diverticulum, which appears as a dark, punched-out cavity, which cannot be illuminated with the cystoscope. An obstruction of the neck of the bladder by a median bar or occasionally by an enlarged prostate is also seen.

Treatment

The diverticulum should be excised and any cause of obstruction removed at the same time. Small diverticula can be left untreated.

Cystitis

Acute cystitis

Inflammation of the bladder may be chemical, as the result of accidental instillation of solutions into

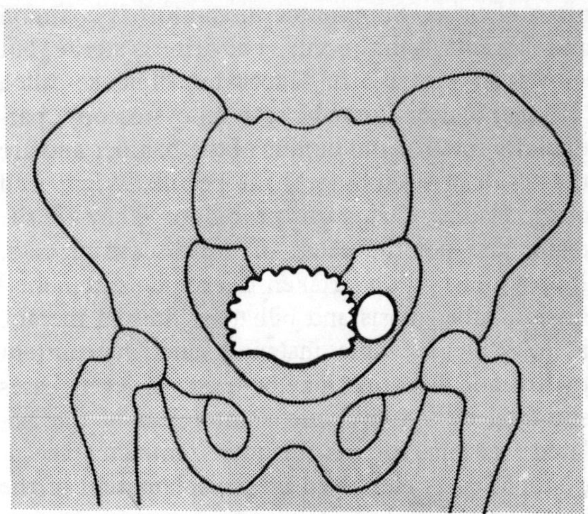

Fig. 23.1 Diverticulum of bladder demonstrated on cystogram which also shows trabeculation of bladder wall

the bladder, or bacterial. The latter type is nearly always accompanied by infection of the upper part of the urinary tract. The basic treatment of bacterial cystitis is similar to that described for pyelonephritis (p. 283). It is important to isolate the organisms in the urine and determine their sensitivities, but with severe symptoms co-trimoxazole—to which 98 per cent of the organisms are sensitive—nalidixic acid or ampicillin can be commenced. These agents should be continued for at least 10 days and a high fluid intake encouraged. Slow resolution, persistent symptoms or recurrence after adequate treatment are all indications to look for an underlying cause such as a lesion higher up the urinary tract, intravesical pathology such as a cystocele, diverticulum, vesico-intestinal fistula or carcinoma and obstructive lesions of the urethra at all ages. Bladder irrigations may be required when excessive amounts of pus or inflammatory debris accumulate. Suitable solutions for this purpose are 1 : 5000 aqueous Hibitane and instillations of Noxyflex.

Chronic interstitial cystitis (Hunner's ulcer)

This uncommon complaint is seen in middle-aged women in whom it may be a type of auto-immune reaction. There is marked frequency of micturition, with urgency, and the passage of small volumes of urine. Suprapubic discomfort is common and haematuria may occur. The urine is sterile, but shows an increase in leucocytes. The so-called 'Hunner's ulcers' may be seen on cystoscopy, particularly towards the fundus of the bladder and are the result of stretching of the peculiar, rigid wall of the bladder during this procedure. They are the result and not the cause of the disease process. Biopsy must be undertaken to exclude carcinoma-in-situ, tuberculosis and bilharzia. Steroid therapy is of value in some instances and intermittent hydrostatic dilatation may be tried. In severe cases sub-total cystectomy with anastomosis of the isolated caecum to the bladder remnant (caecocystoplasty) is employed or transplantation of the ureters to an ileal conduit.

Schistosomiasis

Vesical schistosomiasis is endemic in many tropical and subtropical regions (East Africa, Egypt, Brazil and the Far East). It is due to parasitic infestation of the perivesical veins by adult worms of *Schistosoma haematobium*. Ulceration of the ova through the bladder mucosa produces painless haematuria, but long-standing disease may lead to fibrosis and calcification, and occasionally to carcinoma of the bladder.

Diagnosis depends upon the finding of the characteristic ova, which are oval, with a terminal spine, in the centrifuged deposit of the urine. The infestation responds to treatment with sodium antimony tartrate, which although most efficient does produce toxic side-effects and treatment in hospital is advisable. Ambilhar is a very effective drug. Contracted bladder and severe ureteric disease may respond dramatically with this therapy.

Tuberculosis of the bladder

The bladder lesions are always secondary to tuberculous infection of the kidney and ureter, but are important because they produce symptoms from an early stage. There is marked urinary frequency, particularly by night, and haematuria is common. The urine shows 'sterile pyuria' and tubercle bacilli can be isolated (Renal Tuberculosis, p. 284). Cystoscopy reveals oedema or a group of greyish tubercles around the ureteric orifices; superficial ulcers later appear on the posterior wall of the bladder, characteristically separated by areas of normal mucosa. Advanced disease may produce shortening of the ureter, whilst fibrosis also causes the bladder to become small and contracted. The treatment of urinary tuberculosis has been discussed (p. 286). A small, contracted bladder is difficult to treat and may require plastic enlargement or even transplantation of the ureters.

TUMOURS OF THE BLADDER

Aetiology

Although the cause of most tumours in the bladder is still unknown, prolonged contact with various aromatic chemicals can predispose to neoplasia. In such cases the growth is due to excretion of carcinogens, mainly β-naphthylamine and benzidine, in the urine, these having been previously absorbed over a long period from the skin or food. Workers in the dye industry and those exposed to antioxidants used in rubber processes are susceptible. The majority of patients give no such history and neoplasia appears to be due to an inherent instability of mucosal growth. This produces a tendency towards the development of multiple tumours in the bladder or to recurrence of a previously treated growth. Endogenous carcinogens may develop such as tryptophan metabolites or perhaps by the action of the enzyme β-glucuronidase converting ortho-aminophenols into carcinogenic agents. Non-enzymatic degradation may also take place. Cigarette smoking, schistosomiasis, chronic inflammation, exstrophy and stone are all irritant causes of bladder tumour.

Pathology

Papillary tumours include the so-called 'transitional-cell' papilloma, which is often regarded as a low-grade carcinoma and the malignant tumours which may be divided into (*a*) transitional-cell carcinoma, (*b*) squamous-cell carcinoma and (*c*) adenocarcinoma.

The commonest lesion is the transitional-cell papillary tumour (papilloma). This has a rather delicate structure, consisting of a cluster of vascular fronds, covered by transitional epithelium. The fronds are either long, floating processes or short, squat and nodular. Papillomas are frequently multiple, and generally develop just above and lateral to the ureteric orifices.

The gross structure of malignant bladder tumours may be (*a*) papillary, (*b*) nodular, (*c*) ulcerated and (*d*) flat and infiltrating. Any variety may be altered by necrosis, ulceration or secondary infection.

The extent of macroscopic spread of a malignant bladder tumour is important, since it influences the choice of treatment. It may take place directly through the wall of the bladder into the perivesical tissues; along lymphatics to the paravesical lymph nodes and by the blood stream to the liver, bones and lungs.

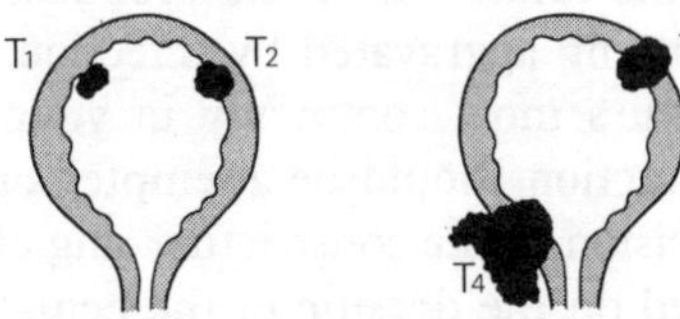

Fig. 23.2 Classification of bladder tumours

The majority of bladder tumours are composed of transitional-celled epithelium, but due to metaplasia, squamous-cell carcinoma (epithelioma) and adenocarcinoma are at times encountered. The degree of differentiation is important in predicting tumour behaviour, since the degree of malignancy varies greatly. Ulceration and infection frequently occur together with an associated cystitis. Obstruction of the internal urinary meatus or of the ureteric orifices may cause hydronephrosis. Pyelonephritis may supervene and lead to renal failure and death.

Clinical features

Men are affected about three times more commonly than women and most cases occur between 50 and 70 years of age. The common initial symptom in all types of bladder tumour is painless haematuria and this is present in over 90 per cent of cases. Frequency and pain on micturition follow later, due to urinary infection. In advanced cases there is strangury, with a constant desire to void and the frequent passage of small, turbid or blood-stained specimens. Infiltration of the sacral plexus by tumour may produce severe pain, both local and referred. Occasionally there may be acute retention of urine, when suprapubic drainage is to be avoided as the tumour can extend on to the anterior abdominal wall.

Physical signs are generally absent in the earlier stages, but the growth may be palpable on bimanual examination, when the degree of fixity should be noted. In later stages gross anaemia is often present, and fistulae into the rectum or vagina and cachexia are at times seen terminally.

Investigations

A mid-stream or catheter specimen of urine should be examined for red blood cells, pus and organisms and cytological examination is helpful. An intravenous urogram may help to demonstrate further proximal tumours or obstruction of the lower end of the ureter by the vesical growth. Alteration of bladder contour may be noted giving the 'bite deformity'. Cystoscopy remains the most important aid in diagnosis and also enables a biopsy to be undertaken. A bimanual examination should follow to assess the presence of a mass and its mobility. The primary tumour (T) can thus be classified: T.1s—pre-invasive carcinoma or carcinoma-in-situ; T.1—tumour not extending beyond lamina propria; T.2—invasion of superficial muscle; T.3a—invasion of deep muscle, b—extension through bladder wall; T.4—tumour fixed or invading neighbouring structures (Fig. 23.2). An attempt may also be made to assess lymph node involvement and metastatic spread where appropriate, and histopathological grading into low grade, medium grade and high grade malignancy is also helpful in assessing prognosis.

Treatment

Where the disease is localised and confined to the mucosa (T.1) *endoscopic diathermy* is to be preferred. Cystoscopy at three-monthly intervals is initially required with later less frequent but regular follow-up, because of the risk of fresh tumours or recurrence. Where the tumour is limited to superficial muscle (T.2) there is a small place for the implantation of *radioactive gold* or *tantalum wire*, generally at open operation, but as in T.3 tumours external irradiation is used. *Partial cystectomy* is employed for local tumours, without any significant infiltration, and preferably towards the fundus of the bladder. *Total cystectomy* with ureteric transplantation is generally reserved for those failing to respond to radiotherapy or those recurring after its use. Multifocal tumours may also need radical surgery, and significant haematuria recurring after radiotherapy may also require cystectomy to control the haemorrhage. Intravesical chemotherapy using ethoglucid and doxorubicin reduces the incidence of recurrence of superficial tumours if instilled at the time of cystoscopy or on the day following. Multifocal tumour not responding to endoscopic diathermy may likewise be brought under control by intravesical chemotherapy. In such cases it is important to consider tumour developing in the upper urinary tract.

URETHRA

Hypospadias

In this common congenital abnormality the external meatus lies ventral to its normal position. The opening is usually near the frenum ('glandular' hypospadias), but may lie anywhere along the under surface of the shaft ('penile' or 'perineal' hypospadias). There is usually a blind dimple marking the normal position of the meatus and the penis may be curved downwards.

No treatment is required for the glandular type, but straightening of the penis by freeing the fibrotic corpus spongiosum is necessary in the other forms. It is generally undertaken between the ages of one and two years and followed by a plastic procedure for the construction of a new urethra between the ages of five and seven years.

Epispadias

This is more serious and often associated with maldevelopment of the urethral sphincters. The meatus lies on the dorsum of the penis. Plastic surgery is necessary to construct a satisfactory urethra.

Phimosis

This is nearly always an acquired condition, as the result of balanitis or ammoniacal burns of the prepuce during infancy. Advice is often sought about the advisability of circumcision. In general, if the prepuce can be retracted far enough to expose the urethral meatus, the skin will eventually become loose enough to retract completely as the infant grows, and treatment is unnecessary. The few filmy adhesions, which are often present between the glans and the prepuce, always disappear and there is no medical necessity for operation in these patients. Circumcision should be strictly avoided in the presence of ammoniacal dermatitis, since the exposed meatus will become excoriated with the development of a meatal ulcer, possibly leading to a meatal stricture.

Paraphimosis occurs from forcible retraction of a tight prepuce over the glans penis. Congestion then prevents reduction of the prepuce, the condition becoming aggravated by infection and oedema. It occurs most commonly in young adults. Manual reduction should be attempted and, if too painful, incision of the constricting ring of prepuce is performed on the dorsum of the penis. Circumcision should be undertaken when infection has subsided.

Injury

Rupture of the anterior urethra is usually the result of a fall astride a bar, with tearing of the bulbous urethra against the bony pubic arch. This produces bruising and tenderness in the perineum and the patient is unable to void. Later extravasation of urine into the scrotum, penis, groins and anterior abdominal wall may occur. Rather than attempt urethral catheterisation, converting a possible partial rupture into a complete one, suprapubic drainage should be established as the bladder distends. After two or three weeks' drainage a urethrogram should be performed. Early surgical interference with anterior urethral injuries may be precipitated by distension of the tissues by haematoma, but this adds the inevitable risk of infection and aggravating subsequent stricture formation.

Rupture of the posterior urethra may complicate a severe fracture of the pelvis. The membranous urethra is an elastic structure which can elongate considerably before it will tear and therefore partial rupture is more likely than a complete one in which the prostate, attached to the pubic symphysis by the puboprostatic ligaments, is torn away from the urethra at its attachment to the perineal membrane. After this injury stricture is bound to result. The condition resembles extraperitoneal rupture of the bladder, and is seen in similar types of injury, but differs from it in that the bladder sphincter remains shut, so that extravasation is uncommon. The patient is unable to pass more than a few drops of blood and attempts to pass a catheter should not be made as this will introduce infection and may convert a partial rupture into a complete one.

Treatment is not urgent in suspected rupture of the bladder or urethra. Providing the urine is sterile there will be no great risk of pelvic cellulitis. When a clinical diagnosis is made a suprapubic cystostomy is performed, a finger being passed inside the bladder to confirm that the prostate is not floating. After three weeks the urethra is inspected with a panendoscope. Repair of the urethra may be necessary at this stage, but when partial rupture has occurred the instrument passes easily. Urethral stricture is common, necessitating regular dilatation and if necessary urethroplasty.

Urethritis

Inflammation of the urethra may be (1) **Bacterial**: (*a*) *gonococcal*; (*b*) *non-specific*, due to *Esch. coli*, *Staph. aureus* or *B. proteus*. (2) **Viral** (**non-specific urethritis**).

Both gonococcal and viral forms are usually acquired by intercourse. The non-specific bacterial variety results from instrumentation and is a common complication of an indwelling urethral catheter, particularly of large calibre.

Clinical features

A muco-purulent urethral discharge is accompanied by a burning pain on micturition. Symptoms may be severe and associated with retention of urine. Diagnosis is made by bacteriological examination of stained films and cultures of the urethral exudate. This persents no difficulty in the bacterial varieties of urethritis. Viral urethritis is probably due to a pleuropneumonia-like organism, so that stained films and culture are apparently sterile. *Trichomonas* infection should be considered. The urine, like the urethral discharge, is liable to contain 'sterile' pus. Co-existent syphilis must always be excluded by serological tests.

Treatment

The appropriate antibiotic should be administered and the patient encouraged to pass urine frequently. In gonococcal infection penicillin is usually adequate, but sensitivity must be determined. Viral urethritis may respond to tetracycline and erythromycin. *Trichomonas* infection should be treated with a 7-day course of metronidazole. Non-specific infection due to an indwelling catheter is mainly prevented by using latex or polythene, which should be of the smallest diameter commensurate with efficient drainage. The urethral meatus should be protected by a sterile dressing, which is changed daily.

Complications

1. *Urethral stricture* only occurs in neglected cases or following prolonged urethral catheter drainage.

2. *Reiter's syndrome* consists of intractable abacterial urethritis, bilateral conjunctivitis and iritis, polyarthritis, dysentery and skin lesions (keratodermia blennorrhagica). Treatment is often unsatisfactory.

Urethral syndrome

In the second and third decades and in the post-menopausal period, many women present with recurrent frequency of micturition and dysuria, the so-called 'urethral syndrome'. There are many contributory factors and careful attention to hygiene, treatment of pathological vaginal discharges and advice on technique in intercourse may help. Senile vaginal changes can be improved by small doses of oestrogen or local hormone cream. Many patients achieve relief by urethral dilatation or urethrotomy.

Urethral stricture

1. Congenital stricture

Pin-hole meatus.
Posterior urethral valves.

Both conditions may cause chronic urinary obstruction in infancy, with bilateral hydronephrosis and uraemia.

2. *Traumatic stricture.*

Injuries to the urethra.
Following prostatectomy; indwelling urethral catheters are often responsible.
Following urethral instrumentation at all ages.
Following hypospadias repair.

3. *Inflammatory stricture.*

Chronic gonorrhoea.
Urinary tuberculosis.
Non-specific urethritis.

The narrowing is generally in the posterior urethra.

4. *Neoplastic stricture.*

Carcinoma of the urethra is rare. It is a squamous-cell lesion of high malignancy.

Clinical features

A previous history of infection or of trauma may be obtained. There is increasing difficulty of micturition, with deterioration in the stream, and finally dribbling. This may be complicated by symptoms due to (*a*) renal failure, (*b*) urinary infection, (*c*) extravasation of urine, (*d*) periurethral abscess, (*e*) urethral fistula or (*f*) acute retention of urine. Bleeding and fistulae particularly occur in the neoplastic type.

The diagnosis rests upon urethrography and when possible micturating cysto-urethrography, with the injection of contrast medium such as diodine along the urethra. It can be confirmed by panendoscopy.

Treatment

Repeated dilatation is adequate for the majority of cases, the urethra being dilated up to its normal calibre (about 25 Charrière), initially once per month and later at gradually increased intervals until the affected area stabilises. Internal urethrotomy is the treatment of choice in established strictures, being performed under direct vision. The stricture may be catheterised with a filiform bougie and in this stricture the affected area endoscopically incised throughout its whole length at the '12 o'clock' position. Localised strictures may be excised. Strictures which are difficult to dilate or require frequent dilatation are treated by *urethroplasty*. The operation is staged, after excision of the stricture, and scrotal skin inlays are used. The malignant lesion necessitates amputation of the penis or wide excision and ureteric transplantation in the female.

TUMOURS OF THE PENIS

Benign skin tumours (papilloma, fibrolipoma or angioma) occasionally occur. The common malignant tumour is carcinoma (epithelioma).

Carcinoma of the penis

The usual macroscopic lesions are the *papillary type* which grows slowly and the *malignant ulcer*, with rolled edges and an indurated base. Histologically the growth is a squamous-cell carcinoma, but various degrees of cellular differentiation occur. The methods of spread are direct infiltration, lymphatic and blood stream. Local infiltration is most marked in the ulcerative variety; the corpora cavernosa become indurated and the distal part of the penis is eventually destroyed. Lymphatic spread takes place to the superficial inguinal and iliac lymph nodes, usually on both sides. Bloodstream metastasis to liver, lungs and bones is less common.

Clinical features

The majority present with a warty growth on the glans or with a grossly infected, sloughing discharge from beneath the prepuce. The inguinal lymph nodes are usually enlarged through infection, or due to metastasis. The differential diagnosis is from simple balanitis, traumatic ulcer, Queyrat's erythroplasia, syphilitic chancre and benign papilloma. A biopsy must always be taken.

Treatment

The most satisfactory method is partial or total amputation of the penis. Where lymph node enlargement is thought to be due to infection it is justifiable to wait for this to settle. Lymphograms may help in the assessment of tumour involvement of lymph nodes. When involvement is present bilateral inguinal block dissection is performed. Regular follow-up is essential, particularly if a conservative policy is adopted towards inguinal nodes. Irradiation is used when the histology is anaplastic and when the patient declines surgery. The local reactions are severe and painful and there is a high incidence of late irradiation necrosis and external meatal stenosis. Bleomycin, an anti-cancer agent, is an alternative where surgery is refused.

Peyronie's disease

This is an unusual condition, also known as 'plastic induration of the penis'. The cause is unknown, but it is probably comparable with Dupuytren's contracture of the palmar fascia. A plaque of dense fibrous tissue appears in the tunica albuginea of one corpus cavernosum, on the dorsum of the penis. This produces curvature of the organ during erection (*chordee*). Treatment is usually unnecessary, but local injections of hydrocortisone may cause improvement. Plastic surgery is occasionally employed.

FURTHER READING

Ashken, M. H. (1982). *Urinary Diversion*. New York: Springer.

Brown, R. B. (1982). Genito-urinary trauma. In *Clinical Urology Illustrated*. Ed. Brown, R. B. Australia: Adis Press.

Riddle, P. R. (1976). Carcinoma of the bladder. *Brit. J. Hosp. Med.* 16, 468–78.

Riddle, P. R. (1981). Urothelial tumours. *Hospital Update* 7, 909–20.

24

Prostate

SIMPLE ENLARGEMENT OF THE PROSTATE

Pathology

The glandular enlargement, which occurs in the majority of men over the age of 40 years, takes place in both lateral and middle lobes. Growth is mainly upwards because of the resistant perineal membrane, and the effects are primarily due to urinary obstruction. Glandular hyperplasia and overgrowth of fibromuscular tissue result in the formation of dense nodules, the peripheral parts of the gland becoming compressed as a false capsule. In some cases hyperplasia of the fibrous tissue similarly results in obstruction, but without glandular enlargement, producing a small fibrous prostate. Lateral lobe enlargement allows a recess of stagnant urine to develop behind the prostate (Fig. 24.1A) and causes lengthening of the prostatic urethra, which may also be flattened from side to side; angulation of the posterior urethra is likewise increased. The middle lobe tends to enlarge into the bladder, the posterior lip of the internal meatus is pushed anteriorly and a post-prostatic recess forms.

The effect of prostatic obstruction upon the bladder is one of gradual hypertrophy and trabeculation. This initially overcomes the obstruction but later dilatation follows, allowing urine to remain in the bladder after micturition. Infection of residual urine is common and calculi may form. Reflux takes place up the ureters with dilatation and loss of contractile power. The bladder pressure is then transmitted to the renal pelves which dilate producing bilateral hydronephrosis (Fig. 24.1B), destruction of renal papillae and loss of renal substance. The mechanism permitting the kidney to retain and deal with salt and water is lost, with marked sodium and water depletion, acidosis, anaemia and, when severe, death from uraemia.

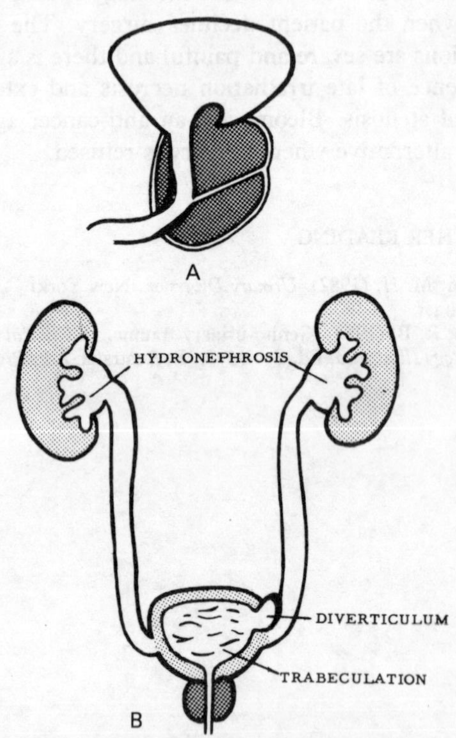

Fig. 24.1 Benign hypertrophy of prostate. **A.** Lateral lobe enlargement producing elongation and angulation of urethra and middle lobe enlargement protruding into the bladder. **B.** The effects on bladder and kidneys.

Clinical features

Mechanical disturbance at the bladder neck and to the urethral outflow causes increased urinary frequency and difficulty with voiding. Frequency is especially troublesome at night, with repeated passage of small quantities, and is particularly characteristic of middle lobe enlargement. Difficulties in micturition include delay in starting, a poor or intermittent stream and dribbling at the end of the act. Haematuria occurs, but is less common. General symptoms, which include loss of appetite, headache, thirst, constipation and lethargy, are frequent and result from the gradual onset of chronic renal failure. A slow development of local symptoms may attract little attention until the general effects become evident.

Examination may indicate signs of renal failure in the dryness and colour of the tongue and skin. Cardiac enlargement or hypertension may also be present. Abdominal examination may reveal a distended bladder or enlarged kidneys. Rectal palpation demonstrates the size and consistency of lateral lobe enlargement, although the former bears little relationship to the severity of symptoms which are mainly due to urethral obstruction. The gland has a firm rubbery feel and the median groove can usually be distinguished. Asymmetrical enlargement may be evident and the looseness of the overlying rectal mucosa in benign hypertrophy is apparent. There is no sign of prostatic enlargement on digital examination when symptoms are solely due to middle lobe obstruction.

Complications

1. *Urinary infection*. Cystitis is common, producing painful, frequent micturition often with haematuria. Acute retention may be precipitated and is liable to recur until the obstruction is relieved.

2. *Acute retention of urine*. This is extremely painful. There is generally a previous history of difficulty and frequency, but the sudden final episode may follow over-distension of the bladder from excessive drinking or voluntary withholding of micturition. The general condition is usually good. The bladder is easily palpable and is both tense and tender.

3. *Chronic retention of urine*. There is generally little or no pain, since the increase in residual urine takes place gradually over many months. The main symptom is urinary frequency, but particularly during sleep some urine may dribble away (overflow incontinence). The general condition may remain good but with gross renal damage pallor and listlessness may be evident. Examination of the abdomen reveals a large bladder, frequently reaching to the level of the umbilicus. Such a swelling is soft, often asymmetrical and is not tender. It should be distinguished from other tumours in the lower abdomen by a fluid consistency, dullness to percussion and an inability to feel the lower limit. If hydronephrosis is present the kidneys may be palpable.

4. *Stone formation*. Phosphatic calculi frequently develop in the bladder in the presence of infection or there may be urate stones. In either case symptoms are unusual, because the calculi tend to lie in the recess behind the elevated trigonal area.

5. *Diverticula of the bladder* may complicate simple enlargement of the prostate, although they are more commonly seen in idiopathic bladder-neck obstruction. By impairing the force of contraction they further impede emptying of the bladder, leading to the early onset of chronic retention of urine.

Investigations

The urine should be examined bacteriologically for evidence of infection. The blood urea, serum creatinine and electrolytes should be determined and an intravenous urogram obtained to demonstrate any associated hydronephrosis. Post-evacuation urography indicates the amount of residual urine in the bladder and is to be preferred to measurement by catheterisation which may introduce infection. The bladder film may also show a filling defect in the lower part due to the enlarged prostate. An important observation is to watch the patient pass water. A more objective measurement of urine flow rate can be obtained by means of a flowmeter. Panendoscopy and cystoscopy should always be performed to demonstrate intravesical prostatic enlargement or associated urethral and bladder pathology and are usually performed immediately prior to surgery. Full urodynamic assessment is necessary where detrusor instability is suspected and the presenting symptoms are of increased frequency of micturition with a normal flow. Prostatectomy will not help such patients.

Differential diagnosis

Idiopathic bladder-neck obstruction produces similar symptoms, but occurs in younger men (25 to 40 years), and the prostate feels normal on rectal examination. *Urethral strictures* can usually be distinguished by a previous history of trauma or urethritis and confirmed by urethrography. *Carcinoma of the prostate* is suggested by a short history of obstruction, and the gland feels craggy, hard and irregular. *Prostatic calculi* occasionally produce obstructive symptoms; they may give rise to a peculiar gravelly sensation on digital palpation, and are invariably radio-opaque. *Neurogenic lesions* affecting the bladder, particularly multiple sclerosis or a prolapsed intervertebral disc, may be suspected from the history and abnormal neurological signs, and urodynamic studies may be invaluable. Late onset *diabetes* in the prostatic age group is a further cause of increased frequency of micturition.

Treatment

Surgical treatment is required for troublesome symptoms and for complications, such as acute retention of urine or renal damage.

Management of retention of urine

Acute retention

Treatment is urgent because of the severity of the pain. Catheterisation by an aseptic technique should be performed in hospital, a closed system of drainage being instituted through a self-retaining catheter and after the appropriate investigations followed within a few days by a prostatectomy. Where symptoms have been minimal prior to the acute episode, it is permissible to remove the catheter after drainage, but if normal micturition is not resumed further catheterisation and surgical treatment will be required. Suprapubic aspiration of the bladder using a long needle is to be preferred when there is delay in admitting a patient to hospital. Where urethral catheterisation proves extremely difficult or impossible, careful introduction of a suprapubic catheter with its associated trocar will give speedy relief. Suprapubic catheterisation is the preferred technique for bladder drainage in some units as urinary infection may be reduced and trauma to the urethra is averted.

Chronic retention

Treatment should preferably be delayed until the completion of a full examination and investigations. If renal function is satisfactory prostatectomy should then be performed, but as some degree of renal failure is usual, preliminary decompression is generally required. When not severe, urethral drainage for two to three weeks, using a self-retaining (*Foley*) or plastic catheter, should be carried out. A sterile dressing around the external meatus is essential and the tubing and plastic container must similarly be sterile and disposable. More pronounced renal drainage may require prolonged drainage for two to three months, a catheter of the silastic type being changed at six- to eight-week intervals. Suprapubic cystostomy is rarely necessary.

Initial decompression in chronic retention should be gradual, about 500 ml being removed every four hours until the bladder is empty. Rapid decompression is not dangerous in acute retention, but may cause bleeding from kidney or bladder in the chronic form.

Methods of prostatectomy

Open methods

Retropubic prostatectomy.
Transvesical prostatectomy.
Perineal prostatectomy.

All 'open' methods of prostatectomy depend upon on the enucleation of the hyperplastic nodules of the gland from the false capsule of compressed prostatic tissue. The approach to the gland varies in the different methods (Fig. 24.2). In the retrophic (Millin) operation the capsule is opened from in front, the nodules enucleated and the capsule resutured. This method has the advantage that micturition is re-established when the urethral catheter is taken out, before the fifth post-operative day. Most of the prostatic urethra is removed at the time of prostatectomy, but the resultant cavity eventually heals by the growth of epithelium from the neck of the bladder. In the transvesical method the bladder is opened and the prostate enucleated from above. It carries the disadvantage that suprapubic bladder drainage may be necessary and there is an increased risk of urinary incontinence. The perineal method is rarely performed as it may result in damage to the rectum or external sphincter of the bladder.

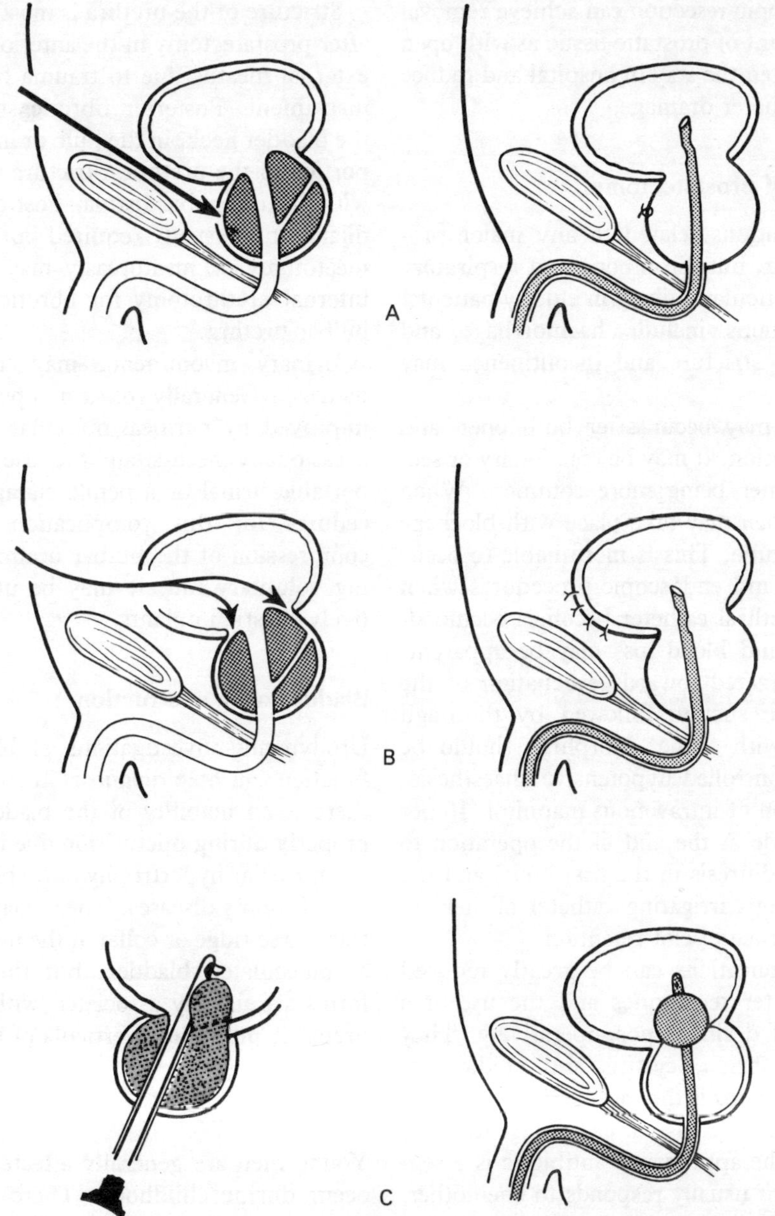

Fig. 24.2 Operations for prostatic hypertrophy showing approach and site of catheter drainage. **A.** Retropubic, with urethral catheter. **B.** Transvesical with urethral catheter. **C.** Perurethral (transurethral) resection of prostate gland.

Endoscopic methods

Transurethral diathermy resection is preferred to the cold punch technique of resection.

Endoscopic methods of prostatectomy are preferable for small fibrous glands, bladder neck obstruction and for carcinoma of the prostate causing obstruction. Transurethral resection of a benign prostate in amounts of 40 to 50 g of adenoma and extending out to the capsule can be performed under direct vision, securing good haemostasis and flushing the chippings from the bladder. Endoscopic resection can achieve removal of the same amount of prostatic tissue as with open techniques, shorten the stay in hospital and reduce the length of catheter drainage.

Complications of prostatectomy

General complications related to any major procedure may occur, but thrombotic and respiratory problems are particularly likely in elderly patients. Local complications include haemorrhage and infection, whilst stricture and incontinence may also result.

Haemorrhage may occur after both open and endoscopic operation. It may be reactionary or secondary, the former being more common. When severe, *clot retention* may take place with blockage of the drainage tube. This is more liable to occur after retropubic and endoscopic procedures when the narrower urethral catheter becomes occluded. Signs of shock and blood loss may be apparent. Treatment is directed towards evacuation of the clot by adequate suction followed by thorough bladder lavage with saline. Morphine should be administered. Controlled hypotensive anaesthesia, the administration of intravenous mannitol (10 per cent) or frusemide at the end of the operation to promote a good diuresis in the first hour, and the use of a continuous irrigating catheter all help to reduce the incidence of clot retention.

Infective complications can be greatly reduced by aseptic catheter techniques and the use of a closed system of drainage post-operatively. They include pyelonephritis, cystitis and epididymo-orchitis. *Pyelonephritis* is the most serious as it may accelerate any renal damage already present. Early treatment with the appropriate antibiotic is essential. Severe *cystitis* usually responds to chemotherapy but may necessitate re-introduction of a catheter to ensure adequate drainage and to permit bladder irrigation. The urine generally contains bacteria for several months after prostatectomy until healing of the prostatic bed is complete and the term 'cystitis' should only be used where there is severe frequency or pyuria. *Epididymo-orchitis* occurs as a result of regurgitation of infected urine into the vas from the prostatic bed and may be present pre-operatively. This sequel is largely eliminated if the vasa deferentia are divided at the time of prostatectomy.

Stricture of the urethra is most commonly found after prostatectomy in the anterior urethra near the external meatus due to trauma from a catheter or instrument. Posterior fibrotic strictures occur at the bladder neck, in the bulb or in the membranous portion of the urethra. Stricture may be associated with a suprapubic fistula. Post-operative urethral dilatation is usually required but in resistant cases meatotomy or meatoplasty may be necessary, or internal urethrotomy for fibrotic strictures in the bulbar urethra.

Urinary incontinence may follow sphincteric damage. Generally of a temporary nature and improved by perineal muscular exercises, it may occasionally necessitate the use of a permanent portable urinal or a penile clamp. Operative procedures for this complication are directed to compression of the bulbar urethra, but surrounding voluntary muscle may be utilised or alternatively silastic implants.

Bladder-neck obstruction

Urodynamic investigations of bladder neck dysfunction can help diagnosis in conditions in which there is an inability of the bladder neck to open properly during micturition due to (*a*) median bar, (*b*) muscular hypertrophy or (*c*) bladder neck fibrosis (Marion's disease). There may be a prominent transverse ridge or collar at the internal meatus and a trabeculated bladder, but the more advanced forms are usually associated with bilateral hydroureter or multiple diverticula of the bladder.

Clinical features

Young men are generally affected, although cases occur during childhood. There is usually a long history of difficulty of micturition, but infection or retention of urine is the common presenting symptom. Signs of obstruction similar to those of prostatic hypertrophy occur, but the gland is not found to be enlarged on rectal examination. The diagnosis is confirmed by the presence of a large residual urine and by the cystoscopic appearance. Intravenous urography may provide evidence of bladder outflow obstruction, but normal appearances cannot exclude it. Post-voiding residual urine, a thick-walled trabeculated bladder and the presence of diverticula or even associated hydronephrosis and hydroureter may be present, but many of these are late manifestations. Recording the flow rate is clearly a most important clinical finding of outflow obstruction but urodynamic assessment of both the detrusor function and the outflow pattern, combining flow rate studies with a micturating cysto-urethrogram, is of value. On occasions vesico-ureteric reflux when voiding and failure of opening of the bladder neck on micturition may be seen.

Treatment

The bladder neck should be incised by endoscopic diathermy incision or endoscopic resection performed. Large diverticula, when present, may require an open operation for their removal.

Acute prostatitis

The responsible organism is generally *Esch. coli* or the staphylococcus, less commonly the streptococcus or gonococcus. Infection may be blood borne or spread from the urethra or bladder. The condition may resolve or proceed to a prostatic abscess or chronic prostatitis. Such an abscess may burst into the urethra or bladder, or it may extend outside the capsule and rupture into the perineum or rectum.

Clinically there is frequency and painful micturition with occasional terminal haematuria. Difficulty in micturition or acute retention may occur. Perineal and rectal pain, malaise and pyrexia are encountered. On rectal examination an extremely tender prostate gland is found, with fluctuation when there is abscess formation.

Treatment consists of bed-rest and antibiotics, preferably when the sensitivity of the organism has been determined from examination of the urine. Catheterisation is required for acute retention and occasionally results in the rupture of an abscess. Drainage may be effected by endoscopic resection.

Chronic prostatitis

A persistent low grade inflammation with occasional exacerbations may follow acute prostatitis or appear without previous symptoms. There may be associated prostatic calculi, but it is unwise to ascribe symptoms to their presence. It may be due to immuno-active causes, and it is of value to check the urinary flow rate. Clinically there may be lassitude and persistent pain in the perineum, genitalia or inner aspect of the thigh. At times recurrent attacks of painful micturition, frequency and pyrexia may be noted. Rectal examination may reveal a firm or irregular prostate and calculi may be palpated or determined by radiography. Iritis or arthritis may be associated. Examination of the urine may reveal no abnormality except when there is an acute exacerbation when pus and organisms may be found but culture of the seminal fluid may help. Tuberculosis and neoplasia require exclusion by complete investigation. Antibiotic therapy may suffice to clear symptoms but perurethral resection may be required in resistant cases.

CARCINOMA OF THE PROSTATE

Pathology

Carcinoma of the prostate is the third commonest cancer occurring in men, being only surpassed by neoplasms of the lung and stomach. Although it may arise in any portion of the gland, in 75 per cent of cases it commences in the posterior lobe. It is a firm nodular tumour which invades at an early stage to become adherent to the surrounding structures, particularly the anterior rectal wall. Spread upwards and outwards involves the seminal vesicles producing the characteristic 'winging' felt on rectal examination. Sectioning of the growth gives a gritty sensation similar to breast cancer. Histologically it is an adenocarcinoma showing various degrees of differentiation, generally in a well-marked fibrous tissue stroma, although anaplastic forms occur.

Direct spread laterally and upwards into the pelvic cellular tissues is frequent and may cause obstruction of the iliac veins and peripheral oedema. Lymphatic spread is initially to the iliac and para-aortic nodes, but occasionally the inguinal group may be involved. Lymphatic obstruction may further contribute to oedema of the lower limbs. Blood stream spread occurs to liver and bones and sometimes produces skin nodules. Bony metastases occur in vertebra, pelvis, rib and femur and are frequently osteosclerotic. An important connection exists between the vertebral veins and those of the prostatic plexus. Involvement of the latter by spread from the posterior lobe accounts

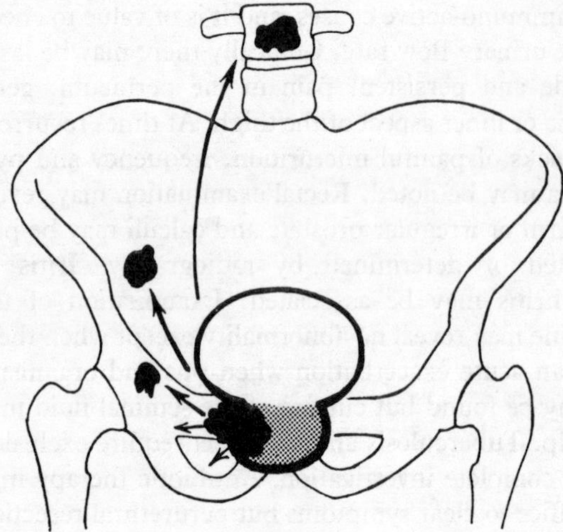

Fig. 24.3 The spread of carcinoma of the prostate locally and by the blood stream to bone

for an early appearance of osseous secondaries (Fig. 24.3).

Clinical features

The disease is most common between 60 and 85 years of age and is rare in men under 50 years. The history is usually shorter and more progressive than that of simple enlargement, but the symptoms of increased frequency, difficulty in micturition and sometimes painless haematuria are similar. Sacral sciatic or perineal pain is fairly common, due to infiltration of the sacral nerve roots. Both acute and chronic retention of urine may occur. Bilateral oedema of the lower limbs due to infiltration of the pelvic lymphatics is often seen. General symptoms are usually the result of bony metastases, which may produce a pathological fracture, occasionally paraplegia, or anaemia due to marrow replacement. The growth may be entirely symptomless and unsuspected areas of carcinoma are discovered in the histological examination of about 10 per cent of enlarged prostates removed by operation.

Examination may reveal pallor, skin nodules, oedema of the lower limbs, a palpable bladder or enlarged inguinal lymph nodes. More commonly the only physical signs are discovered on rectal examination, which usually reveals a craggy, irregular hardness of the prostate. The median groove may be obliterated, there may be fixation of the rectal mucosa, and palpable lateral spread may be noted outside the gland. In advanced disease the prostate feels fixed in the pelvis and there may be infiltration extending around the wall of the rectum. Occasionally the tumour lies in a portion not palpable on rectal examination or the primary lesion may be very small. Under these conditions the prostate may feel normal despite widespread metastases.

Investigations

In advanced disease, anaemia is common and primitive red blood cells may be seen in the stained blood film. Radiographs of the lungs, lumbar spine and pelvis may reveal metastases. The bony deposits are characteristically sclerotic, resembling Paget's disease, but osteolytic metastases also occur. Intravenous urography may reveal bilateral hydronephrosis. The serum acid phosphatase (formol stable) is raised above 3 King-Armstrong units in about 25 per cent of cases, but this only occurs when metastases are present and has little value in early diagnosis. The serum alkaline phosphatase is also raised when there are osseous metastases, but this is a non-specific effect of osteoblastic activity and also occurs in Paget's disease. Needle biopsy of the prostate through the perineum or the transrectal route may be diagnostic. The resectoscope may be used for biopsy and therapy.

Other causes of obstruction at the bladder neck such as benign prostatic hypertrophy, bladder neck obstruction, granulomatous prostatitis and prostatic calculi must be excluded. When skeletal metastases are present, other types of primary carcinoma spreading to bone must be considered such as those of the lung, breast, kidney, thyroid and adrenal, whilst osteitis deformans may give a similar radiological picture.

Treatment

This is directed towards the control of growth of primary and secondary tumours, towards the relief of any urinary obstruction and pain relief. Radical removal of a cancerous prostate by total prostatectomy is rarely performed because of the difficulty in diagnosis before spread has occurred.

Medical management is employed in the majority of cases, 90 per cent showing considerable improvement with oestrogen therapy. This was initially employed by Huggins in Chicago in 1941 and was the first clinical application of the synthetic hormonal control of cancer. The probable mechanism is that oestrogen suppresses pituitary gonadotrophin activity and thereby reduces androgen production in the testis; both factors cause regression of the prostatic neoplasm. Dosage of stilboestrol of 1 mg t.d.s. is thought to be adequate and has less thrombotic side effects. Improvement is rapid, symptoms of primary or metastatic tumour frequently disappearing in a few weeks. Rectal examination reveals a prostate of softer consistency and radiography may show marked regression of pulmonary or osseous deposits. Acute retention should be treated by catheterisation and after confirmation of the diagnosis, by endoscopic resection and bilateral orchidectomy. Resection of the prostate provides an adequate outflow by the removal of tumour bulk. An alternative is catheterisation followed by stilboestrol therapy or by the use of intravenous phosphorylated oestrogen (Honvan) 0.5 to 1.0 g by slow injection after catheterisation. Drainage should be maintained until there is shrinkage of the prostate. Side-effects may follow oestrogen therapy and include nausea, enlargement of the breasts, atrophy of the testes, pigmentation of nipples and genitalia and loss of libido. Lower limb oedema and heart failure may occur from water and salt retention.

Surgical treatment is aimed at relieving urinary obstruction and endoscopic resection is a valuable palliative measure, although it may require to be repeated. When infiltrating carcinoma is discovered on histological examination of a resected prostate oestrogen therapy should be applied. Bilateral orchidectomy causes tumour regression and is often preferred, having fewer side effects than oestrogen therapy, which can be used if orchidectomy fails to control the growth. Orchidectomy is also of use in patients with heart disease when stilboestrol may be contra-indicated.

Radiotherapy is of value in relieving pain or pressure effects in some instances of primary tumour or localised secondary deposits in bone. In some centres radical radiotherapy is the preferred method of primary treatment.

FURTHER READING

Blandy, J. P. (Ed.) (1976). *Urology*. Oxford: Blackwell.
Chisholm, G. D. and Williams, D. I. (Eds.) (1982). *Scientific Foundations of Urology*. 2nd. ed. London: Heinemann.

25

Testis and epididymis

IMPERFECT DESCENT OF THE TESTIS

The testis usually reaches the scrotum at birth, but in about 3 per cent of infants this fails to occur. It is more common in premature infants. The diagnosis in such cases may be an undescended, ectopic or retractile testis.

In the condition of **undescended testis** the gonad on one or both sides remains within the abdomen or becomes arrested in the inguinal canal. The right side is more commonly affected and in unilateral cases the testis is smaller than the normal one. Spermatogenesis is prevented, which may be due to a higher local temperature; bilateral non-descent persisting after puberty causes infertility. The interstitial cells generally develop normally and secondary sexual characteristics appear. An undescended testis is liable to the complications of trauma, torsion or tumour. Although 10 per cent of malignant testicular tumours occur in an undescended testis, these growths are rare, hence the risk of malignant change is not of great practical importance. Seminoma is commoner than teratomatous change.

Ectopic testis usually occurs in the superficial inguinal position, although perineal, penile, femoral and pubic sites are described. The normal descent of the gonad is apparently guided by the gubernaculum testis. When this mechanism fails the testis may migrate to an ectopic position. In the common superficial inguinal position it can be felt anterior to the external oblique aponeurosis. A co-existent inguinal hernia is common in both ectopic and undescended testis.

Retractile testis occurs frequently, the organ being drawn back into the inguinal canal by the cremaster, in which position it may not be possible to feel the testis. In warm surroundings and with co-operation the gonad can generally be manipulated into the scrotum. When enlargement occurs at puberty, descent is permanent.

Treatment

Operation is required when one or both testes have not descended by the age of six years and also when the testis is in an ectopic position. The necessary steps include adequate mobilisation of the cord, fixation of the gonad in the scrotum (orchidopexy) and the removal of any co-existent hernia. Freeing of the testicular vessels on the posterior abdominal wall or the vas in the pelvis may be necessary. The testis is fixed in the scrotal sac either to the scrotal skin or within a subcutaneous scrotal pouch. If the testis does not reach the scrotum it should be fixed at the lowest suitable point and re-explored 9 to 12 months later when it is usually possible to lengthen the cord to allow full descent. If bilateral orchidopexy is required the second operation should be deferred for six months.

The results are particularly satisfactory in the ectopic variety, due to the adequate length of the cord structure. Hormonal treatment using gonadotrophins is only necessary when there is evidence of other endocrine dysfunction, such as extreme fatness or delayed onset of puberty. It is of no value when the testis is ectopic and unnecessary when it is retractile. It may produce precocity in young boys and may even cause tubular damage in excessive dosage.

HYDROCELE OF THE TUNICA VAGINALIS

Accumulation of fluid within the tunica vaginalis of the testis may be primary or secondary, the former being more common.

Primary hydrocele is due to unknown causes, although it has been suggested that it is the result of an insufficiency of lymphatics in the tunica (Fig. 25.1, C). The swelling may appear in infancy, but it is more usual in adults. Those observed in infancy often disappear spontaneously after a few weeks, but this is rare in adults.

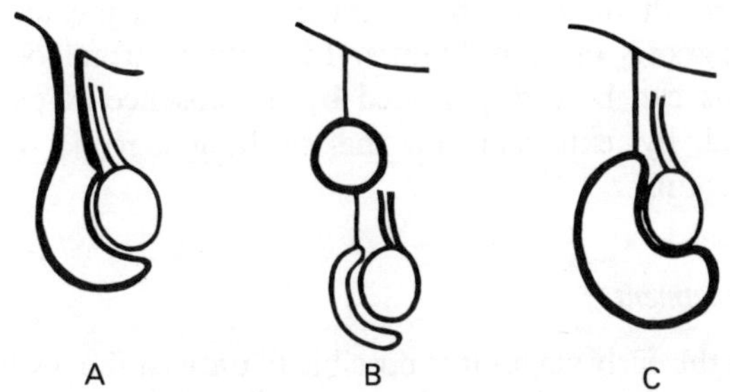

Fig. 25.1 Varieties of hydrocele. **A.** Congenital. **B.** Encysted hydrocele of cord. **C.** Primary vaginal.

The fluid is pale yellow in colour and may contain cholesterol crystals. The amount is variable, but large proportions may be reached. The wall becomes thickened in long-standing disease and flattening of the tesits may follow in severe cases. A hydrocele may be complicated by haemorrhage either from trauma or attempted aspiration, with the formation of a *haematocele*.

Secondary hydrocele is due to a new growth or to an inflammatory condition of the testis or epididymis. It may accumulate rapidly after injury or acute infective lesions such as gonorrhoea or mumps, or more slowly in tuberculosis, syphilis and neoplasm. It also occurs in filariasis. The fluid collection is often smaller than that of the primary type.

Clinical features

A hydrocele is a smooth, pear-shaped swelling which is confined to the scrotum. It may be tense or lax, but fluctuates on pressure and can be transilluminated unless it is thick-walled. The testis cannot be felt distinctly, being completely surrounded by fluid, a useful point in differentiating it from a cyst of the epididymis.

Congenital hydrocele is an uncommon form which occurs in infants (Fig. 25.1, A). There is a small communication with the peritoneal cavity which allows the swelling to vary in size, being often larger at the end of the day. It is sometimes designated a fluid hernia. The majority of hydroceles found in infancy do not show this feature.

Encysted hydrocele of the cord is a cyst in a portion of the obliterated processus vaginalis (Fig. 25.1, B); it forms a swelling in the inguinal canal which moves when traction is applied to the testis.

Treatment

In adults, aspiration may suffice to relieve the symptoms. Preliminary transillumination is important to avoid injury to blood-vessels or to the testis. The gonad should be carefully palpated following aspiration to exclude any underlying pathology. Operative treatment is required for recurrence when repeated aspiration fails or as primary treatment. Part of the tunica vaginalis should be excised and the remainder everted and sutured behind the testis. Haematoma formation should be avoided and good results can be obtained. In secondary hydrocele the underlying disease process should always be treated. In infants, if spontaneous disappearance does not occur after a year, ligation of the processus vaginalis at the internal ring is advisable. The hydrocele may be aspirated but it generally disappears.

Cysts of the epididymis

1. Congenital cysts

These arise in vestigial structures in the epididymis or mesorchium. They are usually small, but may undergo torsion and contain crystal-clear fluid.

2. Acquired cysts

The most common form is a *spermatocele*, which is a retention cyst of the vasa efferentia. A unilocular or multilocular swelling is apparent lying above and behind the testis, and may be distinguished from a hydrocele by the fact that the body of the testis is easily palpable and separate from the swelling (Fig. 25.2). Although transilluminable it contains opalescent fluid in which there are numerous spermatozoa.

A common variety is of small thin-walled multiple cysts containing clear fluid scattered through the epididymis.

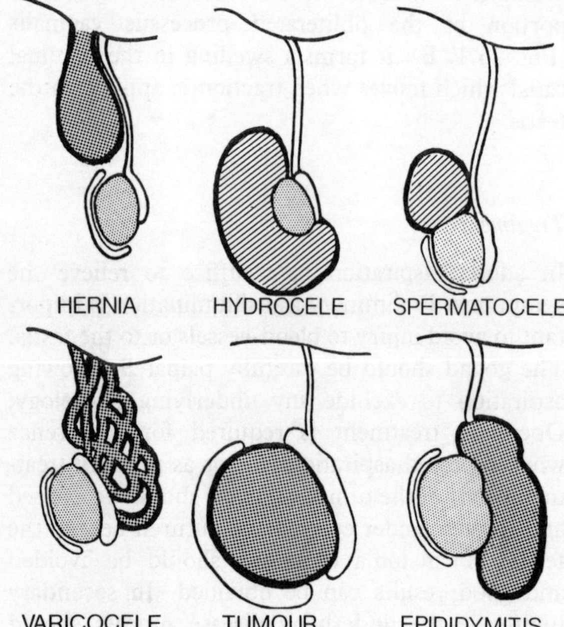

Fig. 25.2 Varieties of scrotal swelling

Treatment

When the cyst is small treatment may be unnecessary, but the majority of spermatoceles require excision. Aspiration is likely to be followed by recurrence. Multiple cysts may require partial or complete epididymectomy.

Torsion of the testis

This condition usually occurs in schoolboys about the age of puberty, often during sport but it may occur at rest. The testis is generally maldeveloped, having a long mesorchium or lying horizontally within the tunica vaginalis. Torsion may also occur in an inguinal ectopic testis.

Clinical features

There are often repeated, minor episodes before the main attack, which takes the form of a sudden severe pain initially in the iliac fossa, later in the testis accompanied by nausea, vomiting and sweating. More frequently there is a gradual rather than abrupt onset. The testis appears drawn up, the scrotum may be oedematous and there is marked local tenderness. Many testes undergo necrosis as a result of delay in treatment due to a mistaken diagnosis of epididymitis. Idiopathic scrotal oedema can be differentiated by the absence of pain and by extension of the swelling beyond the scrotum.

Treatment

In the early stages it is possible to untwist the testis, but unless pain is relieved quickly, urgent operation is essential as infarction occurs after only a few hours. The testis is exposed, untwisted and anchored to prevent recurrence. Orchidectomy is required when the organ is no longer viable. As the abnormal predisposing anatomy may be bilateral, orchidopexy of the opposite side is advisable at the same or subsequent operation.

Varicocele

This condition is usually *primary* but may be *secondary*. The former is generally left-sided and commonly occurs at puberty. The cremasteric system of veins may be primarily involved, but the pampiniform plexus is now thought to be the more usual form. Communications occur between both systems of veins and through collateral channels with the opposite venous system, both within the pelvis and retroperitoneal structures, and the lower limb veins. Secondary varicocele affects either side at any age and is due to invasion or compression of the intra-abdominal portion of the spermatic vein by a renal or retroperitoneal tumour, occasionally by a large hydronephrosis. The veins of the pampiniform plexus become distended.

Clinical features

The condition may be asymptomatic or there may be a complaint of dragging discomfort or aching pain. The left side is more frequently affected, mainly due to the internal spermatic veins draining into the left renal vein and some incompetence in the valvular mechanism, but bilateral varicocele may be seen. The swelling becomes more prominent on standing and disappears during recumbency. When distended, palpation of a varicocele gives the feel of a bunch of worms. There may be associated sub-fertility or low sperm count.

Treatment

A suspensory bandage and reassurance suffice in nearly every case, but ligation of the veins is occasionally required when symptoms are severe or infertility exists.

ACUTE EPIDIDYMO-ORCHITIS

Infection of the epididymis is a common condition, often associated with urinary infection. Organisms generally reach the epididymis from a focus in the prostate gland but regurgitation of urine along the vas deferens or occasionally blood stream infection may occur.

Infection may remain in the epididymis but usually spreads to involve the testis, sometimes producing a small secondary hydrocele. The common organisms are *Esch. coli*, the gonococcus or *Myco. tuberculosis*. The urine may appear sterile on culture. The condition often occurs in young men with a full bladder after sudden muscular effort.

Acute epididymo-orchitis may also follow instrumentation of the urethra, prostatectomy, urethritis and cystitis. Acute orchitis, in which the testis is mainly affected, occurs in mumps and other infectious diseases, including infectious mononucleosis.

Clinical features

Increasing pain in the region of the testis is the initial symptom, often becoming very severe. A swelling is noted which increases with the pain. Malaise, anorexia and general constitutional symptoms are apparent with a pyrexia which may persist for several days. The scrotum is usually red and swollen. On palpation both testis and epididymis are tender and often cannot be distinguished separately in the swelling. There is usually urinary frequency, due to an accompanying infection, and there may be obvious urethritis. Pain and swelling generally subside after four or five days with resolution of the process, but thickening may persist for several weeks. Necrosis and abscess formation may occur.

When urethral discharge is present it should be examined bacteriologically and the urine cultured to determine the underlying organism. Torsion of the testis requires exclusion and evidence of mumps should also be sought when orchitis is present. Rarely a tumour may present as an inflammatory episode.

Treatment

Rest in bed is important with the scrotum well supported. Analgesics should be given, and after a urine sample has been taken for culture and sensitivity, co-trimoxazole (Septrin) or ampicillin should be started and continued for at least 3 to 4 weeks if response is obtained. Incision and drainage of abscesses should be performed, but at times orchidectomy may be required.

Chronic epididymo-orchitis

Two varieties occur: (1) non-specific and (2) tuberculous.

The *non-specific* type is encountered in elderly men with recurrent urinary infection, as a result of which the epididymis becomes irregular, craggy and enlarged. It can only be distinguished from the tuberculous type by careful examination of the urine.

Tuberculous epididymitis is rarely seen unless the kidneys and bladder are also infected. which is suggestive that the route of infection is generally along the vas. As a result the common site is in the tail of the epididymis, which becomes hard and attached to the posterior scrotal skin, where a sinus may eventually form. The spermatic cord and sometimes the vas deferens may feel thickened. The testis is later involved and there may be a small hydrocele. The urine may reveal a 'sterile pyuria' and tubercle bacilli are usually demonstrated; they may also be isolated from the purulent discharge from a sinus.

Treatment of the non-specific type is by a scrotal support; in the specific form it is that of urinary tuberculosis in general (p. 286). Removal of the epididymis (*epididymectomy*) is occasionally necessary when caseation and sinus formation occur, as those rarely heal with chemotherapy alone. In advanced disease *epididymo-orchidectomy* is required. It may also be advisable when a tumour cannot be excluded.

TUMOURS OF THE TESTIS

Most tumours of the testis are malignant, and there are two main varieties, *teratoma* and *seminoma* (Fig. 25.3). Lymphoma is a rare cause in old age. Benign tumours are rare and include the *interstitial-cell tumour*. which secretes androgens and may cause precocious puberty in young children and gynaecomastia in later life.

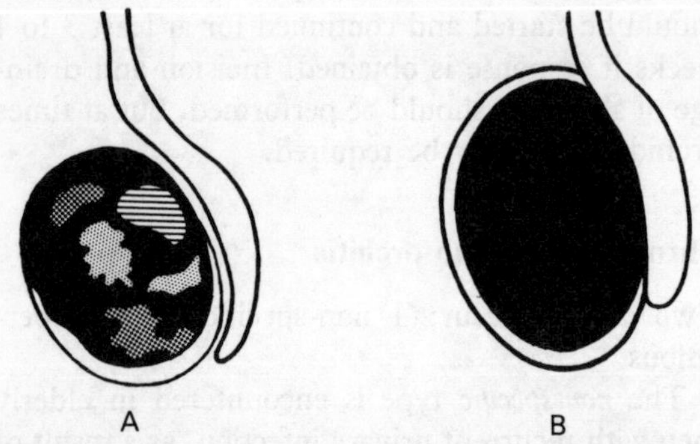

Fig. 25.3 Tumours of testis. **A.** Teratoma. **B.** Seminoma.

Pathology

Teratoma of the testis

This is a highly malignant tumour containing a variety of tissues not found in the normal testis. It is thought to arise in cells retaining a primitive pluripotent character, these being probably derived from the embryonic genital ridge. Ectodermal, endodermal and mesodermal structures may thus be formed or there may be a preponderance of one or more elements.

Considerable variation in size and rate of growth occurs, and some teratomas appear to have almost a benign pattern. A number of different macroscopic types exist, the common one resembling a honeycomb of cystic cavities, lined by various forms of epithelium and often containing portions of cartilage; this variety is called 'fibrocystic disease' of the testis. Dermoid cysts and intestinal glandular masses are also encountered. The least common variety is the differentiated teratoma (TD), containing well-differentiated tissues but without histologically malignant areas. It looks like a dermoid cyst but arises away from the rete testis and contains tissues other than squamous epithelium. The malignant teratomas which are of an intermediate type contain organoid tissue amongst some anaplastic areas, whilst the undifferentiated variety is also called embryonal carcinoma. The trophoblastic malignant teratoma is an uncommon variety which exhibits the undifferentiated histology of a primitive syncytial type.

Spread is mainly by the bloodstream, although it may occur by direct infiltration or by the lymphatics. Vascular metastasis tends to take place early, first to the lungs and liver, later to the skeleton.

Seminoma

This is a carcinoma of the seminiferous tubules. The macroscopic structure is that of a well-defined, rounded, uniform, fleshy tumour. The cut surface is pink or grey and usually bulges outwards. The junction with normal testis appears well delineated. Histologically the normal structure is replaced by clumps of rounded cells similar to spermatocytes, with large spherical nuclei. The stroma is frequently heavily infiltrated with lymphocytes. Direct spread to the epididymis or spermatic cord is common, but lymphatic dissemination is more important. The first group of lymph nodes to be involved is usually the upper lumbar. The supraclavicular group may be implicated later due to spread along the thoracic duct. Bloodstream metastasis is less frequent and not as early as in teratoma.

Clinical features

Teratoma is most common between 15 and 40

years, seminoma between 30 and 50 years. The usual presenting symptom is the gradual appearance of a testicular swelling, although there is considerable variation in the rate of enlargement, and occasionally the onset is rapid. Gynaecomastia occurs rarely and is due to the production of gonadotrophic hormone by the teratomatous tumour. The first symptoms may occasionally relate to the presence of metastatic disease such as haemoptysis or pathological fracture. Slow resolution of apparent inflammation may indicate the presence of a tumour.

Examination reveals a swelling in the body of the testis which is smooth and uniform, with a firm consistency. A small secondary hydrocele is sometimes present and the spermatic cord may be thickened, duc more often to vascularity than to neoplastic invasion. Abdominal masses from involvement of the para-aortic nodes or an enlarged liver, ascites, lower limb oedema and supraclavicular swellings are all indications of extensive disease. Chest radiography should be performed to exclude enlarged mediastinal nodes and an intravenous urogram may demonstrate kidney or ureteric displacement. Lymphography and CT scanning may indicate retroperitoneal node involvement and should be performed prior to radiotherapy.

In the differential diagnosis it is uncommon to encounter a gumma, but a history of syphilis may be obtained and testicular sensation is absent. Serological tests are usually positive, but there may be co-existent tumour. Other conditions to be considered include a haematocele and tuberculous epididymo-orchitis, whilst spontaneous necrosis in a neoplasm may simulate non-specific orchitis. Exploration and orchidectomy may be required in some instances as it is important not to delay diagnosis and treatment. There is no place for biopsy.

Treatment is by orchidectomy with removal of the cord as far as the internal ring, followed by radiotherapy to the para-aortic nodes. The prognosis in seminoma is favourable, an 80 per cent five year survival rate being obtained in patients without metastases. Radiotherapy has also improved the survival figure in teratoma but the latter is not as radiosensitive as seminoma. Chemotherapy in the form of vincristine, bleomycin and cisplatin has improved the prognosis of the primary disease and is helpful in palliation.

FURTHER READING

Blandy. J. P. (Ed.) (1976). *Urology*. Oxford: Blackwell.

Newsman, J. E. (1982). Genito-urinary surgery. In *Essential Surgical Practice*. (Eds.) Cuschieri, A., Giles, G. R. and Moossa, A. R. Bristol: Wright.

26

Skull, brain and spinal cord

SKULL AND BRAIN

CONGENITAL ABNORMALITIES

Defects of the skull with protrusion of the cranial contents are rare. **Meningocele** or **encephalocele** occur in the occipital region. Operative treatment to repair a meningocele may be feasible and should be undertaken soon after birth. **Dermoid cysts** occur in fusion lines, the most common being the external angular dermoid which presents as a cystic swelling at the lateral side of the orbit. Communication with the subarachnoid space is rare. Excision is indicated.

Hydrocephalus

Distension of the cerebral ventricles of the infantile type usually develops soon after birth. The *internal* (non-communicating) form may involve the lateral ventricle due to obstruction of the interventricular foramen or the foramina in the fourth ventricle. Inflammatory and vascular adhesions in the Arnold-Chiari malformation are accompanied by downward displacement of the cerebellar vermis through the foramen magnum. The condition is often associated with *spina bifida* (p. 325) and cerebrospinal fluid does not escape into the subarachnoid space. The *external* (communicating) form may be due to the faulty absorption of cerebrospinal fluid by the arachnoid villi, which become occluded either by damaged red cells in subarachnoid haemorrhage or by chronic inflammation. Obstruction of the basal cisterns may prevent cerebrospinal fluid from reaching the supratentorial subarachnoid space. Overproduction of cerebrospinal fluid by a choroid plexus papilloma is a further rare cause of this form of hydrocephalus. The precise reason and site of the block is often difficult to identify even at autopsy.

The increased intracranial pressure is manifest by progressive enlargement of the head and bulging of the fontanelles. The rate of growth of the head should be measured for comparison with a chart of normal development. Mental retardation, spasticity and minor epileptic attacks are probably associated with underlying brain damage from birth trauma. Vomiting and dehydration as well as increased susceptibility to infection may lead to death. Approximately 25 per cent of cases diagnosed before the age of three months reach adult life, the majority of deaths occurring within 18 months. Natural arrest of the condition without treatment takes place in 50 per cent, but some of these will have mental and physical defects. The diagnosis is confirmed by plain film radiographs which show separation of the sutures and by computerised tomography.

Treatment is not required for the mild type which undergoes spontaneous arrest. Internal hydrocephalus due to aqueduct obstruction may be treated by an operation to drain fluid from the lateral ventricle into the cisterna magna (Torkildsen). Communicating hydrocephalus may be relieved by the drainage of cerebrospinal fluid into the bloodstream. A shunt is formed between the lateral ventricle and atrium via the internal jugular vein. Plastic tubing is used incorporating a valve (Spitz-Holter) which prevents reflux of blood. This is now widely practised and is successful in over 80 per cent of cases. A complication rate exists of about 20 per cent due to thrombosis, infection and blockage of the tube which necessitates revision of the shunt; subdural haematoma may also occur and require treatment.

Neurological investigations

Detailed investigation for space-occupying lesions in the skull may employ many techniques as outlined below; the most appropriate investigation for each condition is indicated later in the text.

Plain skull radiography may demonstrate a fracture, erosion of bone from meningioma and acoustic neuroma, while expansion of the sella turcica may indicate a pituitary tumour.

Computerised tomography scanning (*CT scan*) has radically changed the approach to investigation, mainly because it is a non-invasive technique which provides clear demonstration of many lesions. Repeat scanning after intravenous injection of iodine-containing medium further increases the diagnostic accuracy.

Spinal myelography with injection of myodil or metrizamide outlines the spinal subarachnoid space and serves to outline a tumour or prolapsed intervertebral disc.

Cerebral angiography is performed by injection of radio-opaque medium into the carotid or vertebral arteries, usually under general anaesthesia. The cerebral vessels are outlined in arterial and venous phases and may provide accurate information of distortion of vascular patterns or outline an aneurysm or show atheroma of a vessel wall. The procedure carries a slight risk, for instance of arterial thrombosis, dissemination of emboli and aggravation of cerebral ischaemia.

Air encephalography is performed by removing some CSF via lumbar or cisternal puncture and inserting air. The arachnoid cisterns and ventricles become air filled and distortion of these spaces is found in certain tumours. It gives accurate information of lesions around the pituitary fossa, but is now not widely used.

Isotope scanning with technetium is not as accurate as CT scanning and is used in the detection of cerebral metastases in cases of known malignant disease or non-availability of a CT scanner.

HEAD INJURIES

A convenient classification is under the following headings, one or all of which may be present simultaneously:

1. Scalp wounds.
2. Fracture of the skull.
   - Vault.
   - Base.
3. Brain damage.
   - Concussion.
   - Contusion and laceration.
   - Compression.

Scalp wounds

Although incised wounds occur, blunt trauma is generally responsible, causing contusion and laceration, bleeding being a prominent feature. Infection of the loose areolar space lying beneath the occipitofrontalis aponeurosis readily occurs and may spread inside the skull via the emissary veins with serious consequences. Scalp wounds should therefore be thoroughly cleansed, devitalised tissue excised and all foreign matter removed. The underlying bone, if exposed, should be examined for the presence of a fracture, the wound being then closed by sutures passing through the whole thickness of the scalp. The abundant blood supply promotes rapid healing.

FRACTURES OF THE SKULL

A fracture may involve the vault, more commonly the base or both portions of the skull. The degree of fracture of the skull bears little relationship to the severity of cerebral damage. Severe brain laceration may even be present without fracture of the skull bones.

Fractures may be *simple* or *compound*, *linear* or *comminuted*, whilst *depressed* fragments of bone at the site of a direct injury are common.

Differentiation of the latter from a haematoma of the scalp with a firm edge of organised clot and central soft area may at times be difficult.

Linear fractures may run for several centimetres across the vault, cross the suture lines, pass down to the base of the skull and may be accompanied by separation of suture lines (Fig. 26.1, A).

Compound injuries may be associated with a linear, comminuted or depressed fracture, more commonly the last. Depression of bony fragments due to a localised blow on the skull may lead to pen-

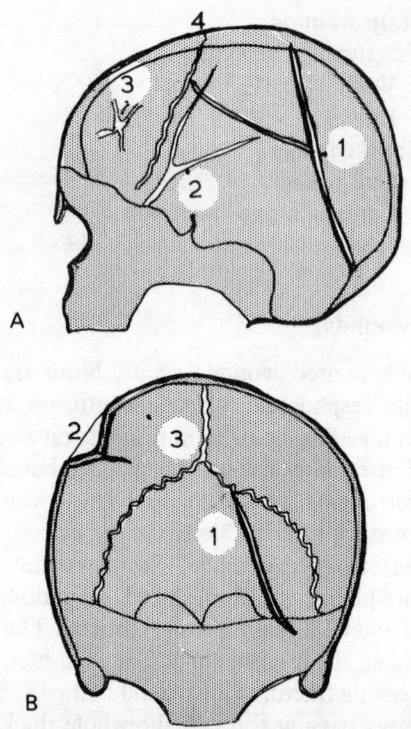

Fig. 26.1 Fractures of skull, and other linear markings.
A. Lateral view showing fracture line (1); meningeal vessels (2); diploic channels (3); frontoparietal suture (4).
B. Anteroposterior view showing linear fracture line (1); depressed fracture (2); suture line (3).

etration of the dura or brain by spicules of bone (Fig. 26.1, B).

Fractures of the base of the skull usually pass irregularly between foramina, often the result of severe trauma, and may be associated with marked cerebral damage, particularly to the brain stem. Bleeding from the ear or nose is a significant feature. Leakage of cerebrospinal fluid from the nose may follow fracture of the cribriform plate. Subconjunctival blood spreading over the eye from behind is indicative of a basal fracture and should be differentiated from a localised haematoma caused by direct injury to eye or orbit, and which has a posterior limit. Bruising in the region of the mastoid process may also be noted after several days.

Basal fractures may be complicated by cranial nerve injury. The olfactory nerves are most commonly affected resulting in anosmia. Facial nerve palsy may result from direct trauma to the nerve or from bleeding into the facial canal. Deafness due to auditory nerve damage may, like facial palsy, occur immediately or be delayed in onset due to involvement of the nerve in scar tissue. Injury to the optic nerve is rare, but may lead to permanent blindness. Oculomotor paresis is not uncommon and is the result of rising intracranial tension causing pressure on the nerve in the tentorium. The trochlear, trigeminal and abducent nerves may each be injured whilst the maxillary division of the fifth nerve may be damaged by fracture of the maxilla.

Skull radiography in all cases of head injury is essential. A depressed fracture in particular may not be recognised by clinical examination.

Treatment

Linear fractures do not require treatment. Cerebral damage constitutes the principal feature and attention should be directed to this aspect.

Elevation of a simple depressed fracture is advisable if the depression is more than the full thickness of the skull vault, particularly in an area where a cosmetic defect may be evident. The onset of post-traumatic epilepsy is not related to the bony depression but to associated cerebral damage. A compound depressed fracture carries a severe risk of infection of the subarachnoid space, and early treatment is essential to deal with the scalp wound, remove debris and elevate the fracture.

Basal fractures of the anterior fossa may involve a nasal air sinus or cribriform plate and allow communication with the subarachnoid space. This should be suspected if there is cerebrospinal rhinorrhoea or radiographs show air in the skull. Antibiotic therapy with penicillin and sulphonamides is given to lessen the risk of infection of the subarachnoid space. Nose blowing should be avoided as it may lead to the development of an aerocele from air forced through the dural defect around the anterior lobes of the brain. Blood exuding from the external auditory meatus should be wiped away, syringing being avoided to lessen the risk of introducing infection. Persistent cerebrospinal fluid leakage or development of an aerocele may require operative closure of the dural defect by craniotomy or through the nasal sinuses.

BRAIN INJURY

Concussion

Concussion is the vague term applied to the transient effects of a mild head injury. It is thought that slight neuronal damage occurs in the mildest brain trauma if a period of amnesia is present. The difference between mild and severe damage may be one of degree rather than of differing type. A period of retrograde amnesia usually exists but is variable in duration and of no prognostic significance. The duration of the 'post-traumatic amnesia' is more important and serves as a guide to the severity of brain damage. If up to one hour it can be considered as mild, 1 to 24 hours as moderate and over this as severe damage.

Cerebral contusion and laceration

This is a more serious pathological state resulting from direct trauma associated with a fracture of the skull or by disruption of the brain due to its rapid movement in relation to the skull. The most severe injuries occur by sudden deceleration of the skull in falls or motor accidents. The brain can be likened to a jelly in a mould where sudden movements of the mould readily produce breaking of the jelly. The contusions and laceration may be spread over the whole brain, and in particular involve the under surface of the frontal and temporal lobes. Contrecoup injury of parts remote from the obvious site of skull injury are not uncommon (Fig. 26.2).

Haemorrhage from torn vessels may cause direct cerebral destruction or lead to compression by accumulation of blood clot. Oedema of the damaged brain produces further compression and provides one of the most serious developments of head injury. Repair may follow due to proliferation of glial tissue, and an ingrowth of blood-vessels from the meninges may produce adhesions. Damage to the vital centres in brain stem and medulla is the common cause of death. Autopsy reveals widespread small haemorrhages associated with generalised oedema of the brain.

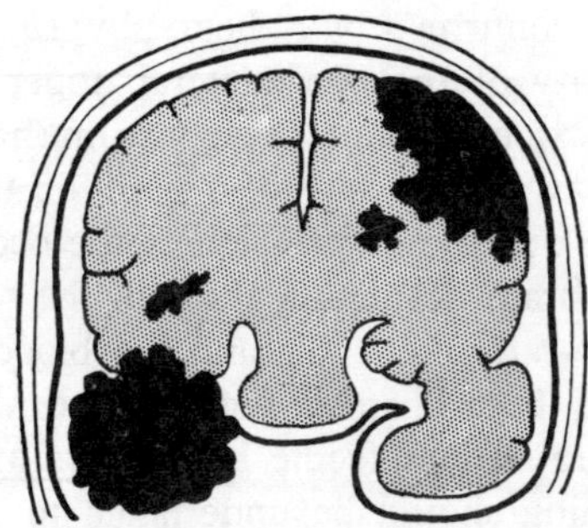

Fig. 26.2 Cerebral contusion and laceration of inferior surface of temporal lobe and contrecoup injury

Clinical features

Early detailed examination in cases of head injury is important because the detection of focal signs at this stage suggests that these are the direct result of trauma. Subsequent development of such signs indicates the onset of cerebral compression by oedema or blood clot.

Attention should be paid to the level of consciousness, signs of paralysis of cranial nerves, spasticity or paralysis of limbs and the state of the reflexes. Observation of the pupils may give useful information. If originally equal and reacting, but with later unilateral dilatation, an intracranial haematoma is probable. Bilateral fixed, dilated pupils soon after injury denote very extensive damage, which is often fatal. A unilateral dilated pupil at the time of injury suggests damage to the eye or optic nerve. Restlessness and photophobia occur with many severe injuries, but are indicative of cerebral oedema and are not of value in localising a lesion. The pulse-rate should be recorded half-hourly, but the development of bradycardia is a late sign of cerebral compression. Stertorous respiration is indicative of severe damage to the brain stem. Alcoholic intoxication must be excluded as a cause of coma. Plain radiographs of the skull are required.

Careful observation and repeated examination with accurate recording of the findings are necessary to detect the development of cerebral compression. Deterioration of the level of consciousness or the appearance of a focal lesion, often accompanied by stertorous respiration and slowing of the pulse, are generally the result of intracranial haemorrhage for which early operation may prove life-saving. CT scanning is indicated at this stage. Detailed examination of the entire body must be made as multiple injuries are common in road traffic accidents. The association with chest injuries is most important as alteration of respiration may be confused with the effects of the head injury.

Treatment

Restlessness should be controlled by mild restraint in quiet surroundings. Drugs should not be given in the early stages because of their depressant effect on respiration and ability to mask physical signs. Paraldehyde and hyoscine may be used when restlessness is extreme.

A clear airway must be maintained by frequent aspiration of blood and mucus, combined with regular changes of posture to lessen the risk of pulmonary infection. Tracheostomy is occasionally necessary to allow easy aspiration of secretions. The development of cerebral oedema may be limited by dehydration, and the fluid intake should be restricted to 1500 ml per 24 hours, given orally or by nasogastric tube, with measurement of daily urinary output. Intravenous infusion of 20 per cent mannitol may prove beneficial. The administration of steroids has little beneficial effect in head injuries. The reduction of cerebrospinal fluid pressure by lumbar puncture can be dangerous in the early stages by causing tentorial herniation of brain, but in the recovering patient it often relieves headache and stupor.

Prolonged unconsciousness calls for attentive nursing to avoid pressure sores, the employment of an alternating pressure mattress being helpful. Urinary retention requires catheterisation and the administration of urinary antiseptic drugs to control infection. Fluid intake and feeding are carried out by means of a nasogastric tube. It is feasible to maintain life for one or more years by this regime, but full recovery is not usual, marked mental deterioration being common. Prolonged hypothermia may be of benefit in certain cases of brain stem injury.

TRAUMATIC INTRACRANIAL HAEMORRHAGE

Intracerebral haemorrhage is not generally amenable to surgical treatment. Extradural and subdural haemorrhage present definite features, the latter being more common though less dramatic in onset (Fig. 26.3).

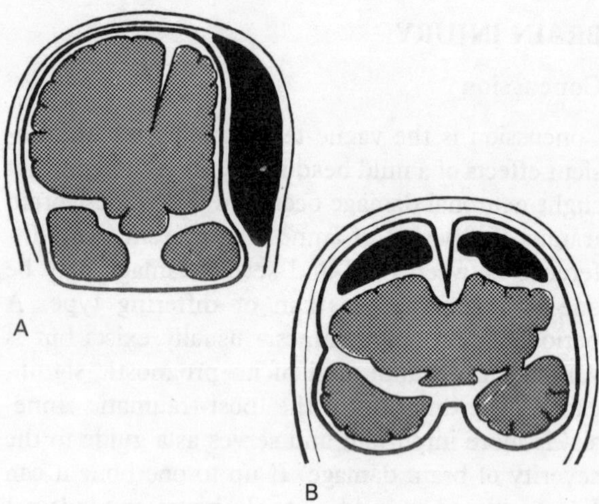

Fig. 26.3 Intracranial haemorrhage. **A.** Extradural. **B.** Subdural.

Extradural haemorrhage

This variety usually follows damage to the middle meningeal vessels by fracture of the skull, the clot lying over the temporo-parietal area. The initial injury may be slight and produce only a short period of unconsciousness. It is often followed by gradual deterioration of the level of consciousness, the classical 'lucid interval' not always occurring. The development of focal paralytic signs is strong indication of a developing haematoma. The affected side may be localised by the following features: (*a*) the presence of bruising or oedema of the scalp over the suspected skull fracture which should be confirmed by radiography; (*b*) weakness or spasticity of the contralateral upper or lower limb and extensor plantar response on that side; (*c*) a dilating or dilated and fixed pupil on the side of the lesion due to compression of the occulomotor nerve by brain herniation through the tentorium. The pulse-rate often falls and the blood-pressure rises, but these changes may be late. The pulse becomes rapid and feeble in the terminal stages. CT scanning should be undertaken to determine the site and size of a haematoma.

Surgical exploration through burr holes in the skull may be required urgently if rapid deterioration occurs. Otherwise CT scanning and possibly angiography should be performed first. Exploration is then undertaken through a correctly-sited bone flap, to evacuate the haematoma and secure haemostasis. Some degree of intradural bleeding is found in a third of cases and may require evacuation.

Subdural haematoma

Haemorrhage into the subdural space usually results from laceration of the veins connecting the cerebral cortex and the venous sinuses. Acute, subacute and chronic forms are recognised. The **acute** form is usually associated with laceration of the brain and accompanies severe injury which is often fatal and rarely amenable to surgical treatment. **Subacute** subdural haemorrhage presents within seven to ten days of injury as a gradual onset of compression and deterioration of level of consciousness. Investigation with CT scanning is usually diagnostic, but angiography may be required. Evacuation of the clot through an osteoplastic flap is often beneficial.

Chronic subdural haematoma often results from slight head injury sustained several weeks or months previously and is found in infants, the elderly and alcoholics. It is usually caused by the tearing of cerebral veins without damage to the brain substance. The clot is surrounded by a well-defined membrane. It then liquefies and slowly increases in size, perhaps by osmotic attraction of water from the cerebrospinal fluid. The clinical presentation may be vague but the history of persistent headache after injury should arouse suspicion. Increasing drowsiness, confusion and dementia may develop. Mild hemiparesis, cranial nerve paresis and papilloedema are often present but localising signs are uncommon. Diagnosis is aided by electroencephalography, cerebral angiography, ultrasonic encephalography and CT scanning. Exploratory burr holes are often required and the haematoma evacuated through these by irrigation.

Complications of head injury

Post-concussional syndrome of headache, dizziness, poor concentration and irritability may arise after mild head injury but varies considerably in severity and duration. It was thought to be an accident neurosis but is more likely to have an organic basis. Treatment in the early stages should be adequate rest and reassurance with gradual resumption of normal work.

Epilepsy in the first week following injury occurs in 5 per cent of cases and is best treated with phenytoin. Late epilepsy has a higher incidence after severe injuries, particularly if there has been an intracranial haematoma, compound depressed fracture or missile injury. Treatment with anticonvulsants should be maintained for 2 to 5 years depending on the severity of the injury, or longer if fits persist.

Neurological defects after head injury occur in 20 to 30 per cent of cases. Hemiparesis may follow intracranial haematoma but it usually improves after 6 months. Cranial nerve damage may involve the olfactory nerves, causing anosmia; the majority recover but some have permanent disability. The seventh nerve is damaged by fractures of the petrous temporal bone and results in facial palsy, which usually improves. Oculomotor nerve dysfunction is common in the early stages after injury but rarely persists.

Subarachnoid haemorrhage

The condition commonly arises from rupture of an aneurysm of the intracranial portion of the internal carotid artery or circle of Willis, but may be due to a tumour or vascular malformation. The primary defect is a lack of the elastic lamina at the bifurcation of the artery which, when associated with hypertension, leads to the development of an aneurysm; they are therefore not congenital in origin. The bleeding varies considerably in amount, entering the subarachnoid space or destroying brain substance and entering the ventricle. It occurs mainly betweeen 40 and 60 years of age with a female preponderance.

Clinical features

The onset is sudden with headaches and pain in the neck and back, accompanied by vomiting and irritability. Neck stiffness is found and Kernig's sign is positive. The patient may become stuporous or unconscious; hemiplegia, dysphasia or other focal neurological signs indicate the development of an intracerebral haematoma. Death occurs immediately in about 10 per cent but the rate rises to 50 per cent in the first month. Lumbar puncture reveals blood-stained cerebrospinal fluid in the early stages but after 7 to 10 days the fluid becomes yellow without any cells. Investigation involves CT scanning, which may outline blood in the basal subarachnoid cisterns and an intracerebral or intraventricular haematoma. Angiography is necessary to outline the exact site and size of the causative cerebral aneurysm.

Treatment of the mild case may be conservative. Bed rest is combined with analgesic drugs and antiemetics, whilst the reduction of intracranial pressure is obtained with steroids and mannitol. Depletion of serum sodium levels may require the administration of sodium chloride, preferably orally. Vasospasm of the cerebral vessels is a serious development, occurring 5 to 10 days after onset, and results in diminished cerebral circulation. It is difficult to treat but may respond to systemic vasodilator drugs. The tendency to recurrent haemorrhage usually necessitates surgical intervention, which should be undertaken at an early stage after the aneurysm is confirmed if the condition of the patient permits. It is not indicated where the patient is in a deep coma, or exhibits severe hemiparesis or decerebrate rigidity. The vessel bearing the aneurysm is exposed by craniotomy and a metal clip applied across the neck of the aneurysm. Indirect reduction of pressure in the aneurysm is obtained by ligature of the common carotid artery on the affected side. This operation is undertaken in a limited number of selected cases but carries the risk of interference with the cerebral circulation.

INFECTION

Scalp

Infection of the scalp does not usually constitute a serious problem since the introduction of antibiotic therapy. The importance of early treatment in any infective lesion and thorough surgical toilet of scalp wounds should be emphasised.

Osteomyelitis of the skull

This is not a common lesion. It generally results from staphylococcal infection and may follow a compound fracture, sinus infection, or be blood-borne from a distant focus. Bone destruction and pus formation occur. The latter may collect under the scalp or form an extradural abscess, the dura being an efficient barrier in preventing subarachnoid involvement. Infective thrombosis of an emissary vein may lead to intracranial venous thrombosis and suppuration.

The condition presents as a painful indurated swelling of the scalp with fever, toxaemia and leucocytosis. Radiographs of the skull show rarefaction and bone destruction after the lesion has been present for two or three weeks. Antibiotic treatment should be given for at least eight weeks after the organism has been identified by aspiration of the pus. Incision is rarely called for and is better avoided.

Extradural abscess

The dura is particularly resistant to the passage of infection, and an abscess lying outside the dura is rarely followed by intracerebral infection. Osteomyelitis of the skull and infection of the nasal sinuses are the usual causes. Increased intracranial tension may arise with the development of papilloedema and focal signs. Drainage by bone removal is required in conjunction with antibiotic therapy.

Subdural abscess

Inflammation in the subdural space results from the spread of infection from osteomyelitis, sinusitis and mastoiditis. The clinical picture is one of severe toxaemia; widespread cortical paralysis produces hemiplegia and hemianaesthesia. Lumbar puncture rarely shows involvement of the subarachnoid space. Antibiotic therapy should be combined with drainage through burr openings, but the prognosis is grave.

Brain abscess

Infection reaching the brain by direct spread from

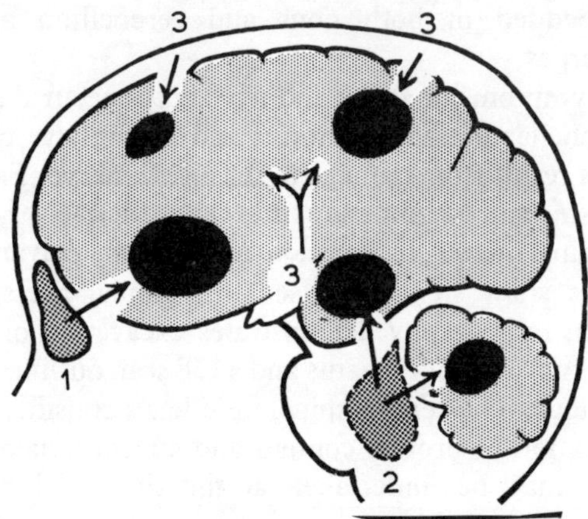

Fig. 26.4 The common sources of brain abscess. Frontal sinus (1); mastoid (2); blood borne from lungs (3).

the frontal sinus or mastoid accounts for the majority of cases (Fig. 26.4), and the temporal lobe or cerebellum are most frequently involved. Haematogenous spread from infective lesions of the lungs may result in single or multiple abscesses in the parietal or frontal regions. *Staph. aureus*, *Strept. haemolyticus* and the pneumococcus are the organisms most frequently responsible. The abscess is initially surrounded by an area of gliosis which later forms a firm capsule containing necrotic brain tissue and pus. Localisation may not be complete and spread of infection may lead to meningitis, while rupture into the ventricle may be rapidly fatal.

Clinical features

Initial symptoms of headache and malaise from meningeal infection are followed by those of a rise of intracranial tension from the development of a space-occupying lesion. Hemiplegia, disturbance of vision and cranial nerve paralysis may be present. Papilloedema is often seen. A frontal lobe abscess produces few signs, alteration of mentality often being the only change. Cerebellar abscess generally causes ataxia and nystagmus. Detailed examination for the primary source of infection is essential, but the clinical picture of a brain abscess may be obscured when antibiotics have been administered for the causative condition.

Lumbar puncture may reveal a rise in cerebrospinal fluid pressure, with a slight rise in protein and polymorph leucocyte content of the fluid. Radiographs of the skull may demonstrate mastoiditis, sinus infection or osteomyelitis. Electroencephalography shows abnormal slow wave activity; a CT scan demonstrates the abscess well and angiography will localise the lesion and determine its size.

Treatment

Antibiotics have lowered the mortality by limiting the spread of infection and the onset of meningitis. Surgical treatment comprises repeated aspiration. A needle is inserted through a burr hole. pus aspirated and penicillin or other appropriate antibiotic injected, combined with a radio-opaque medium. The latter enables the size of the abscess to be followed radiologically. When a small size has been reached and the infection has become quiescent operative removal of the residual glial mass with its enclosed abscess cavity is undertaken. Treatment of any primary lesion in chest or sinuses may be required concurrently. Anticonvulsants should be maintained for at least 3 years as the incidence of epilepsy is high.

Sinus thrombosis

Thrombosis of the intracranial venous sinuses is usually secondary to infection of face, scalp or middle ear. Marked toxaemia, headache and drowsiness are present.

Cavernous sinus thrombosis more commonly follows a boil on the nose or upper lip. It is characterised by exophthalmos and ophthalmoplegia. Marked conjunctival oedema develops. It should be differentiated from orbital cellulitis in which severe toxaemia and ophthalmoplegia are absent.

Lateral sinus thrombosis was a common sequel of mastoiditis, but is now infrequent. Spread of thrombosis to the internal jugular vein may make this structure readily palpable in the neck. Sixth nerve palsy is an occasional accompaniment.

Treatment includes antibiotic and anticoagulant therapy. Surgical drainage of the lateral sinus may be necessary in conjunction with drainage of the mastoid air cells.

TUMOURS

Primary tumours of the skull such as osteoma, plasmacytoma and eosinophilic granuloma, are not common. Secondary deposits from malignant disease of the thyroid, breast, kidney and adrenal are more frequently encountered. Multiple myeloma produces a characteristic 'punched-out' appearance.

Intracranial tumours may arise from the meninges, cranial nerves, pituitary gland, cerebrum or cerebellum.

Meningioma

The meningioma forms 10 to 15 per cent of all intracranial tumours, arising most frequently near the sagittal sinus, the olfactory plate, the sphenoidal ridge or the foramen magnum. It originates in islands of arachnoid cells, which lie on the deep surface of dura, and arachnoid granulations. The tumour is sessile, grey-red and often highly vascular. It may compress the brain but does not invade it. Indentation of the skull occurs with localised hyperostosis of the overlying bone, recognised as a smooth swelling on the skull. The histological picture is of spindle-shaped cells resembling fibroblasts, often arranged in circles around a central blood vessel. Calcification may be present. The tumour is slowly growing and benign, although it may recur locally after removal.

Symptoms are produced by local pressure on the underlying brain and also by the rise of intracranial tension. Plain radiography of the skull may demonstrate calcification in the tumour and localised osteoblastic reaction, a CT scan will outline the lesion readily whilst abnormal vascular patterns are seen on angiography. The results of excision are favourable, though this may prove difficult because of severe haemorrhage.

Acoustic neuroma

This benign tumour arises from the sheath of the eighth cranial nerve in the region of the internal auditory meatus. It may exist as a single entity or be a manifestation of generalised neurofibromatosis. The tumour has a definite capsule, the centre being composed of soft yellow material. It becomes embedded in both pons and cerebellum as it enlarges.

Symptoms of ataxia and nystagmus occur due to cerebellar pressure; tinnitus and progressive deafness result from damage to the eighth nerve. Facial spasm and weakness, and paraesthesiae of trigeminal nerve distribution may occur. Advanced cases show signs of raised intracranial pressure. Plain radiography demonstrates excavation of the internal auditory meatus and a CT scan outlines the tumour. The cerebrospinal fluid has a considerable elevation of protein content and air encephalography may be undertaken at the time of lumbar puncture.

Treatment

Complete removal results in cure, but technical difficulties may preclude this and partial excision may have to suffice. The latter has the effect of relieving symptoms.

PITUITARY TUMOURS

Three benign forms may develop from the anterior lobe of the gland. The *chromophobe* adenoma accounts for the majority of lesions and is composed of clear cells arranged in alveoli. It may grow to a large size and produces its effects by compression of the remaining pituitary substance and by pressure on surrounding structures. Extension occurs principally through the diaphragma sellae to involve the optic nerves and chiasma, but the hypothalamus and midbrain may also be affected, and the third ventricle can become blocked producing hydrocephalus. Spread to the nasal and sphenoidal sinuses may take place. Cystic and degenerative changes occur in the tumour.

Clinically the endocrine picture is one of hypopituitarism, manifested by lassitude and a gain in weight. Loss of sexual libido, testicular atrophy and disappearance of secondary sexual characteristics occur in the male, and the skin becomes soft and the hair scanty. Amenorrhoea takes place in the female. Headache may be pronounced and extension of the tumour to the optic chiasma may produce blindness or failing vision, typically bitemporal hemianopia. Pallor of the optic discs is observed, but papilloedema is rare. Where the lesion involves the nasal passages epistaxis may occur and extension to the orbit can produce unilateral proptosis. Somnolence and polyuria arise with implication of the hypothalamus. Radiographs may show enlargement of the pituitary fossa and erosion of the clinoid processes. Measurement of pituitary hormone levels should be undertaken and detailed assessment made of visual acuity and fields. Investigation with CT scanning, air encephalography and angiography is usually undertaken.

The *eosinophil* adenoma is characterised by acidophil-staining properties. It may also become large and extend upwards. The male is more commonly affected, and the endocrine abnormality results in gigantism in early life and acromegaly in the adult. Enlargement of the hands, mandibular hypertrophy, macroglossia and kyphosis are common in the latter. Pressure effects similar to those of the chromophobe type may be noted.

The *basophil* adenoma is smaller, less common and may be associated with Cushing's syndrome. Pressure effects seldom occur, but an endocrine state similar to that of hyperadrenocorticism may be produced (p. 269).

Treatment is indicated for increasing blindness or severe headache, and operative removal of the tumour is frequently followed by improvement. The gland may be approached by the transfrontal or trans-sphenoidal route, the former being necessary for a large tumour producing marked optic tract pressure. Complete removal of the growth is difficult and recurrence within five years takes place in 30 to 50 per cent of cases. Destruction of the pituitary by trans-sphenoidal insertion of the radioactive yttrium pellets is an alternative procedure giving good results.

CEREBRAL TUMOURS

The **glioma**, which may be benign or malignant, accounts for about half the primary intracranial tumours. There are several varieties.

The *astrocytoma* is usually benign and slowly growing, but may be highly malignant. It develops mainly in the cerebellum of children and young adults and may reach considerable size. Initially solid, cystic degeneration is common, a nodule of tumour tissue lying in the wall.

The *spongioblastoma multiforme* is more common. It arises between 30 and 50 years of age and is a highly cellular widely infiltrating tumour with necrotic areas, affecting principally the frontal, parietal or temporal lobes. Haemorrhage into the tumour is common, but cyst formation rare.

Medulloblastoma arises in the cerebellum of children. It is soft, friable and highly malignant. Projection into the ventricle may lead to the development of hydrocephalus. Invasion of the meninges is common. The histological picture resembles the adrenal neuroblastoma with rosette formation.

Metastatic carcinoma in the cerebral hemisphere or vermis of the cerebellum may be single or multiple. The bronchus is the most common primary site, but the breast and kidney are frequent sources.

Clinical features

Symptoms of intracranial tumours may be due to increased intracranial tension or arise from direct pressure on neighbouring structures.

Raised intracranial pressure results from obstruction to the flow of cerebrospinal fluid or from the increasing volume of a large tumour. Headache, nausea and vomiting are prominent symptoms. The headache, often worse in the morning, is of a throbbing character and gradually becomes more severe, but its situation is of no localising value. Increasing drowsiness, mental deterioration and dementia are common. Visual disturbance often progresses to complete blindness. Menstruation may become irregular, and the male is sometimes impotent.

The local effects may be due to pressure on or destruction of neural elements. Epileptiform attacks, either momentary or full convulsions, are frequent. A focal attack may indicate the side of a tumour, such as spasm of an arm resulting from a lesion of the motor cortex. Temporal lesions produce visual and auditory hallucinations. Aphasia indicates a tumour near the left lateral cerebral sulcus in a right-handed individual. Frontal lobe tumours may be silent or lead to intellectual impairment or dementia. Brain stem tumours cause early multiple cranial nerve palsies with involvement of motor and sensory tracts. Cerebellar tumours produce early signs of raised intracranial pressure followed by nystagmus and ataxia. Detailed neurological examination may help in localising the lesion, but is often unreliable, and ancillary investigations are valuable.

Investigations

Plain radiographs of the skull demonstrate bone erosion, calcification of a tumour, displacement of the pineal gland, or enlargement of the pituitary fossa. Separation of sutures and a 'beaten brass' appearance of the skull occur with raised intracranial pressure. Neuroradiological investigation is undertaken principally by CT scanning, but angiography, isotope scanning and air encephalography are indicated in certain instances.

Treatment

The type of tumour has considerable bearing on the treatment. *Complete removal* is feasible in certain forms of benign tumour, such as meningioma, astrocytoma and acoustic neuroma. *Incomplete removal* is indicated where radical excision is likely to destroy vital structures or produce serious disability. It is employed in certain pituitary adenomas and some acoustic neuromas. Malignant glioma may show temporary relief of intracranial tension, but partial excision may only prolong the illness. *Decompression* by removal of part of the skull is now employed less often as a palliative procedure for the same reason. Ventriculocisternostomy may be necessary in certain cases of third ventricle and midbrain tumours to relieve hydrocephalus. *Irradiation* after decompression may benefit certain gliomas, particularly medulloblastoma.

Trigeminal neuralgia

This condition of unknown aetiology generally arises after the age of 50 years, more commonly in women, and is characterised by paroxysmal attacks of intense pain in the distribution of one or more divisions of the trigeminal nerve. The attacks may be precipitated by any external stimulus, particularly cold, applied to a localised 'trigger' area on the face or gums. The maxillary and mandibular divisions on the right side are more commonly affected. Hyperaesthesia may be present during and between the attacks. Intracranial tumour and aneurysm, by causing pressure on the nerve, may give rise to a similar pain, but usually lead to diminution of sensation on the face. Dental and paranasal sinus infection can be excluded by the more constant nature of the pain and by radiography.

Treatment of mild cases by analgesic drugs is often effective. Carbamazepine may be highly effective but may cause severe vomiting or marrow depression. Severe pain may be relieved by an injection of alcohol into the Gasserian ganglion via a needle passing through the cheek to reach the foramen ovale, or by section of the sensory root of the nerve. Anaesthesia of the face is produced, but is of little significance compared with the original attacks. Relief is usually temporary, but may last for six to twelve months. Division of the sensory root, performed by an intradural approach through the middle cranial fossa, has the advantage of permanency and preserves the corneal nerve supply.

SPINAL CORD

Anatomy

The spinal cord is 45 cm in length and extends in the vertebral canal from the upper border of the atlas to the lower border of the first lumbar vertebra. The lower tapering extremity is termed the conus medullaris. The cord in early foetal life occupies the whole canal, but with growth it becomes relatively shorter. Spinal segments do not thus lie at the same level as the corresponding vertebrae and the lower lumbar and sacral nerve roots pass almost vertically to enter their foramina. A cervical enlargement is present from the third cervical to the second thoracic vertebrae, and a lumbar enlargement from the ninth to the twelfth thoracic vertebrae, at which levels the cord almost fills the spinal canal. Small tumours in these sites therefore produce their effects at an early stage. The cord is surrounded by pia mater, arachnoid mater and dura mater, the last forming a strong membrane which acts as a barrier to infection and tumour

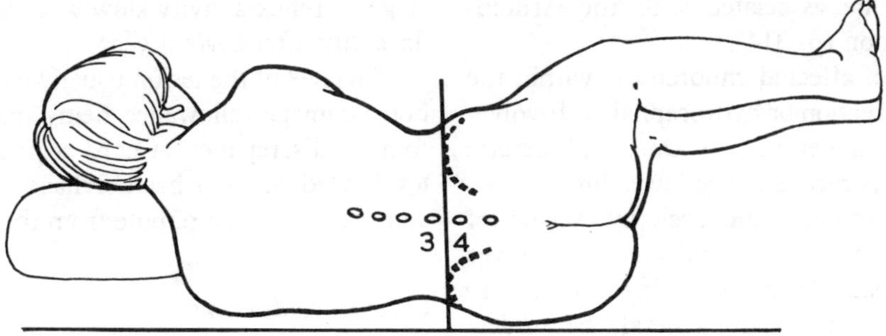

Fig. 26.5 Lumbar puncture. The needle is inserted through the space between the 3rd and 4th spinous processes which lies on a line joining the uppermost part of the iliac crest.

growth. It is separated from the bony walls of the canal by fat and a venous plexus. The subarachnoid space extends to the second sacral vertebra and contains cerebrospinal fluid. The cord is attached to the dura by pointed fibrous bands called dentate ligaments.

Lumbar puncture may be required for diagnostic or therapeutic reasons. It is performed by inserting a needle in the midline between the spinous processes of the third and fourth lumbar vertebrae. This point may be defined by a line joining the superior limit of both iliac crests (Fig. 26.5). Penetration of the dura is readily detected, and with the patient in the lateral position fluid flows readily and its pressure can be measured by a glass manometer (Fig. 26.6). Compression of both jugular veins raises the intracranial pressure, and in the normal subject this is transmitted to the spinal theca and can be recorded (Queckenstedt phenomenon). The resting value is 130 mm of fluid; it rises to about 200 mm on compression and falls quickly on release. Blockage of the spinal canal by tumour or arachnoid adhesions prevents this change and the test is therefore of considerable diagnostic importance. Stagnation of fluid is followed by a rise in protein content above the normal (200 to 400 mg per litre).

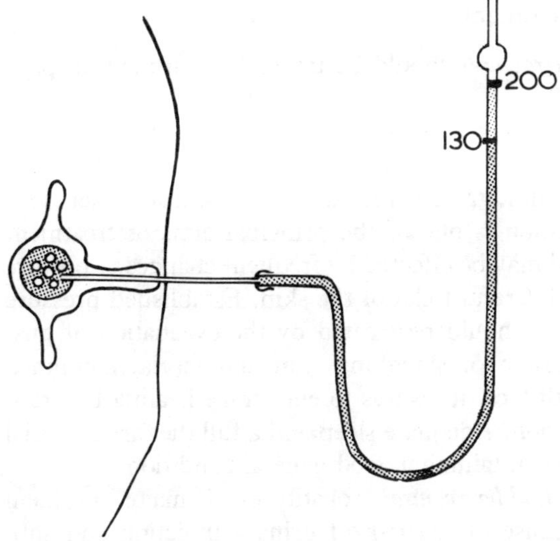

Fig. 26.6 Spinal puncture manometry; jugular compression causes the pressure to rise from 130 to 200 mm

Cerebrospinal fluid may also be obtained by puncture of the cisterna magna with a needle inserted between the spine of the axis and the occiput, care being taken to avoid damage to the underlying medulla. Penicillin and streptomycin may be inserted into the subarachnoid space by either of these routes for the treatment of meningitis, neither drug being normally excreted into the cerebrospinal fluid following systemic administration.

Congenital anomalies

Meningocele and myelomeningocele

Protrusion of the meninges occurs as the result of a defect in the vertebral laminae (*spina bifida*). It is more common in the lumbosacral region and when composed of meninges alone is known as a **meningocele**. A sac is formed which may be unilocular or multilocular, communicating with subarachnoid space of which it is a dilated portion. More frequently elements of the cord are found crossing the cyst cavity and are adherent to the skin, the condition being known as a **myelomeningocele.**

The latter may be associated with the Arnold-Chiari phenomenon (p. 314).

The majority of affected children die within the first year from infection or hydrocephalus. Involvement of the sacral nerves may cause sphincteric disturbance and paralysis of the lower limbs.

Treatment of simple meningocele by excision of the sac and closure of muscle and skin defect gives good results. Repair of a myelomeningocele is more complicated, but should, in general, be undertaken. The management of limb paralysis and rectal or urinary incontinence presents many problems which require the combined care of a surgeon in each specialty. Resection of the bladder-neck or its reconstruction by plastic procedures may result in urinary control. Diversion of the urinary flow by transplantation of the ureters or uretero-ileostomy is an alternative.

INJURY OF THE SPINAL CORD

Spinal cord damage arises most commonly in fracture dislocation of the cervical spine, but may also occur in the thoracolumbar region. The extent of the lesion varies from slight bruising to complete transection. In the former the neural damage may be minimal with only transient loss of function, or there may be degeneration of the axis cylinder and death of the nerve cells; recovery of unmyelinated fibres does not occur.

Clinical features

The effect of an injury depends on its severity and its level. A state of *spinal shock* develops in all cases and results in cessation of cord function. This is manifest by complete muscular paralysis, loss of sensation below the lesion, abolition of reflexes and retention of urine. Improvement within a short period of up to three weeks indicates minor injury, but if paraplegia or tetraplegia persists for a longer period permanent damage must be assumed.

In the permanent state reflex activity slowly returns, automatic micturition and defaecation develop, and limb reflexes may be elicited after three or four weeks. A mass reflex may be present at this stage consisting of flexor spasms of the lower limbs, involuntary micturition and sweating. The stage of reflex activity slowly passes into complete flaccidity after several years.

The level of the lesion usually corresponds to the bony damage, allowance being made for the anatomical discrepancy of cord segments to vertebral level. Oedema and haemorrhage may occasionally compress the cord remote from the site of fracture.

Cervical cord lesions

A complete lesion above the fourth cervical vertebra produces respiratory paralysis and death; below this level diaphragmatic respiration can maintain oxygenation even if the thoracic muscles are paralysed. Paralysis of upper and lower limbs results when the lesion is above the first thoracic segment. Pulmonary infection due to poor respiratory movement is a frequent complication and is often fatal.

Thoracolumbar cord lesion

The twelfth thoracic and first lumbar vertebrae are most commonly involved resulting in paralysis of the lower limbs, with loss of sensation of thighs and legs. Movements of the hip are maintained. Injury of the nerve roots of the cauda equina is uncommon but results in variable defects of muscular power and sensation of the lower limbs and in sphincter disturbances.

Treatment

Fractures should be treated as outlined on page 378.

Bedsores, due to pressure on anaesthetised areas, usually arise over bony prominences such as the sacrum, greater trochanter, heel and shoulder. Prevention is one of the principal aims of treatment and may be effected by frequent changes of posture and careful toilet of the skin. Established pressure sores should be treated by the evacuation of pus, excision of sloughing skin and fascia, combined with local measures to encourage healing by granulation. Adequate sleep and a full diet are essential in maintaining a good general condition.

Bladder control constitutes a major problem because of the risk of urinary infection and subsequent fatal pyelonephritis. Repeated catheterisation is better avoided, and continuous tidal drainage combined with antibiotic therapy offers the best results. Suprapubic cystostomy is sometimes employed but does not necessarily prevent urinary infection. The development of automatic micturition may follow after five to six weeks, emptying being aided by manual suprapubic compression by the patient. Prolonged recumbency and immobilisation should be avoided as they encourage the stagnation of urine and lead to stone formation.

Contractures should be prevented by intensive physiotherapy and splintage. Painful muscle spasms may require temporary paralysis of nerves by alcohol injection or their section for permanent results.

Rehabilitation is of considerable importance and the morale must be maintained. Graduated exercises will lead to an improvement in recovering muscles. Power in intact muscles can be further developed to compensate for paralysis and may allow reasonable activity. Re-education may permit walking with the aid of a caliper or crutch, and such treatment is preferably carried out in a spinal injury centre where association with other paraplegics leads to a keen spirit of competition and an improved mental outlook.

Epidural infection

Acute infection is uncommon. It may arise subsequent to osteomyelitis of the spine or from an infective focus elsewhere in the body. Back pain and later weakness of the lower limbs is rapidly followed by their complete paralysis. Lumbar puncture demonstrates spinal block and an increased leucocyte count in the cerebrospinal fluid. Laminectomy and drainage produce complete recovery if performed early, but if delayed poor spinal function results from thrombosis of cord vessels.

Chronic infection is usually tuberculous and is now rare. The presence of granulation tissue and caseous material under tension in the epidural space is secondary to a vertebral lesion. Paraplegia may arise early in the course of the disease or be delayed for many years. Chemotherapy, spinal immobilisation and drainage of the abscess by removal of a rib and transverse process is necessary. Laminectomy may result in weakening of the vertebral column.

TUMOURS

The majority of tumours affecting the spinal cord are *intrathecal* but extramedullary (Fig. 26.7, B); they comprise meningioma and neurofibroma and generally arise in the thoracic region. Commonly oval in shape, extension outside the vertebral canal may occur with the production of a dumb-bell tumour. In neurofibroma the posterior nerve root is more usually affected. Calcification may take place. *Extradural* tumours include plasmacytoma, lipoma, angioma, osteoma and secondary neoplasm (Fig. 26.7, A). *Intramedullary* tumours are gliomatous lesions similar to those already described (p. 323 and Fig. 26.7, C).

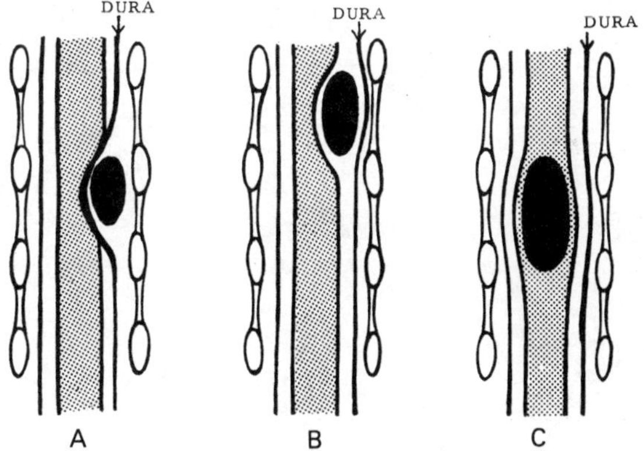

Fig. 26.7 Tumours in the spinal canal causing pressure on the spinal cord. **A.** Extradural. **B.** Intrathecal. **C.** Intramedullary.

Clinically the common tumour is manifest by pain radiating along the distribution of the compressed spinal nerve root. Gradual paralysis and sensory disturbance follow and may eventually become complete. The Brown-Sequard syndrome may develop from compression of one side of the cord. It consists of spastic paralysis and loss of vibration and joint sense on the same side below the lesion. On the opposite side there is loss of pain and thermal sensation. Sphincteric disturbance affecting bowel and bladder may occur with the development of automatic micturition and faecal incontinence. Radiography of the vertebrae may show bony erosion from pressure of a tumour, and the diagnosis of a spinal block can be made by lumbar puncture and myelography.

Laminectomy is indicated. Removal of the tumour is followed by slow recovery of paraplegia in most instances. Decompression of the spinal cord followed by irradiation may be of benefit for malignant secondary deposits.

Chordotomy

Division of the spinothalamic tract on the anteromedial aspect of the spinal cord is performed for the relief of intractable pain (p. 446). The section is made in the thoracic or cervical region above the upper limit of the pain.

FURTHER READING

Hayward. R. (1980). *Essentials of Neurosurgery*. Oxford: Blackwell.

Hayward, R. (1980). *Management of Acute Head Injuries*. Oxford: Blackwell.

Jennett, B. and Teasdale, G. (1981). *Management of Head Injuries*. Philadelphia: F. A. Davis Co.

27

Orthopaedic surgery

DEFINITIONS

To facilitate subsequent description, the following definitions of orthopaedic terms are included.

A. Words used to describe parts

'Cubitus' refers to the elbow.
'Coxa' refers to the hip.
'Genu' refers to the knee.
'Talipes' refers to the heel and foot together.
'Pes' refers to the forefoot alone, although these last two are often used synonymously.

B. Words used to describe deformities

'Valgus' describes a deformity where the part is directed away from the midline of the body.
'Varus' describes a deformity in which the part is directed towards the midline.
'Equinus', derived from the vertical position of the tarsus in a horse's foot, is used to describe limitation of dorsiflexion of the foot.
'Calcaneus' is used to describe deformities where the calcaneum assumes a more vertical position than normal.

C. Words used to describe spinal changes

'Kyphosis' describes abnormal forward curvature.
'Lordosis' is excessive backward curvature.
'Scoliosis' denotes lateral curvature from the midline.

D. Words used to describe operative procedures

Osteotomy is the division of a bone.
Tenotomy is the division of a tendon.
Arthrodesis is fusion of a joint.
Tenodesis is deliberate anchoring of a tendon, perfomed to control an abnormal movement.
Epiphyseodesis is fusion of an epiphysis, undertaken to correct or prevent the onset of deformity in the growing limb.
Arthroplasty is reconstruction of a joint, aimed at restoring movement.
Pseudarthrosis describes a false joint,which may be deliberately sought, as in certain operations on the hip, or result from a pathological process, as when a false joint forms at the site of an ununited fracture.

DEFORMITIES

GENERALISED CONGENITAL DEFORMITIES

These lesions are due to abnormal mesenchymal development. Bony abnormalities are easily recognised but other mesenchymal tissues may also be involved. They may be classified as follows:

1. General errors of mesenchymal development. Osteogenesis imperfecta.
2. Errors mainly restricted to bone.
   (*a*) Cartilage bone:
   Multiple osteochondromatosis.
   Dyschondroplasia.
   Achondroplasia.

(*b*) Membrane bone:
Cleidocranial dysostosis.

3. Errors mainly restricted to muscle.
Arthrogryposis multiplex congenita.

Osteogenesis imperfecta (fragilitas ossium)

In this hereditary condition there are brittle bones, lax ligaments and blue sclerotics, the last due to an abnormal translucency rendering the choroid pigment visible. Occasionally the bones are normal, only blue sclerotics and joint laxity being present.

Clinical features

Two types occur: (1) *Foetal*, in which multiple fractures, deformities and poor ossification in the skull are present at birth. Many survive only for a few days, but in others spontaneous fractures occur with severe deformities of trunk and limbs. (2) *Adolescent*, where the child is normal at birth but develops a tendency to fractures from minor trauma later, which diminishes again as maturity is reached.

Multiple osteochondromatosis

A hereditary abnormality of the epiphyseal plate is present, nests of cartilage cells becoming separated from the edges of the plate in the metaphysis. These continue to grow, forming exostoses bearing a cartilaginous cap until the parent epiphysis fuses. The exostosis points away from the epiphysis becoming, as growth proceeds, left behind on the shaft. As the whole epiphysis is involved some stunting of growth follows. Exostoses causing symptoms from pressure should be removed.

Dyschondroplasia

This developmental abnormality of the epiphyseal plate results in nests of cartilage cells becoming displaced within the bone, forming enchondromata. The condition is not hereditary, is commonly unilateral, and may be confined to one bone. There may be multiple enchondromata of the long bones of the hands and feet. Shortening of an involved major long bone may be considerable.

Achondroplasia

This is a familial condition characterised by uniform aplasia of epiphyseal cartilage. It leads to dwarfing with short limbs and a trunk of normal size, accompanied by a prominent forehead and fingers approaching equal length ('trident hand').

Cleidocranial dysostosis

This condition is a hereditary developmental abnormality affecting mainly membranous bone, with absence of clavicles and a large skull vault in which there is delayed closure of sutures. Rarely there is aplasia of the pubic bones.

Arthrogryposis multiplex congenita

In this rare condition there is widespread fibrosis of muscle leading to multiple secondary deformities such as dislocated hips, club feet and hands, and generalised joint stiffness. The deformities are markedly resistant to treatment.

LOCALISED CONGENITAL DEFORMITIES

Two main groups exist: (1) those due to arrested development, which occurs in three forms, and (2) those due to abnormal development.

Arrested development

1. Failure of fusion

Spina bifida. The neural canal may fail to fuse, the degree varying from a state incompatible with life, with rudimentary nervous tissue lying exposed on the back (myelomeningocele), to a minor laminar defect in the lumbosacral region, accidentally discovered on radiography. The severe defect is associated with hydrocephalus, due to a block in cerebrospinal fluid movement and resulting in raised intracranial pressure. Involvement of neural elements leads to secondary abnormalities in the legs, varying from minor pes cavus to extreme club foot, dislocated hips and complete paraplegia with incontinence (p. 325).

2. Absence of parts

Large portions of limbs may fail to develop. There may be an absence of major bones such as the femur, tibia or radius causing characteristic deformities, or minor lesions such as aplasia of a metatarsal, or absence of a muscle may occur.

3. Failure of one stage of development

Examples include *congenital dislocation of the hip*, where the probable basic error is faulty acetabular development; *Sprengel's shoulder*, the scapula failing to descend from the neck to its final upper thoracic level; *syndactylism*, or webbing of the fingers or toes; and *congenital coxa vara*, due to failure of ossification in the lower portion of the femoral neck.

Congenital dislocation of the hip

Deficient acetabular development permits upwards displacement of the femoral head. Before ambulation subluxation is frequent, dislocation only taking place after weight-bearing has begun. As a result of the displacement there is late appearance of the ossific centre for the femoral *head*, a vertical and forward pointing femoral *neck* (anteversion), a stretched *capsule*, often adherent to the femoral head, and the fibro-cartilaginous limbus (labrum acetabulare) becomes forced into the socket by the abnormally placed head, often preventing full reduction.

Clinical features

Females are predominantly affected. There is a hereditary tendency and it is common in Northern Italy, Austria and parts of France, but is rare in negroid races. It may be unilateral or bilateral. The incidence is higher with increased joint laxity and following breech delivery with extended hips. During the routine examination of all neonates particular attention is given to movement of the hips. Limitation of abduction of the hips in flexion and shortening of limb length are two important signs of unilateral dislocation. If the dislocation can be reduced, a marked click will be felt on abduction of the leg in the fully flexed position and due to the femoral head riding over the edge of the acetabulum. Bilateral dislocations are less readily diagnosed but limited abduction becomes the most important sign. Occasionally hip dislocation is not recognised until after a child has started to walk. A characteristic limp is noted with a swaying movement towards the affected side. This is due to inefficient abductor muscles which have no real fulcrum and is called Trendelenburg's sign (Fig. 27.1).

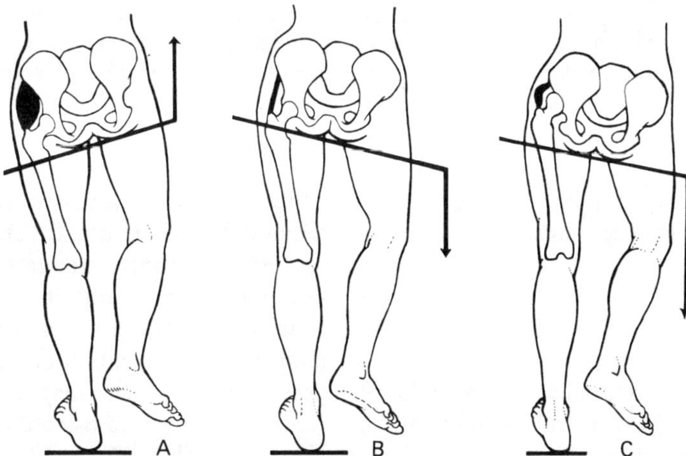

Fig. 27.1 Trendelenburg test. The patient stands on one leg, normally the opposite buttock rises (**A**). A positive result shown by the opposite buttock falling indicates disease. It is found if the abductor muscles are weak as in poliomyelitis (**B**); or if the fulcrum of the hip joint is destroyed as in dislocation (**C**).

Radiographs in young infants may be difficult to interpret because the epiphysis for the femoral head has not yet appeared. Positioning of the lower limb in 45 degrees of abduction demonstrates a break in continuity of a line drawn around the upper margin of the obturator foramen and continued below the femoral neck (Shenton's line) (Fig. 27.2).

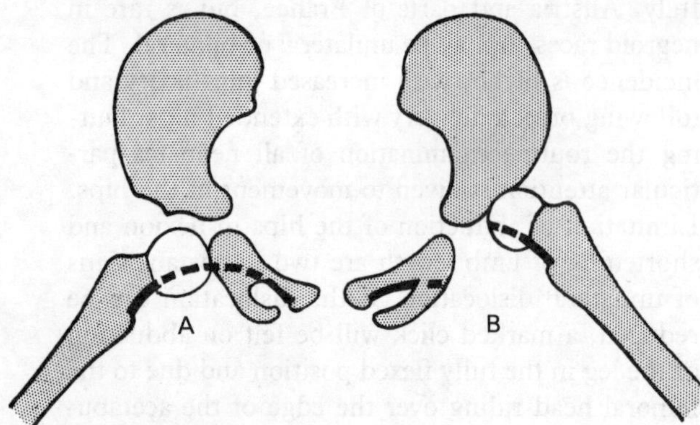

Fig. 27.2 Congenital dislocation of the hip. X-ray outline demonstrates the normal Shenton's line (**A**) and a broken line in dislocation (**B**).

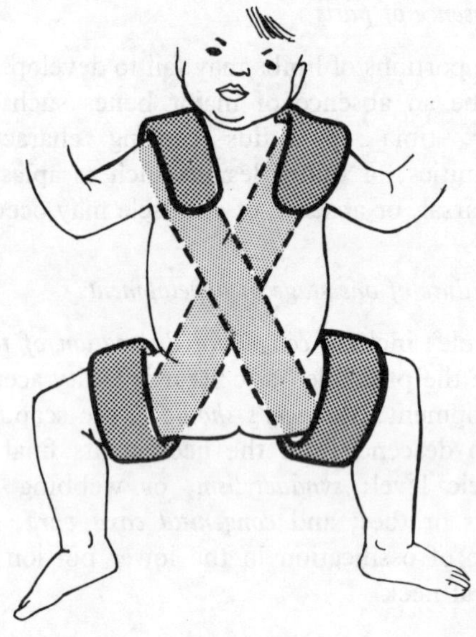

Fig. 27.3 Malleable aluminium splint to maintain abduction in congenital dislocation of the hip

Differential diagnosis

Acute pyogenic arthritis of infancy, by destroying the epiphysis of the head of the femur, leaves an unstable joint indistinguishable from congenital dislocation. A febrile illness in early infancy or scars in the region of the hip joint should raise suspicion whilst radiography reveals a normal acetabulum, with destructive changes in the femur. Congenital coxa vara causes progressive angulation in early childhood and a similar clinical appearance. Paralytic dislocation due to muscle imbalance may occur, but the causal paralysis is unmistakable.

Treatment

In the newborn the abnormal hip must be reduced by full abduction and held in this position by an abduction splint (Fig. 27.3) for several months until the joint is stable. When reduction cannot be easily obtained, the legs should be held in traction using a hoop frame which allows gradual abduction whilst still maintaining traction. During this period the femoral head is brought down to the acetabular margin and allowed to remain in the acetabulum on abduction. When this is satisfactory the position is held in an abduction plaster or harness until hip development is adequate.

If reduction is not thus obtained, open reduction at one year should be undertaken. There is no indication for surgery prior to this age and it can result in necrosis of the femoral head. Whilst waiting the joint is left unimpeded to maintain mobility. The operative aim is to reduce the femoral head by removing all obstructing tissue, the position being retained by a plaster hip spica. Usually the femoral neck is markedly anteverted and the hip can only be properly reduced by full internal rotation, requiring a derotating osteotomy of the femur at an interval of six weeks. There is minimal development of the acetabulum after five years and surgery after this age may include realigning the acetabulum by iliac osteotomy to correct the deficient roof. (Fig. 27.4). It is now uncommon for congenitally dislocated hips to present in adolescence but at this age they are often better left untreated, surgery not then improving function.

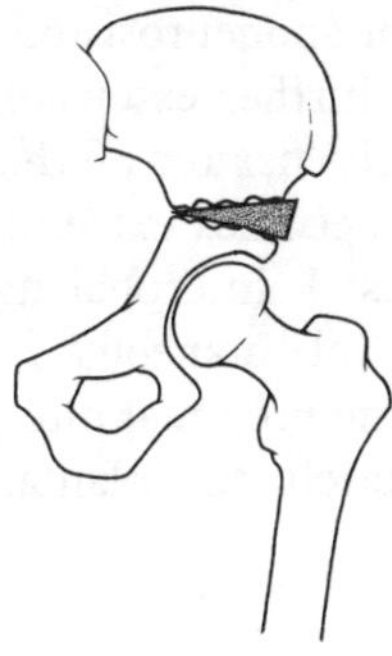

Fig. 27.4 Realignment of the acetabulum by iliac osteotomy and insertion of a wedge-shaped bone graft

Abnormal development

Congenital talipes equinovarus

This deformity consists of three elements—*equinus*, the hindfoot being drawn up with a tight tendo calcaneus, *varus*, the sole facing inwards, and *adduction* of the forefoot, making the inner border of the foot concave and point upwards, often partly masking the equinus element. The head of the talus, which is normally felt just below and anterior to the medial malleolus, forms a prominence in front of the lateral malleolus. This in turn causes internal rotation of the mid-tarsal joint and allows the anterior tibial muscles to draw the foot upwards into adduction.

Talipes equinovarus may also be secondary to congenital neurogenic lesions, such as spina bifida, or be myogenic as in arthrogryposis. Intra-uterine pressure may be an aetiological factor.

Clinical features. Males predominate, often with a familial trend. The condition is frequently bilateral, one foot usually being more affected than the other. Mild forms may be unrecognised, as normal infants tend to hold their feet inverted. When the deformity is restricted to the forefoot it is known as *metatarsus varus*.

Treatment. Early treatment begun immediately after birth results in a useful plantigrade foot. The aim, which is restoration of the normal talo-calcaneal relationship, is accomplished by repeated manipulation and subsequent plaster casts until the deformity has been fully corrected. These are followed by Denis Browne splints (Fig. 27.5), which utilise the infant's natural tendency to kick as a corrective force. Firm boots are worn for the first four or five years to hold correction. If this is not achieved by the age of six to eight weeks then surgical release offers the best results. Soft tissue operations, such as elongation of the tendo calcaneus, division of the contracted tissue on the inner side of the foot, or transplantation of the tibialis anterior tendon to the outer side of the foot are suitable up to six years of age. At a later age a wedge may be excised from the outer side of the foot at the calcaneo-cuboid joint, so that the forefoot may be aligned. Where deformity is severe and symptoms suggest correction, extensive bony procedures such as a triple arthrodesis may be carried out, stabilising the three joints as shown in Fig. 27.6.

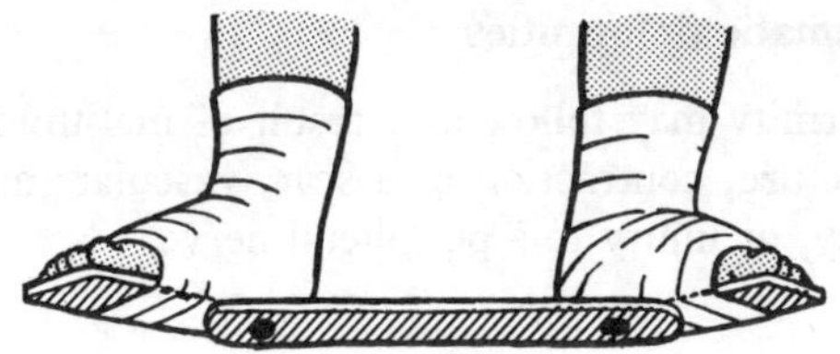

Fig. 27.5 Denis Browne splint applied for talipes equinovarus

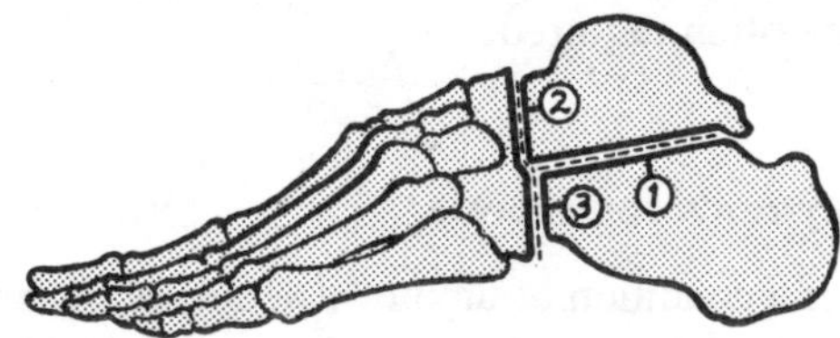

Fig. 27.6 Triple arthrodesis. 1. The subtalar joint. 2. The talonavicular joint. 3. The calcaneocuboid joint.

Congenital talipes calcaneovalgus

The typical club-foot deformity is reversed with the foot held in dorsiflexion and eversion. Intra-uterine pressure is an aetiological factor. Confusion may arise with the rare condition of congenital vertical talus, in which the latter points directly downwards with the navicular articulating with the neck of the talus. In both lesions there is excessive dorsiflexion but in congenital vertical talus the sole of the foot is markedly convex. Simple calcaneovalgus deformity corrects spontaneously whilst congenital vertical talus requires surgical reduction.

Traumatic deformities

Deformity may follow as a result of mal-union of a fracture, contraction of a scar, vascular insufficiency, or injury to a peripheral nerve.

1. Mal-union of fractures

When a bone unites in an unsatisfactory position, improvement can only be obtained by an open operation (osteotomy) or closed manipulation (refracture), the latter only being feasible before consolidation is complete. Both methods can be combined (osteotomy-osteoclasis), the majority of the bone being divided surgically, the remainder being completed by careful manipulation 10 to 14 days later.

2. Contraction of scars

The degree of deformity resulting from a scar depends on its site, direction and the extent of tissue destruction. Scars crossing a joint, particularly the flexor surface, or at right angles to natural skin creases are particularly liable to contract. Plastic operations on the scar or its excision and skin grafting are often required.

Dupuytren's contracture

This is a condition of unknown aetiology, whereby the palmar aponeurosis becomes replaced by fibrous tissue, which subsequently contracts. The slip of aponeurosis to the ring finger is most commonly affected, followed by that to the little and then to the middle finger, the index and thumb being rarely involved. Fibrosis beneath the skin produces bands on either side of the tendon sheath, which cause flexion of the metacarpophalangeal and proximal interphalangeal joints.

Clinical features

The lesion more often affects males, may be hereditary and usually commences in middle life. It is often bilateral and may be precipitated by trauma where a predisposition exists. A small fibrous nodule appears initially at the base of the ring or little finger in the distal palmar crease and spreads to involve the slip of aponeurosis on the ulnar side of the digit. Later, further extension occurs to other fingers. Eventually flexion of the proximal interphalangeal joint becomes extreme, producing dislocation, the distal interphalangeal joint being hyperextended. Subcutaneous thickening of the dorsal aspect of the proximal interphalangeal joints is often seen. Rarely the plantar fascia becomes involved.

Treatment

The early mild lesion may be treated by repeated stretching of the involved finger, but complete excision of all involved palmar fascia, with careful freeing of the skin, digital nerves and vessels is to be preferred in more advanced cases. Where deformity is marked, secondary joint changes are present and amputation may give the best functional result.

Vascular insufficiency

Connective tissue survives interruption of the blood supply and its later restoration more easily than the highly developed muscles and nerves. Volkmann's ischaemic contracture is considered on page 373.

Infantile torticollis

This deformity is due to tightness in one sternomastoid muscle, as a result of interstitial fibrosis and probably follows impairment of its blood supply at the time of parturition. The condition develops during childhood, the muscle failing to lengthen proportionately with growth elsewhere. Soon after birth a fusiform swelling in the sternomastoid may be observed which eventually disappears. Tilting of the head to one side may later be apparent producing finally facial asymmetry. The condition must be distinguished from torticollis due to ocular causes, spasm from adjacent inflammatory lesions such as adenitis, and congenital anomalies or disease of the cervical spine.

Treatment

The mother should be taught to stretch the infant's

sternomastoid several times a day for about one year. Operation at the age of three to four years is required if conservative measures fail. The muscle should be divided near its insertion and regular physiotherapy and stretching should be carried out until full correction is achieved.

NEUROLOGICAL DEFORMITIES

The main causes of neurological deformaties apart from peripheral nerve injures (p. 413) are obstetric paralysis, cerebral palsy, anterior poliomyelitis and spina bifida and peroneal muscle atrophy.

Obstetric paralysis

This is due to traction on the head or arm during a difficult delivery, presenting in three ways depending upon the site of damage to the brachial plexus. The *upper arm* type (Erb-Duchenne) is due to injury to the upper trunk (fifth and sixth cervical roots); the *lower arm* type (Klumpke) is due to injury of the lower trunk (eighth cervical and first thoracic roots); and the *whole arm* type occurs where the complete plexus is disrupted.

The upper arm type is most common, with paralysis of the shoulder muscles, biceps and brachioradialis, together with the extensors of the wrist and fingers in severe cases. The humerus is adducted and internally rotated by the unopposed action of latissimus dorsi, with the hand held in pronation. When the extensors are paralysed, both wrist and fingers are flexed.

Treatment

Spontaneous recovery is usual but daily passive movements particularly external rotation of the shoulder joint should be performed. Assessment is carried out at about the age of one year and when an established clinical pattern is present surgical correction may be indicated at the age of five years.

Cerebral palsy ('spastic paralysis')

Spasticity is associated with an upper motor neurone lesion, which may be at any level from the cerebral cortex to the spinal cord. The following relates to the condition in childhood but much is applicable to other spastic conditions such as hemiplegia following a cerebrovascular accident.

Pathology

The usual cause is a birth injury, either direct damage to the brain substance or the result of intracranial haemorrhage. It may also follow meningitis or encephalitis in early post-natal life. Lesions may be considered at three levels: (*a*) *cortical*, leading to either or both spasticity and mental deficiency; (*b*) *mid-brain*, causing involuntary movements (athetosis); and (*c*) *cerebellar*, which is rare but causes cerebellar ataxia.

Clinical features

The age at which symptoms appear is related to the degree of severity. Delay in raising the head or sitting are early features. Other neurological signs become evident later, and although generally mixed may be considered under three headings.

1. *Mental retardation.* All grades from normal to complete idiocy occur, but the level of intelligence is often higher than the appearance suggests, particularly in athetosis, where lack of muscle control renders speech difficult. Some emotional instability is usually present.

2. *Involuntary movements* (athetosis) vary from a coarse tremor when attempting fine movements to constant writhing affecting the whole body. They are worse when purposeful movements are attempted or on emotional stress and are usually absent in sleep. The upper limbs tend to be more affected.

3. *Spasticity.* Tone and tendon reflexes are increased. Deformities, resulting from the stronger muscles overcoming the weaker ones, tend to follow a pattern. In the upper limb the arm is adducted and internally rotated, the elbow and wrist flexed and pronated, whilst the fingers are flexed over the thumb. In the lower limb the hip is flexed and adducted, hence if both are affected they cross each other when walking is attempted and produce a 'scissors' gait. In severe cases the hips may be dislocated, the knees flexed and the feet in equinus.

Treatment

A cure is not feasible due to the permanent cerebral damage, but much can be done to make the best use of remaining function. Treatment is mainly conservative, consisting of re-education and corrective splinting, with operation as an adjunct in selected cases. The aim in re-education is to teach voluntary relaxation and strengthening of the weaker muscle groups. Corrective splints aid relaxation when spasm is marked, control any tendency to deformity, and assist function. Care must be employed in their use, as a splint to control one deformity may hinder the overall progress.

When one muscle group is stronger than its antagonists, balance may be restored by selective division of nerves, for example, adductor spasm causing the 'scissors' gait may be controlled by division of the obturator nerve. Elongation or division of tendons is useful in correcting established deformities, such as elongation of the tendo calcaneus for equinus of the foot, or division of the hamstrings for flexion contracture of the knee. Arthrodesis of joints may be of value in adults. Operation should be preceded by a trial with the joint splinted in the proposed position of fusion, to ascertain that function will not be retarded. Selective destruction of the globus pallidus may help where athetosis is marked.

Anterior poliomyelitis

Poliomyelitis is caused by a filter-passing virus which attacks the anterior horn cells in the spinal cord and brain stem. It is generally endemic with occasional local epidemics. The virus is excreted mainly in the faeces and respiratory secretions, being chiefly spread by droplet. The incubation period is two to three weeks. In about half of the cases the attack is abortive. Groups of anterior horn cells are affected with surrounding oedema and haemorrhage. Some cells are destroyed, others recovering when the oedema subsides, so that the final disability cannot be assessed from the initial paralysis. Death is usually from respiratory failure.

Clinical features

Children are more often affected than adults. There are three clinical stages.

1. *The stage of onset* consists of an acute febrile illness with the signs of meningeal irritation such as headache, drowsiness and neck stiffness, together with pain in the affected muscles. Flaccid paralysis follows rapidly and is often extensive. The fever is transient, but pain remains for three to six weeks. Lumbar puncture at this stage shows a moderate increase in both cells and pressure.

2. *The stage of recovery*. Improvement of the initial paralysis begins when the pain subsides, and continues for about two years. Related at first to recovery in the anterior horn cells, it is later due to improved efficiency of the surviving neuromuscular units. Recovery is unlikely in a muscle which has remained completely paralysed for six months.

3. *The stage of residual paralysis* is reached when the muscle power no longer alters. Deformities may occur either from stretching of paralysed muscles, gravity or external pressure such as bed clothes. When paralysis is extensive the limb may be cold with associated chilblains, and if the attack occurred before growth was complete, shortening may follow.

Treatment

Active immunity may be established by inoculation with a living attenuated vaccine given orally. The dead virus administrated by injection acts more quickly and is useful in epidemics. Direct treatment of the infection is not of value and management is directed towards the avoidance of complications and assistance in the development of remaining muscle power.

During the stage of onset rest is essential, with careful positioning of the limbs to permit muscular relaxation. The upper limbs are placed with the shoulders moderately abducted, the elbows flexed and the wrists slightly dorsiflexed. The lower limbs are maintained with the knees in slight flexion and the feet at right angles, care being taken to avoid external rotation at the hip. Heat relieves pain, and stiffness can be avoided by gentle daily passive movements. Respiratory failure may develop rapidly and require immediate treatment (p. 119).

Stage of recovery. Graduated exercises and light splintage should be continued to assist the recovering muscles. Gravity-eliminated exercises in warm water (hydrotherapy) are useful for extensive paralysis.

Stage of residual paralysis. The emphasis is directed towards function. This stage is not finally reached for about two years but the ultimate pattern of paralysis can usually be predicted after six to nine months. Exercises aimed at making extra use of the remaining active muscles are performed.

Soft tissue operations may improve residual deformity by elongation or division of tendons, or correct muscle imbalance by tendon transplantation. Arthrodesis of a joint to provide stability as in the foot or shoulder may be of value. Surgical appliances may also be used.

Peroneal muscular atrophy

This condition affects the motor component of the peripheral nerves and produces wasting and weakness of the peroneal group of muscles in the calf and the small muscles of the hands. Typical deformities of claw toes, pes cavus and ulnar claw hands develop with time. The condition may first manifest itself at the age of five to ten years and gradually progresses through life. When severe the deformities can be corrected by surgery to the feet and although they may be considerable actual disability may be only slight.

POSTURE

Postural conditions in the spine

Anatomy

In the sagittal plane the spine has several curves; the thoracic and pelvic which are concave forwards, and the cervical and lumbar which are concave backwards. The former are present at birth and are fixed; the latter develop as the erect position is assumed and are mobile. Postero-laterally the vertebrae articulate by *plane* joints and spinal movements take place by gliding at these joints. Anteriorly the bodies are joined by the strong, continuous anterior and posterior longitudinal ligaments. Between the bodies lie the *intervertebral discs*, which function as shock absorbers and, being elastic, alter in shape with movement of the bones. The discs consist of two parts; the *annulus fibrosus*, attached to the rims of the vertebral bodies and longitudinal ligaments, and the central semigelatinous *nucleus pulposus*. Between the first and second cervical vertebrae there is no disc, as the odontoid process of the second projects into the first, whose body it replaces.

Acute back strain

Several factors may be responsible. The lumbar fascia may be torn at the musculotendinous junctions or insertions, the intervertebral ligaments may be damaged or the posterior facet joints partly disrupted. These result in severe pain mainly due to protective muscular spasm.

Clinical features

The history of severe backache seizing a young or middle-aged adult when stooping is often preceded by a minor injury two or three weeks previously. It can be initially incapacitating or may gradually increase over 24 hours. The pain is aggravated by spinal movement, coughing and jolting, and relieved by recumbency. The attack gradually subsides, sometimes completely and permanently, but a liability to further episodes and chronic backache may result. The persistence of symptoms for more than a few days is an indication for radiography.

Treatment

Recumbency on a firm mattress with analgesics and local heat usually leads to rapid improvement. Mobilising exercises, short-wave diathermy and friction to the tender area should follow. Manipulation is successful in selected cases.

Chronic back strain

Aetiological factors can be classified as follows:

1. *Muscular*. Faulty posture may impose a strain on muscles and lead to pain.
2. *Ligamentous*. Persistent muscle strain is transmitted to the ligaments which are unable to withstand it and become painful.
3. *Articular*. Minor anomalies, such as unilateral sacralisation of the fifth lumbar vertebra, or asymmetrical intervertebral articulations impair the mechanical efficiency of the spine and predispose to back strain.

Persistent ligamentous strain may eventually cause degenerative joint changes.

Clinical features

The symptom of backache commences in early middle age and often emanates from a debilitating illness or in women from multiple pregnancies. It is aggravated by exercise and stooping and relieved by rest. The onset may be gradual and the pain is usually localised. Examination in most cases shows only local tenderness and mild stiffness in the back. A chronic low-grade septic focus elsewhere is often present. Radiography is indicated in all but the mildest case to exclude more serious causes of backache.

Treatment

Physiotherapy in the form of heat, massage and spinal exercises is employed to mobilise the back and strengthen the musculature. Manipulation in selected cases may be useful. If these measures fail and the pain is disabling, a supporting corset may be necessary. Septic foci should be eradicated and other more serious causes of backache should be excluded.

Prolapsed intervertebral disc

Intervertebral disc degeneration occurs throughout adult life, the nucleus pulposus becoming drier and inspissated, and the annulus fibrosus losing its elasticity. Trauma may split the annulus, the nucleus pulposus extruding backwards to impinge on a nerve root as it enters an intervertebral foramen (Fig. 27.7). In the *lumbar region* the lumbo-sacral disc is most often affected, followed by that between the fourth and fifth and the third and fourth lumbar vertebrae; in the *cervical region* the discs between the fifth and sixth, and sixth and seventh cervical vertebrae are commonly affected, whilst those above and below are also often involved.

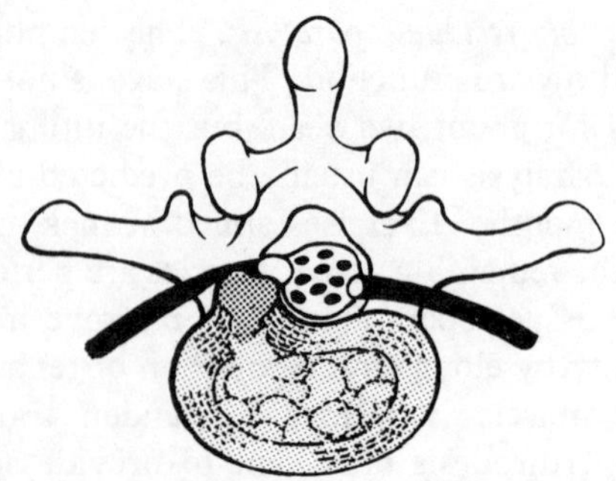

Fig. 27.7 Prolapsed intervertebral disc causing pressure on the spinal nerve root

1. Lumbar region

Clinical features. The condition affects adults of both sexes between 20 and 40 years. It commences as a sudden severe low back pain, which either immediately or a few days later radiates to one limb in an area supplied by a nerve root. The pain is aggravated by any increase in intraspinal pressure, as in coughing, sneezing and straining, or by stretching the root over the prolapsed disc as by stooping. It is usually relieved by lying flat on a firm surface. Examination reveals muscular spasm, often a general tilt to one side with local spinal tenderness, and variable evidence of nerve root irritation such as sensory blunting, selective muscle weakness, and decrease or absence of the tendon

Table 5 Nerve root irritation—lumbar discs

Disc	Nerve Root	Area of Sensory Distribution	Muscle Weakness	Tendon Reflex Alteration	Stretch Test Positive	
Lumbo-sacral	1st sacral	Sole, outer side ankle and foot	Not constant	Ankle reflex absent	Straight leg raising	Sciatic nerve
4th to 5th lumbar	5th lumbar	Dorsum foot and great toe	Toe extensors, (even foot drop)	Ankle reflex often diminished	Straight leg raising	
3rd and 4th lumbar	4th lumbar	Front of knee and shin	Slight—quadriceps	Knee reflex diminished	Femoral stretch test	Femoral nerve
2nd to 3rd lumbar	3rd lumbar	Adductor region of thigh	Slight—quadriceps	Knee reflex diminished	Femoral stretch test	

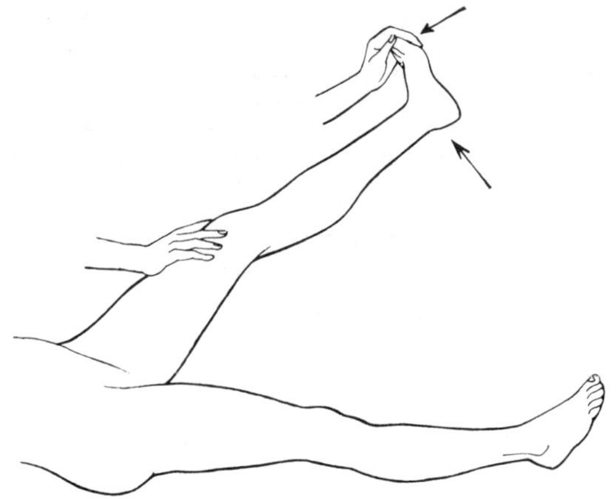

Fig. 27.8 The straight leg raising test (Laségue's sign)

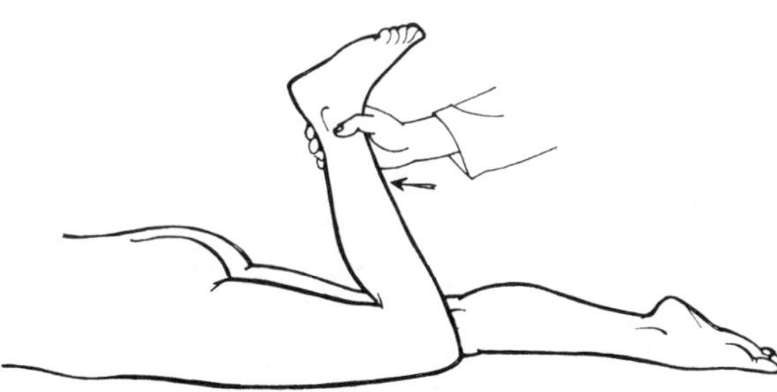

Fig. 27.9 The femoral nerve stretch test

jerk (Table 5). Stretching the affected nerve causes pain in the area of its distribution, for example, the *straight leg raising test* in the sciatic nerve, or in the femoral, by flexing the knee, with the hip extended (Figs. 27.8 and 27.9). The acute attack subsides after a variable interval, but recurrence is common. In some instances low backache results from degenerative changes, or severe sciatica persists, leading to considerable incapacity. Rarely a sudden massive central disc prolapse may impinge on the cauda equina, leading to bladder paralysis and widespread neurological signs in the lower limbs.

Radiography is normal initially, but narrowing of the disc space with lipping occurs later. Lumbar puncture to determine the cerebrospinal fluid pressure and protein content is of value in excluding spinal tumours. Myelography may demonstrate the disc prolapse or a tumour.

Treatment. Conservative measures usually suffice. Bed rest in the supine position on a rigid mattress for 10 to 21 days is followed by heat and exercises.

Operative removal of the disc is reserved for resistant cases with definite evidence of nerve root involvement. Immediate surgery is indicated only in the rare case with a massive central prolapse.

2. *Cervical region*

Clinical features. The age of onset of 40 to 60 years is later than in the lumbar region, symptoms in the neck being due to degenerative changes rather than disc prolapse. The main presentation is of neck pain and nerve root irritation, leading to nocturnal arm pain. The former usually arises suddenly, is commonly unilateral and may be preceded by a minor injury two to four weeks earlier. The neck is often tilted away from the painful side, with tenderness at the level of the lesion, whilst lateral flexion towards the affected side, extension, and to a lesser extent flexion, are limited. Nerve root irritation is shown by sensory blunting, muscle weakness and diminution of tendon reflexes (see Table 6). Shoulder stiffness may be a feature if the sixth cervical root is involved. Rarely quadriplegia follows a sudden massive central prolapse, and reactive new bone formation around a central disc degeneration may cause cord irritation of insidious onset.

Radiography usually shows narrowing of the space and lipping of the vertebral bodies related to the involved disc, oblique views showing distortion of the intervertebral foramina. Lumbar puncture and myelography are indicated when central lesions are suspected. Other causes of nerve irritation must be excluded, particularly cervical rib, ulnar neuritis at the elbow and the carpal tunnel syndrome (p. 342).

Treatment. Except in the rare central lesion, treatment is conservative. Heat, mobilising exercises and friction to the tender areas, combined with traction and manual manipulation are initial measures. A sorbo rubber collar can be used either alone or with physiotherapy, and is particularly valuable at night. In resistant cases a light polythene support is indicated, and in severe instances surgical excision of the disc may be necessary to

Table 6 Nerve root irritation—cervical discs

Disc	Nerve root	Area of sensory distribution	Muscle weakness	Tendon reflex alteration	
5th to 6th cervical	6th cervical	Pain from shoulder down pre-axial border of arm Numbness in thumb	Weakness and wasting elbow flexors	Diminished biceps reflex	No specific "stretch tests"
6th to 7th cervical	7th cervical	Pain midline forearm to middle finger Numbness middle finger	Possible wasting and slight weakness forearm muscles	Slightly diminished biceps and triceps reflex	
7th cervical to 1st thoracic	8th cervical	Pain down postaxial border of forearm	Wasting and weakness small muscles of hand	Diminished triceps reflex	
1st to 2nd thoracic	1st thoracic	Numbness ring and little fingers			

decompress the affected nerve root and relieve symptoms.

Spondylolisthesis

The stability between two vertebrae is partly dependent on the posterior hook formed by the facets, laminae and spinous processes. Severe stress may break the pedicle, allowing the vertebral body and column above to slip forwards; the displacement is called a spondylolisthesis. There may be a predisposing congenital weakness such as an occult defect in the lamina, but often there is no apparent cause.

Symptoms can commence at any age and consist of backache and nerve root irritation. Examination reveals a characteristic 'step' palpable and often visible in the line of the spinous processes, together with marked skin creases below the ribs. The diagnosis is confirmed by radiography, often demonstrated best in oblique views (Fig. 27.10). In mild cases exercises, by improving muscle tone, or a lumbo-sacral corset may suffice, but if the slip is severe and progressive, spinal fusion is indicated.

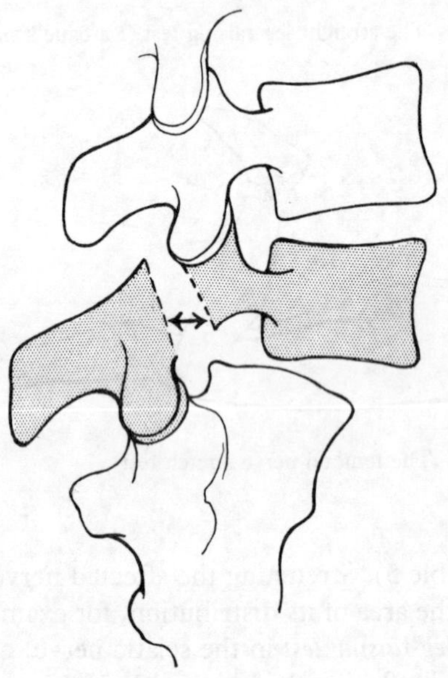

Fig. 27.10 Spondylolisthesis, showing the site of break in the lamina

Scoliosis

Lateral curvature of the spine (scoliosis) may be postural or structural. *Postural scoliosis* is mild, disappears in recumbency, and is seen only in children. Radiologically there is no rotation of the vertebrae, and treatment consists of exercises to correct bad postural habits. In *structural scoliosis*, in addition to the lateral curve, the vertebral bodies are also rotated. In the thoracic region this leads to asymmetry of the ribs, which become flat on the concave side and prominent on the convex (razor-back deformity). In severe cases there is reduction of the vital capacity and general stunting of growth. Structural scoliosis is either primary or *idiopathic*, or secondary to a known cause. The latter may be *congenital*, due to maldevelopment of vertebrae or ribs; *neurological* due to a difference in strength of the spinal musculature, as in poliomyelitis; or *compensatory* to such conditions as a short leg, or severe unilateral pulmonary disease.

Idiopathic scoliosis. The degree of deformity produced by a given curve varies with the level at which it occurs. Thoracic curves, which are usually convex to the right, produce the greatest deformity, while lumbar curves often pass unnoticed until osteoarthritis supervenes in later life. Females are predominantly affected.

Paralytic scoliosis. The appearance is similar to idiopathic scoliosis, except that both sexes are affected equally, and the curve may be in either direction. Deterioration tends to be more rapid and difficult to control. The progression of the curve has to be prevented as far as possible by applying a Milwaukee spinal brace and when growth is nearly complete fusion of the entire curvature is undertaken to prevent further deformity in adulthood.

Congenital scoliosis. This is caused by abnormal vertebral bodies which may be incomplete such as in hemivertebra, thus causing marked curves early in life. Although the curve may be short, it is characteristically rigid and resistant to correction.

Curves which appear early and progress rapidly can be controlled to some degree by a Milwaukee brace (Fig. 27.11) which acts by support, in which the patient has to extend constantly. Treatment is not indicated for mild cases. Most curves are partly mobile, thus can be corrected in plaster and then followed by extensive spinal fusion to maintain the position.

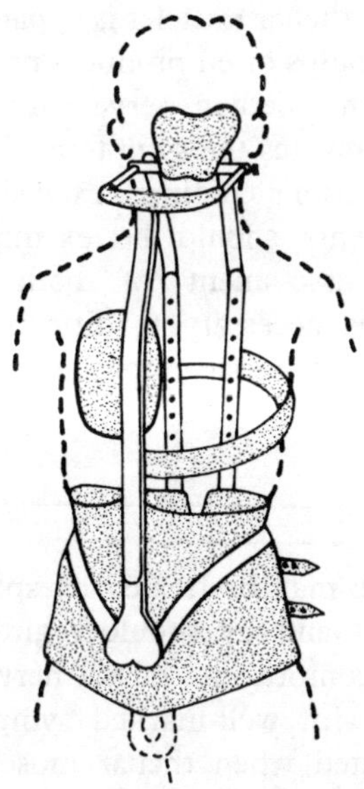

Fig. 27.11 Milwaukee brace for scoliosis of the spine. The principle is of active spinal extension by the patient to prevent progression. Points of contact are the chin, occiput and iliac crests.

Coccydynia

Persistent pain in the coccygeal region may occur after a fall on the buttocks, but can also result from advanced pelvic neoplasms or local infective conditions. Females are mainly affected in two age groups, just after the menarche and near the menopause. The pain is aggravated by adopting or relinquishing the sitting position. Treatment is often unsatisfactory; heat, manipulation and excision of the coccyx are frequently employed. The condition usually subsides spontaneously after several months.

Thoracic inlet syndrome

Pressure on the brachial plexus and subclavian artery by a cervical rib or fascial band in the scalene muscles may result in neurological or vascular changes in the upper limb.

Anatomy

A cervical rib when present articulates with the transverse process of the seventh cervical vertebra and runs laterally and forwards for a variable extent, occasionally articulating with the first rib. The anterior part of an incomplete rib may be represented by a fibrous band. The brachial plexus is stretched over the cervical rib leading to pressure on its lowest trunk. The subclavian artery arches over the rib at a lower level and may be compressed against it by the scalenus anterior muscle or by the clavicle. The syndrome may occasionally be produced by the scalenus anterior muscle compressing the brachial plexus and subclavian artery against abnormal, tense, tendinous fibres in the scalenus medius muscle.

Clinical features

Symptoms develop most commonly in middle-aged

females when descent of the shoulder girdle occurs due to diminished muscle tone. The right side is more commonly affected though cervical ribs are often bilateral. The nervous, muscular or circulatory systems may be affected. Pain in the shoulder, the arm and medial side of the forearm and hand is the predominant feature. It varies in intensity and location from day to day. Weakness, paraesthesiae and changes in colour of the hand are common complaints.

Palpation in the supraclavicular region may reveal a bony cervical rib. The subclavian artery is often prominent, and on occasions has been mistaken for an aneurysm. Weakness of the intrinsic muscles of the hand may be demonstrated, the hypothenar and interosseous muscles being principally affected. Diminution of sensation is frquently elicited over the medial border of the forearm and hand. Obliteration of the radial pulse can often be produced by elevation of the arm or deep inspiration which causes contraction of scalenus anterior, but this sign may occasionally be elicited in normal people. Trophic changes and gangrene of the finger-tips may occur as a result of damage to the subclavian artery with intimal changes and the formation of emboli. Radiographs may reveal a cervical rib or beaking of the transverse process associated with a fibrous band.

Differentiation should be made from the carpal tunnel syndrome. Syringomyelia, progressive muscular atrophy and vasospastic conditions of the upper limb must also be excluded.

Treatment

Exercises to improve the tone in the shoulder girdle muscles may bring relief of mild symptoms. Operative removal of a cervical rib is beneficial in the majority of cases and is always indicated when arterial emboli are occurring. Resection of the medial margin of the first rib may also be performed to allow adequate decompression.

Carpal tunnel syndrome

Aetiology

The condition is due to compression of the median nerve as it passes deep to the flexor retinaculum in its course from the forearm to the palm. The exact cause of the compression is not known in the majority of cases. Occasionally it is due to swelling of the tendon sheaths with a rheumatoid type inflammation or is associated with fractures of the carpal bones or lower end of the radius. It may be that repeated minor injuries alter conduction in the nerve as it is stretched over the lunate bone in hyperextension of the wrist. This view is supported by the fact that excessive use of the wrist during housework aggravates the pain.

Clinical features

Middle-aged women are principally affected. The main complaint is of burning pain and paraesthesiae in the area of hand supplied by the median nerve. The condition is bilateral in 50 per cent of cases. It occurs mainly at night, often awakening the patient from sleep and persisting for several hours. Radiation of pain to the arm is common and swelling of the fingers may occur. Weakness of the hand is frequent and fine movements are poorly performed. Examination may reveal only slight diminution of sensation in the median nerve territory of the hand; in about one-third of cases partial wasting of the thenar muscles is apparent. Pressure on the finger pulps often produces pain, and direct pressure on the median nerve with the wrist in extension aggravates the symptoms.

Proximal lesions require exclusion. Cervical neck movements should be examined. Careful neurological assessment of both upper and lower limbs is necessary to differentiate peripheral neuritis, progressive muscular atrophy and syringomyelia.

Treatment

The mild case may be treated by splinting of the wrist at night and by shoulder girdle exercises. Operative decompression of the nerve is required for patients with well-marked symptoms and is always indicated when thenar muscle wasting is present.

The flexor retinaculum is exposed through a longitudinal incision in the palm from the distal wrist skin crease and is completely divided. This often demonstrates marked flattening of the median nerve where compression has taken place and release rapidly improves the symptoms. Pain disappears and sensation returns to normal but muscle wasting rarely recovers.

POSTURAL CONDITIONS IN THE LOWER LIMB

THE KNEE

The shafts of the femora are directed inwards, making an angle with the tibia of about 15 degrees. The erect posture tends to increase this angle and produce a valgus deformity of the knee, which is resisted by the medial ligament and vastus medialis muscle.

Genu valgum

Mild knock-knee is common in children up to the age of five but can cause considerable anxiety in parents. In the absence of any joint or muscle abnormality reassurance is given of spontaneous correction and an associated tendency towards flat feet also resolves. When deformity is marked, radiography is indicated to exclude abnormal bone development as seen in rickets, either primary or secondary to renal abnormality.

Treatment. This is not indicated where the bone is normal. Many devices such as the 'mermaid splint' and inner shoe raises recommended in the past, have been shown to make no difference. After damage to the femoral or tibial epiphyses from injury or following osteomyelitis there may be marked deformity and osteotomy should be performed. When only part of the epiphysis is fused arrest of further growth may be obtained by curetting the remaining cartilage and stapling the plate (*epiphyseodesis*).

Genu varum

Bow-leg deformity occurs mainly as a result of bending of the bony shafts rather than disability at the knee joints. Minor tibial bowing is common in infants. If more marked it may be due to a condition such as rickets. Postural bowing seldom requires active treatment.

THE FOOT

The foot has two functions, to provide a stable base upon which the body is supported, and as a means of propulsion. The weight is taken by the talus, from which it is distributed backwards to the posterior tubercles of the calcaneum, and forwards to the metatarsal heads. This is the *longitudinal* arch, which is better developed on the inner side. It is supported by: the tendons of tibialis posterior, tibialis anterior and peroneus longus, which act as slings from above; the short plantar muscles which function as a bowstring between the pillars of the arch; and the ligaments which serve as ties between the various segments (Fig. 27.12). The metatarsal heads are held together by the transverse ligaments and weight should be spread more or less evenly through all five to provide a broad platform for balance.

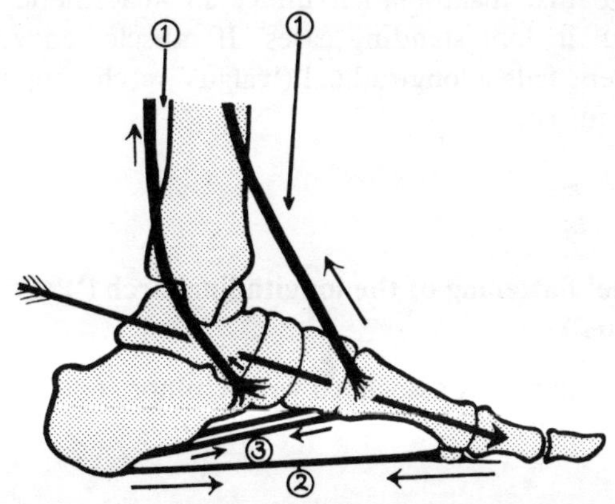

Fig. 27.12 Structures maintaining the longitudinal arch of the foot. **1.** Tendons raising arch. **2.** Short flexor muscles act as bowstrings. **3.** Long and short plantar ligaments act as ties. The long arrow indicates the normal straight line axis of the talus, navicular, cuneiform and first metatarsal bones.

Disorders of stability

Foot strain

If the small muscles of the foot fail to maintain an efficient 'bowstring', strain falls on the ligaments, which become painful. It may occur in a normal foot when muscle tone is lost, as after illness or fatigue, but is more common in 'flat foot', when the muscles, working at a mechanical disadvantage, are less able to protect the ligaments.

Pain, predominantly under the longitudinal arch, is the chief complaint. At first felt only on weight-bearing, it later becomes constant. Slight oedema of the dorsum of the foot, tenderness and general stiffness may be found. If untreated the inflammatory exudate around the ligaments leads to increasing stiffness and eventual structural changes in the joints.

In atypical cases further investigation is required. A raised sedimentation rate suggests an inflammatory lesion, rheumatoid arthritis or ankylosing spondylitis. Radiography may show a local infective condition or a minor congenital anomaly. Gout is excluded by a blood uric acid estimation, and gonococcal fasciitis by the complement-fixation test.

Treatment. Pain may be relieved by rest and contrast foot-baths. Insole supports improve symptoms over the long term. Physiotherapy is helpful, consisting of exercises and faradic and contrast foot-baths; manipulation under an anaesthetic is useful in long-standing cases. If muscle redevelopment fails a longitudinal ('valgus') arch support is required.

'True' flattening of the longitudinal arch ('Pes planus')

This is generally associated with a minor congenital abnormality.

1. At the talo-navicular joint

The normal talus slopes gently downwards in the same line as the first metatarsal. If the slope is more vertical the arch becomes flattened. The head of the talus may become prominent and painful requiring a specially moulded insole support to relieve symptoms.

2. At the naviculo-cuneiform joint

Flattening at this level is usually due to inefficiency of the tibialis posterior tendon, and is often associated with a small ossicle in the tendon at its insertion into the tubercle of the navicular—the *os tibiale externum*. Exercises and a longitudinal arch support are usually required. Rarely a large accessory ossicle requires excision, or arthrodesis of the naviculo-cuneiform joint should be advised.

3. At the cuneiform–first metatarsal joint

The first metatarsal may lie in a more horizontal plane than normal (Fig. 27.13), *metatarsus primus elevatus*. Flattening of the longitudinal arch occurs with reversal of the transverse arch, and because the first metatarsal head does not take any weight there is a predisposition to hallux rigidus (p. 346). The first metatarsal may also diverge to produce an unduly wide forefoot (Fig. 27.15), *metatarsus primus varus*, which, in addition to flattening of the longitudinal arch, predisposes to hallux valgus (p. 346).

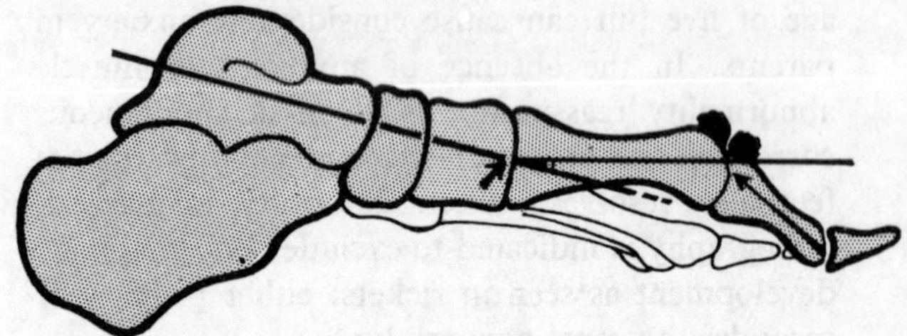

Fig. 27.13 Metatarsus primus elevatus. The resulting stress on the first metatarsal joint is indicated; dorsal exostoses may form.

'Apparent' flattening of the longitudinal arch ('Pes valgus')

Two mechanisms are responsible.

1. Tightness of the tendo calcaneus

The foot as a result of this lesion can only become plantigrade by rolling inwards. Although well demonstrated in mild cases of congenital spastic paraplegia, in minor forms it is one of the commonest causes of flat foot. Treatment includes stretching of the tendon, arch supports and raising of the heel. Operative lengthening of the tendon is never justifiable.

2. *Peroneal spasm* ('spasmodic flat foot')

The spasm is a reflex aimed at protective immobilisation of the mid-tarsal joint and is evoked by irritative lesions such as early infective arthritis or minor congenital anomalies. In the latter, spasm is due to excessive strain transmitted to other tarsal joints, and often commences in youths leaving school. Pain is felt in the tarsal region, and the foot is held in rigid valgus, the peroneal tendons being easily visible.

Treatment

Where an infective lesion has been excluded, six to eight weeks rest in a plaster of Paris cast, applied in the relaxed position under an anaesthetic, followed by an arch support may suffice to prevent recurrence. In severe cases triple arthrodesis is often necessary.

Elevation of the longitudinal arch ('Pes cavus')

Pes cavus may be idiopathic or secondary to a neurological disorder, such as poliomyelitis, spina bifida or Friedreich's ataxia. Shortening of the muscles and fascia in the sole of the foot causes in mild cases dropping of the forefoot, and in the more severe a vertical 'calcaneus' position of the heel, which may be also inverted. Associated clawing of the toes is due to inefficiency of the interossei and in most instances is followed by their dorsal subluxation. The lesion is usually bilateral but not necessarily symmetrical.

Clinical features

In the idiopathic group the condition is usually first noticed between the ages of 5 and 10 years, is more common in boys and may be familial. Mild cases may remain symptomless, but when severe, painful callosities develop under the metatarsal heads, corns occur on the clawed toes and there is an ache in the tarsus. Clawing of the toes is also associated with rigid flat feet in the elderly and may follow a fracture of the tibial shaft, disuse atrophy of the intrinsic muscles being responsible.

Treatment

In adults a metatarsal support (Fig. 27.14) and altered footwear may suffice. Advanced cases may require excision of the proximal phalanges to correct the toes and trimming of the metatarsal heads. *In children* mild degrees respond to foot exercises and a metatarsal bar, but surgery is indicated for marked deformity. It consists of division of the plantar fascia, and either fusion of the interphalangeal joints or transplantation of the flexor tendons into the extensors on the dorsum of the toe. In the hallux the long extensor is transplanted to the metatarsal neck and the interphalangeal joint fused. In adolecents when the arch is extremely high a wedge of bone with the base upwards is removed from the tarsus.

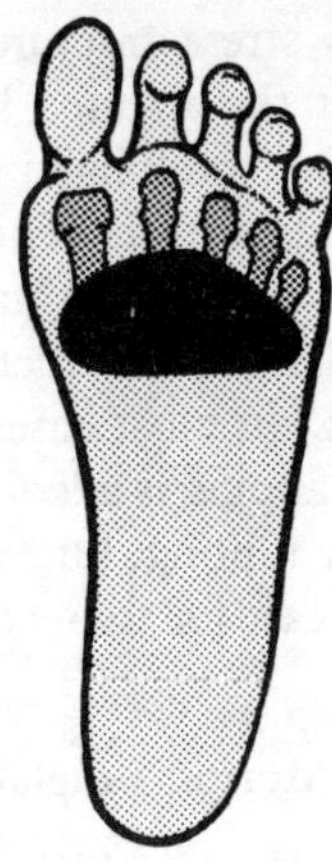

Fig. 27.14 The correct position for a metatarsal support

Metatarsal abnormalities

Metatarsalgia

Failure to bear weight on the first metatarsal head produces callosities under the heads of the second, third and fourth metatarsals. This imbalance produces pain, metatarsalgia, often likened to standing on pebbles. The toes are frequently stiff and clawed, and the forefoot may be wide. Conservative measures are employed, consisting of physiotherapy and a metatarsal support. Surgery is only indicated to correct severe clawing of the toes.

Stress ('march') fracture

Shortening of the first metatarsal, by throwing more weight on to the second and third metatarsals, may lead to stress fractures of their shafts. Pain is noted over the affected bone, often occurring suddenly after prolonged or unaccustomed walking on a hard surface. The radiograph may show a hair-line crack with minimal periosteal reaction or abundant callus resembling osteomyelitis or a neoplasm. In most cases a metatarsal pad and elastoplast strapping is adequate treatment, the fracture invariably uniting, but when pain is severe a plaster of Paris cast for two weeks is indicated.

Digital neuroma ('Morton's metatarsalgia')

In this condition there is thickening of the nerve in the interdigital cleft, probably due to ischaemic changes resulting from the excess pressure in reversal of the anterior arch. It is commonest in the third and fourth cleft, and is not a true tumour. Periodic shooting pain radiates between two adjacent toes. Tenderness localised to the affected cleft is present and lateral metatarsal compression produces pain at the same site. Treatment is excision of the thickened portion of the nerve.

Pain in the foot from vascular insufficiency, rheumatic plantar fasciitis, and neurological disorders should be excluded by careful examination and investigation.

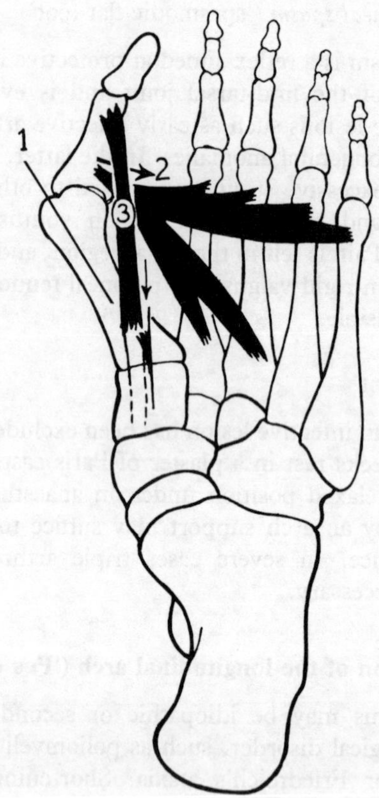

Fig. 27.15 The causes of hallux valgus. **1.** Metatarsus primus varus. **2.** The action of adductor hallucis. **3.** Bowstring effect of long tendons to the toe.

Disorders of propulsion ('Disorders of the toes')

Great toe

Mal-position of the first metatarsal is a predisposing cause of both hallux valgus and hallux rigidus.

Hallux valgus. In addition to metatarsus primus varus a further predisposing factor is the insertion of the adductor hallucis muscle into the base of the proximal phalanx, and with the appearance of deformity accentuation by the bowstring action of the long flexor and extensor tendons (Fig. 27.15). Unsuitable shoes by compression aggravate the condition. In severe cases the second toes may either develop a hammer deformity or be dorsally subluxated at the metatarsophalangeal joint, due to pressure from the great toe. There may be associated metatarsalgia. Clinically the condition is common in females, often presenting as an inflamed bursa over the prominent first metatarsal head (*bunion*).

Treatment is dependent on the severity of the condition and the symptoms. Hallux valgus at an early age should be given adequate treatment as the deformity is likely to increase with time. Osteotomy of the first metatarsal is carried out to realign the big toe and the exostosis is excised at the same time. The foot has to be held in a plaster cast for six weeks after surgery until the metatarsal is stable. When the first metatarsal joint shows degenerative changes an excision arthroplasty is carried out, removing the base of the proximal phalanx and the exostosis to allow a fibrous pseudarthrosis to develop which should allow pain-free movements (Fig. 27.16).

Hallux rigidus. Osteoarthritis of the first metatarsophalangeal joint is known as hallux rigidus. It usually follows abnormal strains on the joint in association with metatarsus primus elevatus (p. 344); less often it is due to direct trauma. Pain occurs in the joint, particularly on forced dorsiflexion. Enlargement of the metatarsal head with dorsal osteophyte formation may cause pressure symptoms. It can be differentiated from gout by the absence of nocturnal pain and a normal blood uric acid.

Treatment. Pain on walking may be relieved by attaching a metatarsal bar to the shoe beneath the metatarsal heads thus preventing extension of the big toe on walking. When severe, arthrodesis of the metatarsophalangeal joint in younger patients, or arthroplasty (Keller's operation (Fig. 27.16)) should be performed.

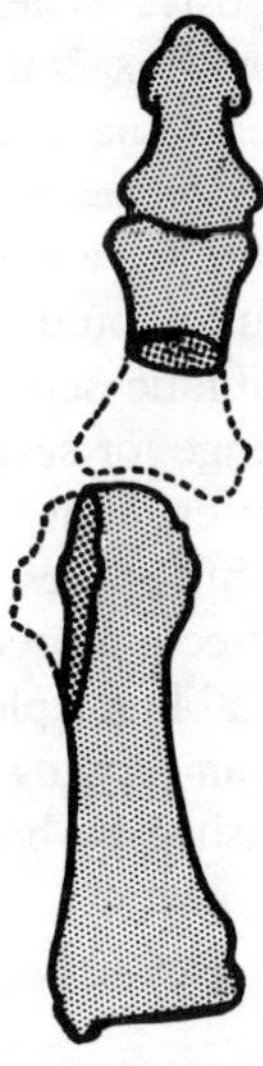

Fig. 27.16 Keller's operation for hallux valgus. The base of the proximal phalanx and the exostosis on the first metatarsal are excised.

Lesser toes

Hammer toe. This consists of a flexion deformity at the proximal interphalangeal joint, with compensatory hyperextension of the distal joint. It may occur in conjuction with hallux valgus, but often no cause is found. The second or third toe is usually affected. Arthrodesis or excision of the proximal interphalangeal joint should be undertaken.

Mallet toe. This is a flexion deformity of the distal interphalangeal joint, leading to a painful corn either at the tip of the toe or directly over the joint. Surgical correction and arthrodesis of the distal joint gives good results.

Dorsal displacement of the fifth toe. The fifth toe may lie above and across the fourth, causing symptoms from pressure. Although the skin is tight, release of the extensor tendon is required in addition to a plastic procedure on the skin, in order to ensure satisfactory correction.

Toenails

Ingrowing toenail. The edge of the nail, usually of the great toe, becomes turned into the skin and leads to infection. It is caused by injudicious trimming of the nail, and too tight hosiery and shoes.

Treatment. In early cases plugs of wool placed beneath the edges until they have grown clear, followed by cutting the nail straight to the corners, is sufficient. When infection is marked the nail should be avulsed but recurrence is common. In moderate cases wedge resection of the ingrowing edge, base and hypertrophied skin may be successful, but in severe instances the nail, together with its bed, must be excised.

Onychogryphosis. This is horny hypertrophy of the nail, usually seen in the elderly, or where the nail has been previously injured. Chiropody may control growth, but the only cure is excision of the nail bed. Recurrence follows simple avulsion of the nail.

Subungual exostosis. A small exostosis growing from the tip of the terminal phalanx, usually of the great toe, may raise the nail and cause pain. Treatment consists of excision, either through the tip of the toe, or where larger, after removal of part of the nail.

INFECTIONS

Acute osteomyelitis

Pathology

Infection reaches a bone either by the bloodstream or directly through a wound, the former being more common. It occurs mainly in children when growth is active and the blood supply rich. The bones most frequently affected are those particularly liable to trauma, such as the upper end of the tibia and the lower end of the femur. The organism can often be traced to a distant septic focus, as in a boil, impetigo, tonsils or teeth. It is usually a coagulase-positive staphylococcus, but may be a haemolytic streptococcus or pneumococcus.

The formation of a haematoma in the metaphysis of a long bone provides an ideal culture medium for circulating bacteria. The resulting pus spreads through the Haversian canals, raises the periosteum and produces a subperiosteal abscess. Tension generated within the inelastic bone interrupts blood flow in the nutrient artery and elevation of the periosteum ruptures the subperiosteal vessels. Necrosis of the avascular bone follows; if pressure is not relieved and the periosteal stripping continues, this may become widespread. Later dead bone which may include the whole diaphysis separates, forming a *sequestrum*. Simultaneously new bone is produced by the deep layers of the raised periosteum which ensheaths the sequestrum and is known as an *involucrum* (Fig. 27.17). The periosteum may rupture, producing a superficial abscess, skin necrosis and a *sinus*. The firm periosteal attachments to the epiphysis usually act as a barrier to joint involvement, except in the hip in infants where the synovial membrane is reflected on to the metaphysis.

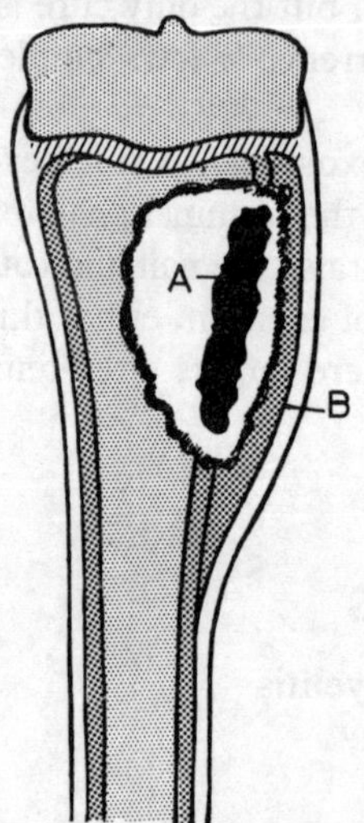

Fig. 27.17 Osteomyelitis. The fully developed lesion showing an abscess cavity with sclerotic lining containing a sequestrum (**A**). Involucrum (**B**).

Clinical features

The condition is most common in boys under the age of 10 years. Pain of sudden onset, aggravated by movement, occurs in a limb. It may be preceded by a history of sore throat or other septic focus and recent minor injury. Marked constitutional upset is apparent, accompanied by pyrexia of 39° to 40°C and tachycardia. Bony tenderness is the only initial local sign, but heat, redness and swelling appear later, together with a small serous sympathetic effusion in the neighbouring joint and tender enlargement of the regional lymph nodes. A diagnosis of acute suppurative arthritis may at this stage be suggested, but aspiration of the joint does not reveal pus. Occasionally in infants several bones are affected simultaneously. When osteomyelitis follows an open wound toxaemia is less marked as there is usually free drainage of pus.

Blood examination reveals a polymorph leucocytosis and in severe cases a positive culture. Investigation of any pus should be carried out for organisms and antibiotic sensitivity. Radiographs may show little change for several days after onset and then only slight erosions and periosteal duplication; diagnosis thus relies mostly on clinical signs. Low-grade infection produces sclerotic bone changes which resemble neoplastic lesions such as osteogenic sarcoma and Ewing's tumour and these have to be distinguished by bone biopsy.

Treatment

Two principles of treatment must be stressed. Firstly the infected bone should be decompressed so that inflammation will not spread further and endanger the blood supply. Secondly the causative organism must be identified so that suitable antibiotics can be given early and in correct dosage. A combination of antibiotics should be started at operation, for example, flucloxacillin and ampicillin, and any necessary changes can be made when the sensitivities are known.

Chronic osteomyelitis

This condition follows either acute osteomyelitis which has failed to resolve, or an infected compound fracture. The bone is sclerotic and thickened and may contain infected cavities in which there may be small sequestra. A thickened involucrum and sinuses may be present as well as puckered scars. Evidence of healed sinuses may be found.

Clinical features

The disease can remain quiescent for years, or existing sinuses may continue to discharge without constitutional disturbance. Sudden reactivation with heat, swelling and abscess formation may occur, sometimes resolving spontaneously. In severe cases there may be anaemia and loss of weight due to low-grade toxaemia. Joint stiffness and contractures may be found and even bony deformity due to interference with growth. Amyloid disease is a late complication.

Radiography shows the extent of the disease and the presence of sequestra. Tomograms may be helpful if sclerosis is marked and sinograms will demonstrate the ramifications of a sinus.

Treatment

In the quiescent stage a persistent sinus should be accepted. Surgery is advisable when discharge is profuse, a large cavity or sequestrum found, or attacks of pain and pyrexia frequent. The cavity is laid open and curetted and overhanging edges of bone removed (saucerisation).

Brodie's abscess

This is a type of chronic osteomyelitis of insidious onset, consisting of an abscess in the end of a long bone, often near the knee, surrounded by dense sclerosis. It may or may not contain a sequestrum, and the pus is often sterile. The main complaint is of a deep boring pain, more severe at night, constitutional signs being absent or minimal. Treatment consists of drainage and thorough curettage of the cavity.

Acute suppurative arthritis

Pathology

This condition is usually blood borne from a focus elsewhere, but may follow a penetrating wound or occasionally spread from an adjacent bony infection. When blood borne, the usual organisms are staphylococci or streptococci, but gonococci may be responsible three weeks after urethritis. The joint fills rapidly with an effusion which remains turbid in mild cases, but becomes purulent in the more severe. Unless the pus is promptly evacuated granulation tissue spreads throughout the joint destroying the articular cartilage. It may extend down to bone and through the capsule into the soft tissues.

Clinical features

The affected joint becomes hot, tender and distended with fluid. All movements are painful and in severe cases muscle spasm may almost completely immobilise the joint. In gonococcal infections several joints may be involved simultaneously, but a large joint, particularly the knee, is usually affected. There is a raised sedimentation rate and leucocytosis, and bacteria can usually be cultured from the effusion. The complement fixation test is generally positive in gonococcal arthritis. Radiographs show changes only when irreversible damage to the articular surfaces has occurred. In untreated cases fibrous or bony ankylosis follows, and external sinuses may persist. The condition must be differentiated form acute osteomyelitis, acute rheumatism and infantile scurvy.

Treatment

Antibiotic thereapy is essential, with the joint splinted in the position of function. The effusion is repeatedly aspirated and the appropriate antibiotic instilled. Thick pus requires open drainage. On subsidence of active disease the joint should be mobilised. Complete resolution may occur, but some permanent damage is common, predisposing to osteoarthritis.

Suppurative bursitis

Adventitious bursae, such as those over the patella, the olecranon and the first metatarsal head in hallus valgus (bunion, p. 346), may become infected with pyogenic organisms directly through a wound or abrasion, often as a result of repeated minor trauma. Antibiotics should be employed together with the drainage of any pus. When suppuration has subsided they may require excision, particularly if repeated attacks have occurred.

TUBERCULOSIS OF BONES AND JOINTS

General features

Pathology

Tubercle bacilli reach a bone or joint by the bloodstream from a focus elsewhere. The organisms settle in areas of local tissue damage following minor trauma and cause hyperaemia and caseation. A cold abscess forms and may discharge to leave a sinus along which secondary infection may occur. In favourable cases the lesion becomes walled off by fibrous tissue, with shrinkage and calcification of any residual abscess but from which tubercle bacilli can be cultured even when the disease is clinically quiescent. In a joint fibrous ankylosis is usual in uncomplicated cases, bony ankylosis only following secondary infection.

Clinical features

Children or young adults in poor general condition are those often affected and there may be a known tuberculous lesion elsewhere. Local features include *pain* of insidious onset and aching character which is aggravated by movement, *spasm* and *wasting* of the surrounding musculature. *Swelling* due to inflammatory thickening and a cold abscess, and *deformity* caused by a combination of tissue destruction, contracture, and muscle spasm are also apparent. Persistent sepsis from secondary infection may lead to amyloid disease. Tuberculous meningitis, genito-urinary lesions, affections of other bones and joints, or miliary spread may occur.

Differential diagnosis

Atypical, non-articular rheumatoid arthritis, subacute infective arthritis, due either to low-virulence pyogenic organisms or bacteria of the Neisserian or coli-typhoid groups, or syphilis may cause confusion.

Investigations

The sedimentation rate is usually raised, serial estimations being of value in assessing progress. Pus should be examined for tubercle bacilli by staining, culture or guinea-pig inoculation. A negative *Mantoux* test suggests that the lesion is unlikely to be tuberculous. Radiography may show decalcification due to hyperaemia, loss of bony trabeculae giving a ground-glass appearance, narrowing of the joint space due to destruction of the articular cartilage, and bulging of soft tissue contours due to the presence of an abscess. Biopsy is indicated in doubtful cases whilst chest radiography, sputum and urine examination should be performed.

Principles of treatment

Treatment is prolonged and must be both general (p. 13) and local.

Local. Conservative treatment consists of local rest by suitable splintage and the aspiration of cold abscesses, streptomycin being instilled at the same time. *Operative* treatment involves drainage or excision of infected material, or fusion of affected joints, preferably by an extra-articular method.

Tuberculosis of the shoulder, elbow, carpal, sacro-iliac and tarsal joints is relatively uncommon today and only disease of the spine, hip and knee will be considered.

Tuberculosis of the spine

The spine is the most common site to be involved in bone and joint tuberculosis, the incidence being maximal in the lower thoracic region. The lesion commences in a vertebral body close to the disc and rapidly spreads to implicate both disc and neighbouring vertebrae. Bony destruction is followed by abscess formation. In the lumbar region a *psoas abscess* may invade the muscle and track down within the sheath to reach the surface below the inguinal ligament. Increasing tension from a *paravertebral abscess* developing in the thoracic region may cause spinal cord compression. A retropharyngeal abscess arising from the cervical vertebrae may extend laterally or rupture into the pharynx.

Gross destruction in several thoracic bodies produces an angular kyphosis (gibbus) which can interfere with the cardio-respiratory systems.

Clinical features

The majority of cases occur in childhood between the ages of three and five years, the sex ratio being equal. The onset is frequently insidious, consisting of mild backache or pain referred along nerve roots, if these are irritated by collapse or pressure from debris. Spasm and wasting of the erector spinae muscles are often marked, whilst kyphosis may appear early and become severe. Abscesses in the groin or loin may be observed. In adults, paraplegia may be the first indication of disease and is an important complication, particularly in the thoracic region.

Differential diagnosis

Crush fractures of a vertebral body, neoplastic deposits and osteochondritis may be distinguished by the absence of involvement of the intervertebral discs. In pyogenic infections sclerosis and new bone formation are more marked whilst in the colityphoid group the agglutination reactions are usually conclusive.

Treatment

Antituberculous chemotherapy has greatly improved the control of infection. Bed rest is advised for a short period initially and only where extensive bone destruction and instability have occurred is surgery indicated. Paraplegia from tuberculous infection is occasionally still seen and if treated adequately the neurological changes can be reversed. Antituberculous drugs are started as soon as the diagnosis is confirmed and should be a combination therapy of more than one drug (p. 13). They should be given for up to two years. Surgical drainage of abscesses is performed early, all necrotic tissues being removed to allow better penetration by drugs. Bone defects are usually filled with a graft to stabilise the vertebral column. Further immobilisation is maintained until the bone is healthy, which is often a period of 2 to 3 months.

Tuberculosis of the hip

The disease is secondary to a lesion elsewhere in the body but usually commences locally as a bony focus in either the femoral neck or the acetabulum, soon spreading to the joint. The synovial membrane is first involved but later bony destruction may allow the joint to sublux, leading to the appearance known as 'wandering acetabulum'.

Clinical features

Boys are affected more often than girls, generally between the ages of 3 and 10 years. Pain and a limp are initial symptoms associated with muscle spasm. Deformity follows, the hip first being held in abduction, external rotation and flexion due to fluid distension of the joint capsule. Later, muscle spasm and bony destruction result in adduction, external rotation and flexion (Fig. 27.18). Wasting, especially of the buttocks, occurs and swelling and induration are often present. A cold abscess may point either below gluteus maximus or anteriorly in the upper thigh and eventually form a sinus. Later in severe cases in young children the epiphyses in the neighbourhood of the knee may fuse prematurely and lead to gross shortening. Early radiological changes are those described on

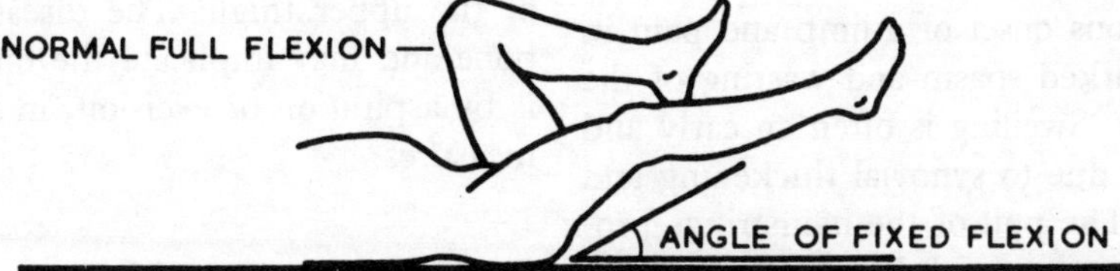

Fig. 27.18 Thomas's test of fixed flexion deformity of the hip. The normal hip is flexed fully so that the lumbar curve is flattened. Deformity is shown as flexion of affected hip.

page 350, whilst in later cases gross destruction of femoral head or acetabulum, or dislocation of the head on to the dorsum ilii may be apparent.

Differential diagnosis

Perthes' disease can be excluded by the absence of wasting or constitutional symptoms and the radiological changes (p. 366). 'Transient synovitis' may be confusing, but both pain and limp disappear rapidly with rest and do not recur. A gradually slipping upper femoral epiphysis and low-grade pyogenic infection also require consideration.

Treatment

General treatment is required (p. 13). Local treatment consists of immobilisation for at least six months. In children a frame and in adults a double plaster of Paris spica should be used. There is usually extensive bony damage, and the ultimate aim should be sound fusion of the joint. Extra-articular arthrodesis should be performed when the active phase is over, but in children should be delayed until after the age of 13 years. Rarely the disease is arrested before there is bony damage, when cautious mobilisation after the condition has become quiescent may be attempted.

Tuberculosis of the knee

The condition as in other joints is secondary to tuberculosis elsewhere. Infection may be initially synovial but destruction of the articular cartilage and subchondral bone can follow later. Sinuses are common because the joint is superficial, but large cold abscesses do not form.

Clinical features

There is an insidious onset of a limp and pain in the joint, with marked spasm and wasting of the quadriceps muscle. Swelling is often an early and prominent feature due to synovial thickening and chronic effusion. The pull of the hamstrings produces a flexion deformity with later backward displacement of the tibia. Culture of the aspirated fluid or biopsy of the synovial membrane confirms the diagnosis.

Treatment

In addition to general management, the knee should be immobilised on a Thomas's splint or in a single hip spica. When there is evidence of significant bony damage, arthrodesis is indicated but if changes are absent or slight, cautious mobilisation should be commenced. If there is marked soft tissue involvement but minimal bone erosion a useful range of movement may be preserved by excision of the diseased synovium (synovectomy).

Other tuberculous lesions

Tuberculous dactylitis

This is tuberculous osteitis affecting the shafts of the 'short' long bones in the hands or feet. It is usually seen in young children, is often multifocal and associated with lesions elsewhere. Syphilitic dactylitis must be excluded.

Tuberculous tenosynovitis

Tuberculosis may affect the flexor tendon sheaths of the hand, which become distended with exudate containing fibrinous melon-seed bodies. Extension occurs deep to the transverse carpal ligament into the forearm, so that fluctuation between the two swellings may be obtained (compound palmar ganglion). Later the tendons become matted together and the hand becomes 'frozen'. Excision of the affected tendon sheath should be performed and general chemotherapeutic measures are essential. A similar condition may be found in rheumatoid arthritis but multiple joint involvement is usual.

Tuberculous bursitis

This may occur in the bursa over the greater trochanter, causing a cystic swelling on the outer side of the upper thigh. The disease later spreads to bone and may implicate the hip joint. Treatment is by aspiration or excision, in addition to general measures.

Syphilis of bones and joints

Congenital lesions

Three conditions are encountered. (1) *Syphilitic*

osteochondritis, in which a plane of granulation tissue forms in several epiphyseal discs, often leading to separation. (2) *Parrot's nodes*, characteristic local areas of periostitis causing thickening of the parietal bones, and requiring no treatment. (3) *Clutton's joints*, which are bilateral, painless effusions involving the knees, rarely other joints, due to syphilitic infiltration of the synovium.

Acquired lesions

Localised or generalised syphilitic osteitis may occur. In the generalised type the tibia is usually affected, subperiosteal new bone being laid down along the anterior border, leading to the deformity known as 'sabre tibia', which must be distinguished from Paget's disease (p. 370). Gummatous lesions of central destruction with surrounding diffuse sclerosis may also affect the tibia and other long bones. Syphilitic dactylitis produces more sclerosis and new bone formation than does tuberculosis. Neurosyphilis can result in a neuropathic joint (p. 363).

Infections of the hand

Pulp infection

Minor wounds are frequent and infection common. The pulp is subdivided into numerous compartments by septa which stretch from skin to bone. Pus is unable to spread freely, leading to a high degree of tension, which interrupts the phalangeal blood supply and causes early bone infection (Fig. 27.19).

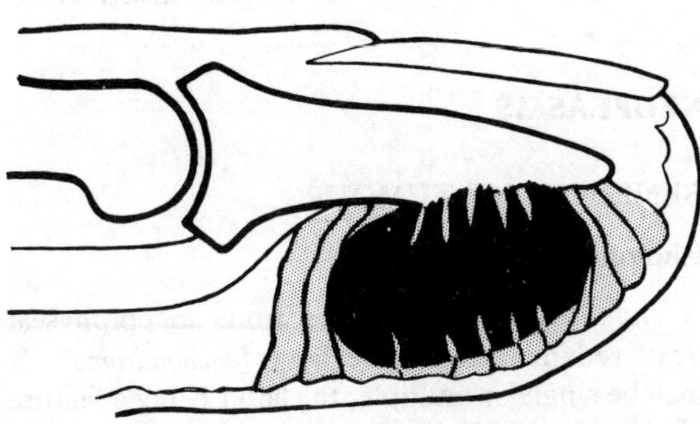

Fig. 27.19 Infection of the terminal pulp space of the finger

Clinical features. A minor puncture wound of the finger-tip may be noted, followed in a day or two by throbbing pain and swelling. A hot, red and tender pulp may be associated with lymphangitis and constitutional upset. Tenosynovitis, bone and joint infection may result if the condition is neglected.

Drainage should be carried out through an incision over the area of maximum localised tenderness. Antibiotics are administered when there is further spread.

Nail bed infection

A minor injury of the nail fold may become infected with spread across the nail bed, and finally deep to the nail (*paronychia*). Tension is not great and pain not therefore severe. Redness, swelling and pus are noted.

In early cases a small vertical incision along the side of the base of the nail suffices, but in more advanced infection the base of the nail should be avulsed. The skin over the bed is raised as a flap by two small lateral incisions and a wick of petroleum jelly gauze inserted (Fig. 27.20).

Deep space infection

A fascial space containing loose areolar tissue is situated deep to the flexor tendons, but superficial to the interossei and adductor pollicis. It is subdiv-

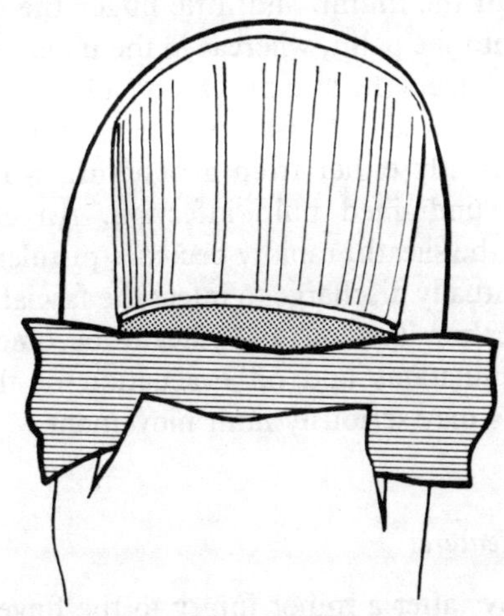

Fig. 27.20 Treatment of paronychia by removal of proximal part of nail and insertion of a petroleum jelly gauze drain

ided by a fibrous septum extending from the third metacarpal to the deep surface of the sheath of the flexor tendon to the index finger. The portion on the ulnar side of the septum is known as the '*mid-palmar space*', and that on the radial side as the '*thenar space*'. Distally this loose areolar tissue surrounds the tendons of the lumbrical muscles forming the lumbrical canals which lead to the base of the fingers. Infection can spread along the lumbrical canals from a lesion at the base of the finger or thumb into these potential spaces, which rapidly fill with pus.

Clinical features. Deep space infections are recognised by ballooning of the palm in a mid-palmar lesion, or the thenar eminence in a thenar space infection. There is often an associated septic focus at the base of a digit. Marked oedema of the dorsum of the hand is usually present. Spread to the tendon sheaths in the hand may follow. Constitutional effects are generally marked.

In a mid-palmar space infection, the web between either the middle and ring, or the ring and little finger should be divided to allow drainage via the lumbrical canal. In a thenar space infection pus should be released by an incision behind and parallel to the web of the thumb (Fig. 27.21).

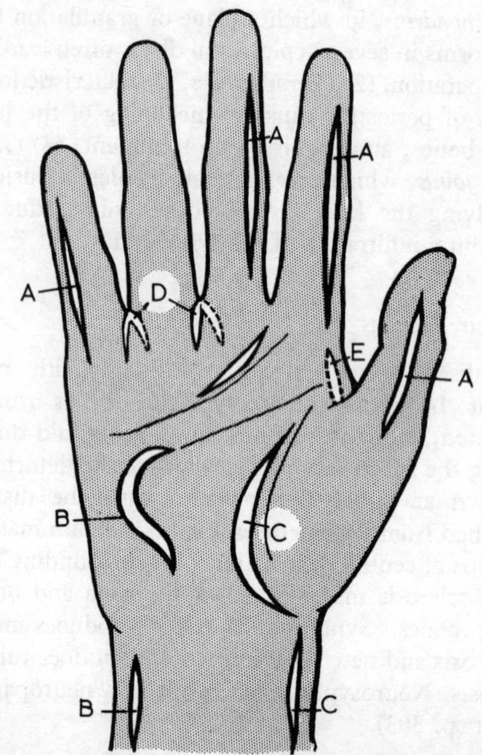

Fig. 27.21 Incisions in the hand to drain infected foci in **A**. Flexor tendon sheath; **B**. Ulnar bursa; **C**. Radial bursa; **D**. Mid-palmar space by splitting web; **E**. Thenar space on dorsum of web.

Suppurative tenosynovitis

Infection can occur in any tendon sheath, but the most common and important are those of the finger flexors. In the thumb and little finger the sheaths extend into the palm, whereas in the index, middle and ring fingers the sheaths end on a level with the metacarpal heads. Organisms reach the tendon sheath directly either from a puncture wound or from an undrained pulp infection. An effusion forms in the sheath, rapidly becomes purulent, and may eventually discharge to infect the fascial spaces of the palm. Tendon and sheath become lined with granulations and on evacuation of the pus adhesions may seriously limit movement.

Clinical features

A few days after a minor injury to the finger pain rapidly develops. The digit is held semiflexed, active or passive movement being extremely painful. In advanced cases the whole finger becomes swollen, hot and exquisitely tender.

In the early stages antibiotics may cause resolution, but unless marked improvement occurs within 24 hours the tendon sheath should be opened proximally and distally, and irrigated with an antibiotic solution (Fig. 27.21). When infection subsides gentle active movements are instituted.

NEOPLASMS

BENIGN BONE TUMOURS

Chondroma

A chondroma usually arises from an epiphyseal 'rest' retained within the bone (*enchondroma*). It may be single or multiple, the latter being a feature of dyschondroplasia (p. 330). A solitary enchondroma is generally found in the 'short' long bones of the hand, often being discovered incidentally or after a fracture. Treatment is only indicated where the swelling is large, and consists of curettage and the insertion of bone chips. Fracture usually leads to spontaneous cure.

Osteochondroma

An osteochondroma arises from an epiphyseal 'rest', which remains on the outside of the bone. When mainly cartilaginous it is known as an *ecchondroma*, and if mainly bone as a *cancellous exostosis*. It may be single or multiple, the latter being referred to as multiple osteochondromatosis (p. 330). When solitary it may arise from the growing end of a large bone, more commonly in the region of the knee. It is directed away from the bone end, has a cap of epiphyseal cartilage, and ceases to grow when the parent epiphysis fuses (Fig. 27.22). Clinically there may be an incidental finding of a swelling, tendons may be obstructed in surmounting the growth, pressure on adjacent nerves may occur, or pain result from fracture of the base. Malignant change, recognised by an increase in size or pain after the parent epiphysis has fused, is rare. Removal is indicated only when symptoms are present.

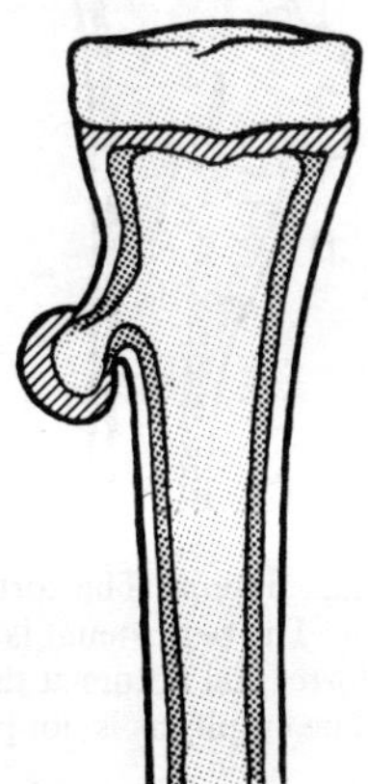

Fig. 27.22 Osteochondroma. The cartilage cap develops as a 'rest' of epiphyseal cartilage left behind as the bone grows.

Osteoma

A true osteoma is composed of hard compact bone (*ivory osteoma*). It generally arises in the skull where it may cause symptoms from local pressure.

Solitary bone cyst

This is a cystic condition which occurs in long bones, particularly the femur or humerus, commencing near the epiphysis, but eventually situated in the shaft as growth progresses. It is lined by fibrous tissue, contains brown fluid and slowly expands the bone (Fig. 27.23). A fracture often produced by minor trauma may be the first indication. Biopsy should be performed. Spontaneous healing may follow a fracture, but curettage and the insertion of bone chips may be necessary.

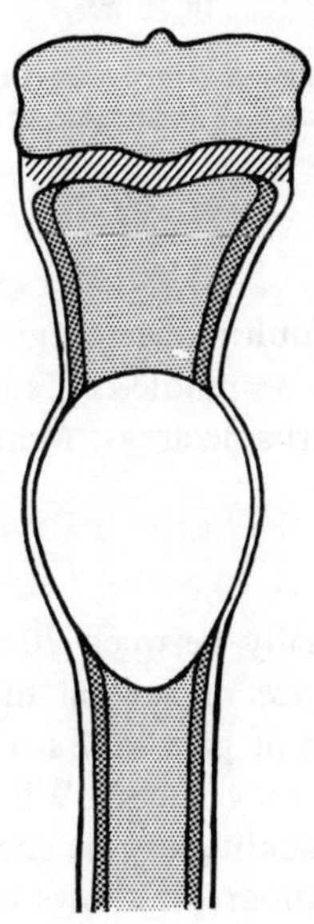

Fig. 27.23 Solitary bone cyst. The oval central cyst expands and thins the cortex.

INTERMEDIATE BONE TUMOUR

Osteoclastoma ('Giant-cell tumour of bone')

Pathology

Several different types occur, both benign and malignant forms being included in the group. The growth originates in the metaphysis of a major long bone and spreads into the epiphyseal area (Fig. 27.24). Seventy-five per cent occur in the region of the knee joint, in femur or tibia. Macroscopically it is a soft, reddish-yellow tumour which is loculated and possesses a well-defined wall. The histological picture is characteristically one of

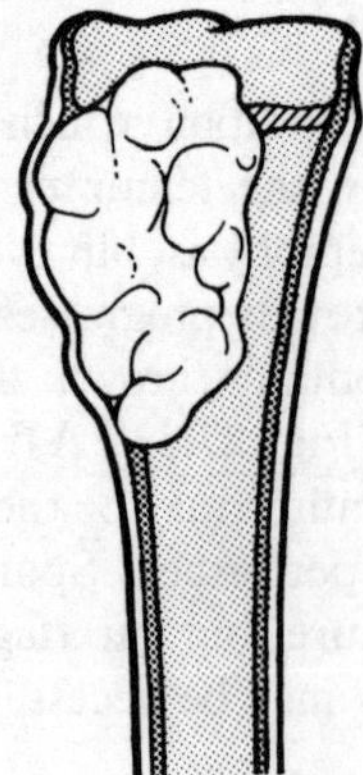

Fig. 27.24 Osteoclastoma. The cortex is expanded and thin. There is a typical soap-bubble appearance.

numerous large multinucleated giant cells, similar to osteoclasts, in a spindle-cell stroma containing scattered haemorrhagic areas. Metastasis is rare.

Clinical features

The onset is usually between 20 and 35 years of age. Symptoms are of several months duration, mainly consisting of pain and swelling, but spontaneous fracture may occur. When the cortex is thin, egg-shell crackling can be elicited in the bony hard mass. A radiograph shows an encapsulated, multilocular, cystic lesion, expanding the cortex, often eccentric and near the end of a long bone.

Biopsy is indicated to exclude other bony lesions. These include a *solitary bone cyst*, more often seen in a younger age group; *osteitis fibrosa cystica*, in which the lesions may be multiple and the serum or urinary calcium levels raised; *osteogenic sarcoma*, where the history is shorter and the lesion less well defined with some periosteal reaction radiologically; *metastatic tumours*, where the bone outline is not enlarged, and a *chronic bone abscess* when pain, perhaps associated with induration and constitutional disturbance, is a feature.

Treatment is by surgery. Radical excision of the entire lesion without impairing limb function should be carried out because of the tendency to recurrence. Occasionally amputation is the only effective means of cure.

PRIMARY MALIGNANT BONE TUMOURS

Osteogenic sarcoma

Pathology

Osteogenic sarcoma is so named because it arises in bone-forming cells (osteoblasts). It may be predominantly osteolytic with bone destruction, or sclerosing with excessive bone formation. It usually occurs in the actively growing metaphysis. There is irregular extension along the shaft and through the cortex. The periosteum is raised, but provides a barrier to local spread until late in the disease, whilst the epiphysis is seldom penetrated (Fig. 27.25). The tumour is composed of numerous spindle-shaped or spheroidal cells lying in a stroma consisting of bony, osteoid, myxomatous, fibrous or cartilaginous tissue, in which are included vascular spaces. Any bone may be affected but the region of the knee is the common site. Spread is mainly by the bloodstream to the lungs.

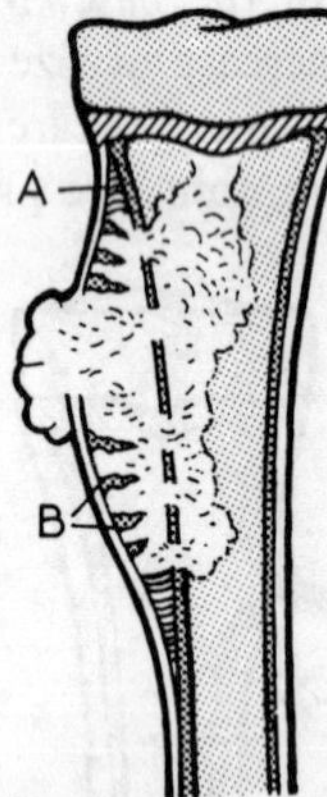

Fig. 27.25 Osteogenic sarcoma. The cortex is penetrated though vestiges remain. The periosteum is raised and later ruptured. New bone formation occurs at the angle (**A**) and spicules form at (**B**). The epiphysis is not penetrated.

Clinical features

Males are affected more often than females and the usual age incidence is in the second decade. In later life the condition may follow Paget's disease of bone. The presentation is by pain, swelling or pathological fracture, sometimes with a history of a mild traumatic incident. Pain is rarely noted for longer than one year and its character is often deep and well localised. Examination shows a diffuse, tender, bony swelling which may be hot, with dilated veins coursing over its surface. Rarely fungation through the skin occurs in late cases. The prognosis is poor; pulmonary metastases are often present before the primary lesion is noted and are at times responsible for the initial symptoms.

Radiological changes include irregular extension along the shaft and into the soft tissues, with a 'ghost' of the cortex still visible, deposition of new bone at the edge of the tumour where the periosteum is being raised, and 'sun-ray' spicules of bone arising from the raised periosteum. A radiograph of the chest may demonstrate secondary deposits and examination of the blood shows a high sedimentation rate and a raised alkaline phosphatase due to bone destruction. The differential diagnosis includes subacute osteomyelitis, syphilitic and typhoid osteitis, other bone tumours and march fractures. An adequate biopsy is always necessary.

Treatment

The management of this aggressive tumour has been improved by the introduction of cytotoxic drugs. Survival following amputation alone has been poor because of the frequency of metastases. Extensive spread of tumour tissue to the endothelial lining of blood vessels is an early feature, but this can be controlled by cytotoxic drugs if the main tumour mass is removed by amputation. Thus immediate amputation followed by combination chemotherapy for several months is advised. Radiotherapy may be added where indicated.

Parosteal sarcoma

This rare tumour arises from the fibrous layer of the periosteum, often near the lower end of the femur. Lobulated ossifying masses are formed alongside the parent bone and composed histologically of fibroblasts or spindle cells. It occurs in the 30 to 40 age group, grows slowly, is relatively benign, but may later metastasise to the lungs. Treatment is by amputation or resection, followed by radiotherapy.

Chondrosarcoma

This not uncommon tumour may arise as a result of malignant change in a pre-existing benign chondroma or may be malignant from the beginning. The long bones, pelvis and ribs are chiefly affected. The growth has a lobulated structure often commencing within the bone, and consists of cartilage with areas of cystic and haemorrhagic degeneration. Histologically well-differentiated cartilage cells may be apparent or a more pleomorphic picture obtained. Spread is generally slow with chiefly local invasion but vascular dissemination may occur.

Clinical features

Adults between 30 and 50 years are mainly affected, the sex distribution being equal. A slowly growing hard swelling is apparent, often altering little in size for years, but rapid increase and associated pain may be noted. Radiography demonstrates a diffuse mass with irregular calcification, related to the affected bone.

Treatment

Wide excision is essential together with the affected segment of bone. Amputation may be required. The tumour is radioresistant.

Ewing's tumour ('Malignant endothelioma')

This uncommon tumour arises from the diaphysis of a long bone generally in childhood. It is soft and greyish in colour, containing the remains of bone undergoing erosion (Fig. 27.26). Histologically it is composed of sheets of small round cells similar in appearance to a neuroblastoma and many cases of apparent Ewing's tumour have been metastatic neuroblastomas from a primary adrenal lesion. In some instances the condition is one of primary reticulum-cell sarcoma. Spread is both vascular and lymphatic. Clinically, in addition to pain and swelling, febrile attacks are common, causing confusion with subacute osteomyelitis. Radiography demonstrates the deposition of layers of new bone beneath the elevated periosteum, giving an 'onion-peel' appearance. Biopsy confirms the diagnosis.

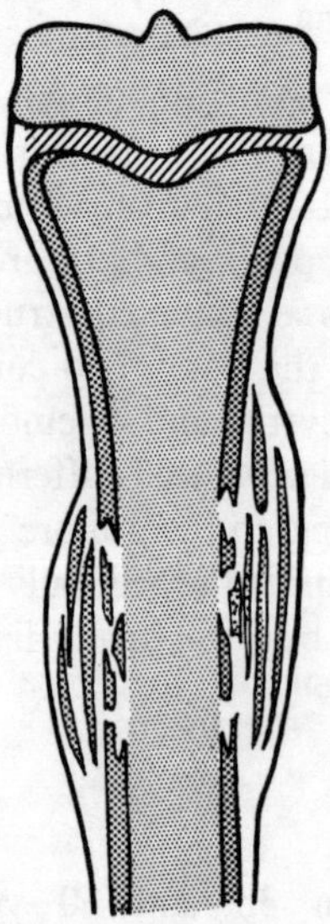

Fig. 27.26 Malignant endothelioma. The tumour arises centrally in the metaphysis. The periosteum is raised with alternating layers of bone deposition and destruction ('onion-peel effect').

Treatment is by amputation and cytotoxic therapy. The prognosis is poor but the use of chemotherapy has improved results.

Myelomatosis

These tumours, arising from plasma cells, are usually multicentric in origin, the condition being known as multiple myelomatosis. Rarely a single growth called a solitary plasmacytoma occurs. Bones which contain red marrow become involved, the ribs, vertebrae, skull, pelvis, sternum, femora and humeri being affected. Deposits appear as small greyish punched-out areas, initially circumscribed but later replacing the whole marrow cavity. Microscopically the lesion consists of small round cells similar to lymphocytes or plasma cells with little intercellular substance. The liver, spleen and lymph nodes may be later implicated.

Multiple myelomatosis

This usual manifestation of the condition occurs in the middle-aged or elderly, with a male predominance. The presenting symptom is pain, which if due to vertebral collapse may be both local and referred. Vertebral disorganisation may later lead to cord compression and paraplegia, whilst marrow destruction produces anaemia. 'Spontaneous' fracture may occur.

An immature proteose is liberated from the plasma cells resulting in a rise in the serum globulin, diminution of the albumin fraction and a markedly raised sedimentation rate. Such proteose molecules are small enough to pass through the glomeruli appearing in the urine as 'Bence-Jones proteose', which precipitates out on heating, disappears when boiling point is reached, reappearing on cooling. Sternal puncture permits the demonstration of plasma cells in the marrow. Radiography shows multiple punched-out areas in the affected bones, including the skull.

Treatment is palliative, but chemotherapy using nitrogen mustards may prolong life for several years. Radiotherapy may relieve pain, and blood transfusions are required for anaemia.

Solitary plasmacytoma

In this rare manifestation of the condition a single myelomatous deposit occurs in one bone, often in a vertebral body, leading to its collapse. Radiotherapy causes rapid disappearance of the lesion. If there is no recurrence for a year, the prognosis is good, but often a solitary plasmacytoma is the prelude to the onset of generalised disease.

The reticuloses

Generalised diseases of the reticulo-endothelial system, such as Hodgkin's disease and the leukaemias, also produce widespread bony deposits.

The skeletal involvement is principally vertebral and may produce paraplegia. Pain and tenderness at the affected site may be noted or a pathological fracture occur. Radiography demonstrates lesions which may be both osteolytic and osteosclerotic. Radiotherapy may relieve local pain and chemotherapy should also be employed (p. 434).

Secondary tumours of bone

This is the most common form of malignant disease in bone, and is blood borne. The common primary sites are the breast, prostate, lung, kidney and thy-

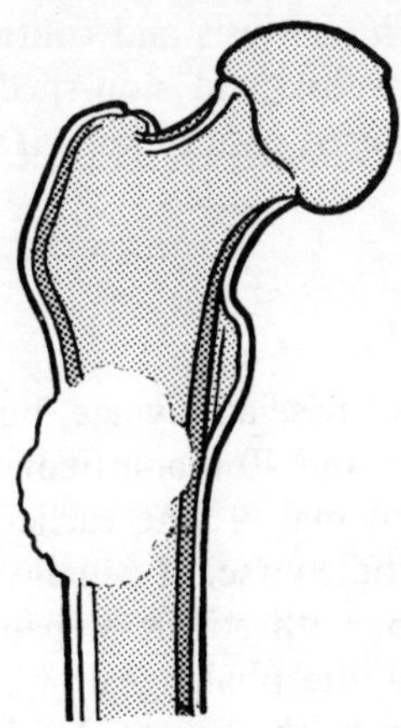

Fig. 27.27 Secondary carcinomatous deposit in bone. This is a destructive lesion of the whole bone including cortex with no periosteal reaction.

roid. Deposits occur most frequently in areas of red marrow such as the vertebral bodies, pelvis, and upper ends of the femora or humeri (Fig. 27.27). Radiography reveals a destructive lesion and biopsy may indicate the primary site. Investigations should be directed towards finding the origin of the initial tumour.

Treatment

Palliation alone is feasible but relief of symptoms can be obtained by radiotherapy, chemotherapy and in some instances hormonal therapy. Vertebral deposits may require suitable supports, and peripheral fractures can be treated by internal fixation followed by radiotherapy.

Tumours of soft tissues

These are relatively uncommon, and only the more important will be considered.

Benign

A **fibroma** may occur in muscle or tendon, producing a small, firm, localised mass. In the abdominal wall, where it is known as a 'desmoid tumour', it tends to be more infiltrative and may recur if not widely excised. **Giant cell tumour of tendon** (benign synovioma) is a small yellow encapsulated tumour arising from the tendon sheaths in the extremities. Histologically, foreign body giant cells and cholesterol-laden xanthoma cells are found. Treatment is by local excision.

Malignant

Malignant synovioma (synovial sarcoma) is a highly malignant neoplasm arising from synovial membranes, tendon sheaths, or bursae. It forms a large fleshy mass spreading widely and infiltrating bone and soft tissue. It may arise in association with any joint, but is more common in the lower limb. Microscopically there are large numbers of spheroidal or spindle cells with numerous mitoses, among which are clefts, representing attempts to form synovial spaces. Spread is both lymphatic and vascular. It usually occurs in middle life, the main complaint being of pain or swelling of the involved part. The tumour is radio-resistant, and wide local excision or amputation is thus required. **Fibrosarcoma** may arise from any structure containing fibrous tissue. It usually spreads rapidly in a local direction and metastasises by the bloodstream. When well differentiated, growth may be slow. Treatment is by wide excision or amputation, as they are radio-resistant. **Rhabdomyosarcoma** is a rare malignant tumour of skeletal (striated) muscle. It generally involves the lower limb and is radio-resistant.

Ganglion

Although not a true tumour, such a cystic swelling can be conveniently considered at this stage. A common lesion, generally arising from a joint, it appears on becoming superficial to be closely associated with a tendon sheath. It is filled with clear viscous jelly-like material, and may become very tense. Usually occurring in smaller joints, it is often found on the dorsum of the hand or foot, or arising from the palmar aspect of a metacarpophalangeal joint. In the latter site it can produce a small tender lesion sufficiently tense to suggest bone or cartilage. In the foot symptoms may be caused by pressure from shoes. Impingement on the median or ulnar nerves in the palm may lead to paraesthesiae in the fingers or weakness of the interossei. Spontaneous regression may occur, but the majority persist or increase in size.

Treatment. Direct manual pressure or an injection of hyalase may cause dispersal, but complete excision is the most certain method of avoiding recurrence.

ARTHRITIS

In addition to trauma and specific infection two main groups of joint lesions produce permanent structural changes.

1. Specific generalised joint diseases characterised by widespread joint involvement, proliferation of synovium and rarefaction in the bones ('atrophic arthritis'). The most important are: (*a*) *rheumatoid arthritis*, in which the peripheral joints are first affected, the disease spreading towards the centre; (*b*) *ankylosing spondylitis*, in which the central spinal and costal joints are first affected and only later, in severe cases, spreading peripherally.

2. Those due to senile changes in the joints, characterised by degenerative changes in the articular cartilage, with sclerosis and hypertrophy of bone, leading to marginal osteophyte formation ('hypertrophic arthritis'), and known as *osteoarthritis*.

Rheumatoid arthritis

Pathology

This is a generalised disease of unknown aetiology. The basic lesion is proliferation of synovial membrane, which usually fills the joint and spreads over the articular cartilage. There is associated hyperaemia, resultant osteoporosis and often an effusion. Changes are reversible until the cartilage is destroyed. Later the synovial proliferations undergo fibrosis thereby limiting movement and by their contraction producing severe deformities. When destruction exposes raw bone, ankylosis takes place. Lesions also occur in tendon sheaths, bursae and subcutaneous tissue, the latter forming nodules usually over bony surfaces such as the ulna. The disease finally remits, affected joints being left either ankylosed by bone or fibrous tissue, or damaged, in which case degenerative changes follow and osteoarthritis is superimposed. A type of polyarthritis akin to rheumatoid arthritis also occurs with psoriasis and colitis, and in association with uveitis and non-specific urethritis, making a recognised pattern known as Reiter's syndrome.

Clinical features

The disease may arise at any age, but is most common between 30 and 40 years. Females are affected more often than males. The earlier the onset the more acute is the course. It usually commences in the upper limb, with stiffness, pain and swelling in the proximal interphalangeal or metacarpophalangeal joints or in the wrists. In the lower limbs the feet, ankles, or knees may be first involved, both sides often being symmetrically affected. Tendon sheaths become thickened, particularly of the wrist extensors, where bilateral effusions are often seen. Systemic manifestations such as anaemia and lassitude are common and muscle wasting is marked. Progress is by a series of exacerbations interspersed with spells of comparative quiescence. In advanced cases almost all joints become affected, and subcutaneous nodules are frequent.

Some degree of deformity is common and is usually of a characteristic pattern. In the hands fibrosis of the intrinsic muscles causes ulnar deviation and flexion at the metacarpophalangeal joints, the interphalangeal joints becoming hyper-extended. The elbows become flexed, and the shoulders adducted and internally rotated. The toes tend to be severely clawed with dislocation at the metatarsophalangeal joints. The feet become valgoid, the knees flexed, and the hips flexed, adducted and externally rotated. Bony ankylosis, particularly when occurring bilaterally in major joints, is disabling. Tendon rupture may occur in the hand due to a combination of attrition over a roughened bony point and weakening associated with tenosynovitis.

Radiography confirms osteoporosis, may demonstrate areas of 'punched-out' trabecular absorption, and may reveal varying degrees of joint destruction. The sedimentation rate is raised, and serial estimations can be used to estimate progress. Specific agglutination tests are useful in diagnosis. Aspiration is helpful in excluding chronic infective arthritis, whilst biopsy may be required in atypical cases.

Treatment

General treatment requires the co-operation of a physician. Rest, a well-balanced diet, salicylates and steroids may be employed. Local treatment may be conservative or operative. The former is directed towards the relief of pain and the prevention of stiffness and deformity. Stiffness is minimised by active movements and the alleviation of muscle spasm by heat, including wax baths for smaller joints. Deformity is prevented by splintage, particularly when worn at night. When pain is severe complete rest on a splint may be required. Operative measures are used either to restore movement by arthroplasty or to correct deformity and relieve pain by arthrodesis. Arthroplasty is preferable in the hip to enable a patient with stiff lower limbs to sit and stand, whereas in the knee, where stability is required, arthrodesis is more satisfactory.

Still's disease

Rheumatoid arthritis occurring in childhood tends to be rapidly progressive, and is known as Still's disease. It is accompanied by fever, sweating and anaemia, often with enlargement of the spleen and lymph nodes. The joints become hot and swollen, and muscle wasting may be extreme. In severe cases most joints are involved, leading to gross crippling.

During the acute phase rest is imperative, whilst steroid therapy is also useful. When the disease has died out a prolonged course of rehabilitation and reconstructive surgery may be necessary to enable the patient to be self-supporting.

Ankylosing spondylitis

This condition of unknown aetiology generally commences in the sacro-iliac joints and spreads upwards to involve the intervertebral and costovertebral joints. Later the hips, shoulders and knees may be affected. Initially there is peri-articular thickening, followed by destruction of the articular cartilage and ossification of the capsule, leading to bony ankylosis. Finally the whole spine may be converted into a continuous rod of bone.

Clinical features

Most cases occur in young adult males, being rare after the age of 50 years. Progress is by a series of exacerbations and remissions, becoming quiescent after a number of years. The first complaint is of low back pain, followed by stiffness, symptoms being most marked on rising in the morning and decreasing with activity. Deformity, consisting mainly of flexion in both spine and hips, occurs later, and is due to a combination of unequal muscle power and gravity. In extreme cases the patient may be so bowed that forward vision is difficult. Stiffness may also affect the costovertebral joints, diminishing chest expansion and resulting in abdominal-type respiration. Iritis is a common complication.

The sedimentation rate is raised, its fluctuations being a guide to the activity of the disease. The first radiological changes are seen in the sacro-iliac joints, which show irregularity of their margins with patchy sclerosis, later becoming completely obliterated. Ossification in the longitudinal spinal ligaments produces the appearance known as 'bamboo spine'.

Differentiation must be made from postural backache, where stiffness is less marked and the sedimentation rate and radiographs of the sacro-iliac joints are normal; from a prolapsed intervertebral disc, where a sudden episode is common; and from tuberculosis of the lumbar spine or sacro-iliac joints. Recent studies of histocompatability antigens have demonstrated links between this type of spondylitis and rheumatic conditions. Clinical surveys have shown that over 90 per cent of patients with ankylosing spondylitis possess the antigen known as HL-A 27 as compared with only four per cent of the normal population, but the full significance of this finding has yet to be determined.

Treatment

Attention to improving the general state of health is important, whilst exercises are useful in controlling deformity and stiffness. The mainstay of treatment is with anti-inflammatory therapy, either phenylbutazone or indomethacin, given in regular doses over an extended period. With an intensive course of physiotherapy it is usually possible to reduce joint stiffness and long-term deformities. When hip disease is established arthroplasty is often indicated. Severe spinal kyphosis may occasionally require correction by spinal osteotomy.

OSTEOARTHRITIS

Osteoarthritis may be primary or secondary. In the former, symptoms occur as a direct result of senile changes and several joints may be affected. Secondary osteoarthritis follows a local abnormality which increases joint wear, as in mal-united fractures, Perthes' disease, or from loose bodies. In both types the changes are similar.

Pathology

The articular cartilage is first affected, becoming softened and worn away to expose the underlying bone. The latter becomes sclerotic and ridged (eburnation) whilst at the edges of the articular surfaces marginal bony hypertrophy occurs, producing lipping and osteophyte formation. Loose bodies may arise from their detachment. At first the synovial membrane is normal; later thickening and fibrosis are usually found.

Clinical features

The initial symptom is generally pain, often precipitated by minor injury, at first present only on movement, later becoming constant. Stiffness and deformity follow. The typical appearance in the hip is one of flexion, adduction and external rotation, whereas in the knee loss of flexion occurs, with muscle wasting and often palpable marginal osteophytes. Finally only a minimal range of painful movement persists in the joint.

Radiography reveals a narrow joint space with sclerosis of the subchondral bone, most marked in the region of maximal weight-bearing. Later disorganisation, deformity and osteophyte formation are seen. When several joints are involved rheumatoid arthritis must be excluded. Tuberculosis or neoplasm are to be considered when a single joint is affected.

Treatment

Conservative management comprises the avoidance of further trauma, weight reduction, and local heat and exercises which maintain muscular protection and minimise joint stiffness. Intra-articular hydrocortisone may relieve pain for a period of six months, whilst supports such as a corset in spinal lesions may be of considerable help.

Operative treatment. When a single joint is affected arthrodesis is advisable. In the spine, fusion of a single segment is helpful in young adults. In unilateral disease of the hip, where the back is mobile, arthrodesis gives a satisfactory result. In older patients, or those with bilateral lesions, movement must be preserved, either by displacement osteotomy where pain is relieved but the range of movement is unaltered (Fig. 27.28), or by arthroplasty which aims at reconstruction of the joint (Fig. 27.29). Arthrodesis is occasionally useful in unilateral disease of the knee, ankle, wrist and tarsus.

Total joint replacement. This procedure has become widely accepted and practised for degenerative joint disease, whether due to trauma, inflammation or primary osteoarthrosis. The development of satisfactory mechanical designs and materials which give both good fixation and long-term wear has enabled advances to be made. The hip joint has received the main focus of research and the prostheses now commonly used are those in which friction has been shown to be low. Designs employ dissimilar materials at the joint interface; the cup is made of high density polythene and the stem of either stainless steel or cobalt-chrome alloy. A small femoral head usually less than 3 cm in diameter also produces less friction. Fixation is performed with a special methacrylate cement which sets extremely hard within ten minutes of being mixed. The materials are also used for other replacements, such as the knee, shoulder and elbow. Where hinge joints are inserted, the stems are of metal but polythene bushes are used to reduce friction and wear. Complications of artificial joints are not uncommon and consist mainly of infection due to the large foreign body and looseness of the components. Sensitivity to the implants in some patients is thought to occur but definite evidence has yet to be found.

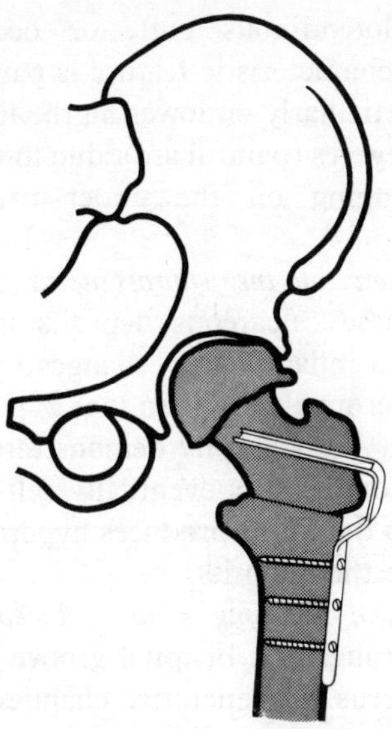

Fig. 27.28 Osteotomy of the hip to produce varus angulation of the femoral neck. The tendency of the head to extrude laterally is corrected.

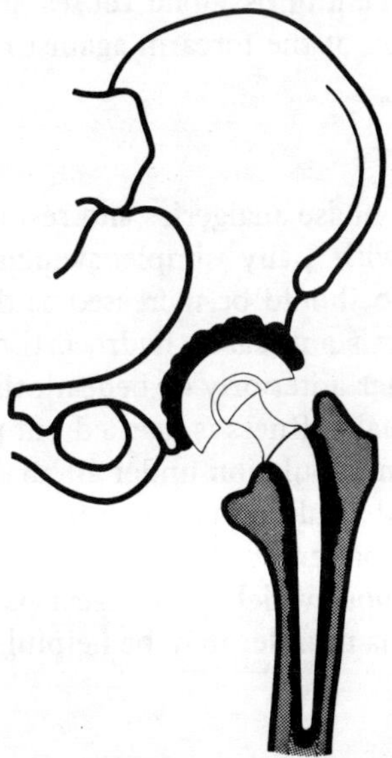

Fig. 27.29 Total replacement of the hip joint with a low friction type of prosthesis, employing a polythene cup and steel stem. Fixation is by methacrylate cement.

Chondromalacia patellae

In this condition there is swelling followed by fissuring of the articular cartilage of the patella. Later bare bone may be exposed and osteoarthritis eventually supervenes. Young adults, with a female preponderance, are affected. The chief symptom is of pain deep to the patella aggravated by movement, particularly when descending steps, together with painful crepitus as the patella moves on the femur. An earlier history of direct trauma to the knee is at times obtained. Mild cases respond to rest in plaster, followed by gentle mobilisation. Advanced cases require surgery, consisting either of removal of the damaged articular cartilage from the patella or excision of the bone itself.

Neuropathic arthritis ('Charcot's joints')

This is an exaggerated form of osteoarthritis, occurring as the result of a loss of pain sensation. Normal protective muscle spasm is not evoked, consequently degenerative changes progress with great rapidity. In the spine and lower limbs, the neurological lesion is generally tabes dorsalis, whereas in the upper limbs, where neuropathic joints are uncommon, syringomyelia is the usual cause. The joint most frequently affected is the knee. The clinical picture is one of a painless but grossly disorganised and unstable joint, together with evidence of the underlying neurological lesion. Treatment is unsatisfactory. Arthrodesis is usually unsuccessful, and a supporting appliance gives the best result.

Haemophilic arthritis

Repeated haemarthroses damage the articular cartilage and lead to a stiff and deformed joint with marked muscle wasting and periarticular thickening. Operative treatment is contra-indicated and advanced cases require suitable supports.

Gouty arthritis

Repeated attacks of acute gout lead to deposits of sodium biurate crystals in the subcutaneous tissues and subchondral bone, with later destruction of articular cartilage. The metatarsophalangeal joint of the big toe is most frequently involved. Treatment is usually by medical means, as surgery may provoke further attacks.

LOCAL PAINFUL CONNECTIVE TISSUE LESIONS

The shoulder

Abduction of the joint is obtained by a combination of scapulo-humeral and scapulo-thoracic movement, the former taking place first. In painful shoulder lesions the rhythm is reversed. Due to the shallow glenoid, stability of the joint is maintained by the flat muscles arising from the scapula and inserted by a common musculotendinous cuff into the tuberosities around the humeral head. The supraspinatus is more vulnerable than subscapularis and infraspinatus, as in reaching the humerus it passes beneath the acromion where, to ensure its smooth gliding, lies the subacromial bursa.

A similar clinical picture may be produced in rupture of the tendinous cuff, subacromial bursitis, calcification in the supraspinatus tendon and tendinitis of the long head of the biceps muscle. An aching pain is prominent, felt maximally over the deltoid near its insertion but with tenderness over the humeral head. It becomes aggravated at night due to relaxation of the protective muscle spasm. Stiffness is a common feature, varying from minimal to complete absence of scapulo-humeral movement (*frozen shoulder*), rotation and abduction being chiefly restricted. Wasting is rarely marked.

Differentiation must be made from other causes of localised shoulder pain such as tuberculosis, where wasting is marked, and osteoarthritis which is uncommon. Referred pain from the fourth and fifth cervical nerve roots may originate in cervical spondylitis, diaphragmatic irritation or coronary disease.

Rupture of the musculotendinous cuff may be partial or complete, and follows forced adduction of the abducted shoulder. It is more common in a tendon with degenerative changes. If only partial rupture occurs the joint is painful, but injection of local anaesthetic will allow active movements to return. Complete rupture is not painful but active abduction is grossly limited and the arm cannot be held in abduction, falling to the side if released. Acute rupture of the cuff should be repaired in young patients, the results being usually satisfactory.

Subacromial bursitis. Chronic inflammation of the bursa may be associated with partial rupture of the musculotendinous cuff, or occur spontaneously. A characteristic feature is pain on abduction and particularly on lowering the limb through 120 to 45 degrees (painful arc), due to the irritative focus impinging on the under-surface of the acromion.

Calcification in the supraspinatus tendon. The cause of these calcareous deposits is unknown. They lead to inflammatory changes by impinging on the subacromial bursa, so that a 'painful arc' is often found. Radiography demonstrates the opacities. The condition is eventually self-limiting, as rupture into the bursa produces hyperaemia which may remove the deposits.

Tendinitis of the long head of biceps occurs as it passes through the bicipital groove in the head of the humerus. Degenerative changes in the tendon and roughening of the groove may lead to spontaneous rupture which may pass unnoticed, producing a characteristic bunching of the lower half of the muscle when the elbow is flexed against resistance. Tendinitis alone causes shoulder pain on supination of the forearm against resistance.

Treatment

In the acute phase analgesics and rest in a sling are indicated, with daily simple swinging exercises whose tempo should be increased as the pain subsides. In resistant cases hydrocortisone may be injected either anteriorly or beneath the acromion. When residual stiffness is marked but pain is minimal gentle manipulation under an anaesthetic may be employed. Calcareous deposits causing symptoms should be removed surgically. Rarely excision of the acromion, which allows freer passage for the supraspinatus muscle, may be helpful.

The elbow

Tennis elbow

Local pain situated over the outer side of the elbow is known as 'tennis elbow', a similar complaint over the inner side being called 'golfer's elbow'. A minor tear of the common extensor origin may be the causative factor when the pain follows a sudden or repetitive movement, but the onset is often insidious and the aetiology unknown. The pain is of an aching character and aggravated by gripping, especially with the arm extended. Marked local tenderness is present over the radial head or lateral humeral epicondyle. Stretching of the common extensor origin by flexion and pronation of the wrist as the elbow is extended aggravates the pain. Symptoms often subside over a period of several months up to two to three years. Early rheumatoid arthritis or referred root pain from a degenerate cervical disc should be excluded.

Treatment. A local injection of hydrocortisone often gives rapid relief, and where there has been a definite predisposing cause manipulation may be curative. In resistant cases three to four weeks' rest in a plaster cast may be helpful whilst rarely operative stripping of the common extensor origin is required.

Wrist and fingers

Stenosing tenovaginitis

Chronic inflammation in the tendon sheath produces constriction and reactionary thickening in the tendon. It occurs at two sites.

In the wrist, where the abductor longus and extensor pollicis brevis tendons cross the radial styloid. Pain is felt in the radial side of the wrist on moving the thumb and a fractured scaphoid may be suspected.

In the fingers or thumb, where the long flexors enter their fibrous tunnels opposite the metacarpal heads. The thickened tendon passes through the constriction with a sudden snap ('trigger finger' or 'trigger thumb'). When several fingers are affected rheumatoid arthritis may supervene.

In both the condition is self-limiting, symptoms subsiding after six months to two years.

Treatment. In early cases hydrocortisone injected into the tendon sheath causes resolution. Later cases require division of the constriction.

Foot

Plantar fasciitis

This is a painful area on the inferomedial aspect of the calcaneum corresponding to the point of attachment of the plantar fascia. In long-standing cases an associated bony spur may be found. Middle-aged males are chiefly affected, although in younger patients it may be the prelude to ankylosing spondylitis. Gout, gonococcal fasciitis and chronic tarsal osteomyelitis must be excluded.

Treatment. When well localised a hydrocortisone injection into the tender area is effective. Alternatively local support consisting of a full-width sponge rubber insole raising the heel from the shoe gives palliative relief.

AFFECTIONS OF THE EPIPHYSES

The epiphysis is concerned with longitudinal bone growth. It consists of a nucleus, initially surrounded by cartilage. Later the whole epiphysis becomes bony except for a narrow cartilaginous plate which separates it from the metaphysis. When growth is complete the epiphysis fuses with the shaft and the cartilaginous plate disappears.

Osteochondritis juvenilis

Pathology

This condition occurs when the epiphysis temporarily loses its blood supply. The cause is unknown, trauma, infection and endocrine disturbance having been suggested. It has been described in almost every epiphysis, being common in some and rare in others. A characteristic cycle takes place, lasting 12 to 18 months. First the epiphysis loses its blood supply and radiologically appears more dense than normal. It then softens, radiologically fragmenting and becoming granular, and may become deformed. Finally revascularisation follows, the bony structure returning to normal, but any altered shape is maintained. When centres not concerned with joint surfaces (apophyses) are affected it is of little significance, but in the weight-bearing epiphyses the articular surfaces become distorted leading later to osteoarthritis.

Osteochondritis of the upper femoral epiphysis ('Perthes' disease')

This is the most important site for osteochondritis and occurs mainly in boys of five to 10 years of age.

The first symptom is a limp followed by pain, which is rarely severe. Slight limitation of abduction and internal rotation is found in the early stages, followed by shortening due to deformity of the femoral head. Spasm is unusual and wasting does not occur. If untreated, symptoms disappear after about one year, but slight limitation of movement and shortening persist. Osteoarthritis is common in later life.

The cycle of changes may be followed radiographically. Initially the capital epiphysis appears denser and smaller with apparent widening of the joint space. This is followed by epiphyseal fragmentation, irregular rarefaction of the metaphysis and broadening of the femoral neck.

The condition must be distinguished from tuberculosis, where wasting and spasm are usually obvious, and slipped upper femoral epiphysis which is characterised by an external rotation deformity.

Treatment. The extent of damage to the femoral epiphysis can be graded either mild or 'at risk' and treatment planned accordingly. The mild cases do not require treatment, whilst gross changes indicate later joint problems due to deformity of the femoral head. This tends to bulge laterally out of the acetabulum and realignment of the upper femur by osteotomy is carried out to ensure better containment, thus providing a more stable joint when the epiphysis has finally healed.

Osteochondritis of the vertebrae

The epiphyseal plates in the vertebral body appear about puberty and fuse at about 18 years of age. Osteochondritis affecting these centres occurs during this period, several epiphyses being involved simultaneously. The main complaint of round shoulders occurs insidiously without more than a minor ache. Radiographs show irregularity and slight anterior wedging of the vertebral bodies, with fragmentation of the plates. If changes are more marked in a single vertebra, tuberculosis may be suspected. In later life degenerative changes, often symptomless, occur in the affected segment of the spine.

Treatment. In mild cases exercises alone are required. Where backache is troublesome a plaster bed for night use is helpful. Rarely, in severe cases, recumbency on a plaster bed, followed by a supporting brace, may be required.

Osteochondritis of the tibial tubercle

This common condition generally occurs in boys between the ages of 10 and 14 years. Pain of a mild nature is noted with some enlargement of the tibial tubercle which may be slightly warm. The opposite tibial tubercle may also be enlarged but is painless. Radiographs show irregularity and fragmentation of the apophysis. Treatment is only necessary for the relief of pain as the lesion is self-curing. The avoidance of trauma is usually sufficient, but if symptoms are troublesome protection by a plaster of Paris cylinder for a few weeks is helpful.

Apophysitis of the calcaneum

The apophysis at the postero-inferior angle of the calcaneum appears about the eighth year, fusing soon after puberty. During the time it is present pain in the heel may occur. Density and fragmentation of the apophysis are noted on radiography. Organised sport should be avoided.

Osteochondritis of the tarsal navicular

This condition affects the bony nucleus of the navicular in children aged three to five years. Pain and a limp are apparent, radiography showing flattening and density of the bone. During the painful phase a walking plaster cast is required for two to three months.

Osteochondritis of the metatarsal head

This is an affection of the head of one of the outer four metatarsals. It is most often seen in the second and least common in the fifth. Symptoms arise in adolescence, and consist of pain, stiffness and enlargement of the metatarsal head. Females are more commonly affected.

In the early stages pain may be relieved by a metatarsal bar, but in adults, if osteoarthritis develops, the metatarsal head should be excised.

Avascular necrosis of the lunate

This condition cannot be regarded as true osteochondritis as it occurs in young adults, but the lunate may undergo a similar cycle of changes. Severe carpal osteoarthritis may follow. Symptoms are of pain in the dorsum of the wrist, worse after exercise, leading to weakness and stiffness. Radiographs initially show increased density with later deformity.

In the early stages prolonged plaster immobilisation may permit revascularisation of the bone. Later, after deformity has occurred but before the onset of osteoarthritis, excision of the lunate may give good results. When osteoarthritis is severe arthrodesis of the wrist is to be preferred.

Slipped upper femoral epiphysis ('Adolescent coxa vara')

In adolescence the upper femoral epiphysis lies at an angle of 45 degrees to the horizontal and is therefore vulnerable to shearing strains. There may be sudden or gradual displacement of the epiphysis. The former results from trauma, but the latter is due to an unknown abnormality in the epiphyseal cartilage, usually seen in hypogonadal children but sometimes occurring in association with renal osteodystrophy (p. 369). It is commonest when growth is most rapid between the ages of 11 and 13 years in girls and 14 and 16 years in boys. The epiphysis displaces downwards and backwards, the latter predominating initially.

Clinical features

Males are affected rather more frequently than females. Sudden displacement follows a rotational twist of the lower limb. There is severe pain in the hip and thigh associated with inability to bear weight, the limb lying in full external rotation with loss of active movement. Gradual displacement occurs in fat and sexually under-developed individuals. The history is of pain, often most marked in the knee, and of a limp. Examination at first shows limitation of internal rotation of the hip, the limb characteristically turning into external rotation as the limit of flexion is reached. Later, movements become increasingly restricted, with an external rotation deformity and shortening. Displacement may follow in the opposite hip, at times occurring whilst the patient is recumbent under treatment. Severe stiffness of the hip joint due to avascular necrosis of the femoral head may be encountered as a complication of treatment.

Radiography of both hips is essential as the condition may be bilateral. Lateral views demonstrate early displacement and in the pre-slipping stage there is widening of the epiphyseal line, with irregularities on the metaphyseal side. A break in Shenton's line (Fig. 27.2) becomes obvious later. Renal function tests should be performed when renal disease is suspected. Other lesions to be excluded include early Perthes' disease, tuberculosis and undiagnosed congenital dislocation of the hip.

Treatment

In cases of sudden displacement encountered within a few days of injury, gentle manipulative reduction followed by internal fixation is indicated. Where displacement is gradual but slight, internal fixation in the position of deformity with fine circular nails inserted along the femoral neck gives the best result. If displacement is severe an osteotomy of the femoral neck below the epiphysis is occasionally carried out, but this may result in avascular necrosis of the epiphysis. More usually an osteotomy of the intertrochanteric region of the femur is done to realign the femur when epiphyseal fusion has occurred in the displaced position.

Osteochondritis dissecans

In this condition there is avascular necrosis of a segment of the articular surface of a bone, the cause of which is not clearly understood. It is most common in the knee joint from the medial femoral condyle and in the elbow joint from the capitellum. The avascular segment dies and separates, the articular cartilage initially remaining intact. Later it disintegrates allowing the loosened bony fragment to become dislodged into the joint cavity as one or more *loose bodies* (Fig. 27.30). The articular cartilage remaining on the loose fragment survives and proliferates to encircle the dead bony nucleus. Osteoarthritic changes finally supervene.

Clinical features

Adolescent males are most often affected. Early symptoms include indeterminate pain and weakness in the joint and there is tenderness over the

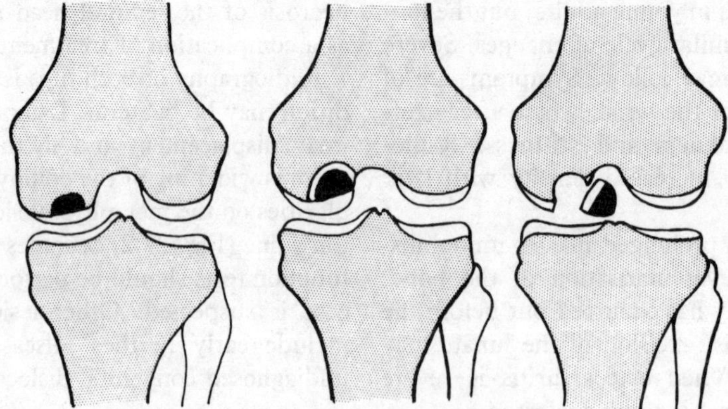

Fig. 27.30 Osteochondritis dissecans with development of a loose body in the knee joint

affected area. Later the features of a loose body such as locking, instability and recurring effusions become apparent. Radiography demonstrates a dense fragment lying either in a depression in the bone or free in the joint. Arthrography may give additional information.

Treatment. In the early stages, before the fragment has separated, immobilisation of the joint in a plaster cast may permit revascularisation. When separation has occurred any loose body should be removed.

Osteochondromatosis is a rare condition in which many cartilaginous loose bodies are formed by proliferation of the synovium. They are often large so that locking may not be a prominent feature. It is important to distinguish loose bodies arising from this cause, as synovectomy is necessary to prevent their further formation.

GENERAL SKELETAL DISEASES

Congenital conditions with widespread skeletal changes have already been discussed (p. 329). Acquired conditions may be considered under deficiency, metabolic and endocrine diseases, together with generalised disorders of unknown cause. Skeletal changes in endocrine disease include those of hyperparathyroidism (p. 92), cretinism in which the appearance of ossification centres is delayed, the pituitary lesions of gigantism and acromegaly (p. 323) and Cushing's syndrome (p. 269).

DEFICIENCY DISEASES

Scurvy

Vitamin C is a water-soluble substance, destroyed by heat, and found mainly in fresh fruit and vegetables, which is essential for maintaining the health of tissues having a mesodermal origin. Deficiency causes changes in the blood-vessels resulting in a tendency to bleed and subperiosteal haemorrhages are common. Deficient matrix formation produces cortical thinning and a tendency to epiphyseal separation.

Clinical features

Scurvy may occur at any age, but is most important in infancy and childhood. In the former it is usually due to artificial feeding deficient in vitamin C. Pain and swelling of the limbs may occur and if severe suggest acute osteomyelitis. The limbs may be held rigid in pseudo-paralysis to mimic early poliomyelitis. Bleeding from the gums near erupting teeth and bruising are common. In older children or adults poverty, dietary fads, or too strict dieting may be responsible. Bleeding either into the gums or skin is the main complaint. Old scars may reopen and at all ages anaemia may be marked. Vitamin C in large doses is rapidly effective in producing a cure.

Rickets

This condition is due to a deficient intake or utilisation of vitamin D. The latter is synthesised in the body when the ergosterol present in the skin is exposed to ultra-violet light, rickets being rare in hot climates. Its absence impairs phosphorus absorption, which prevents calcium phosphate deposition in osteoid tissue. In an attempt to overcome the lack of calcium phosphate, osteoid tissue is formed in excess with diffuse and irregular proliferation of the cartilage cells in the epiphyseal plate. The bones, being poorly calcified, bend as a result of gravity and muscle traction.

Clinical features

Maternal vitamin D is transmitted and rickets is rare during the first six months of life. Affected infants show abdominal distension, irritability and epiphyseal enlargement recognised at the costochondral junctions as a 'rickety rosary'. Traction on the lower ribs by the diaphragm leads to a well-defined sulcus, and the lower limbs bend when walking commences. The fontanelles remain open, and dentition is delayed. Scurvy may also be present.

Coeliac disease in children and idiopathic steatorrhoea in adults, causing failure in absorption of vitamin D, must be considered in the diagnosis, together with chronic renal disease, whilst congenital syphilitic epiphysitis may produce a similar picture.

Treatment

Adequate vitamin D produces a rapid cure, but residual deformities may require surgical correction.

Osteomalacia

This is the adult equivalent of rickets, being due either to deficient intake or absorption of vitamin D. It is rare in Western countries, and usually affects pregnant or lactating women because of extra maternal demands. The softened bones bend under the body weight and a triradiate pelvic deformity may obstruct labour. It must be distinguished from osteoporosis in which osteoid tissue is absent.

METABOLIC DISEASES

Renal osteodystrophy ('Renal rickets')

Chronic renal disease in childhood may alter calcium and phosphorus metabolism, producing bone changes similar to rickets. Two types occur:

1. When the kidneys are unable to excrete phosphorus, which enters the bowel combining with calcium and preventing its absorption. A high serum phosphorus results, and also nitrogen retention.
2. When the kidneys are unable to retain phosphorus, due to a failure of reabsorption from the tubules, leading, like true rickets, to a low serum phosphorus. A failure to reabsorb glucose and amino-acids produces glycosuria and amino-aciduria.

Acidosis occurs in both forms with secondary parathyroid hyperplasia in the first type.

Clinical features

The onset is later than in true rickets, with dwarfing and deformity, often with coxa vara, knock-knees and valgoid feet. When there is phosphorus retention, evidence of chronic renal failure such as excessive thirst, a sallow complexion, polyuria and a high blood urea, may occur. The prognosis is serious. The radiological appearances are similar to true rickets, whilst albuminuria is common in the retention type.

Treatment

High dosage of vitamin D, calcium and phosphorus is indicated, together with management of the acidosis and the renal lesion. The general state seldom permits surgical correction of deformities.

Lipoid granulomatosis

This forms a group of rare conditions in which there is histiocyte proliferation in the reticulo-endothelial system, often leading to a foam-cell appearance. The cause is not known but three groups are recognised.

1. *Eosinophilic granuloma* is an isolated lesion of bone, often of a vertebral body, which may lead to wedging of the body. Lesions may be seen in the

pelvis, femur or humerus and commonly present with pain in males between 15 and 30 years.

2. *Hand-Schüller-Christian disease* involves histiocyte infiltration of several bones, often being most marked in the skull. The onset is in early childhood and radiotherapy may slow the disease process. Extensive lesions do not have a favourable outlook.

3. *Letterer-Siwe's disease* is a rare form of histiocyte infiltration of bone and soft tissues, in particular the liver, spleen and lymph nodes. Progression is rapid with little response to any treatment.

Hypertrophic osteoarthropathy

Clubbing of the fingers is characteristic of chronic pulmonary or cardiac disease, but may also occur in long-standing peripheral circulatory insufficiency and in toxic states. Subperiosteal thickening of distal long bones may be evident.

GENERALISED SKELETAL DISORDERS OF UNKNOWN CAUSE

Osteitis deformans ('Paget's disease of bone')

In this condition there is a gradual change in the structure of several bones. It does not affect the whole skeleton. There is initial hyperaemia, decalcification and softening of the bone with loss of differentiation between cortex and medulla and generalised bony enlargement. Recalcification occurs later, the bone becoming chalky in consistency. The femur, tibia, pelvis, skull, clavicle and spine are most commonly involved.

Clinical features

Both sexes are affected in middle and late life. Symptoms may initially relate to a single bone but become widespread later. Pain of a deep, boring nature is present together with deformity. The latter follows softening, the enlarged and thickened bones bending as a result of gravity and muscle traction. It is most obvious in the legs and spine, but enlargement of the skull is an occasional early symptom. Pathological fractures are common when the bones commence to recalcify and are brittle, the upper femoral shaft being a frequent site. Sarcomatous change may occur in a single bone, and carries a serious prognosis. Rarely it is multicentric in origin. Widespread hyperaemia may be associated with a large arteriovenous shunt and eventual heart failure.

Radiologically there is widening and bowing of the bones with marked cortical thickening. Normal density is diminished with alteration in trabecular structure. Cyst-like areas are common in the pelvis, whilst the skull becomes thickened and woolly. Metastatic disease, particularly prostatic, and myelomatosis may cause confusion, whilst syphilitic and non-specific chronic osteomyelitis must be excluded. Hyperparathyroidism may result in a similar radiological picture in the skull.

Treatment

Uncomplicated Paget's disease is a benign condition for which only symptomatic treatment, such as analgesics and adequate support, is required. Fractures usually unite with routine management.

Senile osteoporosis

Bones in the elderly, particularly females, have a tendency to become porotic due partly to general retarding of metabolism and partly to decreasing hormonal activity. This process may become exaggerated and cause symptoms. There is marked rarefaction and cortical thinning, and in the spine vertebral collapse may occur. The more resilient discs bulge into the vertebral bodies, the latter becoming biconcave in shape. Microscopically there is an absence of osteoid tissue in addition to trabecular thinning.

Clinical features

An increasing stoop and loss of height due to multiple vertebral collapse may be observed. Backache, aggravated by standing and relieved by rest, may occur or sudden severe pain if there is immediate collapse in one bone. Fractures of the femoral neck in elderly women and other fractures following comparatively minor trauma are also partly due to senile osteoporosis. Differentiation should be made from metastatic malignant disease, parathyroid hyperplasia and osteomalacia.

Treatment

Fractures unite readily and should be treated along orthodox lines. Backache can be improved by the use of a light corset.

Polyostotic fibrous dysplasia

This curious disorder of bone is probably a developmental fault. One or more bones are affected, the characteristic feature being patchy replacement by fibrous tissue. The onset is in childhood, but symptoms may not appear before adult life. They are due either to deformity or fracture through an area of fibrosis. Radiologically fibrotic areas exhibit a 'ground-glass' appearance with thinning of the cortex, the bone itself sometimes being enlarged. Rarely such bony changes are associated in females with sexual precocity and areas of skin pigmentation, the combination being known as Albright's syndrome.

Treatment is palliative, the deformed bones being given adequate support. Extensive lesions may require curetting and bone grafting to prevent further symptoms whilst deformity can be corrected by osteotomy.

FURTHER READING

Apley, A. G. and Soloman, L. (1982). In *Apley's System of Orthopaedics and Fractures*. 6th ed. London: Butterworths.

Lloyd-Roberts, G. C. and Ratcliff, A. H. C. (1981). *Hip Disorders in Children*. London: Butterworths.

28

Limb and trunk injuries

BONE INJURIES (FRACTURES)

A fracture is a break in the continuity of a bone. Various adjectives are used to describe certain types.

Simple fracture. A closed injury with intact skin.

Compound fracture. A skin wound communicates with the fracture.

Comminuted fracture. The bone is broken into more than two fragments. It may be either *'simple'* or *'compound'*.

Greenstick fracture. The bone is partly broken and partly buckled, the fracture being peculiar to children.

Pathological fracture occurs in a bone which is more fragile than normal. This may be due either to generalised weakening of bone throughout the skeleton as in osteoporosis or to a localised lesion in the bone, such as a neoplasm.

Stress fracture is encountered at a site where a bone is subjected to repeated similar strains and resembles the 'fatigue' fractures which occur in metals.

Fractures may be caused by *'direct'* or *'indirect'* violence. Those due to the former result from a blow or angulating force applied directly to the bone, whereas those due to indirect violence usually follow a transmitted strain. Soft tissue damage tends to be more extensive in fractures due to direct trauma. Compound fractures due to direct violence are more heavily contaminated than those caused by indirect violence, where the fracture becomes compound as a result of bursting through the skin.

Union of fractures

A haematoma forms around the bone ends following a fracture. This is later replaced by granulation tissue into which osteoblasts grow, producing strands of bone. The resulting tissue, known as *callus*, slowly changes into normal bone and when the process is complete the fracture has united.

Clinical features of fractures

The most constant symptom is pain, aggravated by movement and experienced at the fracture site. It can be elicited by longitudinal percussion of the bone. Localised tenderness at the site of injury is always present. Abnormal mobility is found in fractures of long bones, but is more difficult to demonstrate in smaller and deeper bones. Crepitus is pathognomonic of a fracture, but can only be elicited when the bone ends are disimpacted and freely mobile. It should never be deliberately sought as it may cause further injury to bone and soft tissue. Damage to the surrounding parts, evidenced by bruising and swelling, is usually present.

COMPLICATIONS OF FRACTURES

These may be related directly to the fracture, as in mal-union or non-union or there may be infection when the fracture is compound, leading to osteomyelitis. Alternatively complications may involve the surrounding blood vessels, nerves and tendons, or more remotely, fat embolism may occur.

Mal-union

This is due to two factors which may be present together, (*a*) shortening, due to overlap of the fragments and (*b*) angulation due to their malalignment. Rarely in children premature fusion of an epiphysis which has received a crushing injury occurs, leading to later angular deformity.

Non-union

This is described as 'established' when all attempts by the body to achieve union have ceased and the fracture has not united. When progress is slow 'delayed union' is said to be present. Non-union is distinguished clinically by persistent mobility at the fracture site and radiologically by sclerosis of the bone ends accompanied by a gap. Pathologically the latter is bridged by mature fibrous tissue and a false joint cavity ('pseudarthrosis') may form. Non-union is caused by a combination of two factors.

1. *An inadequate blood supply*. Certain sites are prone to proceed to non-union and in these the blood supply to one of the fragments is likely to be impaired. Examples are high fractures of the femoral neck, fractures of the waist of the scaphoid and fractures of the shafts of the radius, ulna, and tibia. Extensive soft tissue damage may interfere with the blood supply and predisposes to non-union.

2. *Inadequate immobilisation*. Without adequate splintage callus may be unable to bridge the gap between the bone ends. This is particularly likely to occur at sites where the blood supply is also poor. Soft tissues may also prevent union by interposition between the fractured bone ends.

Blood vessels

A main artery may be injured by a sharply divided bone. The damage to the vessel may be small, but spasm of the artery and its collaterals may cause serious ischaemia. Unless circulation is restored within three to four hours permanent damage to muscles and nerves may result in the development of Volkmann's ischaemic contracture. Prolonged failure of circulation may lead to the development of distal gangrene. The application of inelastic encircling bandages and splints may be followed by swelling of a limb and interruption of blood flow.

Volkmann's ischaemic contracture

Striated muscle and nerve fibres are more sensitive to hypoxia than other peripheral structures. Temporary interruption of arterial blood flow to a limb causes early muscular death and subsequent contraction of the resulting infarct. All or part of the muscle may be involved and similar changes may affect major nerves.

Common sites for arterial injury are at the knee and elbow. Early recognition is essential and signs include poor circulation of the nail beds, marked pain on passive extension of the digits and loss of peripheral pulses. Later changes produce fixed contracture of the forearm or calf muscles with severe impairment of function.

Treatment. At the onset of muscular spasm, prompt reduction of the causative fracture with avoidance of all tight encircling dressings is imperative. Failure to obtain immediate relief is an indication for surgery. Exposure of the vessel which is in spasm and the direct application of papaverine is essential (p. 417). In the established condition lengthening of contracted tendons combined with excision of the muscular infarct may be carried out. In several cases tendon transplants and nerve grafting may be required.

Nerves

Nerve trunks may be injured either by the sharp end of a bone at the moment of fracture or later by involvement in callus. Usually damage consists of bruising (neurapraxia), in which case spontaneous recovery in a few weeks can be expected. Complete division is much less common. Late irritation of a nerve due to pressure or stretching may follow malunion of a fracture. It occurs most frequently with the ulnar nerve at the elbow.

Tendons

Tendons may be trapped between bone fragments

as in ankle fractures, causing non-union, while later problems arise from adherence of tendons to bone at the fracture site with loss of movement.

Fat embolism

Occasionally fat globules from the marrow are released into the circulation and produce sudden ischaemia by blocking the smaller end-arteries either in the brain, leading to unconsciousness, or in the lungs, producing dyspnoea and cyanosis. Fat embolism may be a complication of any serious injury, in particular long bone fractures. The combination of confusion, pyrexia and petechial rashes should lead to the diagnosis at an early stage before unconsciousness occurs. Radiography of the chest shows a 'snow storm' effect and the sputum and urine are found to contain abnormal amounts of fat. The basic defect is anoxia due to poor lung perfusion and requires immediate supportive therapy either by oxygen inhalation using a mask, or if this is inadequate, by mechanical ventilation through an endotracheal tube.

GENERAL TREATMENT OF FRACTURES

Management falls into three parts, reduction, immobilisation in the reduced position and final rehabilitation. Reduction may not be required if the bone ends are in good position and impacted into each other. Immobilisation may be omitted at certain sites near large joints where ready union is the rule and a better functional result obtained if some displacement is accepted and early movement encouraged. Examples are fractures of the upper end of the humerus and of the calcaneum.

Reduction

Normal bony relations may be restored either by *closed* manipulation or open reduction. The former is divided into two parts—traction to pull the bone ends opposite one another, followed by manipulation, which in case of injuries caused by indirect violence consists of a manoeuvre in the reverse direction to that which caused the fracture. *Open* reduction is required where it is not feasible either to obtain reduction by closed manipulation or to maintain good position subsequently. It is generally accompanied by *internal fixation* with screws, a plate, an intramedullary nail or encircling wire (Fig. 28.1).

Immobilisation

Apart from the occasions where intramedullary fixation is used, immobilisation is obtained by *external* fixation either by a plaster of Paris cast (p. 376), which to be effective should hold the joints above and below the fracture, or by special methods, such as the Thomas's splint and traction for fractures of the femoral shaft.

Rehabilitation

Residual stiffness following immobilisation is inevitable but may be minimised by the use of the limb in plaster. When the cast is removed a period of mobilising exercises and functional re-education is required to restore normal movement and muscle power in the injured part and to increase the general confidence.

Treatment of non-union

Ununited fractures necessitate bone grafting. A period of immobilisation is then required until union is sound. Preliminary measures, directed towards mobilising the joints and improving skin health are usually advisable for two to three weeks pre-operatively. The scar of a compound fracture may be thin and adherent to bone, so that before embarking upon major bone surgery it may be necessary to provide full thickness skin cover by a plastic procedure such as a pedicle flap from the opposite limb (p. 59).

Method of grafting

Either cortical or cancellous bone may be employed.

Cortical. The osteogenic properties of cortical bone are relatively low, but being hard and strong it provides some internal fixation. The fractured bone may be freshened and the graft, usually from the tibia, fixed to it as an *onlay* graft. Alternatively the graft may be counter-sunk into the recipient

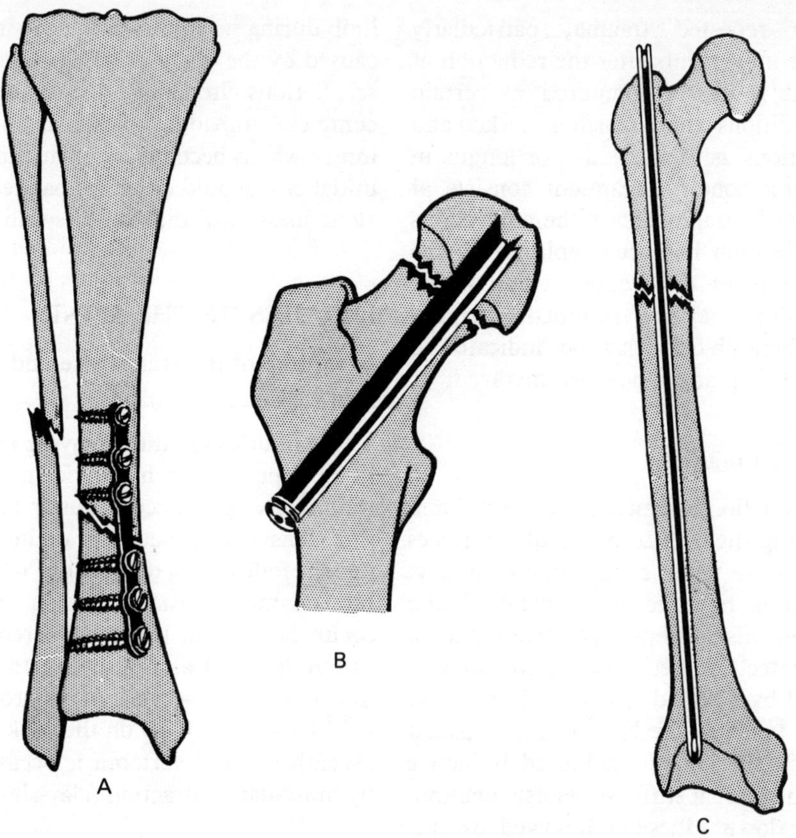

Fig. 28.1 Internal fixation of a fracture. **A.** Plate and screws. **B.** Intramedullary nail (Smith-Petersen type). **C.** Intramedullary nail (Küntscher type).

bone as an *inlay* graft. In the tibia it is often possible to fashion a *sliding inlay* graft by extending the bed below the fracture site and moving the graft downwards to cross it.

Cancellous. Although soft and mechanically weak, cancellous bone is highly osteogenic and provides a good scaffold on which new bone can form and consolidate. Fragments of the ilium are packed around the fracture site, often in combination with some form of metallic internal fixation.

JOINT INJURIES

These are either dislocations or subluxations. A *dislocation* implies complete separation of the articular surfaces, with extensive capsular and soft tissue damage. When the articular surfaces are displaced but still in contact, a *subluxation* has occurred, with soft tissue damage being proportionately less. When there is also a fracture of one of the bones forming a joint a *fracture-dislocation* is said to be present. If the capsular tear fails to heal, *recurrent dislocation* may follow trivial trauma; this is common in the shoulder (p. 381). A *pathological dislocation* is that which takes place spontaneously as in paralytic dislocations due to muscle imbalance.

Complications of joint injuries

Surrounding structures such as major nerve trunks or blood vessels may be damaged in joint injuries. Residual stiffness, due either to adhesion formation within the joint or to scar contraction of the capsule and surrounding structures, may be troublesome. Rarely, *traumatic myositis ossificans* in which bone is laid down in the soft tissues, occurs due to avulsion of the periosteal attachments of a muscle or tendon producing a haematoma into which osteoblasts are liberated. Calcification in this haematoma usually follows repeated trauma, particularly excessive passive movements after the reduction of a dislocation. It is also encountered in certain neurological conditions where spasm is marked and in some occupations as in the adductor longus in horsemen ('rider's bone'). Treatment consists of strict rest until radiography shows the amorphous shadow of calcification has been replaced by the clear sharp outline of ossification, when gentle active mobilisation may be resumed. Surgical excision of a bone block may be indicated if joints such as the hip and elbow are involved.

Treatment of joint injuries

Manipulative reduction is generally successful and consists of causing the displaced articular surfaces to retrace the course taken at the time of injury. Open reduction is required when manipulation fails. In recurrent dislocations, operative repair of the capsular defect is necessary. Reduction is usually followed by a period of two to three weeks immobilisation to allow healing of the capsular tear, after which the joint is mobilised by active exercises. When residual stiffness persists manipulation to break down adhesions followed by further active exercises may be useful.

Plaster of Paris

This substance (anhydrous calcium sulphate) is extensively used as a method of splintage. When moistened it combines with water to form hydrated calcium sulphate, which becomes hard on setting. Muslin bandages impregnated with plaster are commonly used.

Technique of application

The bandages are completely soaked, and applied evenly and rapidly. Any delay during the application of a cast may allow one layer to set before the next is applied, leaving films of air between layers and reducing the overall strength.

Complications of plaster casts

Pressure sores may occur, due either to ridges within the cast resulting from movement of the limb during its application, or to indentations often caused by the operator's fingers before the cast has set. Serious circulatory disturbance may occur if a complete, unpadded plaster is applied to a recent injury which becomes swollen. For this reason the initial cast should either be padded, split, or a slab alone used until the risk of swelling has subsided.

INJURIES OF THE SPINE

Fractures of the transverse and spinous processes

These injuries of adults may be regarded as of soft tissue type, in which the violence of the causative trauma also produced a minor break. Fracture of the transverse process is limited to the lumbar region, following a direct blow to the loin, and visceral damage, particularly of the kidney, may occur. No specific treatment is required, but observation for at least 24 hours to exclude visceral injury is advisable. A spinous process can be damaged by a direct blow on the back. The spine of the seventh cervical vertebra is occasionally fractured by muscular contraction (clay-shoveller's fracture).

Crush fracture of the vertebral body

This injury can occur throughout adult life but the causal violence decreases with age in proportion to the degree of senile osteoporosis. It may occur at any level in the thoraco-lumbar spine, the lower dorsal region being the most common, and follows forced spinal flexion. The collapse is wedge-shaped and when marked produces an angular kyphosis (Fig. 28.2). In multiple injuries, particularly after a fall from a height on to the feet, crush fractures of the vertebral bodies are common but easily overlooked.

Differential diagnosis

Vertebral collapse following minimal trauma or found on incidental examination requires the exclusion of generalised or localised skeletal disease. The former includes senile osteoporosis, hyperparathyroidism, Cushing's syndrome, myelomatosis and widespread secondary carcinoma. Local conditions are either neoplastic, usually secondary deposits,

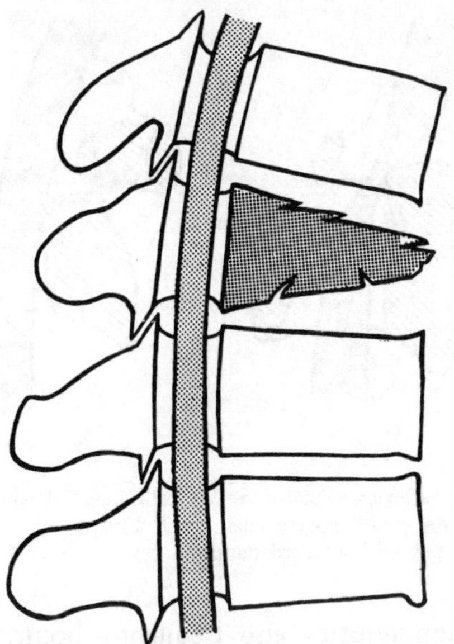

Fig. 28.2 Wedge-shaped fracture of body of lumbar vertebra

or infective, particularly tuberculosis. In young children osteochondritis of a vertebral body occasionally occurs.

Complications

Paralytic ileus commonly follows fracture of the lumbo-dorsal spine and may even occur after the application of a plaster jacket in the absence of any bony injury. Nerve root irritation with referred pain and occasionally injury to the spinal cord are further complications.

Treatment

This is governed by the degree of displacement and the general condition of the patient.

Moderate deformity may be accepted, the spinal musculature being developed to provide compensation. Strict recumbency for four to six weeks on a rigid bed is followed by extension exercises in the prone position as soon as the initial pain has subsided. More intensive mobilisation avoiding flexion is often best carried out in the competitive atmosphere of a rehabilitation centre.

In the frail or elderly bed rest should be limited to a few days, exercises being commenced early and in most cases a supporting corset should be prescribed.

Fracture-dislocation of the spine

While such injuries may occur at any age they are most common during the active working life, and as they are often associated with industrial accidents, they predominate in males. Fracture-dislocations of the spine are caused by a combination of flexion and shearing forces of considerable violence, such as occur in mining accidents due to a collapse of the roof, or in road accidents when a cyclist or motor-cyclist is flung over the handle-bars. In most instances the upper vertebra is displaced forwards with disruption of the posterior intervertebral joints, the articular facets often being locked one beneath the other (Fig. 28.3). The lumbo-dorsal region is most frequently affected, the incidence decreasing as the thoracic spine is ascended.

Neurological damage is common, varying from mild weakness to complete cord transection and paraplegia. Early clinical assessment and recording of the signs present are of utmost importance in management and prognosis.

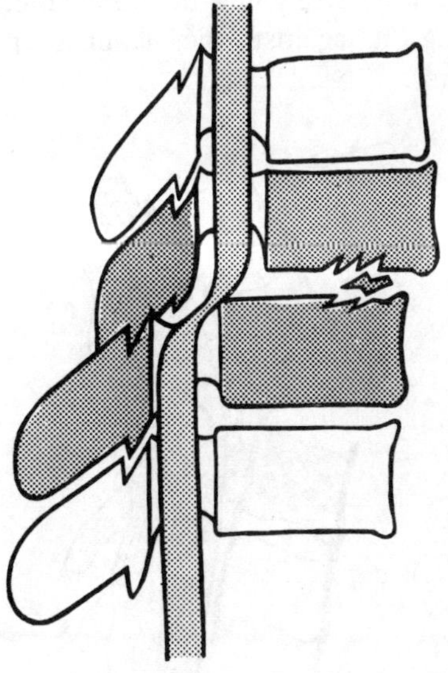

Fig. 28.3 Fracture-dislocation of lumbar vertebrae with spinal cord damage

Treatment

This is dominated by the neurological condition (p. 326), management of the spine being directed towards preventing further damage. All potentially serious spinal injuries should be moved with care to avoid both flexion and extension of the back. Unstable injuries, such as occur where the articular facets are locked, are often better treated surgically. Occasionally internal fixation by plates bolted to the spinous processes is employed.

Injuries of the cervical spine

The cervical region differs from other parts of the spine in three ways. Firstly, the articular facets lie further forward in relationship to the vertebral bodies, which are relatively small; secondly the neural canal is larger than elsewhere so that the cord has a better prospect of escaping serious damage should displacement occur; and thirdly, extension injuries are common due to the mobility of the neck allowing the head to be thrown back by a blow or sudden jolt.

Extension injuries may occur at any level, with or without bony damage, but in the latter rupture of the anterior and posterior longitudinal ligaments occurs. There may be associated cord damage even where there is no radiological evidence of injury. This is due to stretching the cord anteriorly and impinging it against the laminae posteriorly (Fig. 28.4).

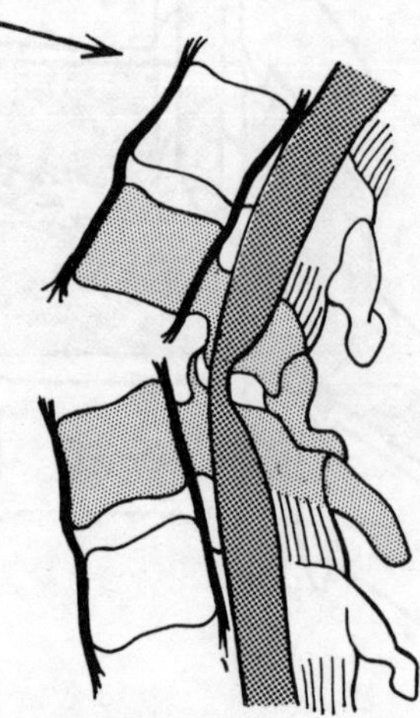

Fig. 28.4 Extension injury of the cervical spine may show no radiological damage yet produce severe cord lesion

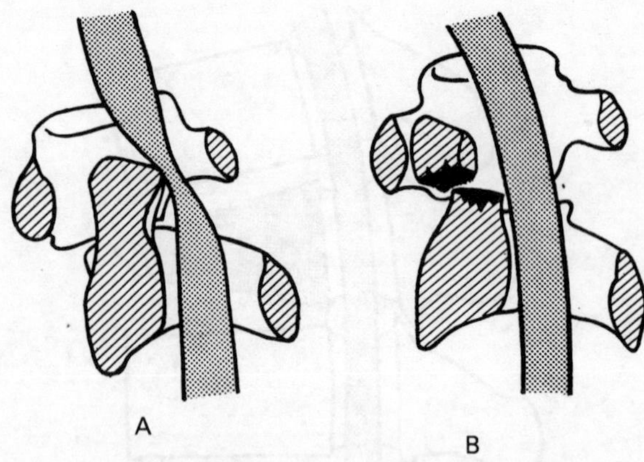

Fig. 28.5 Flexion injury of the cervical spine. **A.** Dislocation of odontoid peg producing cord damage. **B.** Fracture of odontoid peg without cord damage.

Flexion injuries also frequently occur. Dislocation of the odontoid process associated with rupture of the transverse ligament is usually fatal, but fracture may allow the cord to escape injury (Fig. 28.5). Subluxation or dislocation of other cervical vertebrae may result in cord damage, nerve root irritation being usual at the level of injury. Cervical fracture should be considered in all unconscious patients, particularly those with injuries to the face or forehead, suggesting extension of the head.

Treatment

First aid. Care must be taken to maintain the head in a neutral position, particularly during radiography, as damage to the cord may be precipitated or aggravated by careless handling after the accident. An extensible collar is useful for this purpose.

Definitive treatment consists of traction, obtained by a caliper apparatus applied through trephine holes in the outer table of the skull. Dislocation of the intervertebral articulations may be reduced by traction in this way or by manipulation under anaesthesia, but if these fail, then open operative reduction and stabilisation must be undertaken.

Injuries of the pelvis

Pelvic injuries are usually seen in adults and may consist of a single fracture, or multiple fractures with or without displacement.

Isolated injuries

These always follow direct violence and may affect any part of the pelvis, such as one or both pubic rami on a single side, or one iliac bone. In the absence of visceral complications they are of minor significance. If the fracture line involves the acetabulum, haemarthrosis of the hip joint develops and light traction applied to the lower limb for about two weeks is advisable.

Double injuries

Such fractures are due to a crushing force, the direction of which governs the pattern of injury and displacement. The pelvic ring may be broken in two positions: (*a*) *anteriorly*, the pubic rami on both sides being fractured and the central segment displaced posteriorly; (*b*) *laterally*, when the ring is broken both in front and behind. The anterior fracture may be either through the pubic rami or the symphysis pubis, whilst posteriorly it is through the ilium, the sacro-iliac joint, or the ala of the sacrum. In these injuries the weight of the limb rolls the unattached portion of the pelvis outwards (Fig. 28.6). The mobile portion of the pelvis in some cases may displaced upwards (Fig. 28.7). The bladder and urethra are frequently damaged (p. 292) and injury to the bowel or major blood vessels may also occur.

Treatment

The displacement should be reduced as far as possible, and as the pelvis is often moved proximally on one side, traction to one leg by tibial pin and balanced weights will effect adequate reduction. When the symphysis has been widely separated a pelvic sling may help to close the gap.

Injuries of the sacrum and coccyx

All such injuries follow direct violence, and if pelvic injuries with a fracture of a sacral ala are excluded, displacement is unimportant and symptomatic treatment alone is required.

A fall on the coccyx, whether there is a fracture or not, may lead to coccydynia (p. 341).

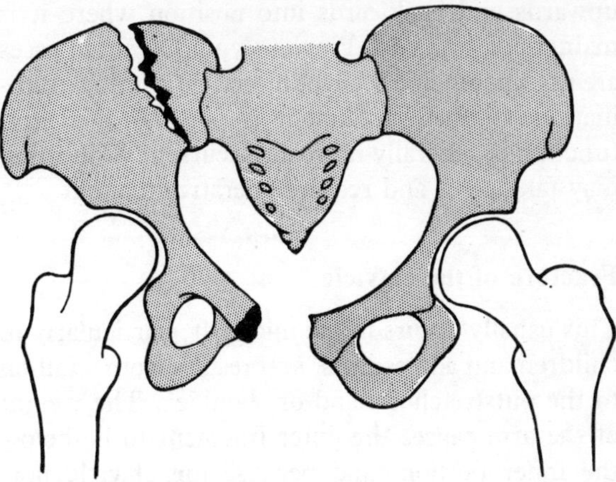

Fig. 28.6 Fracture of the pelvis with outward displacement

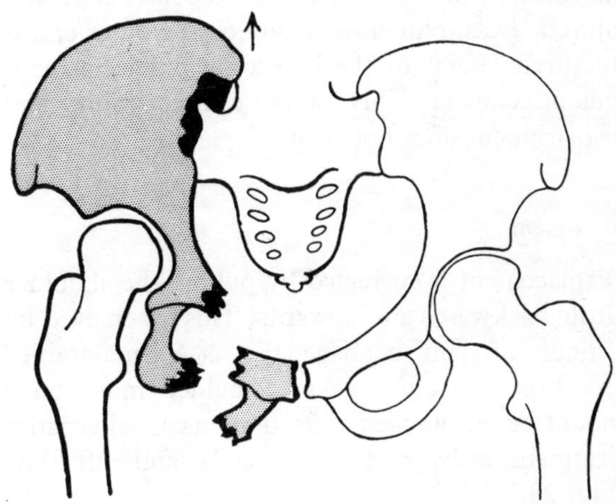

Fig. 28.7 Fracture of the pelvis with upward and outward displacement

INJURIES OF THE UPPER LIMB

SHOULDER GIRDLE

Dislocation of the sternoclavicular joint

This is an injury of adults and usually the result of a fall on the shoulder. The inner end of the clavicle moves anteriorly and downwards. Rarely it may ride upwards and posteriorly, occasionally obstructing the trachea.

Treatment

The prominent inner end of the clavicle is pressed

upwards and backwards into position where it is maintained by a pad. Previously undiagnosed cases are not uncommonly encountered on routine examination; in these treatment is not indicated and function is generally normal. Recurrent dislocation may take place and require operative fixation.

Fracture of the clavicle

This usually occurs in the midshaft, particularly in children and adolescents, and results from a fall on to the outstretched hand or shoulder. The weight of the arm causes the outer fragment to lie below the inner portion, and because the clavicle normally acts as a strut to hold the shoulder away from the trunk there is overlap. Complications are uncommon; only rarely are the subclavian vessels injured. Less frequently in adults, the outer end is fractured lateral to the coracoclavicular ligamentous attachment. This follows a direct injury and displacement does not occur.

Treatment

Displacement is corrected by pulling the shoulder girdle backwards and upwards. This is achieved by a 'figure-of-eight' bandage (Fig. 28.8), maintained for three to four weeks. Shoulder movements should be encouraged from the outset. Alternative treatment is by means of a collar-and-cuff sling (Fig. 28.15).

Injuries to the acromioclavicular joint

This is a plane joint and dislocations and subluxations both occur. Young adults are mainly affected, the causal injury being a fall on to the point of the shoulder which forces the scapula and humerus downwards.

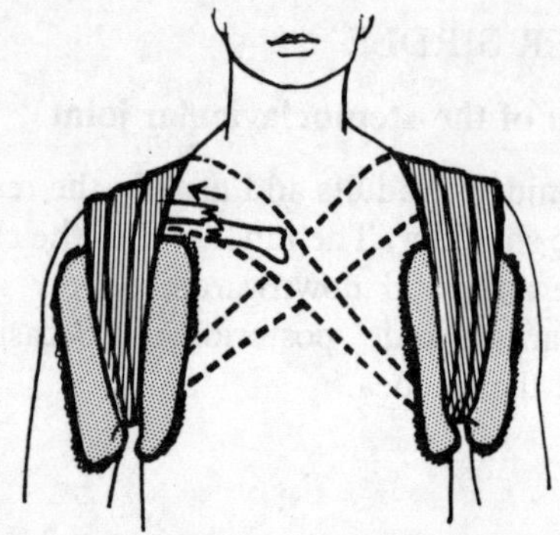

Fig. 28.8 Figure-of-eight bandage for fracture of the clavicle

Dislocation

Significant displacement occurs only if the coracoclavicular ligament is disrupted, the clavicle becoming elevated and the point of the shoulder lowered. Tenderness and bruising are found in the region of the acromioclavicular joint and coracoid process.

Treatment may be either conservative or operative.

Conservative. The outer end of the clavicle must be depressed and the upper limb elevated by either non-stretch zinc oxide strapping or a canvas brace (Fig. 28.9). Splintage should be maintained continuously for four to six weeks.

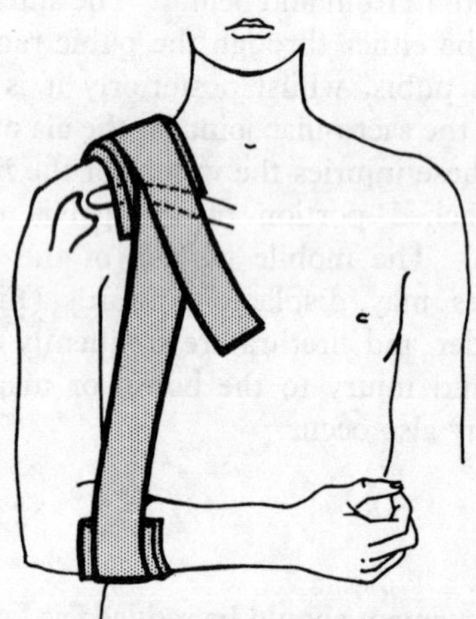

Fig. 28.9 Zinc oxide strapping for treatment of dislocation of acromioclavicular joint

Operative. The clavicle may either be screwed or wired to the coracoid process, or a longitudinal wire may be introduced through the acromion into the medullary cavity of the clavicle. In later cases, where inconvenience is caused by the prominent outer end of the clavicle, the bone may be excised without disturbing normal function.

Subluxation

The mechanism is similar to that of complete dislocation, but the coracoclavicular ligament remains intact, so that significant displacement cannot occur and tenderness will be limited to the joint itself. Treatment consists of the use of a triangular sling to support the limb for two to three weeks.

Dislocation of the shoulder

This common injury occurs throughout adult life. A fall on to the outstretched hand levers the head of the humerus downwards and out of the glenoid fossa, from which position ('subglenoid') it slips forwards. The humeral head is at times driven directly forwards, producing a tear of the glenoid labrum which does not heal, leaving a tendency to recurrence.

Displacement

The head of the humerus comes to lie in one of three positions:

Anteriorly. This is the most frequent, the head being displaced beneath the coracoid process (*subcoracoid*).

Inferiorly (*subglenoid*). This is unusual, as the head normally slips up into the subcoracoid position.

Posteriorly. This is rare, with the head lying behind the glenoid. A lateral radiograph may be essential for diagnosis.

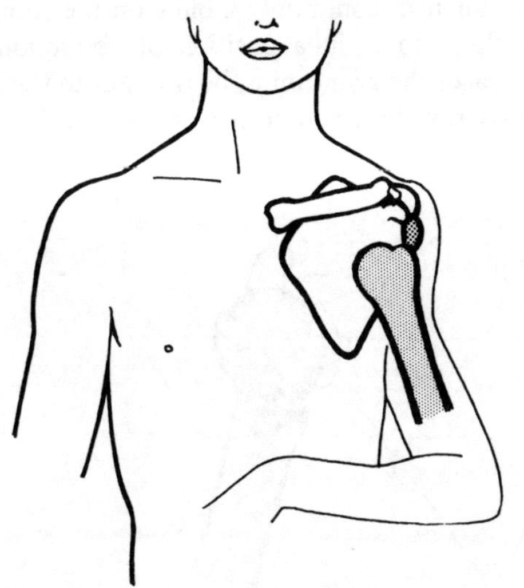

Fig. 28.10 Dislocation of the shoulder, showing displacement in the subcoracoid position

The clinical appearance is characteristic (Fig. 28.10). There is loss of the normal fullness under the deltoid, and the arm abducted by about 30 degrees and internally rotated cannot be brought to the side.

The main complication, apart from recurrent dislocation and persistent stiffness, is damage to the circumflex nerve with deltoid paralysis. Injury to the posterior cord of the brachial plexus and to the axillary vessels may also occur.

Treatment

Two manipulative methods are employed:

Kocher's, in which the arm is externally rotated, adducted across the body, and then internally rotated, traction being maintained throughout.

Hippocrates', where using the surgeon's unbooted foot in the axilla as a fulcrum and with traction on the hand, the arm is slowly adducted.

In young adults two to three weeks of immobilisation with the arm bound to the side allows the capsular tear to heal without the shoulder becoming too stiff, but in older patients cautious mobilisation should be commenced early.

Recurrent dislocation of the shoulder

Following certain dislocations there is a tendency to redislocation with diminishing trauma. In these the head of the humerus has been driven directly forwards by the injuring force, tearing the anterior part of the glenoid labrum from the bone, and leaving a deficiency in the front of the joint through which the head may slip when the arm is externally rotated. As a result of repeated trauma to the humeral head, a depression forms on it which can be seen on radiographs taken with the arm externally rotated (Fig. 28.11).

Treatment. Two operative measures can be employed. Either the torn fibrocartilaginous labrum is reattached to the bone (Bankart's operation) or a pleat is made in the anterior capsule and subscapularis muscle, reinforcing the front of the joint and restricting external rotation (Putti-Platt operation).

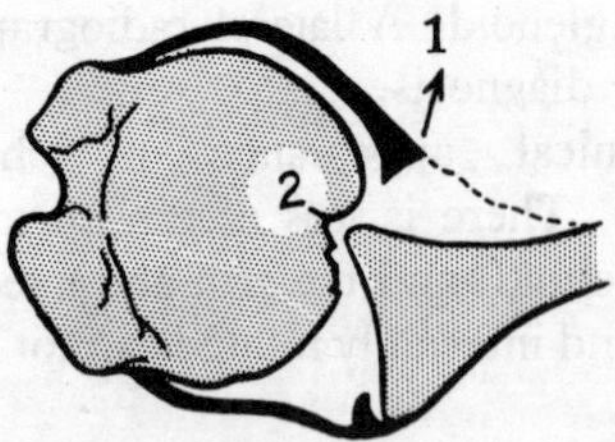

Fig. 28.11 The shoulder joint in recurrent dislocation as viewed from above showing, (1) the tear of the glenoid labrum in front and (2) the depression in the humeral head

Dislocation associated with fractures of the head of the humerus

Two forms are seen. The greater tuberosity may be avulsed, which is common but usually of little significance, and rarely the surgical neck of the humerus may be fractured, preventing reduction.

Fracture of the scapula

This injury follows direct violence, either a fall on to the point of the shoulder fracturing the scapular neck or a blow on the bone itself, fracturing the body. Displacement is rarely significant.

Treatment aims at preventing stiffness, the injury being regarded as to soft tissues only, the bony damage merely emphasising the degree of violence. Early active mobilisation should be employed.

Fractures of the upper end of the humerus

These can be considered according to the degree of displacement.

Fractures without significant displacement

These fractures are common injuries of the elderly, the bone often being comminuted. They result from direct violence, such as a fall on to the point of the shoulder.

Treatment. Union invariably occurs and the principle of treatment is to minimise residual stiffness. The weight of the forearm is supported by a sling, and as soon as the initial pain has diminished, and always within 10 days of the injury, active movements are commenced.

Displaced fractures

Persistent displacement usually implies impaction of the fracture which is either adducted or abducted. They occur in younger age groups than the undisplaced variety, many of the adduction type being fracture-separations of the upper humeral epiphysis.

Adduction fractures (Fig. 28.12,A) result from a blow which adducts the arm during active abduction. Minor displacement should be accepted and early mobilisation commenced. With moderate displacement the fracture may be disimpacted by downward traction followed by early mobilisation. In young patients marked displacement may require open reduction and internal fixation.

Abduction fractures (Fig. 28.12, B) are due to direct violence, commonly a blow on the shoulder when the arm is in a position of abduction. In severe cases the arm cannot be brought to the side. Disimpaction by traction in a downward direction

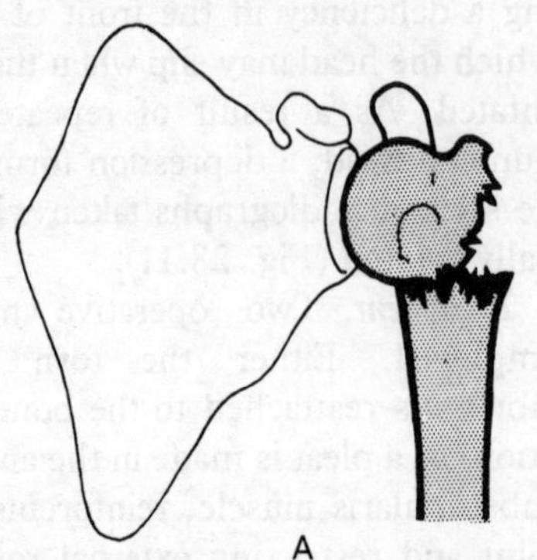

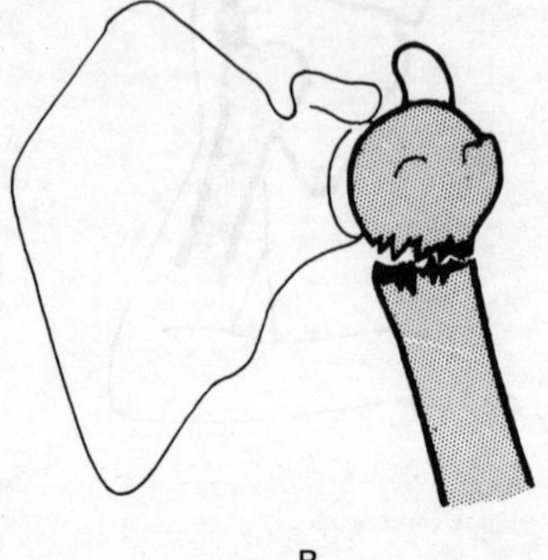

Fig. 28.12 Fracture of the surgical neck of the humerus. **A.** Adduction type. **B.** Abduction type.

is required, followed by a period of 7 to 10 days immobilisation of the arm by the side.

Injuries to muscles and tendons

These usually occur in middle age when degenerative changes are present. Two sites are commonly affected:

The **musculotendinous cuff**, discussed on page 364.

The **tendon of the long head of biceps**. Spontaneous rupture may appear to take place as the condition can pass unrecognised, but it is usually due to attrition in a bicipital groove roughened by osteoarthritis. It results in a characteristic bulge of the belly of the biceps, which increases when the elbow is flexed. In most cases mobilising exercises to the shoulder and elbow alone are required. Occasionally, in younger patients with recent injuries, the tendon may be sutured to the humerus at the bicipital groove.

INJURIES OF THE ARM AND ELBOW

Fractures of the humeral shaft

These injuries occur chiefly in adults. The bone may be fractured by either indirect or direct violence. The former, due to a rotational force, produces a spiral fracture, whereas the latter produces a transverse or comminuted pattern, usually in the middle or lower shaft. The radial nerve may be damaged, particularly in injuries due to direct violence. In most cases the nerve is merely concussed (neurapraxia) and recovery follows in three to six weeks. Involvement of the nerve in callus may result in delayed paralysis. Clinically radial nerve damage is recognised by a wrist drop, sensory changes being minimal.

Treatment

The majority unite readily, and the principle of treatment consists of using the weight of the limb to maintain alignment. This is achieved by the application of a long plaster slab passing from the shoulder below the elbow and up to the axilla, with the patient seated and with the limb hanging away from the side. The wrist is supported in a collar-and-cuff sling. Some overlap may be accepted as slight shortening in the upper limb is unimportant.

Radial nerve damage in most cases is treated by a cock-up splint and stretching of the affected wrist. If the nerve is divided, direct suture gives good results. In late cases, where recovery fails to occur, satisfactory function is achieved by tendon transplants such as the pronator teres into the wrist extensors and the flexor carpi ulnaris into the extensors of the digits.

Fractures of the lower end of the humerus

Supracondylar fractures

Two distinct types occur, depending on whether the lower end of the humerus is displaced posteriorly or anteriorly.

Posterior displacement. This is one of the common injuries of childhood, due to a fall on the outstretched hand with the elbow flexed, the lower end of the humerus being driven backwards. Displacement varies from a hair-line crack to complete separation, with the small distal fragment also rotated and tilted into a valgus position (Fig. 28.13).

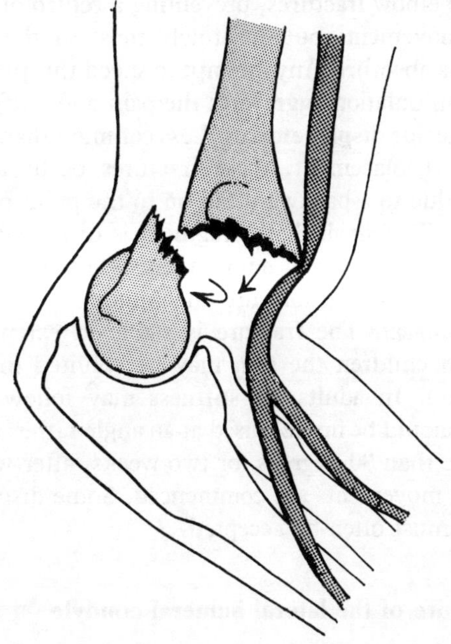

Fig. 28.13 Supracondylar fracture of the humerus with posterior displacement. Damage to the brachial artery may occur.

Treatment. Reduction is stable in flexion. Traction in the position of deformity should be undertaken by an assistant and the elbow flexed by pressure on the olecranon. Reduction is maintained by a collar-and-cuff sling, reinforced if necessary by a plaster of Paris slab. Observation of the hand, finger mobility and the radial pulse are essential following reduction.

Complications. These are not uncommon following severely displaced fractures and demand urgent correction. Redisplacement of the fracture may occur, requiring further manipulation if it is within 48 hours of the injury. Swelling of the elbow and trauma to the brachial artery may result in ischaemia of the forearm muscles, with subsequent contracture. Immediate ischaemia may be relieved by extending the elbow until a radial pulse becomes palpable; loss of position at the fracture has to be accepted. If the blood supply is not improved by this, division of the cubital fascia is performed and the artery exposed. Nerve lesions can occur at the time of injury or follow a difficult manipulation. The median and radial nerves are usually involved but mainly only contused, and recover without surgical intervention. Periarticular calcification (myositis ossificans) is a common complication of severe elbow fractures, preventing a return of normal movement, but eventually most of the new bone is absorbed. Any attempt to speed this process by manipulation aggravates the pain and stiffness.

Anterior displacement. Less common than posterior displacement, these fractures occur at all ages, due to a backward fall on to the point of the elbow. The small distal fragment is displaced and rotated forwards. In adults there is often comminution. Complications are uncommon.

Treatment. The fracture is stable in extension, and in children the arm may be splinted in this position. In adults, as stiffness may follow, the joint should be immobilised at an angle rather more obtuse than 90 degrees for two weeks, after which active movements are commenced. Some displacement must often be accepted.

Fracture of the lateral humeral condyle

This is an injury of childhood, resulting from a fall on to the hand forcing the elbow in a valgoid direction. It can be regarded as a fracture-separation of the capitellar epiphysis, which is displaced laterally (Fig. 28.14). Reduction is difficult to maintain and fibrous union may occur, leading to a slowly increasing valgus deformity and delayed ulnar neuritis.

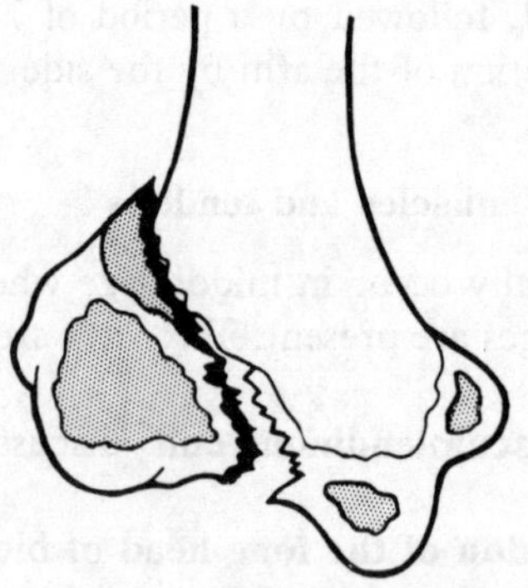

Fig. 28.14 Fracture-separation of the lateral condyle epiphysis of the humerus

Fracture-separation of the medial epicondyle

Avulsion of the medial epicondyle may follow a lateral strain of the elbow in adolescents. In adults the medial ligament may be torn. It can occur in conjunction with dislocation of the elbow, when the fragment may lie in the joint and obstruct reduction. The ulnar nerve may be damaged or delayed neuritis occur.

Treatment

Inclusion of the epicondylar fragment into the joint needs open reduction and fixation with wires, but if displacement is marked and the fragment large, internal fixation is preferable. The arm is supported in a collar-and-cuff sling (Fig. 28.15) for three weeks, when the wires are removed and the elbow mobilised.

Dislocation of the elbow

This occurs at all ages, usually as a result of a fall on the hand. As the elbow joint is mechanically stable, considerable violence is necessary to cause dislocation and the constituent bones are often damaged with associated avulsion of the medial epicondyle, fracture of the coronoid process of the ulna, or comminution of the radial head. Displacement may be posteriorly or laterally, depending on the direction of the injuring force. As with supracondylar fractures, the main nerves or vessels may be damaged or traumatic myositis ossificans can follow later.

Treatment

Manipulative reduction by gentle traction and gradual flexion is generally successful unless a loose fragment such as the medial epicondyle becomes lodged between the bones, when exploration is required. Following reduction the joint is supported in a collar-and-cuff sling (Fig. 28.15) or plaster cast for two to three weeks.

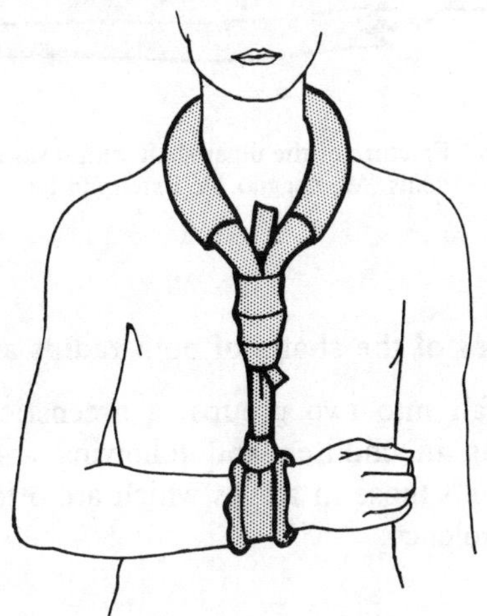

Fig. 28.15 Collar-and-cuff sling. This is worn under the clothes and applied so that the patient cannot easily remove it.

Fracture of the olecranon

The olecranon may be fractured either by direct violence due to a fall on to the elbow, or indirect violence when it is snapped by the contraction of the triceps as the forearm is suddenly forcibly flexed. The contracting triceps causes the small olecranon fragment to become separate (Fig. 28.16).

Treatment

Operation is essential. Where there is no comminution, internal fixation by a circumferential wire

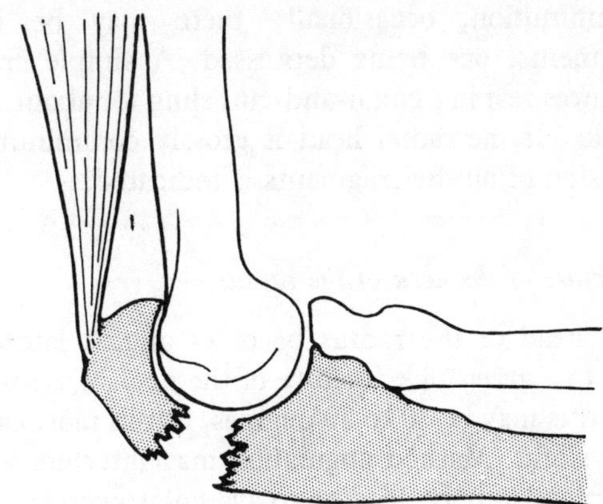

Fig. 28.16 Fracture of the olecranon, showing separation produced by action of triceps muscle

or screw is used. When the fracture is comminuted, excision of the fragments and suture of the triceps of the olecranon stump is preferable.

Fractures of the upper end of the radius

These occur through the head or neck, the former in adults and the latter usually in children. In both the cause is indirect violence, a fall on to the outstretched hand driving the head of the radius against the capitellum. In adults the bone is hard and cracks vertically through the head, whereas in children it is soft and bends at the neck (Fig. 28.17).

Fracture of the head of the radius

This can vary from a fine vertical crack to severe

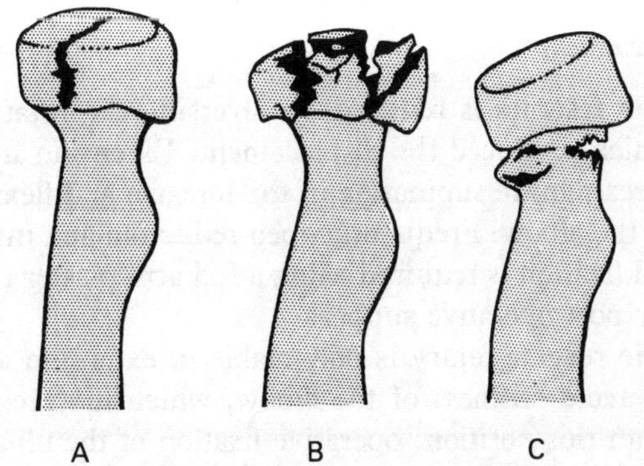

Fig. 28.17 Fractures of the upper end of radius. **A.** Undisplaced crack fracture of the head. **B.** Comminuted fracture of the head. **C.** Greenstick fracture of the neck.

comminution; occasionally there may be two fragments, one being depressed. A simple crack requires rest in a collar-and-cuff sling for about two weeks. If the radial head is grossly comminuted, excision of all the fragments is indicated.

Fracture of the neck of the radius

The head of the radius becomes angled laterally due to a greenstick fracture of the neck. Occasionally this may be 70 to 80 degrees, but in most cases it is slight. Marked angulation may interfere with the blood supply, leading to avascular necrosis and collapse of the bone. In mild cases a collar-and-cuff sling for two weeks is adequate. When displacement is greater than 45 degrees normal relations should be restored by either manual or open reduction.

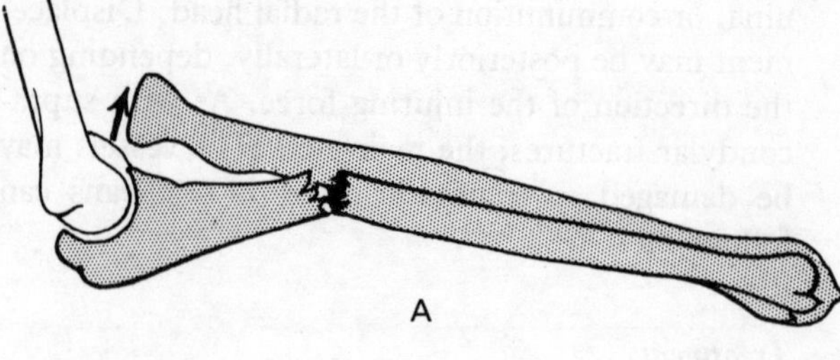

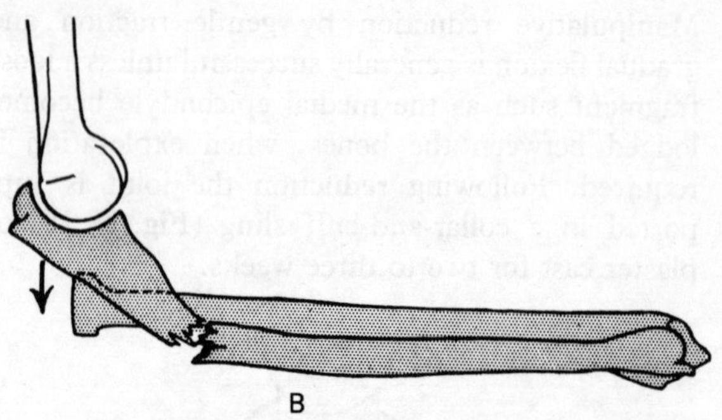

Fig. 28.18 Fracture of the ulnar shaft with dislocation of the head of the radius (Monteggia). **A.** Extension type. **B.** Flexion type.

INJURIES OF THE RADIUS AND ULNA

Fractures of the ulnar shaft with dislocation of the radial head

These injuries occur at any age and are due to a rotational twist. They were first described about 150 years ago by Monteggia. In any displaced fracture of the ulnar shaft alone displacement of the head of the radius is inevitable. The direction of rotation governs the displacement. Pronating forces cause the ulnar fracture and the head of the radius to displace anteriorly (*extension fractures*); with supination the displacement is backwards (*flexion fractures*) (Fig. 28.18).

Treatment

The fracture is reduced by reversing the rotation which produced the displacement. Extension fractures require supination of the forearm and flexion of the elbow. Frequently open reduction and internal fixation is required using a full arm plaster cast for post-operative support.

The reverse injury is only stable in extension and to avoid stiffness of the elbow, which may result from this position, operative fixation of the ulna is indicated. Damage to the superior radio-ulnar joint or fracture of the head of the radius may obstruct reduction, and operation, including excision of the head, may be required to restore rotation.

Fractures of the shafts of both radius and ulna

These fall into two groups, a greenstick variety occurring in children and following a rotational strain, and those in adults which are often due to direct violence.

In children

The force is a rotation-angulation twist and in severe injuries the radial fracture tends to be transverse and complete, lying at a different level from the ulnar fracture which is incomplete and oblique.

Treatment. Manipulative reduction is generally successful, over-reduction being difficult. The position is maintained by an above-elbow plaster cast from the axilla to the metacarpal heads, with the elbow at a right angle.

In adults

Overlap of one or both bones occurs together with rotational deformity due to unopposed muscular action. Fracture of the radius in its upper half results in supination of the proximal fragment and pronation of the distal portion. If this rotational deformity remains uncorrected (*mal-union*) there will be restriction of either pronation or supination. Midshaft fractures of the forearm bones in adults are often slow to unite and may go on to *non-union*. *Cross-union* is a rare complication of compound fractures, generally associated with infection, and is due to fusion of the callus surrounding the two bones. The nerves and vessels may also be occasionally injured.

Treatment. Manipulative reduction may be difficult and internal fixation by a plate is often preferable. Operative alignment of the radius alone may be sufficient.

Fracture of the radial shaft with dislocation of the lower end of the ulna

This is an injury of adults. In children there will be greenstick fractures of both bones. It follows a rotational strain. Disruption of the inferior radio-ulnar joint allows dislocation of the lower end of the ulna when there is a fracture of the radial shaft alone (Fig. 28.19). Clinically, owing to overlap of the radial fragments, there is often marked radial deviation of the hand. Unless normal radio-ulnar relationships are restored some loss of rotation results.

Treatment

Open reduction and internal fixation of the radius is usually necessary to restore the radio-ulnar joint to normality. Persistent subluxation of the lower end of the ulna may be treated by its excision.

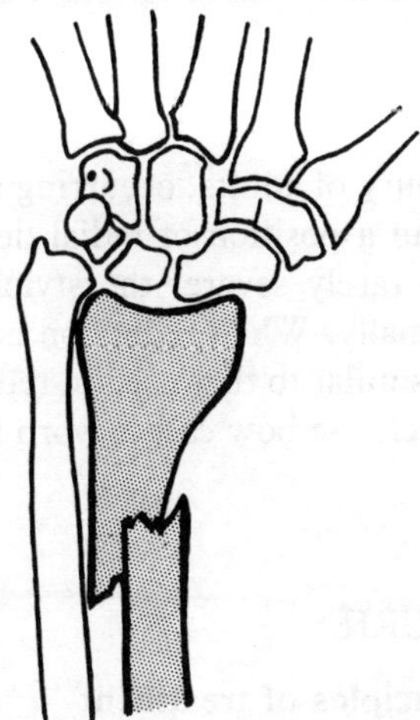

Fig. 28.19 Fracture of the radius with dislocation of the lower end of the ulna

Fractures of the lower end of the radius

Colles' fracture

Abraham Colles, a Dublin surgeon, first described this fracture, which is usually seen in elderly women. It is due to a fall on to the outstretched hand and as the patient is commonly moving forward at the time the hand is also pronated. The lower end of the radius is displaced in three planes—it is rotated backwards, moved backwards as a whole, and tilted to the radial side—producing a 'dinner-fork' deformity. The radius is also often comminuted and its posterior cortex crushed (Fig. 28.20). Some displacement is common, but even considerable residual deformity usually gives a good functional result. The ulnar styloid may also be fractured due to compression from injury.

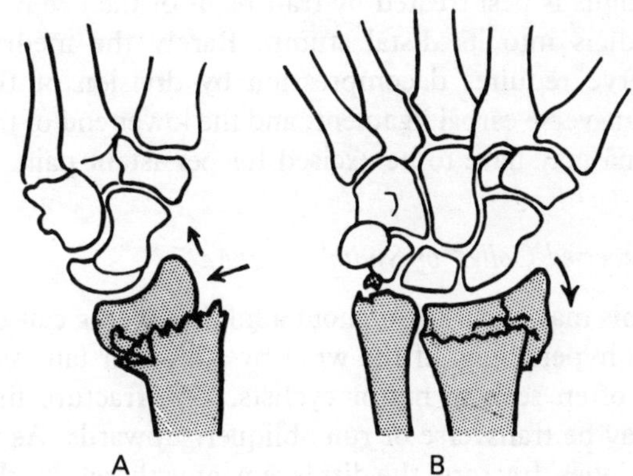

Fig. 28.20 Colles' fracture. Posterior displacement with angulation and lateral tilting of the lower end of radius is present.

Complications. *Joint stiffness* due to simple disuse may occur in the elderly, affecting the shoulder, elbow and fingers. It may also appear in an exaggerated form known as 'Sudek's atrophy', the cause of which is unknown, but is probably due to disuse with an abnormal vasomotor response. In addition to stiffness, the hand is painful, swollen, shiny, and warm. It is most common after a Colles' fracture but may occur at any site. The *extensor pollicis longus* tendon may rupture due to roughening of the bone in the region of the dorsal radial tubercle. It may take place within a few days of injury or after the fracture has united. Deformity of the lower end of the radius occasionally leads to median nerve compression in the carpal tunnel, requiring division of the flexor retinaculum to release the nerve.

Treatment. Manipulative reduction is employed. It consists of disimpaction by traction and gently increasing the deformity, followed by reduction by pressure applied to the smaller fragment in a forward, downward, and ulnar direction. Immobilisation is by a dorsal plaster slab, extending around the radial side of the wrist in order to maintain ulnar deviation, conversion to a full cast being carried out when the swelling has subsided two or three days later. The cast is worn for five to six weeks, during which period shoulder, elbow, and finger exercises are encouraged to prevent stiffness.

Treatment of complications. Sudek's atrophy and shoulder stiffness are treated by a prolonged course of heat and gentle active exercises, aided by occupational therapy. Rupture of the extensor pollicis longus is best treated by transplant of the extensor indicis into its distal stump. Rarely the median nerve requires decompression by division of the transverse carpal ligament, and the lower end of the ulna may have to be excised for persistent pain.

Reversed Colles' or Smith's fracture

This may occur throughout adult life, being caused by hyperflexion of the wrist by a blow or fall, and is often seen in motor cyclists. The fracture line may be transverse or run obliquely upwards. As in a Colles' fracture, the displacement is threefold; the lower fragment being rotated forward, shifted forward, and tilted towards the radial side.

Treatment. Manipulative reduction is employed, consisting of pushing the distal radial fragment backwards and towards the ulnar side, or after disimpaction by fully supinating the hand. In transverse fractures reduction is stable and immobilisation is by a palmar slab, which is completed two to three days later. Oblique fractures are unstable and inclusion of the elbow in the cast may be required. Immobilisation is continued for five to six weeks.

Fractures in children

In childhood posterior displacement injuries take two forms.

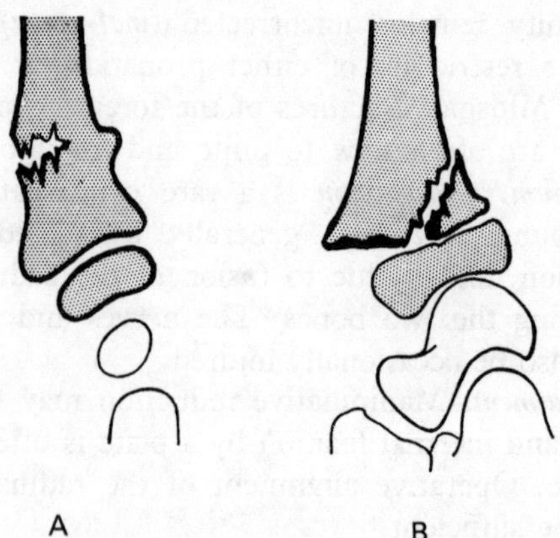

Fig. 28.21 Fracture of the lower end of radius with posterior displacement. **A**. Greenstick fracture in child. **B**. Fracture-separation of epiphysis in adolescent.

(1) **Fracture of the lower shaft**, which occurs in younger children and may be of greenstick type in milder cases, or complete with overlap and an associated greenstick fracture of the lower end of the ulna (Fig. 28.21,A).

(2) **Fracture-separation of the epiphysis**, which is common in adolescents (Fig. 28.21,B). Displacement must be accurately reduced to prevent abnormal epiphyseal growth or partial fusion.

Treatment. Manipulative reduction is sufficient. Where there is complete displacement or in fracture-separations of the epiphysis disimpaction is followed by reduction, as in the management of a Colles' fracture. In simple greenstick fractures the break must be completed. Immobilisation is by a plaster cast worn for three to four weeks.

Fracture of the radial styloid

This is an injury of adults, occurring after a fall on to the hand in a position of radial deviation. Displacement is rarely severe, the styloid being displaced proximally. When reduction is required the technique is similar to that used in reducing Colles' fracture. A below-elbow cast is worn for five to six weeks.

HAND INJURIES

General principles of treatment

In all hand injuries the following points should be observed:

1. *Swelling must be controlled*. Either blood or oedema fluid in the intercellular spaces will lead to adhesions, which will interfere with the smooth working of tendons and small joints.

2. *The fingers must be splinted in flexion*. Ideally the hand should be splinted in the 'position of rest' with the wrist slightly dorsiflexed, the thumb in mid-opposition, and the fingers semiflexed (Fig. 28.22).

3. *Splintage should be minimal*, active movements in the unsplinted portion of the hand being encouraged.

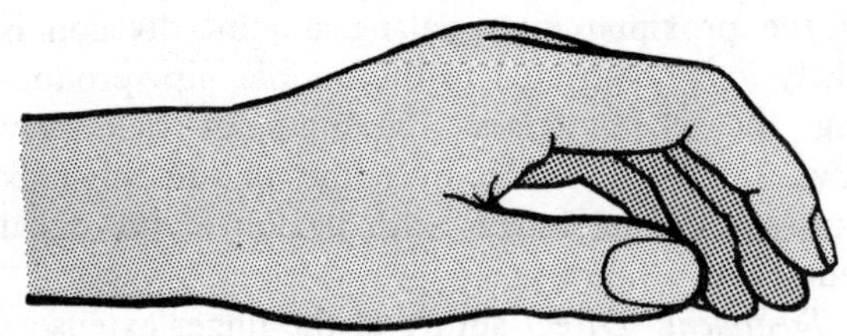

Fig. 28.22 The hand in the position of rest

Injuries of soft parts

Skin injuries

Lacerations may be caused by a sharp object which gives a clean incision, or a blunt object which splits the tissue, with contusion and greater risk of contamination. Devitalisation occurs less frequently than in other parts because of the abundant blood supply. Following cleansing most wounds can be sutured with minimal excision of skin edges. Fine materials should be employed to reduce scar formation, and grafting should be used if direct suture would involve tension. Oedema should be avoided and, except in trivial wounds, a pressure dressing should be applied; in all cases early movements must be encouraged.

Skin loss. Skin defects should be covered early. On the dorsum a split skin graft may suffice, but on the palmar aspect a full thickness graft is necessary to prevent contraction in the scar and to provide a surface strong enough to withstand normal trauma. Small areas may be replaced by free grafts, but larger areas require pedicle grafts (p. 59). Scars crossing flexion creases are liable to contract. When a flexion contracture has occurred correction may be obtained by altering the main direction of the scar so that it is parallel to the flexion crease, as by a 'Z-plasty'. When more pronounced the scar should be excised and replaced by a full thickness graft.

Flexor tendon injuries

Anatomy. The fingers possess two sets of flexor tendons. The flexor digitorum *profundus* arises deep in the forearm, is inserted into the base of the terminal phalanx, and flexes all three finger joints. The flexor digitorum *sublimis* lies in a more superficial plane, splitting distally at the level of the proximal phalanx to be inserted into the base of the middle phalanx, the profundus tendon passing between the two halves. The sublimis flexes the metacarpophalangeal and proximal interphalangeal joints. In addition, the small intrinsic muscles passing from the palm to be inserted into the extensor expansion on the dorsum of the proximal phalanx flex the metacarpophalangeal joints. When the digits are flexed, the tendons pull in a curved direction, and to enable them to work smoothly a gliding mechanism, in the form of a synovial sheath, is provided. The *thumb* contains only two phalanges, and the only long flexor is the flexor pollicis longus. The metacarpophalangeal joint is flexed by the flexor pollicis brevis, which is a component of the thenar eminence.

Clinical features. Division of the flexor digitorum profundus alone results in loss of active flexion at the distal interphalangeal joint. Where both tendons are divided flexion is lost in both interphalangeal joints, although flexion of the metacarpophalangeal joint is preserved. Due to the free movement of the tendons a divided flexor retracts widely, and in recent injuries the proximal end can occasionally be palpated as a tender mass deep in the palm. There may be simultaneous division of digital nerves or fractures of the phalanges, the latter being more likely to follow a crush injury.

Treatment is governed by the cause and site of division (Fig. 28.23).

1. *In incised wounds*. Restoration of tendon function is usually worthwhile, the method of repair varying with the level of division. In the palm direct suture should be performed. Between the metacarpal head and the middle phalanx direct suture is usually indicated as a primary repair but

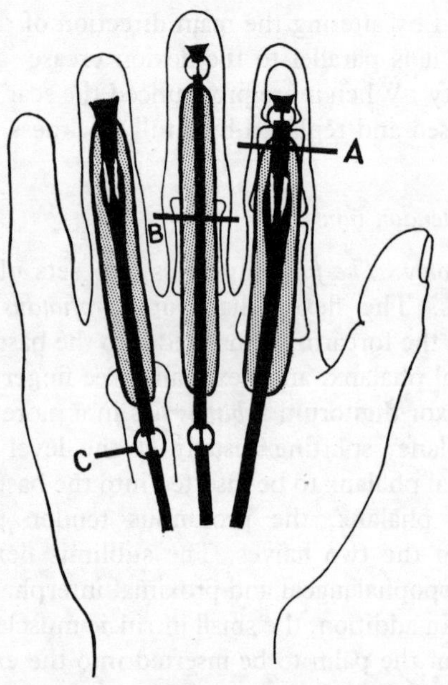

Fig. 28.23 Method of repair of flexor tendons depending on site of injury. **A.** In synovial sheath with profundus tendon alone divided, advancement and suture is performed. **B.** In synovial sheath with both flexor tendons divided, free graft is inserted. **C.** In palm outside the synovial sheath, direct suture is undertaken.

may lead to adhesions in the fibrous sheath. If unsuccessful secondary grafting using a length of palmaris longus tendon is inserted later from the distal phalanx to the mid-palm.

Distal to the proximal interphalangeal joint the profundus alone will have been divided and flexion may be restored either by a tendon graft, or by excision of the distal stump of the tendon with attachment of the proximal end directly to the base of the distal phalanx. In the ring and little fingers function after division of the profundus alone is often barely disturbed and the tendon injury may be better left untreated.

2. *In crush injuries*. The probability of restoring useful movement is remote, particularly if associated with severe skin damage. If both long flexors have been divided, amputation may be the best treatment. If the sublimis is intact and the finger otherwise healthy, arthrodesis of the distal interphalangeal joint gives good function. This particularly applies to the thumb which should never be deliberately amputated. After-care and rehabilitation are particularly important with attention to long-term planning of future employment.

Extensor tendon injuries

Anatomy. The main function of the extensor muscles is to act as antagonists to the flexors. They do not therefore require synovial sheaths and cannot retract widely. In the fingers they act only on the metacarpophalangeal joints, the interphalangeal joints being extended by the intrinsic muscles through their insertion into the extensor expansion. The thumb differs in that the interphalangeal joint is extended by the extensor pollicis longus.

Clinical features. Division on the back of the hand prevents active extension of the metacarpophalangeal joint of the affected finger. At the level of the proximal interphalangeal joint division is likely to be restricted to the middle slip, producing the characteristic 'boutonnière' deformity (Fig. 28.24). Division over the middle phalanx causes a 'mallet finger' with flexion of the distal joint (Fig. 28.25).

Treatment. Direct suture of the finger extensors on the back of the hand is satisfactory; where this is impractical splinting of the metacarpophalangeal joint in hyperextension for three weeks often gives good results. In the thumb division of the extensor pollicis longus is best treated by transplanting the extensor indicis into its distal end. In the finger the boutonnière injury is treated by suturing the two

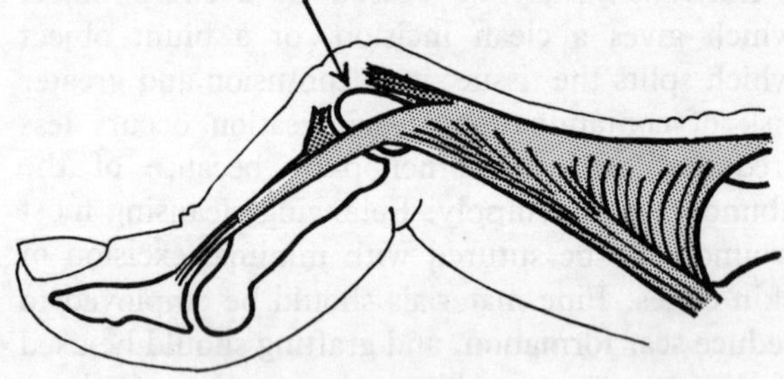

Fig. 28.24 Boutonnière type of extensor tendon injury

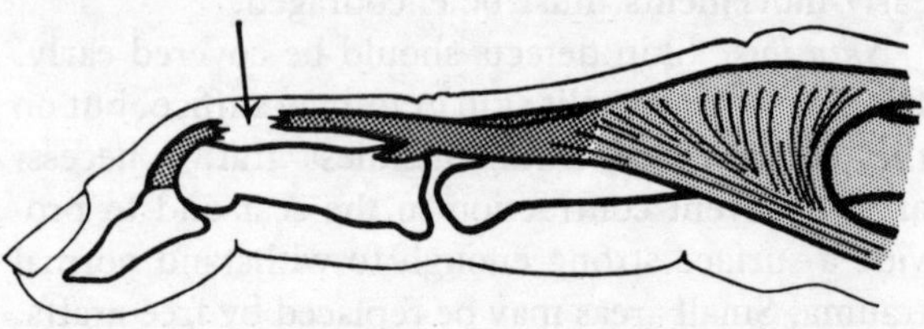

Fig. 28.25 Rupture of the extensor tendon to the distal phalanx producing a mallet finger

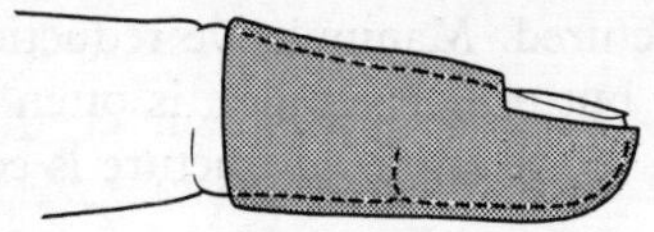

Fig. 28.26 Immobilisation of a mallet finger in plastic finger splint

side slips over the dorsum of the interphalangeal joint, and a mallet finger should be managed by splinting the joint in extension for six weeks (Fig. 28.26).

Injuries of tendons acting on the wrist

The tendons which move the wrist joint function chiefly as synergists to anchor the wrist as the fingers are flexed. They are rarely divided alone, nerves, vessels, and digital tendons usually being injured at the same time. Direct suture is satisfactory.

SKELETAL INJURIES

Injuries of the carpus

Fractures of the scaphoid

Scaphoid fractures are two types, either involving the waist or the tuberosity. The latter, due to a direct fall on the thenar eminence, is unimportant and recovery is rapid.

Fracture of the waist of the scaphoid

This is an injury common between 15 and 30 years of age. Men are affected more often than women for occupational reasons. It results from a fall which forcibly dorsiflexes and deviates the carpus to the radial side, the scaphoid being flexed across the anterior radiocarpal ligament, the strength of which fractures the bone at its waist with flexion of the distal fragment (Fig. 28.27). Radiological appearances show variable degrees of displacement, occasionally failing to show the true injury.

Clinical features. A haemarthrosis of the wrist joint and tenderness over the anatomical snuff-box are important signs, but loss of grip and pinch with marked pain localised to the scaphoid are constant features of the recent injury. Radiography must include oblique views of the scaphoid, but a fracture may not at this time be demonstrated and reliance has to be placed on clinical signs. Repeat radiography 10 to 14 days later may show the full extent of an injury.

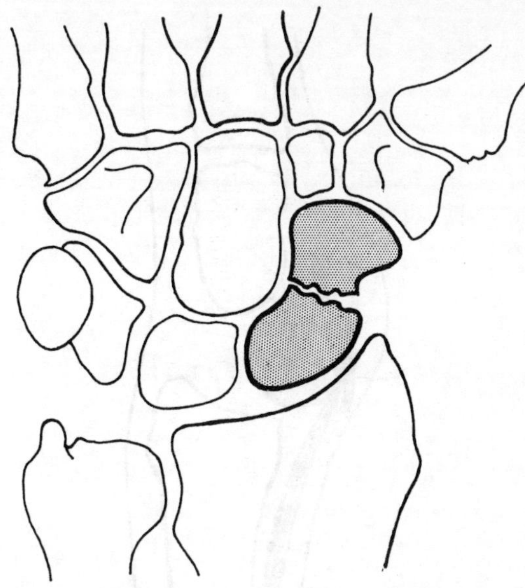

Fig. 28.27 Fracture of the waist of the scaphoid

Complications. *Non-union* and *avascular necrosis* occur and are frequently combined, both being consequent on interference with the blood supply which enters mainly at the distal pole. The degree of trauma affects the incidence of non-union, which is higher in the presence of displacement or comminution.

Treatment. The fracture must be completely immobilised until radiological union has occurred, a period of three months usually being required. This is achieved by using a below-elbow cast which includes the metacarpophalangeal joint of the thumb.

Non-union without signs of avascular necrosis should be treated by stabilisation with a specially designed screw and graft. Avascular necrosis is treated symptomatically and only when pain is marked should any intervention be made. Then either excision of the radial styloid or replacement of the scaphoid by a silastic prosthesis is performed.

Dislocation of the lunate

In this condition the lunate becomes forced out of

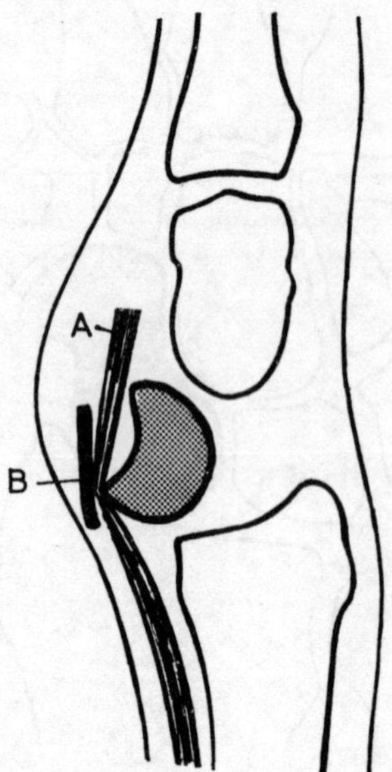

Fig. 28.28 Dislocation of the lunate bone with compression of the median nerve (**A**) against the flexor retinaculum (**B**)

its socket by violent dorsiflexion of the carpus, coming to lie with its concave surface facing forwards. Rarely there is a fracture of the scaphoid in addition, the proximal fragment becoming displaced with the lunate. Pressure on the median nerve is produced, leading to numbness and paraesthesiae in the thumb, index, and middle fingers (Fig. 28.28). Marked swelling and pain are noted. Displacement may be overshadowed by the other carpal bones in the anteroposterior radiograph, but is clearly visible in the lateral view. Avascular necrosis of the displaced bones is a common sequel.

Treatment. Manipulative reduction, by direct pressure on the displaced bone coupled with traction and gradual palmar flexion of the wrist, usually succeeds. Occasionally operation is required. Reduction is followed by six to eight weeks plaster fixation.

Dislocation of the carpus around the lunate

This severe injury usually results from falls on to the outstretched hand in young adults. The lunate, at times accompanied by the whole or proximal pole of the scaphoid, remains undisplaced, while the rest of the carpus comes to lie behind and to the radial side. The radial and ulnar styloids may also be fractured. Manipulative reduction may be successful, but open operation is often necessary. Non-union of the scaphoid fracture is common.

Injuries of the metacarpus

Fracture of the metacarpal shaft and base

This usually follows a blow on the metacarpal head when the fist is clenched. A direct blow on the dorsum of the hand produces a transverse fracture line. In oblique fractures angular displacement is rarely significant but overlap may lead to depression of the metacarpal head.

Treatment. Most fractures unite rapidly and merely require support with strapping or a plaster slab for three weeks. Transverse fractures in which displacement does occur may require fixation with an intramedullary wire.

Fracture of the metacarpal neck

This fracture can occur at any age. In children the injury is a fracture-separation of the epiphysis. This usually follows a blow on the back of the metacarpal head, and is more common in the second and fifth metacarpals. The head becomes angulated forward (Fig. 28.29,A).

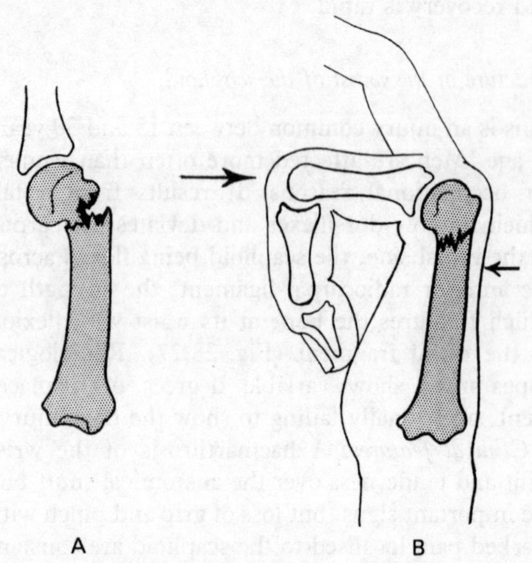

Fig. 28.29 Fracture of the neck of metacarpal bone. **A.** Typical displacement. **B.** Method of reduction.

Treatment. Mild cases may be treated by strapping for two weeks. When displacement is more severe reduction is required and should be fixed with wires to hold the correct length and rotation. Early joint mobilisation is commenced.

Fracture-dislocation of the first metacarpal base ('Bennett's fracture')

This injury is most common in adult males. It is the result of a fall on to the thumb with the metacarpal in an adducted position. This causes a dislocation of the base and shearing off of a small triangular fragment, which remains articulating with the trapezium (Fig. 28.30,A).

Treatment. Thumb traction, abduction of the metarcarpal with pressure at its base, and flexion of the metacarpophalangeal joint reduce the displacement without difficulty (Fig. 28.30,B). Redisplacement is common, due to the obliquity of the fracture line. The position is maintained for four weeks by a cast which includes the proximal phalanx of the thumb, frequent check radiographs being necessary during the first 10 to 14 days. When a fracture is obviously unstable, the fragment should be fixed internally by two wires to ensure that loss of function does not occur. If the fragment is small, mobilisation at an early stage is indicated.

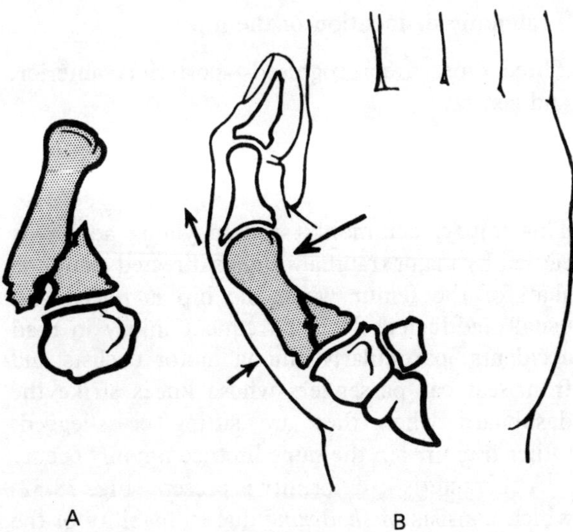

Fig. 28.30 Fracture-dislocation of the base of the first metacarpal bone. **A.** Typical displacement. **B.** Method of reduction.

Dislocation and subluxation of the metacarpophalangeal joints

Dislocation. This takes place in the anteroposterior plane and most frequently affects the thumb, the proximal phalanx being displaced dorsally. The tendons inserted into the proximal phalanx grip the metacarpal head. Reduction is effected by hyperextending the digit while the base of the phalanx is lifted on to the metacarpal head. The joint is held reduced by a Kirschner wire for two weeks and during this time the other joints are actively mobilised.

Subluxation takes place in a lateral direction, the collateral ligament being avulsed. The radiograph often shows that a small fragment of bone has been torn from the base of the proximal phalanx. The thumb is usually affected, but this injury is often unrecognised. When seen early operative repair gives a good result. In later cases mobilisation and active use lead to satisfactory function, although some laxity may persist.

Injuries of the digits

Fractures of the proximal and middle phalanges

Oblique fractures rarely show marked displacement and rapid union occurs. In children the corresponding injury is a fracture-separation of the epiphysis. Immobilisation by strapping the injured finger to its healthy neighbour for two weeks usually suffices (Fig. 28.31).

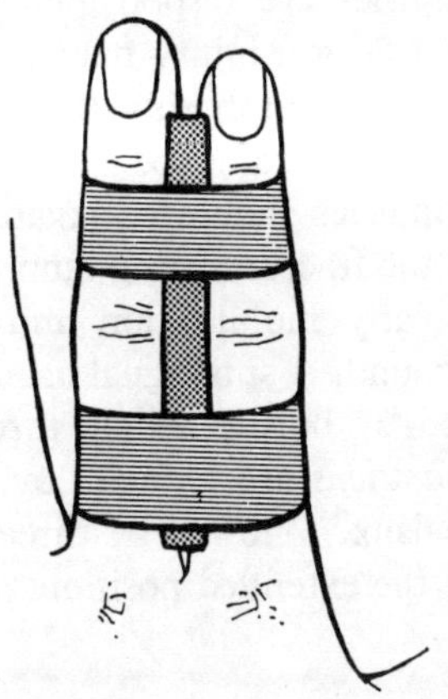

Fig. 28.31 Immobilisation of fracture of phalanges by strapping adjacent fingers. A felt pad separates the fingers and the strapping should not cover the joints.

Transverse fractures develop a characteristic angular deformity, convex forwards, due to the unopposed pull of the flexor and extensor tendons. If this is not fully corrected a sharp ridge is left to which the flexor tendons adhere. If accurate reduction cannot be maintained, then malrotation may occur, leading to considerable loss of function. Unstable fractures of the proximal phalanges are best fixed with wires for three weeks, the remaining joints being kept mobile during this period. Other injuries heal well if the adjoining digits are simply held together (Fig. 28.31).

Dislocation of the interphalangeal joints

This may be either in the anteroposterior or lateral planes. *In the anteroposterior* the more distal phalanx lies either in front of or behind the more proximal. Occasionally the tendon inserted into the base of the dislocated phalanx is avulsed. Reduction is by traction and should be followed by strapping the injured finger to a healthy neighbour for two or three weeks. In *a lateral* dislocation the bone is displaced sideways and there is an associated rupture of the collateral ligament. Treatment consists of reduction followed by strapping the finger to its neighbour on the opposite side to which it inclines for two to three weeks, but full functional recovery is often slow.

Fracture of the terminal phalanges

Crushing injuries are responsible except in children where a flexion injury may cause a fracture-separation of the epiphysis—the equivalent of a mallet finger in the adult (p. 390).

Crushing injuries should be regarded as soft tissue lesions, the fracture being ignored. Treatment consists of early mobilisation and toilet of any associated wound. A subungual haematoma should be evacuated by boring a hole through the nail. *Fracture-separations* are reduced by extending the terminal phalanx, followed by three weeks immobilisation in the extended position.

Reconstructive procedures in the hand

When a hand has been severely injured reconstructive surgery can often restore a considerable degree of function. In severe single digital injuries amputation often yields the best results, but in multiple injuries preservation may be vital. Digits may be reconstructed by using a cancellous bone peg inserted into the base of the remaining phalanx and covered by a tube of skin raised from the abdominal wall, or a useful digit may be fashioned from a metacarpal by deepening an interdigital cleft—a valuable procedure when the phalanges of the thumb have been lost. Function in a stiff deformed finger may be improved by arthrodesis of the interphalangeal joints in the position of function, combined if necessary with arthroplasty of the metacarpophalangeal joint.

One of the most important functions of the hand is opposition. When this is lost due to nerve damage, as in both median and ulnar nerve division at the wrist, such function may be restored by transplantation of the flexor digitorum sublimis from the ring finger into the base of the proximal phalanx of the thumb. If the whole thumb has been lost, the index finger, by shortening and rotation through 120 degrees, may be 'pollicised'. When only one digit remains, function may be improved by a carefully designed prosthesis against which it can be made to work.

INJURIES OF THE LOWER LIMB

Traumatic dislocation of the hip

Three types are recognised—posterior, anterior, and central.

Posterior dislocation

This injury, commonly seen in young adults, is caused by major trauma which is directed along the shaft of the femur when the hip is flexed and usually adducted. It is a frequent injury in road accidents, particularly among motor cyclists and front-seat car passengers whose knees strike the dashboard when they are sitting cross-legged. Other fractures in the same limb commonly occur.

A characteristic deformity is present (Fig. 28.32) which consists of *shortening* due to inability of the abductor muscles to function, and *internal rotation* due to the position of the head behind the acetabulum. Radiography of the hip joint confirms the

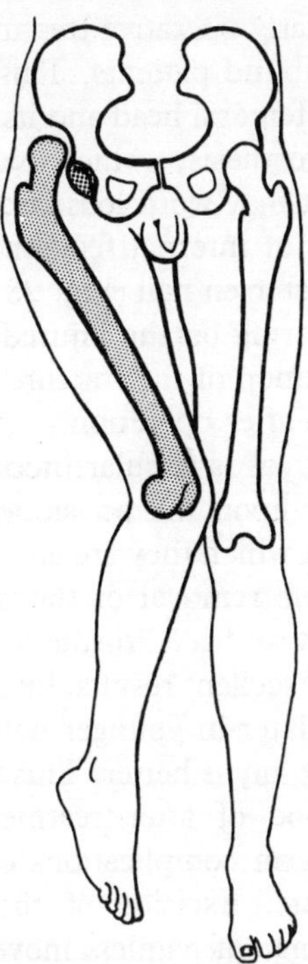

Fig. 28.32 The deformity in posterior dislocation of the hip

displacement, the lateral view often being more helpful.

Immediate complications include damage to the *sciatic nerve*, often only the segment supplying the lateral popliteal nerve being affected. Fracture of the *posterior wall of the acetabulum* or of the femoral head may cause a block to reduction. *Avascular necrosis* of the femoral head may occur later due to stripping of the joint capsule and rupture of the ligamentum teres. It is manifested radiologically by increased density of the head six to eight weeks after the accident and invariably leads to early osteoarthritis.

Treatment. The femoral head must be made to retrace the path it took at the time of the injury. The anaesthetised patient is laid on the floor and, with an assistant steadying the pelvis, the surgeon simultaneously lifts and externally rotates the flexed hip back into the acetabulum. After-treatment consists of light traction for about four weeks until the capsule has healed, weight-bearing being resumed about two weeks later. If a large part of the acetabular margin is fractured, stable reduction may not be maintained and internal fixation will be required.

Anterior dislocation

This uncommon injury is almost the reverse of posterior dislocation, resulting from forcible abduction and external rotation of the hip, as when a heavy weight falls on an individual standing with the legs apart. Reduction is by traction and internal rotation of the flexed limb, followed by four to six weeks light traction.

Central dislocation

This fracture dislocation is the result of the femoral head being driven into the acetabulum. When displacement is minimal, the patient is treated with leg traction for a period of six weeks followed by non-weight bearing for a further six weeks. When displacement is moderate or severe, open reduction of the fragments is necessary to restore acetabular integrity. The fragments may need fixation with a plate and screws to obtain stability. Operative exposure of the fracture is extensive and reduction may be difficult.

FRACTURES OF THE UPPER END OF THE FEMUR

Fractures of the neck of the femur

Two types occur, (1) subcapital, the more common and situated at the junction of the head with the neck, and (2) transcervical, the fracture being in the middle of the neck.

Subcapital fracture

This is an injury of elderly women due to a combination of the shape of the female femoral neck and senile osteoporosis. It is rare in osteoarthritic hips. It may be either *impacted*, when the head is abducted on to the stump of the neck or *displaced*, the head lying free. The latter is the commoner and more important type.

Displaced (adduction) fracture (Fig. 28.33, A). This injury may result from a fall or sudden minimal twist, causing pain on weight-bearing associ-

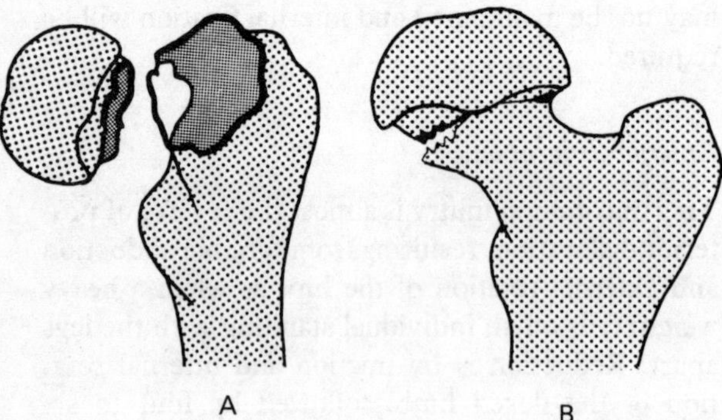

Fig. 28.33 Fracture of the neck of the femur. **A.** Unimpacted (adduction). **B.** Impacted (abduction).

ated with a marked limp. When displacement is severe the leg may rest in external rotation and be obviously short (Fig. 28.34). The blood supply to the femoral head is by retinacular vessels in the capsule and is damaged by gross displacement leading to delayed union, avascular necrosis and non-union. General complications associated with the immobilisation of elderly patients include hypostatic pneumonia, pressure sores, and urinary infection.

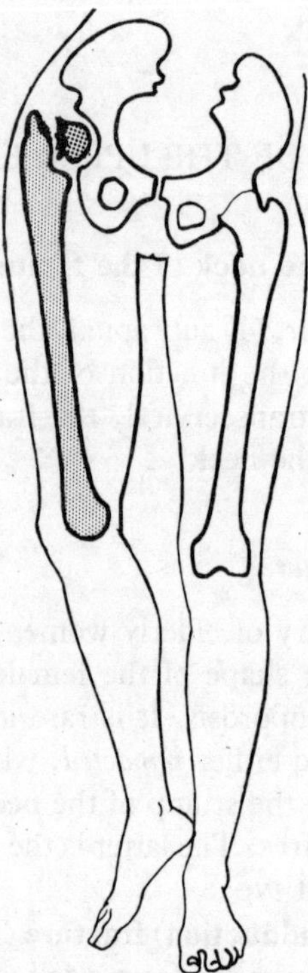

Fig. 28.34 The deformity in fracture of the femoral neck

Treatment. Early operative treatment is indicated in all but moribund patients. This may consist of excision of the femoral head and its replacement by a metallic prosthesis, which will allow early ambulation but may work loose later. The alternative is the use of internal fixation by means of a tri-fin Smith-Petersen nail (Fig. 28.1, B), in which case weight-bearing on the injured limb is usually delayed until union of the fracture has taken place 10 to 12 weeks after operation.

Management of avascular necrosis and non-union depends upon the physique of the patient and the stage at which they are encountered. In the very frail simple removal of the nail under local anaesthetic may suffice. Prosthetic replacement of the head gives excellent results, but as it sometimes becomes loose later in younger patients a sub-trochanteric osteotomy is better. This requires a more prolonged period of after-treatment, but avoids possible long-term complications of prostheses in younger patients. Excision of the femoral head allows a fair range of painless movement but with some instability, and is to be preferred in those who lead a sedentary life.

Impacted (abduction) fracture (Fig. 28.33B). Displacement of the head does not occur and symptoms are minimal. Union is usual, provided that disimpaction does not take place. In the old and frail the avoidance of weight-bearing for four weeks is adequate management. If disimpaction occurs immediate nailing is required. In the younger group primary nailing to prevent disimpaction is to be preferred, early ambulation in about two weeks being allowed.

Transcervical fracture

This occurs in younger patients of both sexes, often following marked trauma, such as a heavy fall on the greater trochanter. Avascular necrosis and non-union are less frequent, and impaction is rare. Treatment is by internal fixation with a tri-fin nail, results usually being satisfactory.

Fractures below the femoral neck

These are of three types, all of which usually occur in the elderly. *Basal fractures* of the neck, which are comparatively uncommon, are the chief fractures of the upper end of the femur to be seen in children; *pertrochanteric fractures*, the line running through the trochanters, a common type which is often comminuted; and *subtrochanteric fractures* at the upper end of the femoral shaft, a relatively uncommon site, except for pathological fractures associated with Paget's disease or neoplastic deposits.

Pertrochanteric fracture

This fracture is common in the elderly, the sex incidence being nearly equal. The leg lies in an adducted and shortened position, with moderate external rotation. Mal-union is common, a diminution of the neck-shaft angle leading to a coxa vara deformity, but non-union is rare owing to the abundant blood supply. Hypostatic pneumonia, bed sores, and urinary infection may result from decubitus unless the patient is mobilised early.

Treatment. Internal fixation with a nail and plate should be performed early to avoid the complications of prolonged bed rest especially in the elderly (Fig. 28.35). Where strong contra-indications to general anaesthesia exist conservative management can be employed and the leg is held in traction for ten to twelve weeks. Pathological fractures should always be fixed early and may be followed by radiotherapy.

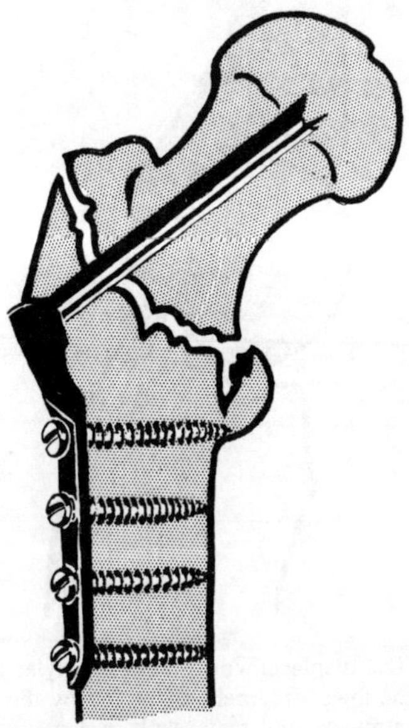

Fig. 28.35 A combined nail and plate used to hold a pertrochanteric fracture of the femur

Fracture of the femoral shaft

In adults the injury is usually due to direct violence, considerable force being required. It is common in motor cyclists, falls from a height, or crushing injuries. Extensive soft tissue damage is often associated. In children the fracture is commonly due to indirect violence in the form of a rotational twist, the fracture line being spiral. Contraction of the long thigh muscles results in shortening, with angulation in any direction. Displacement is less marked in indirect injuries as soft tissue damage and periosteal stripping are not so extensive.

Knee stiffness, due to the quadriceps muscle becoming adherent to the bone at the fracture site, may be troublesome. It is liable to be more marked in comminuted fractures or those near the joint. *Mal-union* may result from overlap or angulation of the fragments. *Non-union* is less common in the femur than other long bones and is usually due to interposition of soft tissues. *Fat embolism*, while a rare complication of fractures, is seen most frequently after femoral shaft injuries.

Treatment

This is either conservative or operative, the former being generally employed. Manipulative reduction is followed by skeletal or skin traction on a Thomas's splint. In the former a wire or pin through the tibial tubercle is used, in the latter adhesive strapping is applied (Fig. 28.36). Skeletal traction is to be preferred, the traction cord either being attached directly to the end of the splint ('fixed traction'), or to a weight with the leg resting in the splint ('balanced traction'), in which case knee movements can be commenced at an early stage (Fig. 28.37). In children skin traction is more satisfactory, as knee stiffness is rare and there is risk of damage to the upper tibial epiphysis by a skeletal pin.

Operative treatment consists of internal fixation by an intramedullary (Küntscher) nail (Fig. 28.1, C). It is indicated when *soft tissue interposition* has prevented reduction; *in multiple injuries*, where internal fixation of major fractures may make the control of the patient as a whole easier; *in the elderly*, in whom the operative risk may be less

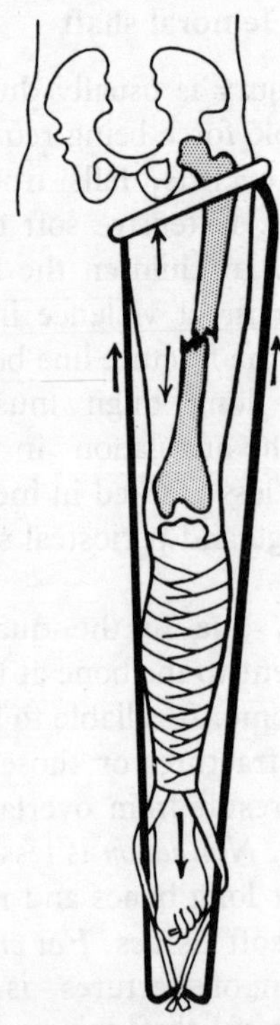

Fig. 28.36 Fixed traction for fracture of the femoral shaft using skin extensions. The pull down the leg is achieved by the counter-pressure of the splint against the ischial tuberosity.

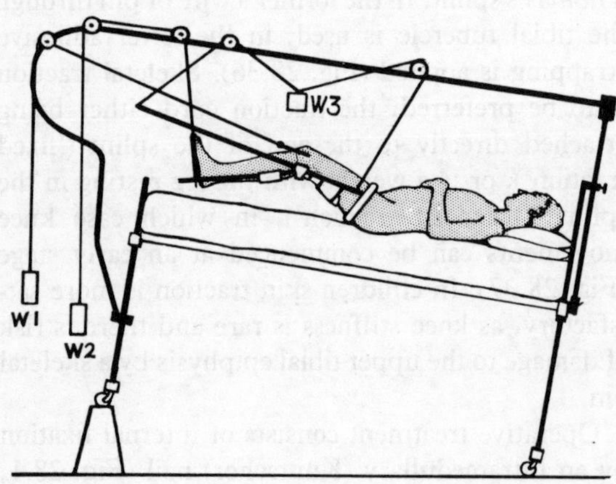

Fig. 28.37 Balanced traction for fracture of the femoral shaft using a pin through the tibial tubercle. The pull is achieved by W1, countertraction being obtained by the body-weight on the inclined bed.

than that of prolonged immobilisation; *in fractures of the upper shaft*, which are difficult to control by conservative means, and for *pathological fractures*.

Fracture of the femoral shaft in infants

A spiral fracture of the femur in infants is not uncommon due to a fall or occasionally to parental violence, and is best managed in overhead traction, suspending both legs vertically for four to six weeks.

FRACTURES OF THE LOWER END OF THE FEMUR

Supracondylar fracture

Adults of any age may be affected, but it is most frequent in the elderly. The fracture may follow direct or indirect violence, the latter consisting of a hyperextension strain of the knee. Deformity is characteristic, with backward angulation and displacement of the lower fragment due to the unopposed pull of the gastrocnemius tendon (Fig. 28.38). The femoral vessels as they pass

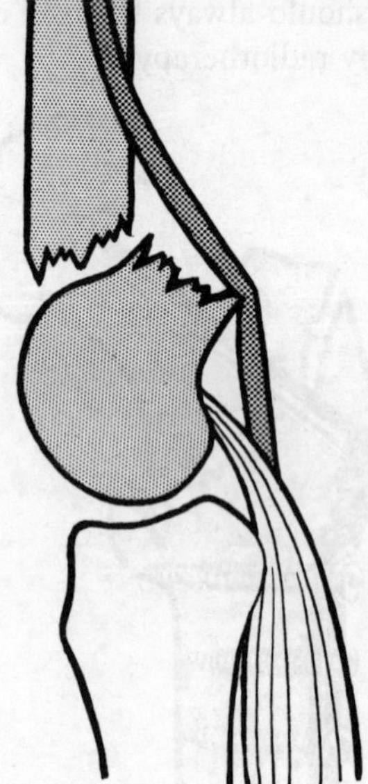

Fig. 28.38 The displacement in supracondylar fracture of the femur. The lower fragment is rotated by the gastrocnemius muscle and may result in damage to the femoral vessels.

through the adductor magnus muscle may be injured by the lower fragment. Extension of the fracture line into the knee may result in a stiff joint and cause difficulty in mobilisation. Minor degrees of residual angulation will cause bow-leg or knock-knee.

Treatment. Skeletal traction through the tibial tubercle is used, the knee being maintained in about 60 degrees of flexion, the hinge of the flexion-piece being placed opposite the fracture rather than the knee joint. Union is rapid and within three weeks cautious knee movements can be instituted. Gross displacement or instability require open reduction and internal fixation. In older patients the risk of immobilisation may be excessive and the fracture can be treated with a plaster cylinder support.

Fracture-separation of the lower femoral epiphysis

This is an uncommon injury of children, mainly adolescents, producing similar features to a supracondylar fracture in adults. Treatment is initial reduction of the displaced epiphysis by manipulation and immobilisation in a plaster cylinder with the knee in flexion to help maintain position.

Fractures of the condyles

These injuries which are relatively uncommon occur in adults of all ages, but are most frequent in older people. A single condyle may be fractured by an angulation strain of the knee, whereas a direct blow on the knee may fracture both condyles ('Y-shaped fracture'). The loose fragment rides upward and is flexed by the gastrocnemius tendon. Complications include damage to the femoral vessels, stiffness and arthritis in the knee, and residual deformity.

Treatment. Conservative management along the lines described for a supracondylar fracture is to be preferred. When satisfactory closed reduction is not feasible, open reduction and fixation of the loose condyle with screws or bolts may be required. In the elderly some deformity may be accepted and a simple plaster cylinder employed.

KNEE INJURIES

Principles of treatment

Stability of the knee is dependent on strong ligaments and the powerful quadriceps muscle which, through its expansions on either side of the patella, supports the joint. Careful examination is essential following all knee injuries with particular attention to ligaments. A haemarthrosis suggests serious disruption of intra-articular structures and needs bed rest even if a gross lesion is not found. When tense it causes severe pain and aspiration of the blood should then be done but under strict asepsis.

The knee can be effectively immobilised after injury by either a wool and non-stretch bandage in two or three layers, and called a Robert Jones bandage (Fig. 28.39), or in a plaster cylinder according to the severity of the injury.

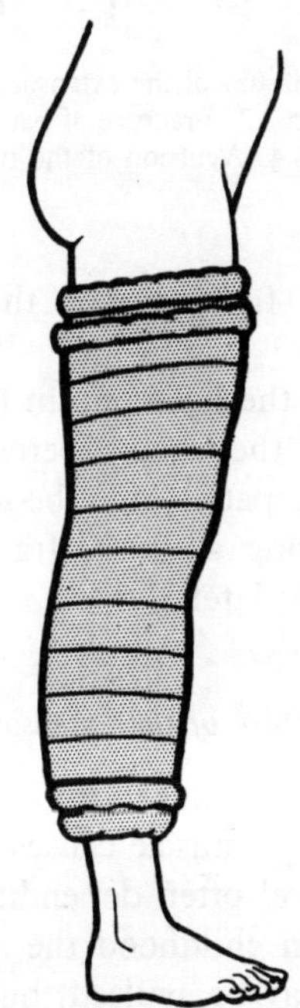

Fig. 28.39 Pressure bandage of two layers of wool and bandage

Injuries of the extensor apparatus

This can be disrupted at four levels (Fig. 28.40).

1. Tear of the quadriceps insertion into the patella.

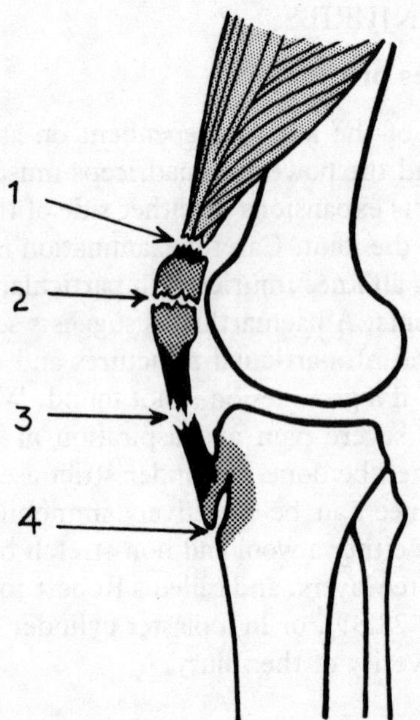

Fig. 28.40 Sites of injury of the extensor apparatus. 1. Rupture of quadriceps. 2. Fracture of patella. 3. Rupture of ligamentum patellae. 4. Avulsion of the tibial tubercle.

2. Transverse fractures of the patella, with separation.
3. Rupture of the ligamentum patellae.
4. Avulsion of the tibial tubercle.

In addition the patella may be injured by direct violence, producing a *stellate* fracture, or it may become dislocated laterally.

Mechanism of rupture of the extensor apparatus

Forced flexion of the knee against an actively contracting quadriceps muscle causes the apparatus to give way, the level often depending upon the age of the patient. In childhood the apophysis of the tibial tubercle may be avulsed, but this is rare. In young adult life the patella may be fractured transversely on the femoral condyles with separation of the fragments, and in later life the ligamentum patellae may be ruptured or the quadriceps insertion be torn.

Clinical features

The knee cannot be actively extended, even against gravity. The level of the lesion can be detected by the point of maximal tenderness and palpation of a gap, although the latter may be masked by haematoma formation. Radiography in rupture of the ligamentum patellae shows the patella to be lying higher than normal, whereas with a tear of the quadriceps the patella lies at a lower level with its upper pole tilted forwards.

Treatment

Operative repair of the defect in the extensor apparatus is essential, and should be followed by a period of about eight weeks immobilisation of the knee in full extension in a plaster of Paris cylinder.

Fractures of the patella

These are of two types: (1) *transverse*, due to indirect violence, with separation and disruption of the quadriceps expansion, and (2) *stellate*, due to direct violence with comminution but without separation. Occasionally there may be a linear fracture without separation.

Treatment

This should consist of reconstitution of the quadriceps mechanism where necessary, and the prevention of irregularities in the patello-femoral articulation. Operation is indicated except where there is no displacement. Transverse fractures are treated either by repair with wire, where a smooth articular surface can be restored, or by excision with repair of the torn quadriceps expansion. Stellate fractures require excision of the patella.

Recurrent dislocation of the patella

Anatomy

Due to the width of the pelvis, when the knee is extended, the femur inclines inward in relation to the tibia and, as the ligamentum patellae is inserted below the level of the joint, the line of pull of the quadriceps lies slightly to the outer side of the knee. These factors are more marked in females because of their wider pelvis. This tendency for the patella to move outwards is normally prevented by the shape of the lateral femoral condyle which is slightly prominent anteriorly.

Mechanism

Recurrent dislocation is liable to occur in a knee, the site of minor congenital anomalies, such as flattening of the lateral condyle, a small high-riding patella, and a genu valgum deformity. Displacement follows sudden quadriceps contraction in a flexed knee. Rarely the normal patella is dislocated laterally by a direct glancing blow with the joint semiflexed.

Clinical features

Adolescent females are commonly affected and may present with the knee locked in semiflexion with the patella displaced, but usually spontaneous reduction occurs and the complaint is of recurrent incidents of locking or insecurity in the joint. Examination, in addition to showing a small, high, and laterally mobile patella, may reveal tenderness to its inner side due to stretching of the medial joint capsule. Discomfort is felt if the bone is pressed gently outward. The condition is often bilateral. In long-standing cases osteoarthritis of the patello-femoral articulation follows. Confusion may occur with other causes of locking in the joint, particularly tears of the medial semilunar cartilage.

Treatment

Persisting displacement can usually be reduced without anaesthesia by pressure on the outer side of the patella. After a single incident recurrence can be minimised by intensive physiotherapy to strengthen the vastus medialis. Operation is indicated in all recurrent cases. It consists of realignment of the muscular pull by moving the tibial tubercle medially, combined with pleating the medial joint capsule.

Injuries due to angulation strains

Three types occur (Fig. 28.41). (1) Ligamentous, in all degrees from a minor collateral ligamentous strain to complete disruption of one collateral and both cruciates. (2) The tibial condyle on the concave side may be crushed and the collateral ligament on the convex side torn. (3) The whole upper end of the tibia may be crushed.

Mechanism

Angulation strains are due either to a fall sideways with the foot anchored on the ground or to a blow on one side of the joint. Such blows and angulation

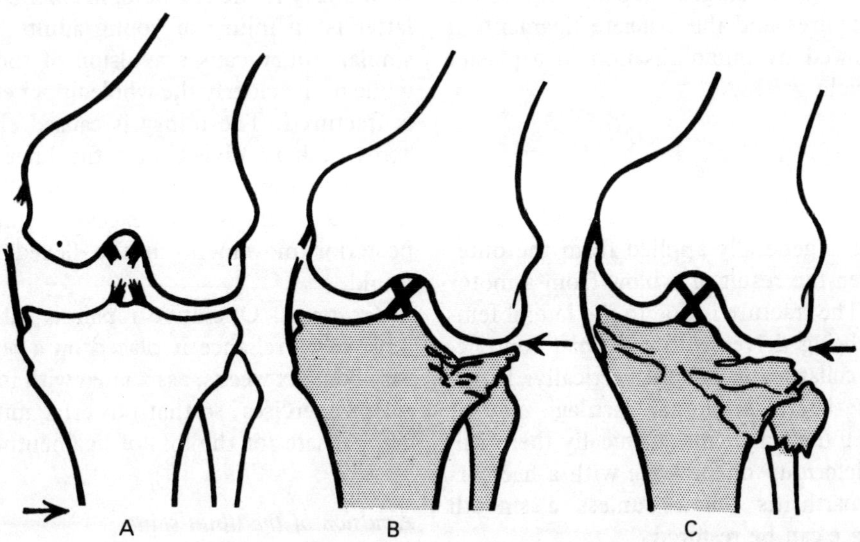

Fig. 28.41 The effects of valgus strain on the knee joint. **A.** Rupture of both cruciate and medical ligaments from angulatory strain. **B.** Collapse of lateral tibial condyle and rupture of medial ligament from a direct blow. **C.** Collapse of upper end of tibia from direct trauma.

strains usually come from the outer side. The nature of the injury is dependent on the age of the patient. In the elderly the bone is softer and tends to collapse, whereas in younger patients the ligaments are more vulnerable. Direct injury generally causes a fracture of one tibial condyle with contralateral ligamentous damage, whilst an angulation strain is more likely to result in pathology to the ligament alone.

Medial ligament injuries

Partial and complete tears occur, the latter associated with rupture of the cruciate ligaments. In the complete variety haemarthrosis, free lateral instability and, about 48 hours later, bruising and oedema of the inner side of the joint are apparent. Incomplete rupture will reveal tenderness, localised above the joint line at the femoral attachment of the ligament, and pain on forcing the leg outwards in valgus strain. Minor injuries may also avulse some of the periosteum, leading to subsequent ossification in the resulting haematoma. A concomitant tear of the medial semilunar cartilage may be present in complete ligamentous disruption.

Treatment. Partial rupture should be treated by pressure bandaging and quadriceps exercises. Complete rupture requires surgical repair both of the collateral structures and the cruciate ligaments if possible, followed by immobilisation in a plaster cylinder for eight weeks.

Fractures of the tibial condyles

The lateral condyle is usually fractured, as the injuring force is generally applied from the outer side. It is often the result of a blow from a motor car bumper. The fracture is due to the lateral femoral condyle being driven into the tibial condyle, which either collapses or is split vertically. In the latter case the lateral semilunar cartilage may be forced between the fragments. Clinically there will be a valgus deformity of the knee with a haemarthrosis. Osteoarthritis follows unless a smooth articular surface can be restored.

Treatment. Early movement is encouraged to avoid stiffness and to obtain a smooth articular surface. In mild cases the haemarthrosis is aspirated and a pressure bandage used to support the knee. Weight-bearing is deferred for eight weeks. In more severe cases manipulative reduction by simultaneous direct pressure on the fractured condyle and angulation to overcome the lateral displacement is employed, followed by about four weeks immobilisation in a plaster cylinder. Mobilisation is then encouraged but weight-bearing is not permitted for 10 to 12 weeks. Operation is reserved for younger patients in whom comminution is not great. If the whole condyle is displaced downwards it may be reattached by a screw, and if a single large fragment of articular bone has been driven downwards it may be elevated, the lateral semilunar cartilage often having to be removed at the same time.

Injuries due to shearing forces

The direction of force may be anteroposterior or lateral. Antero-posterior strains either drive the tibia bodily backwards or rarely forwards, rupturing the cruciates or avulsing the tibial spine. Severe lateral shearing strains are uncommon and cause dislocation of the knee.

Cruciate ligament injuries

The cruciate ligaments are torn either in association with injury to the collateral ligaments or alone. The latter is an injury of young adults; in children a similar injury causes avulsion of the tibial spine, while in the elderly the whole upper end of the tibia is fractured. The injury is caused either by a fall across a hard object with the knee flexed or by hyperextension of the joint. Clinically, in addition to a haemarthrosis, an excessive range of anteroposterior movement in the flexed knee will be found.

Treatment. Operative repair is difficult, and in most cases reliance is placed on a plaster cylinder for about six weeks, associated with intensive quadriceps exercises, so that powerful musculature can compensate for the loss of ligamentous stability.

Avulsion of the tibial spine

This is commonly seen in childhood, when the whole intercondylar eminence is raised. Immobilisation in a plaster cylinder with the joint extended for six weeks is usually adequate for full functional recovery, although the radiograph remains unchanged. Rarely when the bone is entirely avulsed and lies free in the joint surgical replacement is necessary.

Dislocation of the knee

This is an uncommon injury requiring considerable violence. Lateral displacement can only occur when all the collateral and cruciate ligaments have been disrupted. Gangrene may result from injury to the popliteal vessels. Manipulative reduction should be followed by six weeks in a plaster cylinder. Mild residual stiffness and ligamentous laxity are common, but considering the extensive capsular damage they are not often severe.

Injuries associated with rotational strains

Semilunar cartilage injuries

Anatomy. Two semilunar cartilages (menisci) remain of the complete cartilaginous discs which in foetal life are interposed between the tibia and femur and serve to deepen the articular surfaces of the tibial condyles. The medial cartilage is narrow and firmly attached to the joint capsule (Fig. 28.42, A), whilst the lateral cartilage is thicker, and wider, and less firmly attached peripherally. Normal knee flexion is not a simple hinge movement, the femoral condyles rolling on the upper end of the tibia. As the medial condyle is larger than the lateral, towards the end of extension the tibia rotates a few degrees laterally, rendering the medial cartilage more vulnerable.

Mechanism. If during weight-bearing on the semiflexed knee a lateral rotational strain is applied to the foot, the medial semilunar cartilage may be swept between the articular surfaces of the femoral and tibial condyles and be split longitudinally. The site of the tear depends upon the position of the leg at the moment of injury. In midflexion the cartilage may be split longitudinally in the middle, remaining attached at each end—a 'bucket-handle' tear; in full flexion the cartilage is torn posteriorly—a 'posterior horn' tear, and when flexion is minimal the cartilage is disrupted anteriorly—the 'anterior horn' tear (Fig. 28.42, B, C, D).

The lateral cartilage may be injured by a rotational strain in the reverse direction. It occurs less frequently because it is more mobile, and less gliding takes place in the lateral compartment of the joint.

Clinical features. Young adults are most often affected, as in later life osteoarthritic changes lead to atrophy of the meniscus. A sudden severe pain

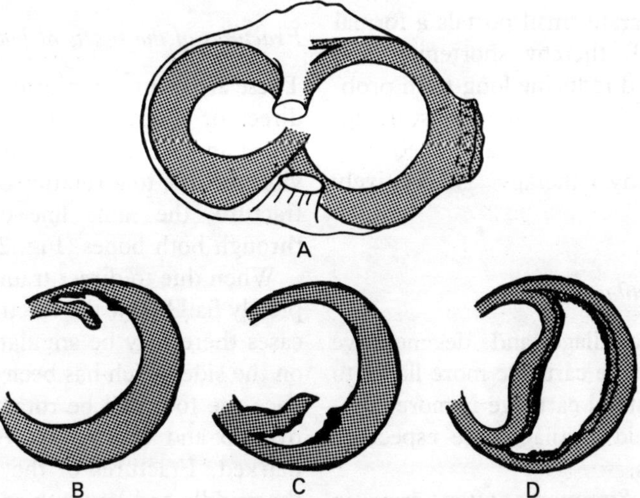

Fig. 28.42 The upper end of tibia and menisci. **A**. The medial meniscus is attached to the medial ligament. **B**. Anterior horn tear. **C**. Posterior horn tear. **D**. Bucket-handle tear.

follows a rotational twist of the flexed knee, often at football. The joint gives way and full extension cannot be obtained. An effusion develops, and recurrent locking or giving way may prevent normal activities. Initially joint recovery takes four to six weeks, but further incidents occur with increasing frequency and less reaction. Posterior horn tears are common in miners; the joint rarely locks but feels insecure, particularly when descending stairs.

Examination between incidents may reveal little abnormality, but terminal limitation of flexion and extension accompanies marked tenderness in the joint on the injured side, particularly at the site of the tear. Quadriceps wasting is also evident. In cases of doubt a characteristic 'click' may sometimes be elicited in medial cartilage injuries by extending the laterally rotated knee, under anaesthesia if the patient cannot relax. The radiograph will be normal, but air or contrast arthrograms may demonstrate a tear.

Other causes of effusion and locking of the knee, such as loose bodies, dislocation of the patella, and strains of the collateral ligaments, must be excluded.

Treatment. Clinical confirmation of meniscus tears is obtained by arthroscopy of the knee. Clear visual inspection of the compartments of the joint reveals the cause of mechanical symptoms. Significant tears of the menisci are excised by arthroscopic surgery, leaving as much of the intact meniscus as possible. By using separate small portals a formal arthrotomy is avoided, thereby shortening and improving recovery, and reducing long-term problems of joint adhesions and tender scarring. Weight-bearing can be encouraged immediately and post-operative physiotherapy is relatively short.

Abnormal semilunar cartilages

Congenital 'discoid' cartilage and degenerative 'cystic' changes render the cartilage more liable to be torn. In both the lateral cartilage is more commonly affected. Discoid cartilages are especially liable to cystic changes.

Discoid cartilage. Symptoms often arise in childhood and consist of pronounced audible and visible clicking in the outer side of the joint progressing until this occurs whenever the knee is extended. It is due to the cartilage becoming bunched up until sufficient tension is present when it suddenly recoils and jolts the knee. Repeated trauma may eventually cause a split in the cartilage. The condition can be suspected radiologically as the outer joint space may appear unduly wide. Treatment is by meniscectomy.

Cystic cartilage. A tense cystic swelling is found on the outer side of the knee in an adult. It may be an incidental finding or there may be an aching pain. It usually lies just in front of or behind the lateral ligament, and as it arises from the cartilage a cyst presenting anteriorly is most prominent when the knee is extended, almost disappearing on flexion as the cartilage is drawn backwards. The cyst, which resembles a ganglion, may herniate through the capsule and come to lie below the joint line.

Other swellings related to the knee which can cause confusion include exostoses of the femur or tibia, a neurofibroma arising from the lateral popliteal nerve, a loose body, and rarely tumours, such as a lipoma of the infrapatellar fat pad, angioma, or synovioma.

Treatment. Meniscectomy is curative but only indicated if symptoms are severe. Recurrence follows removal of the cyst alone.

INJURIES OF THE LEG

Fractures of the tibia and fibula

Fractures of the shafts of both tibia and fibula

These are common injuries which can be caused by direct or indirect violence. Comminution is frequent and the fracture is often compound. Indirect violence due to a rotational twist produces a spiral fracture, the same line often appearing to run through both bones (Fig. 28.43).

When due to direct trauma the leg may be completely flail below the fracture site, or in less severe cases there may be angulation, with the concavity on the side which has been struck. In indirect violence the foot will be rotated, often laterally, with overlap and shortening. Angulation may not be marked. Fractures of the tibial shaft particularly the middle and lower thirds are often seen to have large butterfly fragments. If these become avascular delayed union is likely.

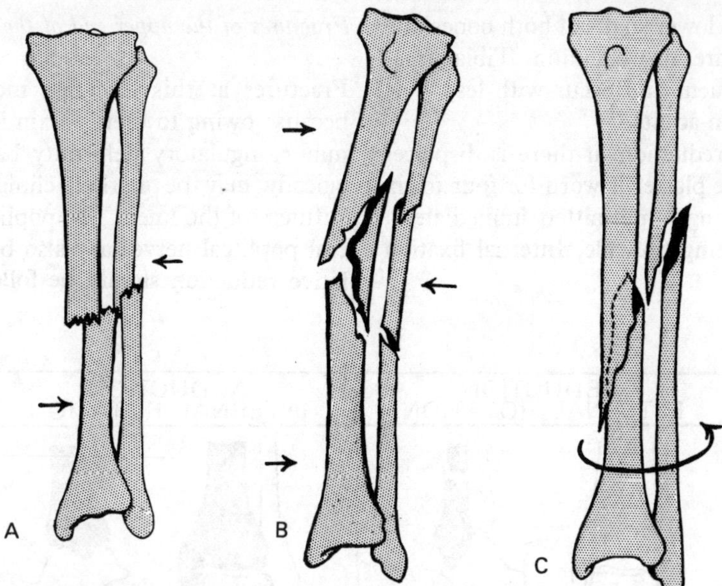

Fig. 28.43 Fracture of the tibia and fibula. **A.** Transverse fracture due to direct violence. **B.** Comminuted fracture due to direct violence. **C.** Spiral fracture due to torsional strain of indirect violence.

Treatment. Management depends on stability after reduction. Transverse fractures tend to be stable and a long leg plaster will maintain position. Comminuted fractures usually lead to shortening and over-riding of the fragments and require traction with a pin inserted into the calcaneum. This is kept for six weeks, when early union should provide enough stability to allow plaster support. Some degree of angulation in plaster can be improved by the insertion of a wedge. Plasters to be wedged should be padded and are unsuitable for weight-bearing. A careful check on the position of tibial fractures should be made at regular intervals and when adequate reduction cannot be maintained internal fixation has to be carried out, using a strong plate (Fig. 28.1A). The skin overlying the fracture may necrose either due to the injury or pressure from plaster, causing an added serious complication.

Reduction is followed by immobilisation in an above-knee plaster cast, extending from the groin to the base of the toes. The knee is slightly flexed to control rotation and the foot positioned at 90 degrees to the leg in both planes (plantigrade). Weight-bearing is permitted in the plaster when the fracture is considered stable. The period of immobilisation is rarely shorter than 12 weeks.

Isolated fractures of the tibial shaft

These are always due to direct violence, such as a kick at football, the force of which, owing to the relatively greater springiness in the fibula, is insufficient to break both bones. The intact fibula by its splinting action prevents severe displacement, but also by holding the fractured bone ends apart may cause delay in union, especially if local soft tissue damage is severe. Conservative treatment with an above-knee plaster is usually adequate.

Isolated fractures of the fibular shaft

These fractures are also due to direct violence from a blow on the outer side of the leg and displacement is minimal. Associated diastasis at the inferior tibio-fibular joint may be present (p. 409). Simple fractures may be treated by strapping, but inferior tibio-fibular joint diastasis requires screw fixation to maintain ankle joint stability (Fig. 28.51).

Fractures of the tibia and fibula in childhood

Indirect violence in the form of rotational strains often causes fractures in childhood, which are usually long oblique cracks of the tibia alone. Greenstick fractures of the lower shafts of both bones due to bending strains are also common. Tibial fractures are more frequent and occur with less violence in children than adults.

Treatment. After reduction, if there is displacement, an above-knee plaster is worn for four to six weeks. Weight-bearing is permitted immediately, uneventful union being the rule. Internal fixation is not employed.

Fractures of the upper end of the tibial shaft

Fractures at this level are mentioned separately because owing to their proximity to the knee joint minor angulatory deformity barely visible radiologically may be marked clinically, with residual stiffness of the knee. The popliteal vessels and lateral popliteal nerve may also be injured. Manipulative reduction should be followed by an above-

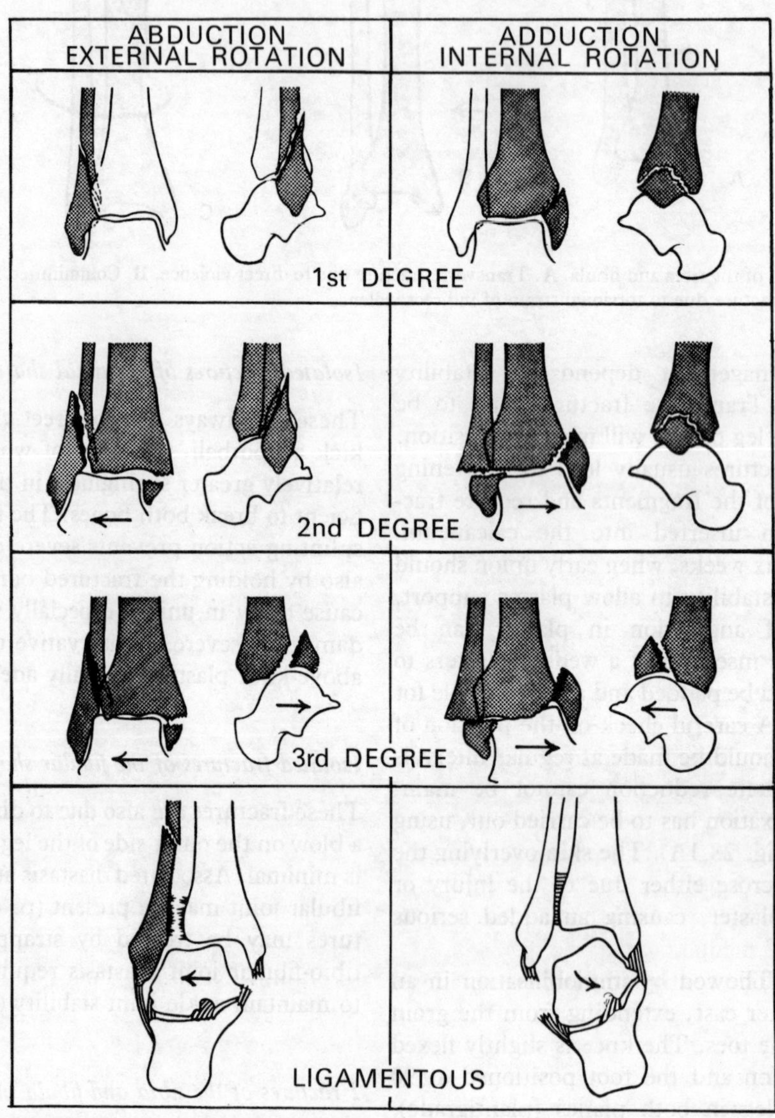

Fig. 28.44 Injuries of the ankle joint

knee plaster cast. This latter should be removed in three to four weeks to allow mobilisation of the knee, but weight-bearing is not permitted until the fracture has consolidated 10 to 12 weeks after the injury.

INJURIES OF THE ANKLE AND FOOT

Fractures of the ankle

Most ankle injuries follow indirect violence and can be classified according to the direction of force (Fig. 28.44). The majority occur in walking or running and are primarily due to rotational strains. They can be divided into five groups:

1. Abduction-external rotation injuries.
2. Adduction-internal rotation injuries.
3. True abduction injuries.
4. Vertical compression injuries.
5. In childhood fracture-separation of the lower tibial and fibular epiphyses.

When the talus is displaced from its normal relationship to the lower tibial articular surface the injury is described as a 'fracture-dislocation'.

Abduction-external rotation injuries (Pott's fractures)

Percival Pott in 1768 described outward fracture-dislocation of the ankle, several years after he himself had sustained a leg injury which was probably a fracture of the tibial shaft.

These injuries are subdivided according to the extent of the damage.

First degree. The lateral malleolus alone is fractured, the line running obliquely upwards and backwards (Fig. 28.45).

Second degree. The talus moves laterally and the lateral malleolus is fractured obliquely, with either a transverse fracture of the medial malleolus or disruption of the medial ligament (Fig. 28.46).

Third degree. The continuation of the rotational force as the patient moves forwards not only rotates the talus laterally but also displaces it backwards, producing fractures of the lateral malleolus, medial malleolus (or the medial ligament), and the posterior portion of the lower tibial articular surface (Fig. 28.47).

Soft tissue interposition, especially a flap of periosteum from the medial malleolus, may impede reduction or prevent union. Later osteoarthritis may follow due either to imperfect reduction or damage to the articular cartilage.

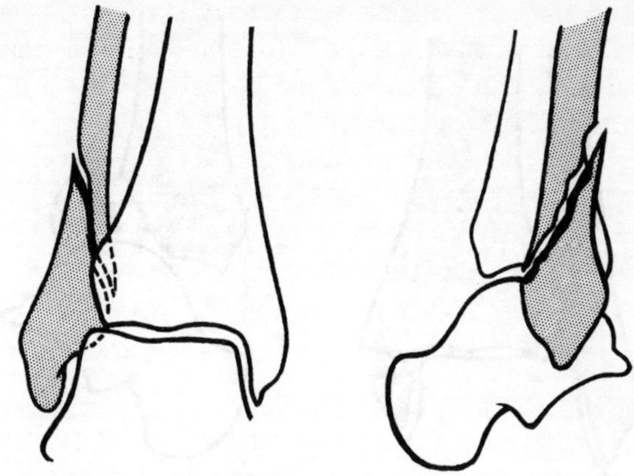

Fig. 28.45 First degree abduction-external rotation fracture of the ankle joint without displacement

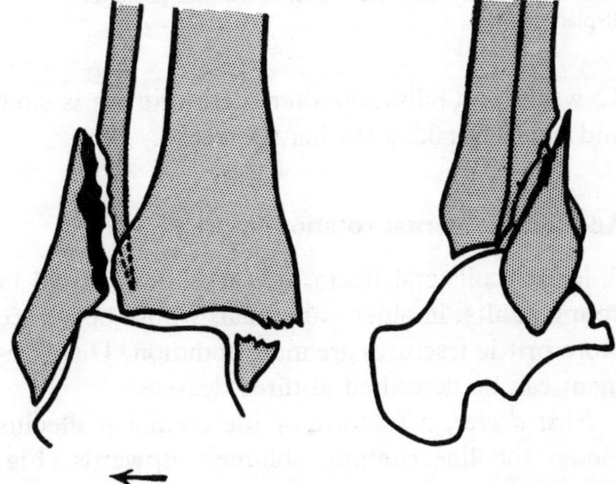

Fig. 28.46 Second degree abduction-external rotation fracture-dislocation of the ankle joint with lateral displacement

Treatment

Manipulation should be carried out urgently to restore position. This is usually adequate for oblique fractures of the distal fibula, and a below-knee plaster will hold reduction. Displaced fractures of the medial malleolus and the articular surface of the tibia always require open reduction followed by internal fixation with screws. This is supported by a below-knee plaster, from tibial tubercle to toes, with the ankle at a right angle for

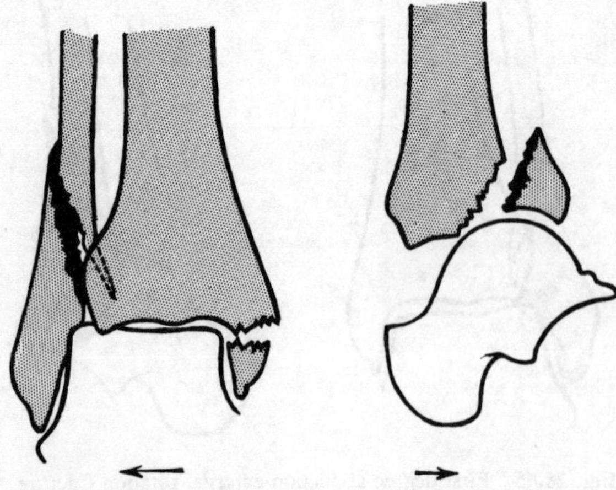

Fig. 28.47 Third degree abduction-external rotation fracture-dislocation of the ankle joint with lateral and posterior displacement

12 weeks. Mobilisation after these injuries is slow and likely to take a further six weeks.

Adduction-internal rotation injuries

A lateral collateral ligament tear is more usual in young adults; in older individuals whose bones are more brittle fractures are more common. Displacement can be described in three degrees.

First degree, a fracture of the medial malleolus alone, the line running obliquely upwards (Fig. 28.48).

Second degree, where both malleoli are fractured, the lateral transversely and the talus displaced medially (Fig. 28.49).

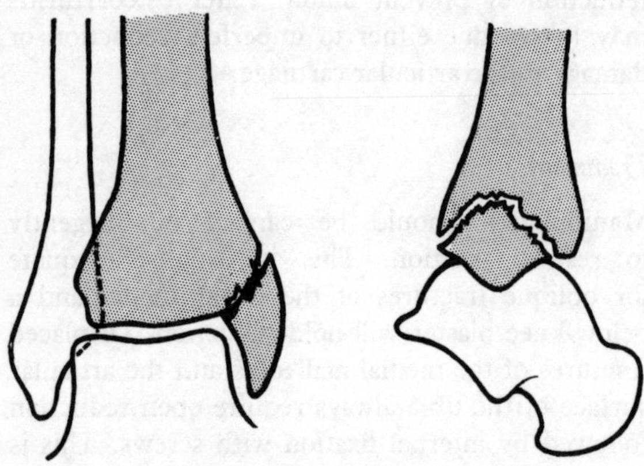

Fig. 28.48 First degree adduction-internal rotation fracture of the ankle joint without displacement

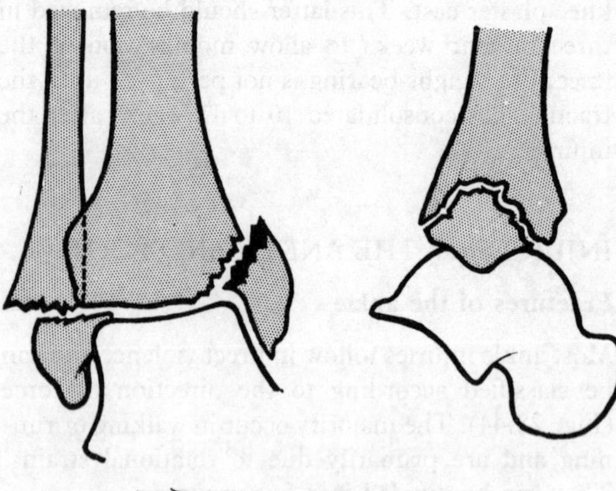

Fig. 28.49 Second degree adduction-internal rotation fracture-dislocation of the ankle joint with medial displacement

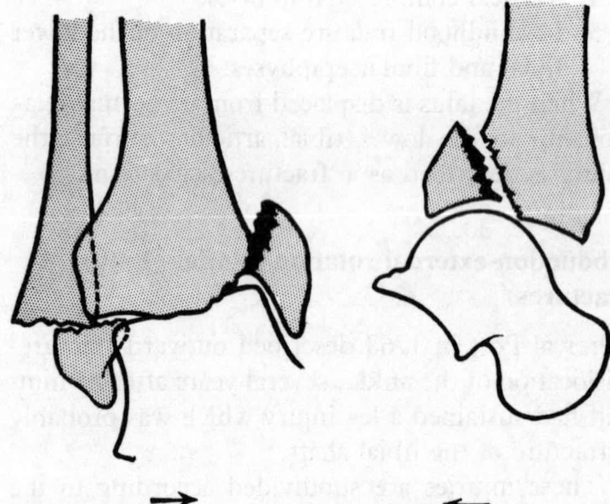

Fig. 28.50 Third degree adduction-internal rotation fracture-dislocation of the ankle joint with medial and posterior displacement

Third degree, where, in addition to the malleoli, there is a posterior marginal fragment from the articular surface of the tibia with medial and backwards displacement of the talus (Fig. 28.50).

Treatment

Manipulative reduction by abduction and external rotation of the foot is followed by immobilisation in a below-knee plaster. Operative reduction and screwing is invariably necessary to achieve satisfactory position and stability.

True abduction injuries

These are less common because the patient is not moving at the moment of injury. Three types occur:

1. The lateral malleolus alone may be fractured, the line running upwards but not backwards.
2. Both malleoli may be fractured in a transverse direction with lateral displacement of the talus.
3. The fibula may fracture at a higher level in its shaft, the talus being displaced laterally and the inferior tibiofibular ligament disrupted (*diastasis*); the medical ligament or malleolus also being injured (Fig. 28.51). The fibular fracture may be easily overlooked when it lies above the level of the routine films of the ankle joint.

Treatment

Reduction of the talar dislocation is often not feasible without direct compression of the disrupted distal tibio-fibular joint by a long transverse screw. This may provide adequate stability but when the medial malleolus is also fractured it requires fixation.

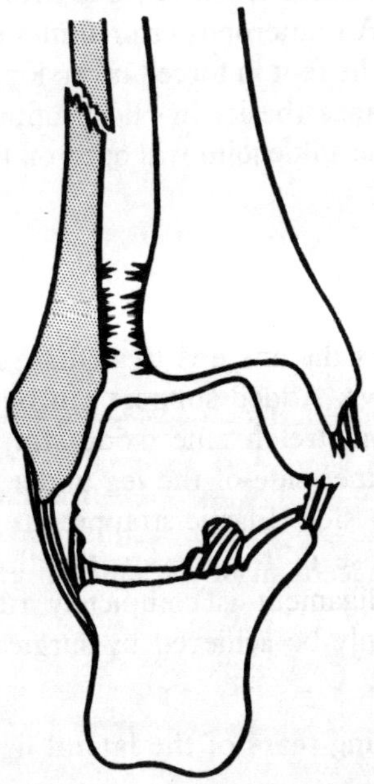

Fig. 28.51 Diastasis of the inferior tibiofibular joint is associated with fracture of the fibula and disruption of the inner side of the joint

Vertical compression injuries

In falls from a height the talus may be driven upwards disrupting the ankle joint. There is no fixed pattern of displacement (Fig. 28.52). Manipulation and immobilisation in a below-knee plaster are usually employed, though comminution may be too great to allow perfect repositioning and some permanent residual stiffness is common. Arthrodesis of the joint after the fracture has united may be more satisfactory in severe cases.

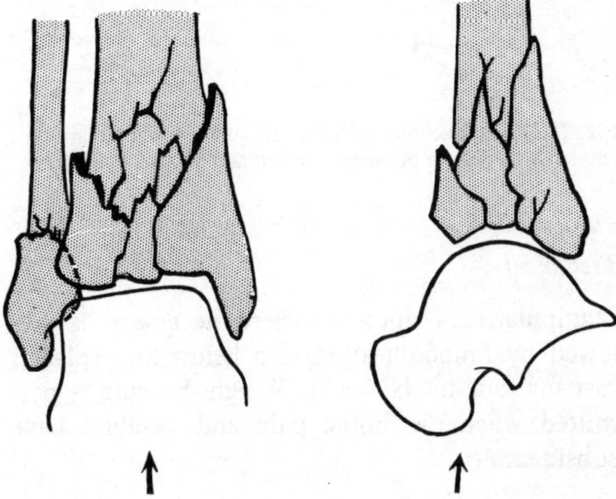

Fig. 28.52 Vertical compression fracture of the ankle joint

Fracture-separation of the inferior tibial and fibular epiphyses

In children trauma which in an adult would cause fracture-dislocation of the ankle may produce either fracture-separation of the epiphyses or a spiral fracture of the tibial shaft. Displacement varies with the direction of force. In abduction-external rotation injuries there is initially minimal separation of the lower fibular epiphysis. Further trauma produces outward and backward displacement of the lower tibial epiphysis, a fragment of the metaphysis usually remaining attached to the epiphysis. Adduction-internal rotation injuries may cause crushing of the epiphyseal plate rather than medial displacement. If this occurs premature fusion of the epiphysis may follow leading to a late varus deformity, caused by the continued growth of the fibula (Fig. 28.53).

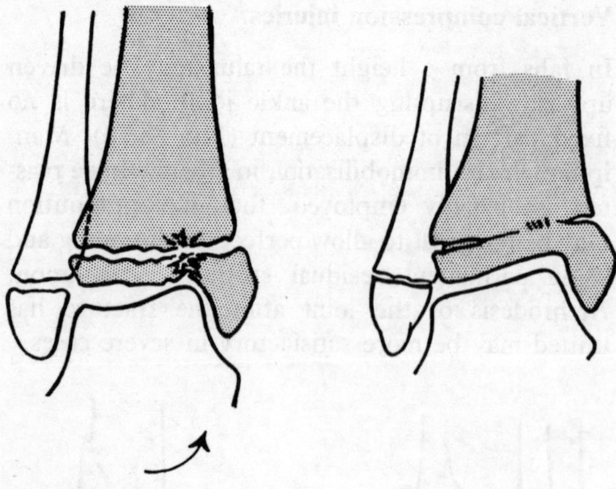

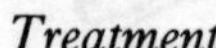

Fig. 28.53 Adduction crush fracture of the lower tibial epiphysis leading to premature fusion and a varus deformity

Treatment

Manipulative reduction where necessary is followed by immobilisation in a below-knee plaster cast for four to six weeks. Weight-bearing is permitted when the initial pain and swelling have subsided.

SOFT TISSUE INJURIES OF THE ANKLE AND FOOT

Tear of the lateral ligament (sprained ankle)

The lateral ligament is in three portions—the anterior talofibular ligament passing forwards to the neck of the talus, the calcaneofibular ligament extending vertically downwards from the tip of the malleolus to the calcaneum, and the posterior talofibular ligament passing backwards to the posterior tubercle of the talus. The ankle is sprained by an internal rotation-adduction twist. The anterior talofibular ligament is first injured, but with continued force the calcaneofibular ligament is also torn, followed by an inward tilt of the talus.

Clinical features

Swelling of the lateral part of the ankle is evident with maximum tenderness over the anterior talofibular ligament in front of the lateral malleolus, or

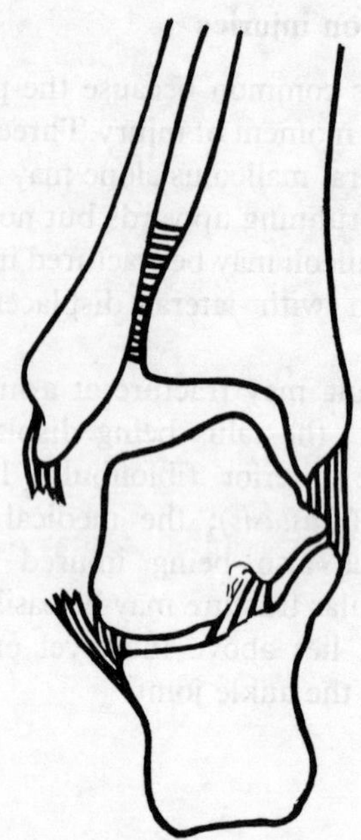

Fig. 28.54 Complete rupture of the lateral ligament allows the talus to tilt

below the tip of the lateral malleolus in tears of the calcaneofibular ligament. Radiography may show a small transverse crack or flake avulsed from the malleolus. An anteroposterior film should also be taken with the foot in forced inversion, if necessary employing anaesthesia. In calcaneofibular ligamentous tears the ankle joint will open on the outer side (Fig. 28.54).

Treatment

In *mild* cases the ankle is treated by strapping for 10 to 14 days. Added support can be obtained by a 'U' of non-stretch zinc oxide strapping passed down the inner side of the leg under the sole and up the outer side. Elastic strapping is then applied from the base of the toes to the tibial tubercle. When the ligament is completely ruptured, stability can only be achieved by surgical repair.

Long-standing tears of the lateral ligament

Symptoms of ankle weakness and instability often originate from a severe sprain inadequately treated several years previously. Forced inversion films will show tilting of the talus. Initially muscle re-education, particularly of the peronei, should be employed to control such tilting. The heel of the shoe may also be increased in width in the lower part on the outer side. In persistent cases with marked incapacity reconstruction of the ligament using the peroneus brevis tendon should be carried out.

Tear of the anterior capsule of the ankle joint

This follows a sudden plantar flexion strain of the foot, when a flake is often also avulsed from the neck of the talus. Strapping for 10 to 14 days is usually all that is required.

Tear of structures in the region of the sinus tarsi

The cause is similar to that of a sprain of the ankle and the bifurcate and subtalar ligaments are often damaged with the lateral ligament of the ankle in an inversion twist of the foot. Occasionally a flake of bone is avulsed from the antero-superior angle of the calcaneum. Strapping for 10 to 14 days is adequate. When swelling and pain are marked, a walking plaster cast should be applied and worn for two to three weeks.

Rupture of the tendo calcaneus

This is an injury most frequently seen in adults of 35 to 45 years and often follows unaccustomed athletic activity. The rupture is caused by a sudden dorsiflexion strain on the foot occurring simultaneously with contraction of the calf muscle. There are usually pre-existing early degenerative changes in the tendon. The common site of the tear is 3 to 5 cm above the insertion into the calcaneum, the plantaris usually remaining intact. Partial ruptures take place at the musculotendinous junction at a higher level.

Clinical features

A sudden sharp pain is encountered behind the ankle after jumping or forced dorsiflexion of the foot. Due to the action of the long toe flexors weak active plantar flexion is present, but inability to raise the heel from the ground results in loss of the normal springing gait on walking. Examination reveals a gap in the tendon in the early stages, later masked by a haematoma, but with tenderness and induration at the site of rupture. On absorption of the haematoma the gap again becomes palpable.

Treatment

Operative repair is required followed by a plaster cast, with the foot in equinus and the knee in 45 degrees of flexion, which is retained for six to eight weeks.

FRACTURES AND DISLOCATIONS OF THE FOOT

The foot can be described in three parts: (1) the hind-foot, consisting of the talus and calcaneum; (2) the midfoot, which is the region of the midtarsal joint and the remainder of the tarsus; and (3) the forefoot consisting of the metatarsals and toes.

Injuries of the hind-foot

Fracture of the neck of the talus

Forced dorsiflexion traps the neck of the talus between the anterior margin of the tibia and the calcaneum. If violence is sufficient the body of the talus may be displaced backwards. The head of the talus lies at a higher level than normal, with the stump of the neck pointing downwards. *Avascular necrosis* of the body of the talus is common, particularly after dislocation, as the blood enters through the sinus tarsi in the region of its neck. Occasionally backward displacement of the body of the talus may injure the posterior tibial nerve and vessels.

Treatment. Owing to the danger of inducing avascular necrosis management is conservative. The fracture is reduced by plantar flexion and a plaster cast applied in this position, the foot being brought to a right angle after four to six weeks. The cast is maintained for 10 to 12 weeks from the time of injury. When the body of the talus has displaced posteriorly, reduction by manipulation and strong traction using a calcaneal pin should be attempted. Avascular necrosis, as shown by increased density of the body of the talus, should be treated by arthrodesis of both ankle and subtaloid joints.

Dislocations around the talus

These rare injuries follow extreme inversion of the foot such as in falls from a height in which the foot becomes caught during descent. The talus itself may be dislocated, coming to lie on the outer side of the tarsus, or it may remain in the ankle mortise, the foot being dislocated round it (*peritalar dislocation of the tarsus*). Avascular necrosis is common and compound injuries frequent. Treatment is by manipulative reduction, but later arthrodesis is often necessary.

Fractures of the calcaneum

These common injuries in adults are due to a fall on the foot from a height and are often bilateral. Comminution is usually severe, the whole bone being flattened and the subtalar articular surface driven into its substance (Fig. 28.55). In many cases the fracture also involves the calcaneocuboid joint.

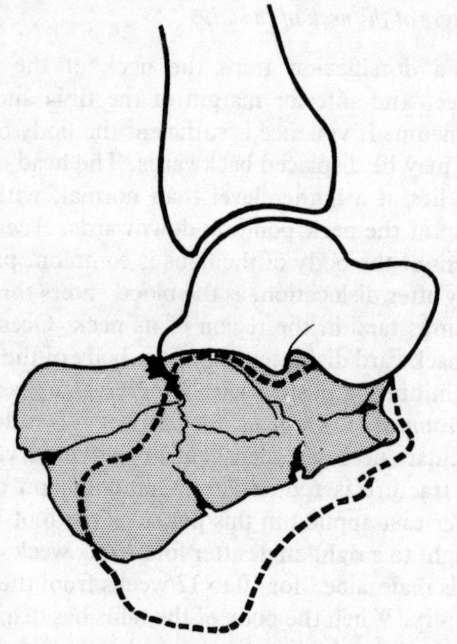

Fig. 28.55 Fracture of the calcaneum. The subtalar joint is disorganised, the dotted line indicating the normal bone outline.

Clinical features

Flatness of the foot is apparent and excessive dorsiflexion is present, due to relaxation of the tendo calcaneus. A characteristic bruise in the sole of the foot is to be found, due to rupture of the plantar fascia and long plantar ligaments. Tarsal osteoarthritis occurs subsequently. In falls from a height the combination of fractured calcanea, crush fractures of the vertebral bodies, and a basal fracture of the skull is not infrequent.

Treatment

Reduction is seldom feasible. Elevation, to control the swelling, and early mobilisation to minimise adhesion formation and to obtain some degree of alignment are preferable. Weight-bearing is delayed for 10 to 12 weeks. In younger individuals, where comminution is minimal and the subtalar joint intact, operative measures may be employed to restore the normal contour.

Injuries of the midfoot

Midtarsal dislocation

This usually follows a severe angulatory strain to the foot and displacement can be either medial or lateral. There may also be a fracture of the cuboid or navicular. Reduction is seldom difficult and is followed by eight weeks in a below-knee plaster. The results are good if the articular surfaces are not damaged.

Tarsal fractures

The navicular is most often involved with a split in the bone, the superficial fragment being displaced medially and upwards. Avulsion of the tuberosity may also occur. Crush fracture of the cuboid is also encountered. Undisplaced fractures require about six weeks in a below-knee plaster cast. Displaced fractures of the navicular are difficult to reduce and many later require arthrodesis of the talonavicular joint.

Tarsometatarsal dislocations

These usually involve either all five or the lateral

four metatarsals. The dorsalis pedis artery may be damaged as it passes between the first and second metatarsals with resulting vasospasm of the vessels supplying the toes. Manipulative reduction is usually successful and is followed by six to eight weeks immobilisation in plaster.

Injuries of the metatarsals and toes

Fractures of the metatarsals

These occur at the base, through the shaft, or through the neck. Stress fractures are considered separately (p. 345). Fracture of the **base** of a metaarsal most frequently occurs in the fifth, where it is avulsed by inversion of the forefoot. Fractures of the **shaft** are common in all metatarsals and are usually due to direct violence. Fractures of the **neck** are also associated with crushing injuries of the foot and often occur with fractures of the toe.

Treatment. Severe displacement in fractures of the metatarsal neck requires reduction, but in other sites malposition is acceptable. In severe degrees of local trauma a below-knee plaster with a toe platform is indicated but, when slight, strapping from the toes to the tibial tubercle with a felt pad under the longitudinal arch suffices.

Fractures of the toes

Symptomatic treatment only is required. In severe and multiple toe injuries a walking plaster cast, with toe platform, is applied for two to three weeks. In other instances an old shoe with a rigid sole in which the toe cap is cut to avoid pressure, should be worn for two to three weeks.

In the *great toe* damage to the metatarsophalangeal joint may lead to the later development of hallux rigidus (p. 346), and injury to the nail bed may cause onychogryphosis (p. 347).

PERIPHERAL NERVE INJURIES

Peripheral nerves are commonly damaged in the forearm and wrist by lacerations and careful testing of their function is necessary. Dislocations may injure nerve trunks by stretching or bone fragments may cause direct damage. Due to their position the radial nerve in the arm and the lateral popliteal nerve at the fibular neck are commonly involved.

Pathology

Mild injury does not cause a definitive change in the nerve structure apart from slight swelling, but temporary loss of conduction may result. When the injury is severe Wallerian degeneration occurs in the nerve fibres distal to the point of injury. The axis cylinder disappears, the myelin sheath fragments and is absorbed, and the neurilemmal sheath shows proliferative changes. Regeneration commences by the downgrowth of axis cylinders. When the sheath has been divided many of these enter the neurilemmal channels of the distal stump, but some are deviated laterally and their function lost. The rate of growth of the axon is 1 to 2 mm per day. Full functional recovery requires re-innervation of the muscle groups and skin areas. Fibrous tissue between the cut ends of the nerve may prevent entry of the new axis cylinder into the neurilemmal channel and the nerve fibres become curled up with the formation of a neuroma. The swelling that appears on the distal cut end of the nerve is due to proliferation of the neurilemmal sheaths.

Clinically it is important to distinguish between a transient block and a complete degenerative lesion. This is only feasible with the aid of electrical testing of the muscle activity and nerve conduction, using measured stimuli. Such stimuli are applied by skin electrodes directly over the muscle to be tested. The effectiveness of any stimulus is dependent on both intensity and duration. Normal muscle has a response to faradic (short duration) and galvanic (long duration) stimuli, whereas denervated muscle will not respond to faradic stimulation and only sluggishly to galvanic stimuli. A strength-duration test is employed and the figures necessary to produce contraction can be recorded graphically. The type of curve of denervated muscle differs markedly from that of normal muscle and the test is valuable in the detection of a complete nerve lesion. It is not applicable within 10 days of injury until Wallerian degeneration has ceased. Complete *reaction of degeneration* is the term applied to the condition of absent faradic response, sluggish galvanic response, and absent nerve conduction; it does not give any information on the likelihood of regeneration.

The *electromyogram* may give valuable help regarding the denervation of muscle. Normal muscle action potentials can be picked up from the motor units by insertion of a needle electrode into the muscle, amplified and then visualised on a cathode ray tube. These are readily distinguishable from the fibrillation potentials found in denervated muscle. Re-innervation may also be detected in some instances by this method. Electrical tests in addition to aiding in the diagnosis of the type of nerve lesion are of use in planning treatment and establishing the prognosis.

Type of nerve injury

Neurapraxia is the term applied to the condition of transient physiological block without degeneration which follows slight injury. The prognosis is good, recovery usually being complete in six weeks.

Axonotmesis is more serious and the result of compression or traction injuries producing damage to the whole nerve or merely to the axis cylinder. The important feature is the maintenance of continuity of the nerve sheath. Wallerian degeneration occurs but recovery follows, often after several weeks or months, by growth within the intact sheath, unless prevented by excessive fibrosis.

Neurotmesis describes the division of a nerve in whole or in part, which occurs with incised or lacerated wounds or as a complication of a fracture. The resulting neuroma is usually a barrier to spontaneous recovery.

Clinical features

Complete interruption of nerve conduction produces flaccid paralysis of the muscles supplied, absence of deep reflexes, and subsequent wasting. Cutaneous sensation is lost over the area supplied by the nerve, the extent of loss to light touch being slightly larger than the loss to pinprick.

Incomplete interruption of conduction may be difficult to distinguish from the complete variety in the early stages. After an interval of three weeks electrical reactions give considerable help in assessing the true nature of the lesion. After six weeks persistence of muscle paralysis indicates a complete lesion.

Partial division of a nerve may be detected by detailed examination of the muscles supplied, aided by the electrical reactions of the individual muscles. The extent of sensory loss may be helpful, but overlap of supply by intact nerves is often present.

The accurate recording of motor and sensory loss at regular intervals is of assistance in assessing recovery. It should be emphasised that careful clinical examination is necessary when a nerve is likely to have been exposed to the risk of damage. Many cases of legal action are due to neglect of this principle.

The median nerve is often injured at the wrist. The loss of sensation in hand and fingers is serious and trophic changes and causalgia frequently result. Wasting of the thenar muscles produces slight deformity, the index finger is extended in the *pointing* position. If the lesion is at or above the elbow there will be weakness of pronation of the forearm, flexion of the thumb and fingers and flexion of the wrist.

Ulnar nerve division is characterised by paralysis of the intrinsic muscles of the hand. The latter is held in a characteristic position with the fourth and fifth fingers in a claw-like deformity. Wasting of the hypothenar and first web-space muscle groups is easily seen. Sensory loss is confined to the little finger and medial side of the ring finger. Traumatic ulnar neuritis arises from irritation of the nerve as it passes behind the medial epicondyle. This may occur due to pressure of callus from a fracture of the medial epicondyle, or be the result of stretching of the nerve due to valgus deformity of the forearm following displacement of a fracture of the lateral condyle of the humerus. The onset is often delayed for many years after injury.

The radial nerve may be damaged in a fracture of the humeral shaft and is occasionally compressed during anaesthesia by the edge of the operating table. The lesion is evident by a loss of muscular power in the extensors of the wrist and fingers causing a wrist drop. Extension of the interphalangeal joints of the fingers can be performed by the interossei which are supplied by the ulnar nerve. Sensory loss on the back of the forearm and hand may be slight due to an overlap from median and ulnar nerves.

Brachial plexus lesions usually result from a traction injury occurring in childbirth or a motor-cycle accident, when the shoulder and neck are forcibly drawn apart. The extent of the damage varies considerably. The presence of a Horner's syndrome indicates that the nerve roots have been torn near the spinal cord. Complete paralysis of shoulder, arm, and hand muscles may be present with loss of sensation over most of the upper limb. The degree of recovery varies, complete return of motor power being unusual. An orthopaedic reconstructive operation may provide a useful limb, but amputation and the fitting of a prosthesis is often necessary.

The sciatic nerve may be damaged in the buttock by dislocation of the hip or in the thigh by gunshot wounds and lacerations. The extent of paralysis and sensory loss depends on the level of injury. A complete lesion in the buttock leaves little power or sensation below the knee, while division of the lateral popliteal branch results in foot-drop. Injury to the medial branch leads to marked disability with loss of active plantar flexion and absent sensation on the sole of the foot.

Treatment

Transient and degenerative lesions with the nerve remaining in continuity require only supportive measures. Management is aimed at keeping the limb mobile, preventing fixed deformity and avoiding injury to the anaesthetic skin. Passive stretching of the muscles and splintage are needed until recovery takes place. Particular attention must be given to care of the skin. Diversional and remedial exercises maintain morale and foster maximum recovery. Restoration of conduction is to be expected within six to nine months, during which time repeated detailed clinical examination and recordings are essential.

Operative treatment is indicated in neurotmesis. Primary nerve suture may be performed when clean open wounds are explored, but where local infection appears probable secondary nerve suture after two to three weeks is to be preferred. Failure of functional recovery in closed injuries after six to nine months also demands exposure of the nerve. Excision of a neuroma may be required, followed by nerve suture or grafting. The development of an irritative nerve lesion by the pressure of bony callus is an indication for exploration and mobilisation of the nerve. Transplantation of the ulnar nerve from behind the medial epicondyle to an anterior position is a common example.

The results of nerve suture are variable and it is uncommon for complete return of function to occur. Permanent use of orthopaedic appliances, such as an ankle back splint, may become necessary. Tendon transplantation and joint arthrodesis are often of value in late cases in restoring useful function to a partially paralysed limb.

Causalgia

Causalgia is the term applied to the severe burning pain occurring in the cutaneous distribution of an injured peripheral nerve. It is an uncommon complication found in less than 5 per cent of injuries but may severely incapacitate the patient and prove resistant to treatment.

Aetiology

The median and sciatic nerves are most commonly involved. The true nature of the lesion is not known and various theories have been put forward, the most probable being that efferent impulses in sympathethic fibres stimulate afferent sensory fibres. Alteration of the pain regulatory centres of the central nervous system or of vasomotor control are less likely causes.

Clinical features

The intense burning pain felt in the cutaneous distribution of the injured nerve may arise within a few weeks or months of injury. Movement and changes in temperature may aggravate it and elevation of the affected part often gives relief. The skin becomes reddish-blue, shiny, and covered with beads of sweat. When the fingers are involved there is atrophy of the pulp. Hyperaesthesia is present and the patient avoids anything touching the affected part.

Treatment

Partial relief may be produced by sympathectomy

but this should be combined with excision of the damaged section of nerve, followed by resuture of the stumps. The pain is very severe and can result in later personality disintegration. The affected limb should not be immobilised and active and passive movements are recommended as far as can be tolerated. Hypersensitive areas should be protected with a guard to reduce external stimuli. Early treatment and rehabilitation are essential.

FURTHER READING

Apley, A. G. and Soloman, L. (1982). In *Apley's System of Orthopaedics and Fractures*. 6th ed. London: Butterworth.

Wilson, J. N. (1983). In *Watson-Jones, Fractures and Joint Injuries*. Vol. 1 and 2. 6th ed. Edinburgh: Churchill Livingstone.

29

Vascular and lymphatic systems

ARTERIES

Congenital abnormalities

Congenital arteriovenous fistula

This condition results from the persistence of connections between the arterial and venous trunks present in the early stages of foetal development. It occurs most commonly in the lower limb and is usually multiple. The limb may increase in length due to overgrowth of bone and become swollen from the presence of fistulae in the soft tissues.

Birthmarks are often present on the skin and enlarged and tortuous superficial veins are a marked feature. Radiographs may reveal erosion of bone by vascular channels; arteriography rarely demonstrates the fistulae because of their multiplicity. Treatment can be by excision of small feeding vessels from adjacent normal arteries. Removal of localised masses of fistulae and dilated veins may be feasible in some cases. Amputation may become necessary if ulceration or gangrene develop in later life, or if the patient develops cardiac failure as a result of the altered haemodynamic state. Control of bone length in the growing child by excision of the epiphyses may become necessary, but the results are not always satisfactory.

Cirsoid aneurysm

This variety of multiple arteriovenous fistulae involves the scalp vessels. Formerly considered to be congenital it probably results from birth trauma. The swelling is present most commonly in the occipital region and on palpation has been likened to a bag of writhing worms. Surgical excision is the treatment of choice.

Arterial injuries

Wounds of the blood-vessels are common in war. A number occur in civilian life and constitute an important aspect of traumatic surgery because of the serious nature of the injury.

Blunt injuries and fractures commonly produce **arterial spasm** which results in marked diminution or even complete cessation of blood flow in the vessel. **Contusion** of the arterial wall may be followed by thrombosis of the affected segment or later by gradual aneurysmal dilatation. **Laceration** is usually the result of an open wound but may complicate a fracture. The arterial wall may be divided partially or completely. A haematoma in the surrounding soft tissues may obstruct the collateral circulation, producing a precarious state of ischaemia.

Early treatment is essential in all forms of arterial injury. Laceration of an artery usually results in free haemorrhage, requiring urgent first-aid measures for its arrest. Local pressure on the wound by firm pads is the most effective method. If a large vessel is damaged a tourniquet may be necessary, but great care must be exercised in its use, as it cuts off collateral circulation completely and if left on for over 30 minutes may impede survival of the limb. Severe blood loss requires urgent replacement.

Surgical exploration of the wound is generally indicated to define the extent of injury. Repair of the arterial wound by suture or anastomosis of the cut ends is the ideal procedure. A segment of vessel which is grossly damaged should be replaced by a graft of autogenous vein or arterial prosthesis. Arterial spasm may be relieved by the local application of a 2.4 per cent solution of papaverine sulphate. Damage to small arteries, such as the radial or ulnar, should be treated by ligature of the divided ends.

After all forms of open or closed injury adoption of the following measures facilitates recovery of the limb by making most use of available blood flow and avoiding tissue damage by local ischaemia. The limb should be supported evenly to avoid localised pressure on the skin, and elevation to about 10 degrees will assist venous and lymphatic drainage and reduce swelling. Tight bandages and plaster of Paris casts should not be applied. The affected limb should be cooled with a fan to lower its metabolism. Anticoagulant therapy with intravenous heparin should be given for 48 hours to prevent extension of thrombosis unless widespread haematoma formation has occurred. Tense haematomas of the soft tissues should be relieved by incision of the skin and deep fascia of the limb. The site of a fracture may require exploration in order to relieve pressure on an artery, for example, in supracondylar fracture of the humerus or in a comminuted fracture of the upper end of the tibia.

Traumatic arteriovenous fistula

Damage to an artery and adjacent vein may result in an abnormal passage being established between both vessels and is often due to a knife wound. A haematoma develops between artery and vein, in most instances leading to the formation of an aneurysmal sac joining the two; less commonly the artery and vein are touching, forming an aneurysmal varix.

A large fistula is followed by ischaemic change in the limb due to short-circuiting of blood. Decrease in the peripheral resistance causes an overflow to the right heart which may be followed after some years by dilatation of the heart and cardiac failure. There is a decrease in the diastolic pressure and increase in the pulse pressure, the extent depending on the size of the fistula. There is also an increase in the blood volume of up to 15 per cent to compensate for the lowered blood-pressure.

The presence of an arteriovenous fistula may be recognised immediately, or the diagnosis may not be made for several years. The site of a fistula is recognised by the presence of a palpable thrill and audible bruit, which are continuous and 'machinery like', and often subjective. Compression of the fistula is followed by a slowing of the pulse-rate and elevation of the blood-pressure. Arteriography may be necessary to define the fistula before operation.

Surgical repair of the defect should be undertaken if possible to avoid the risk of cardiac decompensation. The ideal procedure is separation of vein and artery and repair of the defect in their walls, utilising a graft if necessary. Ligation of the artery proximal to the fistula is dangerous as it permits all blood flow from the collaterals to enter the vein, resulting in gangrene of the extremity. Closure of the fistula is followed by gradual decrease of heart size and of blood volume.

OCCLUSIVE VASCULAR DISEASE

Occlusion of peripheral arteries may occur suddenly due to an embolus or thrombosis, or gradually as in atherosclerosis and thromboangiitis obliterans (Fig. 29.1). These conditions principally involve the lower abdominal aorta, iliac and lower limb vessels. The upper limb may be affected by embolism but only rarely by atherosclerosis.

EMBOLISM

Pathology

This condition is due to transmission of an organised thrombus from one site in the circulation to another where it becomes lodged, generally at the point of division of an artery, thereby obstructing the blood flow. The embolus originates either in the atrium or on an area of myocardial infarction or on an atheromatous ulcer of the aorta. The development of organised clot in the left atrium is common in mitral stenosis, whence it may be dislodged by alteration of heart rhythm such as occurs in atrial fibrillation. Impaction takes place at the site of division of peripheral vessels, the majority occurring in the common femoral at the origin of the profunda. Larger thrombi may become arrested at the bifurcation of the aorta. Embolism in the upper limb is less common and rarely produces severe disturbance because of the more adequate collateral circulation. Cerebral embolism is common and when multiple often proves fatal.

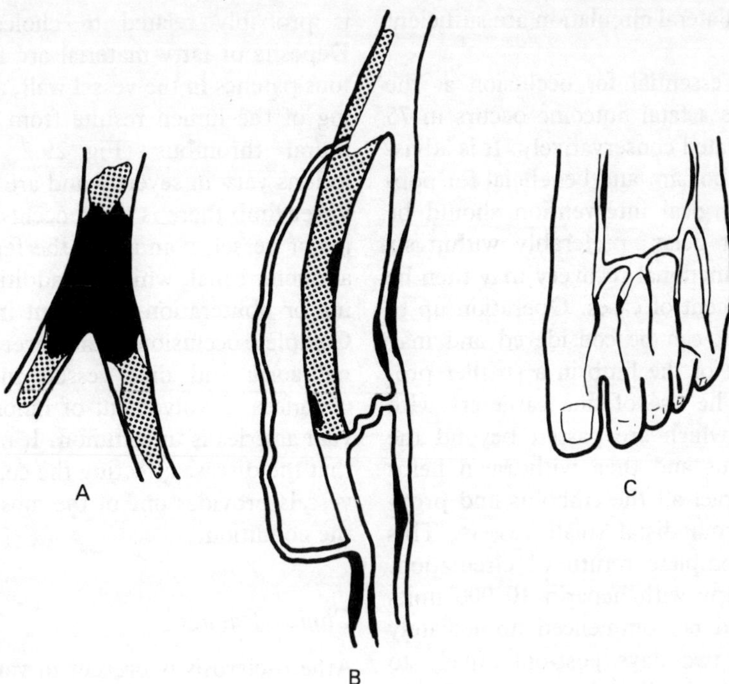

Fig. 29.1 The causes of peripheral arterial occlusion. **A.** Embolism. **B.** Atherosclerosis. **C.** Thrombo-angiitis obliterans in distal vessels.

Obstruction of the circulation produces sudden ischaemia of the affected part, which if not relieved may proceed to gangrene. The degree of ischaemia depends on the efficiency of the collateral circulation, which may also be restricted by arterial spasm initiated by the embolus. Secondary thrombosis occurs in the artery distal to the embolus and may obstruct the collateral circulation still further. In late cases it will also develop proximally.

Clinical features

Pain, pallor and paralysis of the affected limb are the principal symptoms of embolism; they vary considerably in degree and the larger the vessel blocked the greater is the effect. The pain is sudden in onset and usually severe; it results from ischaemia of muscle and nerve. The affected limb becomes pale in the early stages, but after some hours blotchy areas of blue discoloration appear. The level of colour change depends on the site of the embolus and may be helpful in diagnosis. It occurs at the forefoot in popliteal occlusion, at the lower part of the leg in femoral obstruction and in both thighs with aortic bifurcation embolism. The degree of muscular paralysis varies considerably, depending on the efficiency of the collateral circulation. Complete paralysis of the limb is rare and usually only the more distal parts are affected.

The limb appears cold to the touch and loss of sensation is detectable over the distal part. Arterial pulsation is absent in vessels distal to the occlusion, but immediately proximal the pulse becomes exaggerated, a useful point in localisation of the embolus.

Embolism may usually be distinguished from spontaneous arterial thrombosis occurring on an atheromatous plaque by the sudden onset of the former condition.

Treatment

Early diagnosis and treatment are important in saving limb and life. Embolic occlusion of the upper limb vessels and of the smaller leg vessels does not always produce severe ischaemic change of the extremity, and anticoagulant therapy with heparin, and warfarin with conservative measures designed to encourage the collateral circulation are sufficient in most cases.

Embolectomy is essential for occlusion at the aortic bifurcation as a fatal outcome occurs in 75 per cent of cases treated conservatively. It is advisable for femoral embolism, and beneficial for popliteal embolism. Surgical intervention should be undertaken without delay, preferably within six to ten hours; full functional recovery may then be obtained in 85 per cent of cases. Operation up to 48 hours after onset can be considered and may lead to preservation of the limb in a smaller proportion of cases. The use of fine catheters with inflatable balloons which are passed beyond the propagated thrombus and then withdrawn helps considerably to extract all the embolus and propagated thrombus from distal small vessels. This leads to a more complete return of circulation. Anticoagulant therapy with heparin 10 000 units intravenously should be commenced immediately and continued for two days post-operatively to prevent arterial thrombosis. Treatment of any associated cardiac condition is also necessary and long-term anticoagulant therapy plays a significant role in reducing the incidence of recurrent embolism.

ATHEROSCLEROSIS

Pathology

The aetiology of this condition is unknown, but it is probably related to cholesterol metabolism. Deposits of fatty material are found in atheromatous patches in the vessel wall, and further narrowing of the lumen results from the formation of a mural thrombus (Fig. 29.2). The obliterative lesions vary in severity and are widespread. In the lower limb there is often occlusion of a segment of major vessel, commonly the femoral artery in the adductor canal, whilst, in addition, patchy narrowing or obliteration is present in the tibial vessels. Complete occlusion of the lower part of the abdominal aorta and iliac vessels may occur in some instances. Involvement of innominate and subclavian arteries is uncommon. It must be emphasised that the disease affecting the coronary and cerebral vessels provides one of the most serious aspects of the condition.

Clinical features

Atherosclerosis is present in varying degrees in all elderly people. Only in severe cases where the blood flow to the limb is reduced to a critical level does it produce symptoms and these are usually gradual in onset. Sudden deterioration is indicative of thrombosis in a narrowed segment of artery. The development of a satisfactory collateral circulation through muscular branches is sufficient to maintain the leg in a good nutritional state in spite of blockage of the femoral artery over a length of 10 to 15 cm.

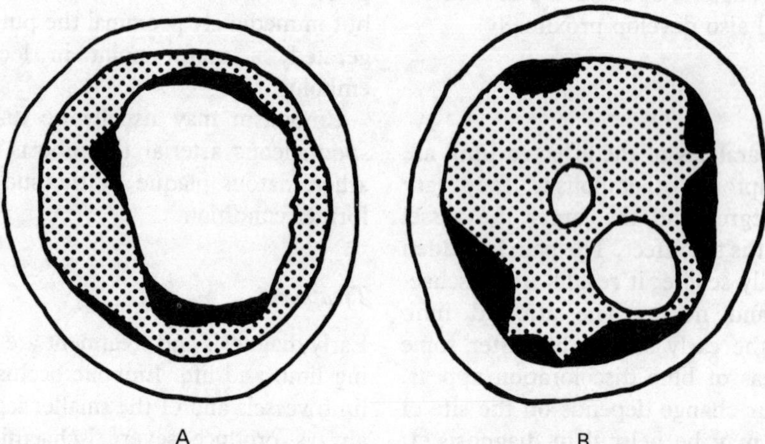

Fig. 29.2 The changes in atherosclerosis. **A.** Atheromatous patches in the intima. **B.** Complete occlusion of artery with recanalisation of thrombus.

Intermittent claudication and coldness of the feet are the commonest presenting symptoms. The former is a condition of severe cramp-like pain produced by walking and relieved by rest. It is generally felt in the calf muscles, but is also experienced in the foot or gluteal region. The walking distance required to produce the pain gradually becomes shorter and may in time prove incapacitating. In many instances this symptom will then improve over several months with the development of a collateral circulation.

Rest pain is a distressing feature. It is often worse at night, causing loss of sleep, and leading to a rapid deterioration of morale. It is indicative of marked ischaemia and is often followed by gangrenous change. Gangrene of a toe is often occasioned by slight trauma or infection or by the sudden obliteration of the artery by thrombosis. It may spread to involve the whole foot and is usually painful. Atherosclerotic gangrene is dry in type and separation of the affected part occurs slowly.

The severity of the ischaemia and the site and extent of the arterial lesion should be assessed. The appearance of pallor on elevation of the limb followed by marked rubor on dependency indicates a fairly severe degree of ischaemia. The temperature of the affected limb may be found to be lower than on the opposite side. The detection of arterial pulsation in femoral, popliteal, anterior and posterior tibial vessels gives valuable information of the level of the obstructive lesion. The presence of a systolic bruit over a vessel indicates partial occlusion, which may also be suggested by the disappearance of ankle pulses after rapid exercise of the legs. This sign is due to deviation of all available blood into the muscles.

Occlusion of the terminal aorta and iliac vessels produces the Leriche syndrome. This is characterised by claudication in the buttocks and thighs, coldness and pallor of the feet, and impotence. Gangrene of the toes and feet occurs in about 30 per cent of cases.

Involvement of the subclavian vessels is followed by pain and colour change in the hands aggravated by use, and usually noticed by workers using the hand above the head.

Careful attention should be given to the condition of the cardiovascular and renal systems, bearing in mind the widespread nature of the disease process and the common association with diabetes.

Investigations

The Doppler ultrasound flow velocity detector is a non-invasive method of determining flow in peripheral vessels and provides a quantitative assessment of vessel patency. Simple probes can be used in clinics and wards. Various refinements of this technique are being developed which enable cross-sectional and lateral scans to be obtained and are particularly applicable to the carotid arteries.

Arteriography performed by the injection of radio-opaque material into the artery is useful in demonstrating the state of the lumen. Irregularity of intimal lining or complete blockage of the vessel may be seen and the extent of the collateral circulation shown. The femoral arteriogram (Fig. 29.3) is most commonly required, but if disease of terminal aorta or iliac vessels is suspected then injection into the aorta becomes necessary. This vessel is punctured by a needle inserted obliquely through the back and passing close to the left side of the vertebral body. The aorta and branches are best demonstrated by retrograde passage of a fine catheter up the femoral and iliac arteries; the tip of the catheter may be accurately positioned in the vessel to be demonstrated. These procedures carry a slight risk of damage to the arterial wall with subsequent thrombosis, and in the case of aortography there is the possibility of renal damage by the injected material.

Measurement of blood flow in the distal part of the limb can be undertaken by *venous occlusion plethysmography*. In this technique obstruction of venous outflow is accompanied by an increase in size of the limb, which can be measured by enclosing it in an airtight measuring chamber, thus indirectly determining the arterial inflow.

The recording of *skin temperatures* of the limb and the vasodilator response to body warming gives information about the skin vessels only; it is not useful in assessing cases of atherosclerosis, but is of value in vasospastic conditions.

Treatment

The slowly progressive nature of this generalised

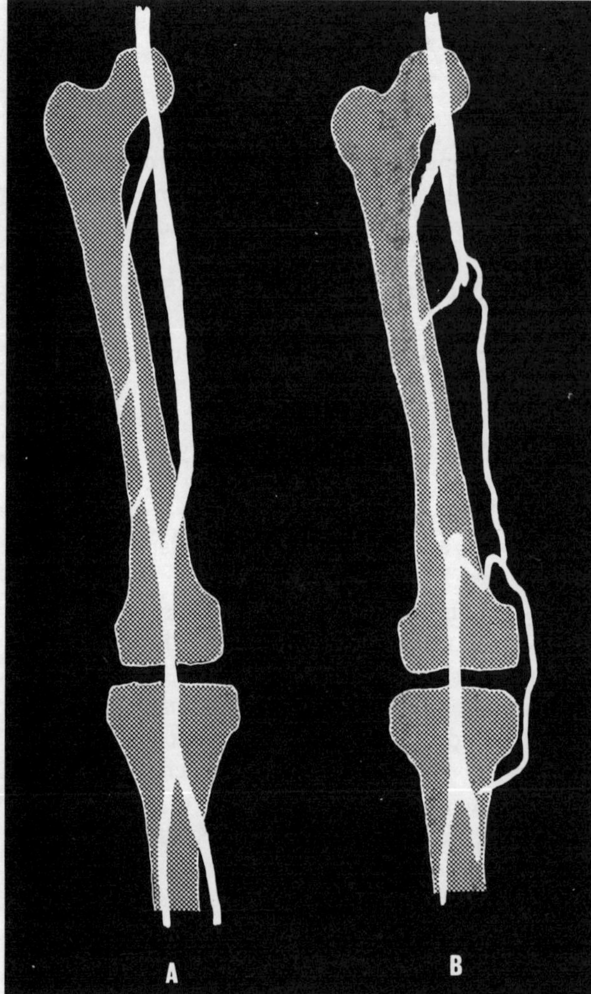

Fig. 29.3 Femoral arteriogram. **A.** Normal. **B.** Occlusion of femoral artery in adductor canal with development of collateral circulation.

disease governs treatment and prognosis. Consideration must always be given to any possible involvement of the coronary and cerebral arteries before advocating major surgery. Attempts at cure of local manifestations are mainly palliative, but much may be done to relieve pain and in some instances preserve a limb. Attention should be directed to improvement in general health and eradication of sepsis. The provision of sound sleep is a valuable therapeutic measure. Careful toilet of the feet is essential and smoking should be discouraged. Vasodilator drugs are prescribed widely but there is no proof that they confer any benefit in increasing peripheral circulation.

The blood flow in the lower limb may be improved by removal of the major vessel obstruction or by increase in the collateral circulation. The latter may be achieved by *sympathectomy*, but the increase in muscle blood flow is insufficient to relieve intermittent claudication. In certain cases of gangrene the blood supply of the skin may be increased sufficiently to allow healing, and rest pain may be relieved, but this result is variable and unpredictable.

The results of direct surgical treatment of the arterial lesion are worthwhile in most instances. *By-pass grafting* is the usual procedure (Fig. 29.4). Alternatively the occluded segment may be recanalised by removing the organised thrombus and intima, a procedure termed *thrombendarterectomy* (Fig. 29.5). This is satisfactory in large vessels, such as the iliac and common femoral, where brisk blood flow prevents post-operative thrombosis, but it is unsuitable for smaller vessels. The diameter of the popliteal artery at the lower end of the endarterectomy may be enlarged by the addition of a patch of saphenous vein. Endarterectomy and reconstruction of the origin of the profunda femoris artery gives good results in carefully selected cases.

Arterial grafts

Excision of the obstructed segment of artery and its replacement by an arterial graft has been practised widely for the femoral vessels, but subsequent thrombosis led to its abandonment. The use of long autogenous saphenous vein by-pass grafts from the common femoral artery to popliteal artery is more satisfactory. Flexible tubing made of Dacron or Teflon is used for the replacement or by-pass of larger vessels such as the iliac artery. Cross-over grafts from one femoral artery to the contralateral artery, or from axillary to femoral artery are used in certain selected instances.

The *selection* of cases for these procedures is critical.

Gangrene of digits and severe pain at rest are definite indications for direct arterial surgery because if successful a major amputation is avoided. Severe intermittent claudication which prevents the patient from following his occupation also justifies surgery. The long-term patency after aorto-iliac reconstruction is about 75 per cent at

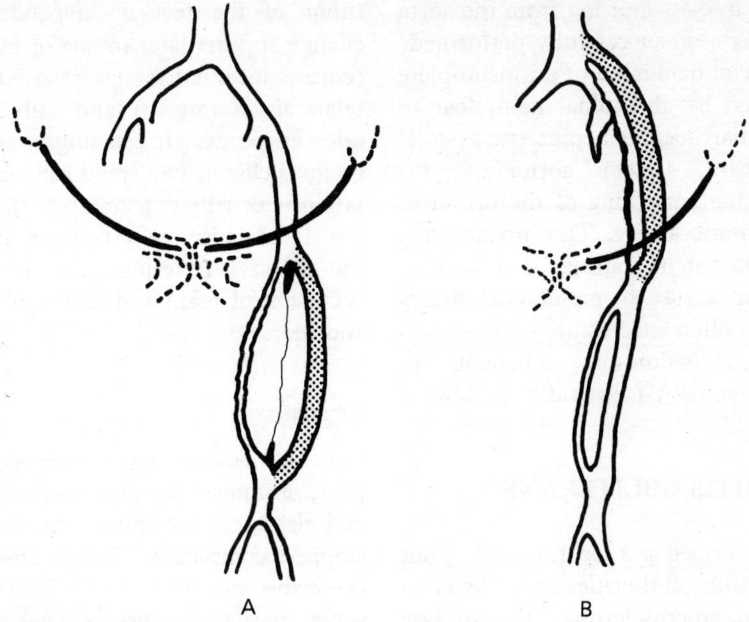

Fig. 29.4 Arterial by-pass graft. **A**. Femoral artery to popliteal artery with vein graft. **B**. Aorta to common femoral artery with synthetic arterial tube prosthesis.

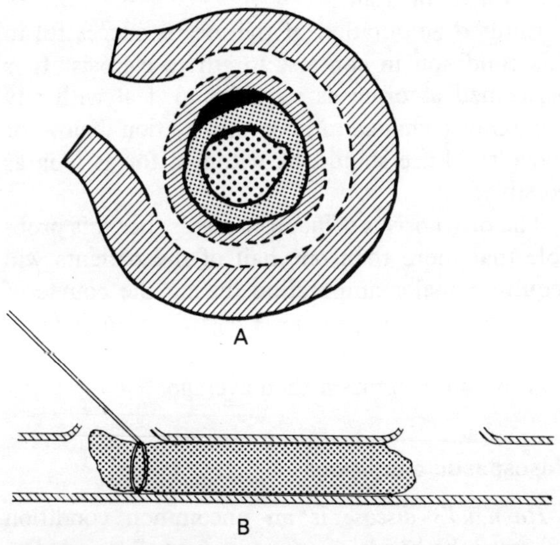

Fig. 29.5 Thrombendarterectomy. **A**. Cross section of artery showing plane of separation in tunica media. **B**. Longitudinal view of artery showing two openings through which the occlusion is removed.

five years, but carries an operative mortality of 5 per cent. The mortality of femoro-popliteal reconstruction is lower, being about 1 to 2 per cent, but the five-year patency is 40 to 50 per cent.

Amputation

Gangrene of the foot not responding to the above measures will, in most cases, necessitate mid-thigh amputation. Preservation of more of the limb may be successful in certain carefully selected cases if the collateral circulation to the leg or knee is good. Gangrene associated with *diabetes* is largely infective in nature but distal small vessel thrombosis occurs. The major arterial supply is often good and limited amputation of the toes or part of the foot is successful if combined with control of both diabetes and infection.

Special sites of occlusion

Internal carotid artery occlusion is usually heralded by transient disturbance of vision or speech and hemiparesis. The treatment of incomplete occlusion at this stage by thrombendarterectomy gives good results.

Renal artery stenosis, which may lead to the development of hypertension, may be diagnosed by auscultation of a bruit in the back and confirmed by aortography and detailed renal function tests.

Endarterectomy or by-pass grafting from the aorta or splenic artery has been successfully performed.

Mesenteric arterial occlusion of an incomplete type is characterised by abdominal pain, fear of food, wasting and diarrhoea. An epigastric systolic bruit may be heard. Lateral aortography is required to define the narrowing of the origin of the superior mesenteric artery. Thrombendarterectomy and venous patch grafting or a by-pass venous graft from aorta to mesenteric artery beyond the block is often successful.

Coronary artery occlusion may be benefited in selected cases by venous by-pass grafts (p. 128).

THROMBOANGIITIS OBLITERANS

This condition is described as a separate entity, but it is contended by some authorities that this is an early form of local atherosclerosis. The disease affects a young age group and may pursue a rapid course to gangrene of toes or leg, but there is a tendency to spontaneous improvement with advancing years. It is rare in women.

Pathology

No definite aetiological agent is known. Excessive smoking aggravates the condition by causing arterial spasm; a possible relationship to fungal infection of the feet has been suggested. The large and small vessels of the limb are involved by a process of intimal thickening and thrombosis. Characteristically this also involves the vein and the whole neurovascular bundle becomes included in a well-marked fibrotic reaction. Recanalisation of the arterial thrombus is a pronounced feature. The condition may be confined to the small vessels of the toes and feet for some years before affecting the major limb vessels.

Clinical features

Pain in the toes and feet is a prominent feature; it may be severe at rest, particularly at night or may occur with exercise. Fibrotic involvement of the nerve accounts for a certain amount of pain. Thrombosis of superficial veins of the feet and legs is an early sign and is accompanied by well-marked rubor of the feet on dependency. Gangrenous change appears later in one or more toes and often remains localised for long periods. It is frequently bilateral. Remission and subsequent relapse is often encountered. The fingers are affected by gangrenous change in a small proportion of cases. Pulsation is usually detectable in the femoral arteries, but distal pulses may become obliterated early in the disease. Arteriography demonstrates patchy occlusion of main and collateral vessels in the leg and foot.

Treatment

General measures which improve nutrition, relieve pain, promote sleep and eradicate sepsis in the feet and elsewhere are important. Smoking should be stopped completely. Vasodilator drugs are often prescribed but their efficacy is doubtful. During an acute phase of the disease when thrombosis is predominating the use of anticoagulant therapy for about six weeks may limit spread. The results of sympathectomy are variable, but if pain is severe it is worthy of trial.

Limited amputation of the toes is successful in this condition in contrast to atherosclerosis. It is performed as often as required to deal with any gangrenous change. Major amputation below or above the knee should be withheld for as long as possible.

The prognosis is difficult to assess, but it is probable that more than one half of the patients will require a major amputation during the course of their disease. The prognosis regarding life is fairly good, cardiac and cerebral thrombosis being only slightly more common than average.

Vasospastic conditions

Raynaud's disease is an uncommon condition affecting the hands of young women. There is frequently an inherited predisposition; the disease may be initiated by childbirth, infection or emotional upset, and there may be a neuro-endocrine factor. The disease is vasospastic and has been attributed to intermittent active closure of the small arteries of the fingers. The underlying fault is a local hypersensitivity to cold. Organic narrowing or closure of the digital vessels develops in the later stages. The attacks are usually precipitated by cold or emotional disturbance and are characterised by blanching of the digits followed by blueness and pain, and later by redness. Sclerodactyly and patches of gangrene or ulcers appear on the finger-tips after some years. Treatment involves protection from cold and administration of vasodilator drugs. Reserpine (0.25 mg twice daily) and tri-iodothyronine (20 μg four times daily) give benefit in a proportion of cases. Sympathectomy is followed by partial or complete relief of symptoms and is advised when the attacks of pain are incapacitating and for the presence of ulcers.

Raynaud's phenomenon is a wider term, embracing all cases in which there are intermittent colour changes in the hands and fingers. It includes Raynaud's disease and is also seen in association with exposure to severe cold, repeated vibrational injury, collagen disease, obliterative vascular disease and ergot poisoning.

Chronic pernio (chilblains). This condition develops as a response to cold and is characterised by purple blotches on the fingers and toes, ulceration occurring in severe cases. Histological appearances are of fat necrosis and giant-cell formation. Protection from cold is essential as a preventive measure. Vitamin D or tolazoline may relieve the condition. Lumbar sympathectomy is often beneficial for the chronic case with severe leg involvement.

ANEURYSM

Aetiology

An aneurysm is a localised dilatation of an artery resulting from weakness of its wall. With the decline of syphilis atherosclerosis is now the commonest cause. Atherosclerotic degeneration of the whole of the arterial wall may give rise to a spindle-shaped enlargement of *fusiform* type. Localised weakness of part of the wall may produce a *saccular* form. Thrombosis in the aneurysm occurs to some extent in each type. The common site for this lesion is the abdominal aorta, below the origin of the renal vessels (Fig. 29.6). The aneurysm is usually saccular in shape and gradually enlarging may become 10 to 12 cm in diameter. Extension may be in an anterior or posterior direction, the latter producing vertebral erosion. Rupture at its posterior border near the spinal column is a frequent complication.

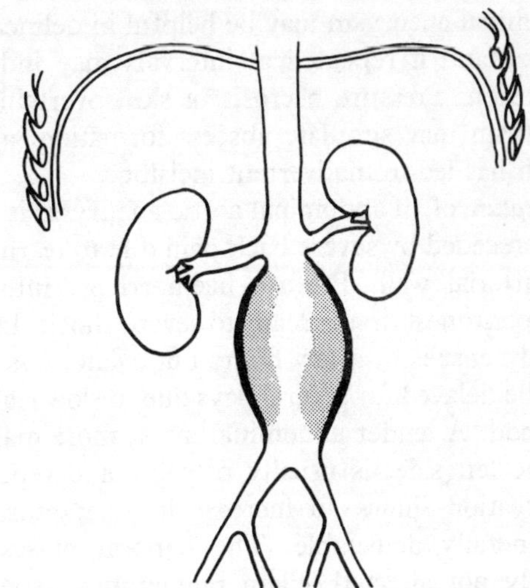

Fig. 29.6 Saccular aneurysm of abdominal aorta with partial thrombosis

A *traumatic* aneurysm is usually a false type with the development of a sac in the haematoma surrounding a damaged artery.

A *mycotic* aneurysm follows weakening of the arterial wall from infection. This may be the result of an infected embolus in bacterial endocarditis or of the artery lying in an abscess cavity.

A *post-stenotic* aneurysm is the result of weakening of the wall of an artery, produced by the increased lateral stress immediately distal to a constriction. It is encountered in relationship to a cervical rib, in which situation embolism in the upper limb may arise from a mural thrombus.

Clinical features

The presence of an expansile swelling, at times asymptomatic but usually painful, is characteristic. Pain is a prominent feature if nerves or bone are compressed. A thrill may be palpable and a bruit audible over the swelling. In the diagnosis of an abdominal aortic aneurysm care must be taken to differentiate it from a swelling showing transmitted pulsation from a normal underlying aorta. Vascular malignant tumours may occasionally appear pulsatile, but proximal arterial occlusion will not lead to diminution in size of the swelling, which is a feature of an aneurysm. Ultrasonic scanning of an abdominal aneurysm may be helpful in delineating its size and if repeated at intervals may indicate expansion. Pressure necrosis of skin overlying an aneurysm may simulate abscess formation, a fact which has led to inadvertent incision.

Rupture of an abdominal aortic aneurysm is usually preceded by severe back pain due to tearing of the arterial wall. Profuse haemorrhage into the retroperitoneal tissues leads to severe shock. Death usually ensues in a few hours but a fatal outcome may be delayed for several days due to slow leakage of blood. A tender abdominal mass, more marked on the left side, is usually palpable and repeated observation shows an increase in size; pulsation is generally detectable. The femoral pulses are usually not affected. Plain radiographs generally show the outline of the aneurysm, calcification in its walls being commonly present.

The thoracic aortic aneurysm is generally syphilitic. It may involve the arch of the aorta or innominate artery and produces chest pain due to pressure on surrounding structures. Oesophageal involvement may cause dysphagia, whilst hoarseness may result from recurrent laryngeal nerve pressure.

Treatment

Complete excision of the aneurysm and replacement by a synthetic woven arterial prosthesis is the ideal procedure. In the thoracic region this presents many problems which have been overcome to some extent by the use of hypothermia, which allows temporary cessation of blood flow to the brain and spinal cord. The maintenance of circulation by temporary by-pass tubes may also be employed while the aneurysm is being excised. Excision of an abdominal aortic aneurysm below the renal vessels presents less difficulty and is the accepted form of treatment (Fig. 29.7). It should be undertaken when pain is a prominent symptom and for all aneurysms over 7 cm in width. Resection and grafting of ruptured aneurysm should be undertaken in all cases if the age and general condition allow because the untreated condition is fatal. Operative mortality is about 10 per cent for unruptured cases but rises to 50 per cent for those ruptured.

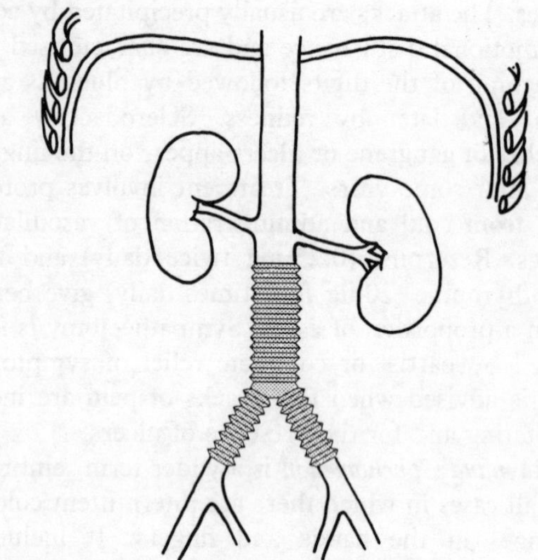

Fig. 29.7 Dacron or Teflon prosthesis inserted after excision of aortic aneurysm

An aneurysm of a peripheral vessel is preferably treated by excision and graft replacement if the general condition of the patient permits.

Dissecting aneurysm

Dissecting aneurysm is an uncommon but generally fatal condition. Separation of the layers of the arterial wall occurs by the passage of blood through an atheromatous ulcer or intimal tear, with permeation in the medial layer. This process usually commences in the ascending portion of the aorta and may spread through the thoracic and abdominal segments but it may also arise in the iliac arteries. It is commonly associated with degeneration of the medial layer. Separation for several centimetres occurs, and the blood under pressure may block peripheral vessels, such as the renal, mesenteric or iliac arteries.

The outcome is generally fatal from rupture or renal failure, but natural cures have resulted from extravasated blood bursting back into the aortic lumen at a lower level, forming a 'double-barrelled' aorta. Surgical treatment by thoracotomy and closure of the internal tear or graft insertion should be undertaken in selected cases with the assistance of a heart lung machine and circulatory arrest. Drug treatment of the associated hypertension is required post-operatively.

VENOUS SYSTEM

Varicose veins

Varicose dilatation occurs in the veins of the anal canal, oesophagus and lower limb, but the term varicose veins is generally applied to the last, which will be considered here.

Anatomy

The long saphenous vein commences at the medial end of the dorsal venous arch of the foot (Fig. 29.8). It passes in front of the medial malleolus, ascends the leg in the subcutaneous tissue just behind the medial border of the tibia to the posteromedial aspect of the knee and then along the medial side of the thigh. It perforates the deep fascia at the saphenous opening and terminates in the femoral vein. Several tributaries enter from the subcutaneous tissues of the leg and thigh, the most constant being the posterior arch vein of the calf which is often in communication with the short saphenous vein. The superficial circumflex iliac, epigastric and external pudendal veins join the saphenous vein near its termination, whilst the deep external pudendal vein enters it deep to the saphenous opening.

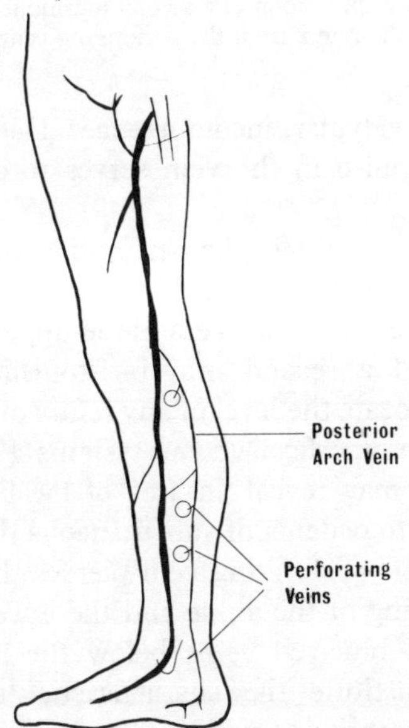

Fig. 29.8 Long saphenous vein with tributaries and perforating veins

Connections with the anterior and posterior tibial and femoral veins occur through branches which perforate the deep fascia. Three ankle perforating veins are present which join the posterior tibial veins with the posterior arch vein. The middle perforating vein is generally the largest. Other perforating veins are found just below the knee, in the lower part of the adductor canal and in the middle of the calf. Inconstant perforating veins are present on the lateral aspect of the ankle.

Blood flow from the leg at rest is slow and is maintained by the arterial pressure and by the negative pressure of the great thoracic veins on respiration. Elevation of the lower limb speeds up the flow to some extent. Exercise produces a marked increase, occasioned by the action of the calf muscles enclosed in a dense fibrous sheath. The soleus muscle contains several large venous spaces which join the posterior tibial and peroneal veins; compression of these by the muscle constitutes an efficient pump action. Blood flow in the deep veins is thus accelerated, the flow from the superficial veins taking place mainly via the perforating veins and aided by the presence of valves at these sites. Reflux outwards only occurs when the valves are damaged.

The venous pressure in the superficial veins in the erect position is equal to the height of a column of blood to the heart. Exercise results in a rapid lowering of the pressure in the superficial veins, the pressure in the deep veins fluctuating widely. Destruction of the valves of the perforating veins or of the long saphenous vein at the groin prevents the pump action, and the pressure in the superficial veins then remains high on exercise.

The short saphenous vein begins at the lateral side of the foot, passes up the posterior aspect of the calf and ends in the popliteal vein. It also receives several tributaries and communicates with deep veins on the lateral side of the tendo calcaneus.

Pathology

Varicosity of the superficial veins of the lower limb may be primary or secondary to an underlying cause. The aetiology of *primary* varices is uncertain, but a familial tendency is often present. The vein wall becomes thinner and loses its elastic fibres. Localised dilatations occur rendering the valves incompetent and leading to persistently high pressure of blood in the vein which causes further dilatation. *Secondary* varices may be due to increased intra-abdominal pressure from a tumour or pregnant uterus, whilst compensatory dilatation of the superficial veins may be seen as a result of persistent thrombosis in the deep veins. An arteriovenous fistula of congenital or traumatic origin usually leads to the development of varices.

Incompetence of the deep valves and perforating vein valves most frequently results from their destruction by thrombosis followed by recanalisation. The resulting development of a high-pressure leak into the superficial veins leads to marked varices and secondary changes in the subcutaneous tissues and skin, often followed by ulceration (p. 430).

Clinical features

The principal symptom is a dull aching pain in the calf aggravated by standing and becoming more severe at the end of the day. Enlargement and tortuosity of the saphenous vein usually commences in the leg where it may form a localised swelling, the distension later involving the thigh veins. Women often complain of the unsightly appearance and of blue dilated skin venules. Enlargement of the vein at the saphenous opening may produce a soft swelling, often 2 cm in diameter, which has a well-marked cough impulse and empties on recumbency.

Examination of the patient in the erect position will define the segment of vein involved. Attention should be given to the short saphenous vein on the lateral side of the leg and in the popliteal space. The degree of competence of the valves in the saphenous and perforating veins is determined by careful inspection and palpation of the leg. Numerous tests are described to demonstrate the efficiency of the venous valves. The Trendelenburg test gives information on the valves in the long saphenous system (Fig. 29.9). It is performed by emptying the vein by limb elevation and then occluding it at the saphenous opening. The presence of retrograde filling from above on resuming the upright posture and removing the tourniquet

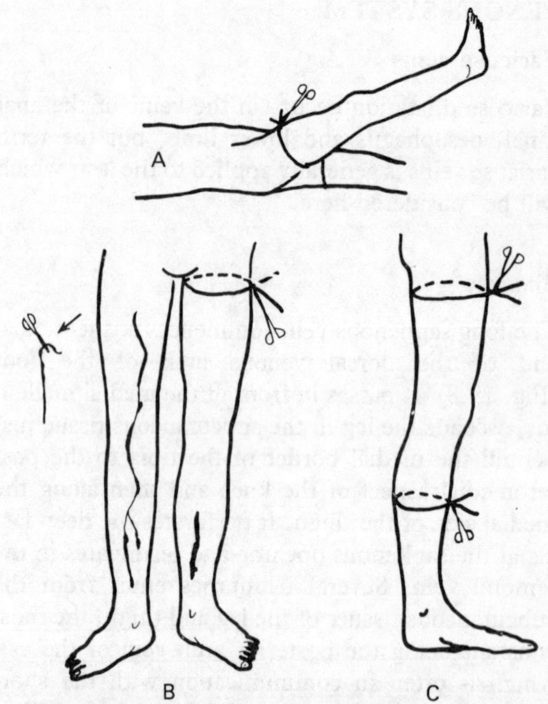

Fig. 29.9 Trendelenburg test for varicose veins: **A.** Leg elevated and saphenous vein then occluded in thigh with rubber tourniquet (both limbs). **B.** Removal of rubber tourniquet (T) on right side allows free retrograde filling of saphenous vein demonstrating incompetence of valves. Filling of veins in lower half of left leg has occurred from perforating veins. **C.** The application of a second tourniquet on left leg will control the reflux from the perforating veins.

indicates valvular incompetence. Detection of a cough impulse in the vein serves to confirm this finding.

Deficient valves in the perforating veins are best demonstrated by the use of a rubber tourniquet to occlude the saphenous vein in the upper part of the thigh, and a second movable tourniquet which serves to locate the level of any reflux of blood from the deep to superficial venous systems (Fig. 29.9,C). Palpation may reveal an area of localised tenderness, due to oedema of subcutaneous tissues at the position the perforating vein pierces the deep fascia. Swelling of the ankle and the development of superficial blue-red veins below the medial malleolus constitute the characteristic 'ankle flare' found in association with incompetence of the perforating veins. It may be followed by ulceration.

Patency of the deep venous channels may be demonstrated by the application of a tourniquet to the thigh to occlude the superficial veins. Subsequent exercise makes the veins less conspicuous and softer due to the action of the muscular calf pump; pain and increased swelling of the veins indicates occlusion of the deep channels. Phlebography may occasionally be necessary to demonstrate the patency of the deep venous system. It also serves to outline perforating veins. It is performed by the injection of radio-opaque material into a vein on the dorsum of the foot.

Complications

Oedema of the lower leg and ankle may be slight in association with primary veins. It is often marked in the presence of incompetent ankle perforating veins, the subcutaneous tissues becoming hard and indurated. *Pigmentation* and *eczema* are also more pronounced with patent ankle perforating veins. Both conditions are precursors of *ulcer* formation, which usually commences on the medial aspect of the lower third of the leg but may extend around the limb. *Haemorrhage* from rupture of a distended varix is common and often profuse until controlled by elevation and pressure. *Superficial phlebitis* is accompanied by localised thrombosis of the superficial veins over a variable area. Marked pain and tenderness are present with reddening of the overlying skin. The thrombophlebitis may extend to the saphenous opening, but only rarely is it followed by thrombosis of the femoral vein or pulmonary embolism.

Treatment

Elastic stockings may be used to provide relief of symptoms in patients unfit for or unwilling to undergo operative treatment, and are useful for the control of varicose veins secondary to pregnancy.

Injection treatment is suitable for the milder varicosities and can be used for the more extensive condition as an alternative to operation. The aim of treatment is to convert the vein into a solid fibrous cord and also cause occlusion of the perforating veins. Sodium tetradecyl sulphate is injected at three or four sites into the vein which is emptied by elevation of the limb. Pressure pads and elastic bandages are applied from foot to thigh and covered by an elastic stocking for a period of about six weeks. It is essential to walk at least two miles daily to develop the musculo-fascial calf pump and encourage good flow in the deep veins.

Surgical treatment provides the most satisfactory means of controlling varicosities and is indicated when the valves are incompetent. The saphenous vein is divided at its termination, care being taken to interrupt all tributaries in the area, thus preventing their subsequent enlargement and the consequent recurrence of varicose veins through collateral channels. The procedure of *stripping* the long saphenous vein in a part or the whole of its course is widely employed; it destroys the principal superficial venous channel, but may not result in division of the perforating veins. If these have been shown to be incompetent they should be carefully marked before operation and divided at the opening in the deep fascia. Recurrence after operation may follow the enlargement of small veins left undisturbed in the initial procedure or failure to divide communications with the deep veins. Injection therapy as outlined above proves very satisfactory in the treatment of such recurrence.

Deep venous thrombosis

Thrombosis in the veins of the calf, thigh and pelvis are common complications of many diseases and may follow childbirth and operation. The condition may cause sudden death by embolism or lead to the development of the post-phlebitic syndrome with distressing swelling of the leg and ulcer formation.

Clinical features

The condition may arise insidiously in patients with malignant disease, cardio-respiratory disease or any chronic debilitating illness, or may follow operation or injury. Slight calf pain may be the only complaint, associated with localised tenderness and on careful measurement slight swelling of the ankle may be detected. Massive venous thrombosis is characterised by the sudden onset of severe pain and marked swelling of the whole lower limb which becomes dusky blue in colour and may be very tender.

The detection of venous thrombosis in the post-operative period requires constant awareness of the problem. Early diagnosis is essential to lower the incidence of pulmonary embolism. Repeated careful examination of the leg is important but only 50 per cent of cases are thus diagnosed and ancillary aids are useful. Ascending phlebography of calf, thigh and pelvic veins is accurate but requires specialised radiology. Fibrinogen labelled with radioactive ^{125}I is incorporated into the thrombi and can be detected by an external scintillating counter. The use of ultrasonic recordings of venous flow provides a simpler diagnostic test but it probably is useful only for main vein thrombosis.

Treatment

The use of anticoagulant therapy is described on page 43. Thrombectomy may be undertaken through an incision in the femoral vein and extraction of the clot performed using inflatable balloon catheters. Plication of the inferior vena cava by clamps or suture is indicated in certain cases of recurrent embolism.

Venous ulceration

An ulcer on the medial aspect of the lower third of the leg, so often labelled 'varicose', is usually the sequel of deep venous thrombosis. It is the result of persistently high venous pressure in the tissues following destruction of the venous valves (p. 428). The exact mechanism of the ulceration is not known, but it is suggested that deposition of an impermeable fibrin cuff around dermal capillaries is caused by prolonged venous hypertension. This leads to a condition of liposclerosis which progresses to dermal ulceration, often initiated by minor injury. The role of dilated perforating veins in aggravating the venous hypertension should be stressed (Fig. 29.10).

A history of previous venous thrombosis, occurring in child-birth or following operation or chronic illness, may be obtained. Examination reveals swelling of the leg with hard non-pitting oedema and areas of blue discoloration. The ulcers, which are often painful, vary considerably in size from a few millimetres to several centimetres, and are most frequently situated just above the medial malleolus but may extend to encircle the limb. The patency of the deep veins should be tested and the

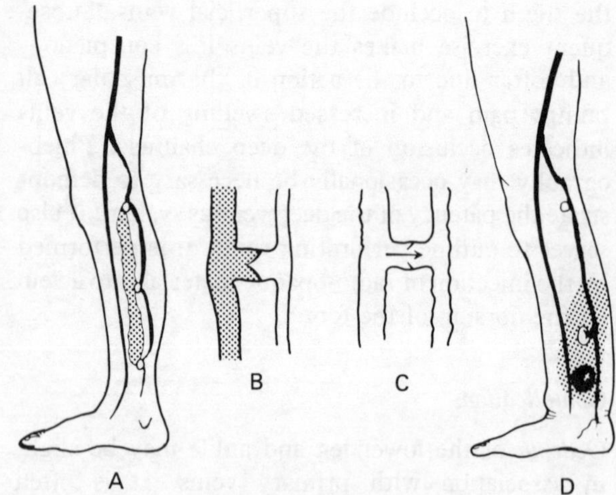

Fig. 29.10 The stages in development of venous ulceration. **A.** Thrombosis of deep venous channels. **B.** Thrombosis of deep vein spreads to perforating vein and destroys its valve. **C.** Free reflux now occurs through the perforating vein from deep to superficial veins. **D.** The enlarged incompetent perforating veins result in oedema of the leg, an ulcer and dilatation of superficial veins.

presence of any perforating veins sought. The middle ankle perforating vein is the most commonly affected. The differential diagnosis includes ulceration occurring in arterial insufficiency and hypertension. Syphilis and tuberculosis are now rare causes. Neoplastic ulceration should be excluded by biopsy.

Treatment

Healing of the ulcer is obtained by lowering the venous back pressure on the subcutaneous tissues. It occurs with bed rest, but this is not always a practicable procedure and relapse is common on resuming the erect posture. *Supportive bandaging* is the most satisfactory treatment and if applied competently from toes to thigh will reduce oedema and aid healing. Localised pressure over the medial ankle perforating veins may be increased by inclusion of a sponge-rubber pad under the bandage. The webbing elastic bandage is most satisfactory for the co-operative patient, but if not applied correctly is of no value. An occlusive bandage of Elastoplast or Viscopaste applied for 10 to 14 days proves more satisfactory in other cases. Physiotherapy helps considerably in dispersing oedema and improving ankle movements. Local applications should be carefully chosen, castor oil and thin zinc cream being most satisfactory. Antibiotic ointment should be avoided as it may lead to skin sensitisation and a worsening of the condition.

Surgical management by division of the saphenous and perforating veins is indicated where these are shown to be incompetent. A long incision near the medial border of the tibia is required to expose all the perforating veins, which are divided in the subfascial plane. Excision and skin grafting of the ulcer may be necessary if the condition has been present for many years. Post-operative supportive bandaging and the permanent use of elastic stockings is usually advisable to prevent the recurrence of ulceration in these cases. Stanozolol may benefit some patients.

Axillary vein thrombosis

Spontaneous thrombosis of the axillary vein tends to occur in young men engaged in strenuous occupations, arising most frequently after rowing or using the arm in the abducted position. It is probably initiated by minor damage to small tributaries. Insidious swelling and blueness of the whole upper limb is accompanied by distension of the superficial veins. Response to anticoagulant therapy is generally good if treatment is continued for at least five weeks.

LYMPHATIC SYSTEM

Chronic lymphoedema

Obstruction of the lymphatics results in swelling due to the accumulation of interstitial fluid. Chronic lymphoedema can be divided into primary and secondary types.

Primary lymphoedema is due to congenital maldevelopment of the lymphatic trunks and particularly affects the lower limb. In most instances hypoplasia of the ducts is responsible.

The condition is of insidious onset and occurs more commonly in women, often commencing at puberty. The distal part of the leg is first affected and initially may be temporarily relieved by elevation, but in the later stages the whole limb becomes grossly oedematous. Discomfort from heaviness and an unsightly appearance are the main complaints. Recurrent cellulitis and thickening of the skin may develop. Lymphography demonstrates the exact form of maldevelopment, the outlook being better where hypoplasia alone exists.

Treatment in mild cases consists of the application of strong, well-fitting elastic stockings during the day, elevation of the foot of the bed by 30 cm at night and courses of diuretics. Severe cases with functional impairment require surgical treatment. The buried dermis flap operation is suitable for most cases and re-routes the lymph from the dermal plexus towards the deep lymphatic trunks.

Secondary lymphoedema is the result of inflammatory or neoplastic involvement of the lymphatics or the nodes. It may also occur after their surgical extirpation in block dissection of axilla or groin or treatment with radiotherapy. Parasitic lymphoedema is due to the presence of filaria in the lymphatics. Secondary lymphoedema appears more rapidly than the primary form, and the inflammatory type may be associated with recurrent infection in the skin, generally streptococcal in orgin. Lymphography demonstrates the site of obstruction and hence differentiates primary and secondary forms. Oedema of venous origin may be distinguished by venography.

Prolonged antibiotic therapy may be necessary in inflammatory lymphoedema and simple measures of massage, elevation and support by elastic stockings should be prescribed intially in neoplastic forms. When the causative disease is inactive, plastic surgery similar to that required in primary lymphoedema can be undertaken.

LYMPH NODE ENLARGEMENT

The detection of enlarged lymph nodes presents many problems in diagnosis. Careful attention should be paid to the clinical history and general examination, aided by specific investigations of the blood and by radiology. In most instances histological examination of the lymph node will be necessary to establish the correct diagnosis.

Lymph node enlargement may be due to the following conditions:

Inflammation—
- Acute
- Chronic

Tumour—
- Lymphosarcoma
- Secondary deposit

Reticuloses—
- Lymphoma (Hodgkin's disease)
- Leukaemia.

INFLAMMATION

Acute infection is often followed by painful enlargement of the regional lymph nodes. It may be associated with the characteristic red streaks of lymphangitis. Intensive antibiotic therapy may produce resolution, but suppuration and abscess formation require surgical drainage. *Infective mononucleosis* is characterised by painful enlargement of the lymph nodes of neck and axilla associated with malaise and fever. The white blood count and Paul-Bunnell reaction may help in the diagnosis.

Chronic inflammation may be the result of non-specific infection, tuberculous or syphilitic disease or lymphogranuloma inguinale. In the non-specific form infection is generally present in the area of lymph node drainage. Improvement occurs with removal of the cause, although antibiotic therapy may be required.

Tuberculous lymphadenitis is generally encountered in the cervical, mediastinal or mesenteric regions. Cervical and mesenteric involvement result from infection with the bovine organism in a poorly nourished child. The incidence is rapidly diminishing due to pasteurisation of milk, improved living conditions and general eradication of tuberculosis.

The lymph node is infected from a primary focus situated in the mouth, pharynx, lung or bowel. It shows the characteristic changes of an accumulation of round cells and giant cells followed by caseation. Tubercle bacilli may be seen on a suitably stained section of node and can be isolated by culture. The nodes surrounded by inflammatory exudate and fibrosis become adherent to adjacent structures. An abscess may form and point on to the skin or discharge into a bronchus. A sinus track from a caseating gland can persist and secondary infection is then common. The diagnosis may be made by the aspiration of pus and culture of the tubercle bacillus on Lowenstein medium.

The clinical features and treatment are discussed under the region involved.

Syphilitic lymphadenitis is encountered as a painless rubbery enlargement of nodes draining the area of the primary chancre and is most frequently seen in the groin. Widespread involvement of small discrete nodes in the neck, axilla and groin is found in the secondary stage. A serological test should always be performed in cases of generalised lymphadenopathy.

Lymphogranuloma inguinale results from a virus infection of venereal origin and is encountered most commonly in Negro races. The primary lesion consists of small vesicles on the genitalia. Three to six weeks later brawny enlargement of the inguinal lymph nodes develops, followed by their breakdown and sinus formation. In the female lymphatic spread from vulva to perirectal tissue leads to the development of a rectal stricture. The diagnosis is confirmed by the intradermal injection of a specific antigen (Frei test). Antibiotics provide the most satisfactory form of treatment.

TUMOURS

Primary tumours of lymphatic origin may be classified into lymphosarcoma and reticulum-cell sarcoma. Many other forms are described with only slight variations, some bearing a relationship with the reticulosis group.

Lymphosarcoma occurs mainly in middle age with male predominance. The cervical, mediastinal and abdominal lymph nodes are most commonly affected, but widespread involvement is usual. Marked enlargement of a group of nodes is characteristic. The histological appearance is of masses of round cells resembling lymphocytes. Widespread visceral metastasis occurs. Treatment consists of irradiation of localised masses and chemotherapy (p. 440) for the diffuse lesions. The prognosis is generally poor.

Reticulum-cell sarcoma is uncommon and

occurs most often in a cervical lymph node, spread to adjacent nodes taking place moderately quickly. Diagnosis is established after biopsy. Radiotherapy offers reasonable hope of regression for a number of years.

Secondary neoplasm. Metastasis from a malignant lesion is one of the commonest causes of lymph node enlargement. It may be the presenting feature in certain sites, such as the pharynx. One or more nodes may be enlarged, but widespread lymphatic involvement is uncommon. The node is characteristically hard and initially mobile, but subsequent fixation and breakdown with skin ulceration may occur. The detection of a hard discrete lymph node should lead to careful examination and investigation for a primary tumour in the appropriate lymphatic drainage area. The treatment of metastatic lymph nodes is considered under the regional sections and may be by surgical, radiotherapeutic, chemotherapeutic or hormonal methods.

RETICULOSES

Lymphoma (Hodgkin's disease)

Pathology

The aetiology of this condition which affects the reticulo-endothelial system is not known. It is classified as a malignant condition affecting the reticulum cell with a tendency to form giant cell systems; the presence of Reed-Sternberg cells is characteristic. The lymph nodes usually enlarge in groups, the cervical area being most commonly affected. They are of soft rubbery consistency, later becoming matted together with fibrous tissue. Involvement of other tissues may occur, the spleen, kidney, liver and bone being principally affected. Four types are recognised histologically. The *lymphocytic predominant* and *nodular sclerosing* carry a favourable prognosis. The *mixed cellularity* have an intermediate outlook and the *lymphocytic depleted* have a bad prognosis.

Clinical features

Males are more commonly affected, with a peak incidence at 25 and 70 years. Painless enlargement of the lymph nodes is noticed, but pain can be induced by ingestion of alcohol. Pressure of nodes on bronchi, bile ducts and spinal cord may produce characteristic appropriate symptoms and signs. Systemic symptoms of pruritus, irregular fever, general malaise and weight loss are present in certain cases. Anaemia may become evident as the disease progresses with development of thrombocytopenia.

Diagnosis depends on histological examination of an enlarged lymph node and biospy should be performed at an early stage in suspected cases. Establishment of the precise extent of the disease leads to the following staging:

- Stage I — Involvement of single lymph node region or single extra-lymphatic site.
- Stage II — Involvement of two or more lymph node areas on the same side of the diaphragm or extra-lymphatic site and lymph node region on same side of diaphragm.
- Stage III — Involvement of lymph node regions on both sides of diaphragm and may be accompanied by extra-lymphatic or splenic involvement.
- Stage IV — Diffuse involvement of extra-lymphatic sites with or without lymph node enlargement.

Careful clinical examination, chest radiography and abdominal lymphography will outline the main lymph node areas. Liver function tests, liver and splenic isotope scans and CT scanning may help in determining abdominal disease but establishment of splenic involvement is difficult. Laparotomy with splenectomy for accurate staging is therefore performed. It will also allow the histological diagnosis of hepatic deposits and intra-abdominal lymph node enlargement. Clinical staging was found to be altered as a result of laparotomy in about 50 per cent of cases in some series thus allowing more radical therapy with improved results.

Treatment

Localised Hodgkin's disease is best treated by radiotherapy. Lesions above the diaphragm are treated by irradiation of the neck, axillae and mediastinum. Irradiation below the diaphragm involves the para-aortic, pelvic and inguinal regions. The result of treatment of Stage I and II lesions is good, 80 per cent living over five years, and there is hope that a significant proportion are cured.

Chemotherapy is the appropriate treatment for widespread disease (Stage III and IV). The agents usually employed are the nitrogen mustard drugs, vinca alkaloids and procarbazine. When used alone remission occurs in about 25 per cent of patients. Combination of all drugs with prednisolone in repeated courses has given remission in 80 per cent of cases with encouraging results at five years.

Leukaemia

Acute and chronic forms must occasionally be considered in surgical diagnosis. Fever, pharyngeal ulceration, anaemia and purpura are encountered in the *acute* form and blood examination determines the type. In the *chronic* form, glandular enlargement, left upper abdominal pain due to splenic infarction, haemorrhage or leukaemic skin or bone nodules may be noted. Blood and sternal marrow examination confirms the diagnosis.

FURTHER READING

Dodd, H. and Cockett, F. B. (1976). *The Pathology and Surgery of the Veins of the Lower Limb*. 2nd ed. Edinburgh: Churchill Livingstone.

Horton, R. E. (1980). *Vascular Surgery*. London: Hodder and Stoughton.

Irving, M. (1979). The surgery of Hodgkin' disease. In *Surgical Review I*. Eds. Lumley J. S. P. and Craven, J. L. London: Pitman.

Jamieson, C. (1982). *The Surgical Management of Vascular Disease*. London: Heinemann.

Kester, R. C. and Levenson, S. H. (1981). *A Practice of Vascular Surgery*. London: Pitman.

Walker, W. F. (1980). *Colour Atlas of Peripheral Vascular Diseases*. London: Wolfe Medical.

30

Principles of management of malignant disease

In 1980 there were 129280 deaths from cancer and the reticuloses, which accounts for one death in every five persons. The corresponding figure in 1970 was 115729, and although the difference is partly due to an increased population, preservation of a greater number of older persons and improvements in diagnosis, the increase indicates the importance of these diseases in society. Cancer is the second commonest cause of death and is accompanied by difficult medical and social problems. Although, in general, the aetiology of the disease is unknown, certain predisposing factors and conditions are apparent and their recognition may result in prevention, an initial step in management.

Prevention

Much has been done to decrease the number of occupational cancers since the recognition that chronic irritation may produce skin and other epithelial lesions. Contact cancers on hands, arms and chest due to coal tar, creosote or petroleum oil are now infrequent in industry. The recognition of the carcinogenic action of the aromatic amines in the urine has eradicated cancer of the bladder in aniline dye workers by regular screening by urinary cytology. Asbestos has been noted to be an important cause of mesothelioma in industry. Adequate protection for radiologists has removed the risk of chronic radiation dermatitis and subsequent carcinoma, and the dangers of radiotherapy in the treatment of lupus, psoriasis and other skin conditions are well recognised. About 20 per cent of children with thyroid cancer in the United States were given irradiation for an enlarged thymus in infancy often prior to tonsillectomy, and this practice has now been discontinued. The use of radioisotopes imposes a risk because of the potential carcinogenic action, and the use of radioactive iodine in non-malignant thyroid lesions is thus often restricted to patients over 40 years. Radiotherapy for lesions such as ankylosing spondylitis may cause leukaemia at a later date. Excessive diagnostic radiology may be a factor in the development of cancer, and repeated examinations should be limited. Atmospheric pollution by radioactivity may also result in increased malignancy in the future.

The role of iron in preventing postcricoid carcinoma is recognised, and its administration is a simple method of treating the anaemia and glossitis and obviating some cancers at this site.

Statistical evidence indicates a relationship between cigarette smoking and lung cancer and to a lesser degree, to cancer of the tongue, pharynx, larynx and bladder. Public education with regard to the risks may eventually lower the incidence.

Cancer may often be prevented by the timely treatment of pathological conditions known to become malignant. Removal of the large intestine in familial polyposis coli is a classical example, and colectomy will also prevent neoplastic change in ulcerative colitis. Adequate excision of benign melanomas, and the correct management of leucoplakia and of urinary and biliary calculi are other means of preventing cancer.

Diagnosis

A full clinical history and examination are important, with particular reference to the age of the patient, the duration of symptoms, the effect on other systems and the overall state of health. The general condition is often affected and the nutritional state, the degree of weight loss, clinical evidence of anaemia or cardiac and pulmonary dysfunction may all influence the final management. The characteristics of any local lesion must be accurately noted and recorded. The degree of involvement of other structures and the extent of spread to adjacent lymph nodes or to more distant sites should be ascertained. Rectal and vaginal examinations should never be omitted or mismanagement may result.

Accessory investigations should commence with the simplest and proceed to the more complicated. Estimation of the haemoglobin may detect a secondary anaemia, and the erythrocyte sedimentation rate is often elevated. Urine examination may reveal red blood cells, bacteria, or even malignant cells in cancer of the bladder, whilst occult blood in the stool may be the sole indication of alimentary growths. Radiography frequently gives valuable additional information. The use of plain films, at times with tomography, may demonstrate lesions in the neck, chest, abdomen of bones and mammography is helpful in breast cancer (p. 138). Contrast media are employed in the alimentary, urinary and biliary tracts. Ultrasound scanning is of great value in abdominal and pelvic tumours as well as those of kidney and thyroid, whilst CT scanning is essential in detecting central nervous system pathology. Both methods are used in follow-up treatment as well as lymphography, which with CT scanning shows the presence of para-aortic node involvement in testicular tumours. These methods are also complementary. Angiography can also be helpful in renal, hepatic and pancreatic tumours. Isotope scanning in bone, thyroid, pancreatic, hepatic and cerebral tumours is at times helpful. Endoscopy using fibreoptic instruments allows direct vision and assessment of the local spread of internal lesions. Laparoscopy has a place in the diagnosis and follow-up of intraperitoneal malignancy, particularly ovarian tumours. Cytological examination of secretions or washings is helpful in the detection of cancer of the bronchus, cervix, stomach and colon. The final diagnosis frequently rests on the histological examination of biopsy material obtained directly or by needle biopsy aspiration, and such confirmation should never be omitted where radical treatment is contemplated. Tumour markers should be measured in specific lesions such as β-HCG (human chrionic gonadotrophin) in chorioncarcinoma and testicular tumours with a chorionic element, and α-feto protein in hepatoma and testicular tumours. As well as being helpful in diagnosis they may monitor complete or incomplete tumour removal, diagnose early relapse and assess response to therapy. CEA (carcino embryronic antigen) has been measured in large bowel tumours but is non-specific, raised levels being obtained in other conditions. Hormone receptor studies in cancerous breast tissue have facilitated a more rational approach to the management of this disease. When present a better prospect of response to hormone treatment can be expected.

TUMOUR CLASSIFICATION

The histological structure of the tumour is of value in assessing prognosis and indicating management. The well differentiated neoplasms such as squamous cell carcinomas are slowly growing and disseminate less quickly than the rapidly progressive adenocarcinomas. Certain poorly differentiated tumours are often markedly radiosensitive and may show temporary remission with such treatment, although they usually carry a bad prognosis. The histological type should always be correlated with the natural history of the disease in a particular site when assessing prognosis.

Tumours may be staged by their histological structure or by their extent. Histological grading by Broder's method has proved useful in estimating prognosis particularly in high-grade tumours. Dukes' classification of the degree of spread of carcinoma of the rectum (p. 229), determined when the specimen has been surgically removed, is also of value in assessing the prognosis.

Clinical staging and classification of a lesion is important in planning treatment and as an indication of prognosis. A satisfactory form with international agreement has been in existence for carcinoma of the cervix since 1929, but the present T.N.M system is more generally applicable. T refers to the primary tumour, N to the regional lymph nodes and M to the distant metastases. This classification is particularly suitable for easily palpable growths. The breast is given as an example.

T—Primary tumour

T1 = Small tumour (less than 2 cm) confined to breast.
T2 = Moderate tumour (less than 5 cm) limited to or with slight extension beyond breast.
T3 = Large tumour (less than 10 cm) with local infiltration reaching neighbouring structures.
T4 = Tumour of more than 10 cm, or widespread invasion of neighbouring structures.

N—Regional lymph nodes

NO = No palpable nodes.
N1 = Mobile homolateral nodes.
N2 = Fixed homolateral nodes.
N3 = Homolateral supraclavicular or infraclavicular lymph nodes, mobile or fixed.

M—Distant metastases

MO = No distant metastases.
M = Distant metastases including local involvement wide of the tumour and contralateral lymph nodes or breast.

Stage I = T1, NO, MO.
T2, NO, MO.
Stage II = T1, N1, MO.
T2, N1, MO.
Stage III = T1, N2 or N3, MO.
T2, N2 or N3, MO.
T3, NO, N1, N2 or N3, MO.
T4, NO, N1, N2 or N3, MO.
Stage IV = Any combination of T and N symbols including M.

TREATMENT OF THE PRE-MALIGNANT LESION

Benign tumours, such as papillomas and naevi in sites exposed to chronic irritation, should be excised with a clear margin of surrounding healthy tissue. Leucoplakia which has progressed to deep fissuring is better treated by excision before cancer supervenes. Bowen's disease of the skin is a pre-malignant state and adequate excision is neccessary. Familial polyposis coli carries a grave risk of carcinoma, and total colectomy is advisable before malignant change occurs. Ulcerative colitis progresses in some instances to cancer, the lesion beginning at the base of a stricture, and surgery should be considered in long-standing cases.

METHODS AVAILABLE IN THE MANAGEMENT OF THE MALIGNANT LESION

There are three principal means of treating a malignant lesion:

1. Surgery.
2. Radiotherapy.
3. Chemotherapy.

Each method may be used individually or a combination of any two or all three may be employed.

Surgical treatment

This is advocated for adenocarcinomas, in particular of the alimentary tract such as stomach, colon and rectum, and for radio-insensitive lesions such as melanomas. It may be preferred in the management of many other tumours, particularly where radiotherapy is inadequate, although in some sites, including tongue, larynx and bladder, it has been largely replaced by irradiation in order to preserve function. Surgery is frequently used in conjunction with radiotherapy for tumours of the breast, thyroid or bone as part of a planned programme. Failure to respond or recurrence after radiotherapy may necessitate excision. Surgery may be employed as follows:

1. Radical excision of tumour and all lymph drainage area.
2. Palliation—
By-pass procedures.
Hormonal control.
Local palliative measures.

Pre-operative management

The general nutritional state should be improved by a high protein and high calorie diet with plentiful amounts of vitamins, if necessary given intramuscularly. The haemoglobin and red cell count, the blood urea, the total protein and electrolytes, and, particularly in the presence of jaundice, the liver function tests are determined. Correction of abnormal levels by electrolyte replacement and blood transfusion is undertaken and where indicated enteral or parenteral alimentation provided. Oral, dental or respiratory sepsis should be treated. Physiotherapy, particularly instruction in breathing exercises, should be given to reduce the incidence of post-operative respiratory complications. Pre-operative emptying of the bowel by aperients and subsequent lavage in non-obstructed cases, is advisable before operation on the large intestine. Gastric and oesophageal aspiration and lavage may be necessary in the presence of obstructive lesions of the upper alimentary tract. Pre-operative parenteral vitamin K_1 should be given to counteract the tendency to bleeding in cases of obstructive jaundice. Antibiotic cover is required in large bowel resection, poor risk respiratory patients and in the presence of a cardiac prosthesis.

Operative management

The following general considerations are important. *Radical excision* should be performed as early as possible to obtain the best result. Even when the lesion is apparently fixed and inoperable a bold approach often allows removal. Subsequent histology may reveal the infiltration to be inflammatory and not neoplastic. The aim is to remove the growth together with an adequate margin of surrounding healthy tissue. Monobloc dissections to include the regional lymph nodes should be performed in alimentary cancer. When the disease is considered curable, the prime responsibility is adequate excision and failure to observe this will result in recurrence. Considerations of reconstruction should not be allowed to interfere with this intention. Control of haemorrhage in extensive procedures of the head and neck or in radical amputation of the limbs is facilitated by preliminary ligation of the main vessels. Dissemination of the lesion may be prevented by gentle handling, by vein ligation before manipulation of the tumour and in colonic growths the placing of ligatures around the intestine proximal and distal to the lesion may lessen the tendency to tumour implantation at the suture line. Cutting into a tumour for diagnostic purposes, such as in a breast lesion or a suspected melanoma, should be avoided and the growth excised with a margin of healthy tissue. The operative use of a diathermy knife reduces the risk of local implantation of tumour cells. Frozen section histology of the tumour edge during operation, particularly in head and neck lesions, is valuable in determining the extent of excision required. Primary skin closure should not be considered a main requisite and free split thickness skin grafts can be employed where necessary. A temporary tracheostomy is often of great value in the post-operative management of head and neck procedures. Accurate and detailed notes should be made of the operative findings and procedure for future reference in planning the full course of treatment.

Post-operative management is similar to that of any major procedure and is discussed in Chapter 2. Emphasis should be laid on the early healing of wounds, in particular where future radiotherapy is required.

Palliative excision. Limited excision of a tumour is often the most satisfactory form of palliation. Removal of the primary lesion may allow a less painful death from progressing metastases. Excision of an ulcerating and fungating breast carcinoma removes an unpleasant spectacle and diminishes toxic absorption from the necrotic area. Local pain and obstructive phenomena, at times of gross severity, are seen in the rectum or oesophagus and may be temporarily relieved by palliative excision. Such removal may also prevent undesirable complications due to continued growth such as perforation, obstruction, haemorrhage and fistula formation. Palliative excision may be employed in conjunction with radiotherapy and chemotherapy to diminish the amount of tumour tissue subjected to irradiation in such neoplasms as a Wilms' tumour, or to allow more concentrated action of radioactive isotopes on the remaining metastases in thyroid carcinoma.

The type of surgery employed may be resection alone, or in superficial tumours may be combined with skin grafting. In alimentary lesions restoration of continuity must be attempted either directly or by the insertion or construction of tubes. Colostomy or even ileostomy may be required, but if possible these should be avoided, even at the expense of a more limited resection. Great care should be taken that the patient is not left in a worse condition as a result of palliative surgery.

Residual tumour should be marked with metal clips to denote the site for future radiotherapy. Liver perfusion with cytotoxic drugs may give some relief and occasionally wedge resection or lobectomy for a solitary metastasis. Finally, the prognosis, even in palliative resections, may be improved by close co-operation between surgeon and radiotherapist.

By-pass procedures. In either alimentary or urinary obstruction a short-circuiting operation may be required as a palliative measure. A nephrostomy or ureteric transplant may occasionally be necessary to relieve pain or back pressure, but the uraemia which results from obstruction causes a painless death, and major surgery is often better avoided. A simple method is the cystoscopic insertion of a pigtail catheter for renal drainage. In pyloric obstruction, gastro-enterostomy may be a more simple procedure than palliative excision, and as it restores continuity is preferable to gastrostomy or jejunostomy.

Pain relief. The presence of pain in an advanced lesion calls for a well-considered plan of treatment designed to bring lasting relief with as few side-effects as possible. Radiotherapy, chemotherapy and surgery, singly or in combination, can produce effective pain control, often assisted by anaesthetic techniques (Chapter 31). The administration of large amounts of drugs, often habit forming, is not advisable until the terminal stages. Where the general health is maintained direct surgical attack on nervous pathways is preferable (p. 446).

Hormonal control. Hormone dependency of certain breast tumours is discussed on page 137. Operative removal of endocrine organs for such lesions may involve oophorectomy, adrenalectomy or hypophysectomy. Bilateral orchidectomy may be employed for prostatic carcinoma, either as an alternative or in conjunction with oestrogen therapy.

Radiotherapy

Indications

The majority of squamous-cell carcinomas respond well, and radiotherapy may be used alone as an alternative to surgery. The superior cosmetic results in cancer of the skin and lip and of functional results in cancer of the tongue, larynx and pharynx, with an equally good prognosis, make it the preferred treatment for these sites. Although used alone in the cure of malignant disease, it plays an important part when combined with surgery, and may be employed pre-operatively, post-operatively or at the time of operation. The main pre-operative use is to decrease the tumour size, to halt progression or to obtain temporary remission in rapidly growing lesions, such as Wilms' tumour, some breast cancers or Ewing's tumour of bone. A number of apparently inoperable neoplasms may become operable, and the risk of dissemination at operation is lessened. Post-operative irradiation is given whenever malignancy is known or thought from the natural history of the disease to have been left behind. In cancer of the breast the axillary, supraclavicular and internal mammary regions may be irradiated, as are the para-aortic nodes for a seminoma. At operation radiotherapy may be employed to irradiate local tumour or residual growth by the implantation of radioactive isotopes.

Technical methods available

1. External radiotherapy—low and high energy units.
2. Interstitial and intracavitary radiotherapy.
3. Systemic radioactive isotopes.

The majority of routine therapy is now carried out with megavoltage units. In the United Kingdom kilocurie *cobalt apparatus* (2000–5000 curies) and *linear accelerators* are more commonly used, whilst in North America and in Europe the *betatron* is more frequently employed. These machines have greater power of penetration of tissue with precise definition of the beam edge. They produce less damage to the vascular and connective tissues with less fibrosis and diminished impairment of the healing process. Skin and bone are protected. Low energy units in the form of superficial radiotherapy are used in skin neoplasms. *Caesium* is used in the form of needles for direct insertion into tissues in cancer of the tongue and floor of the mouth, in the form of moulds for tumours of the maxilla, or in boxes or tubes for intracavitary treatment in cancer of the uterus. Iridium in the form of wire is used for direct implantation into tissues such as the tongue and bladder. Cobalt-60 is also a satisfactory source of radiation and has proved its value in therapy as a unit for irradiating deep-seated lesions with minimal skin reaction. *Radioactive isotopes* suitable for therapy are obtained by exposing stable isotopes such as iodine, phosphorus and gold to the atomic pile, and these may be given by mouth or by injection. Radioactive iodine is of value in treating thyroid cancer, either the primary site or the metastases. Radioactive phosphorus is used in treating polycythaemia vera and occasionally the reticuloses. Radioactive gold may be used by direct implantation for residual tumour at an operative site, or for recurrent skin tumours where radical excision would result in mutilation. Radioactive tantalum wire with physical properties similar to radium may be employed curatively in cancer of the bladder. Radioactive gold may also be instilled in liquid form into the pleural or peritoneal cavities for the control of malignant effusions in a fit patient for whom repeated aspirations are tedious. Hyperbaric oxygen can be used in combination with radiotherapy in an attempt to overcome the resistance of hypoxic malignant cells. Increased sensitivity to X-rays occurs in the presence of excess oxygen. Certain tumours, such as secondary squamous carcinoma in lymph nodes, contain a proportion of anoxic cells and are particularly resistant to conventional radiotherapy. A high rate of local control and marked response to these lesions has been observed when radiotherapy has been employed in the presence of hyperbaric oxygen. Certain drugs are now being used as an alternative to hyperbaric oxygen in an attempt to sensitise hypoxic cells and improve their response to radiotherapy. Fast neutrons produced by a cyclotron have more recently been noted to cause marked regression of large ulcerating tumours, particularly of the head and neck, limbs, breast and inoperable inguinal and axillary lymph nodes, in some instances following failure or recurrence after surgery, chemotherapy, cobalt, X-rays or gamma irradiation.

Side effects

These may be general or local, but with modern forms of treatment both are unusual. Lassitude, malaise, or anaemia may occur. Nausea and anorexia may be apparent but can be alleviated by such drugs as prochlorperazine (Stemetil) and metoclopramide (Maxolon). Local erythema and skin desquamation commonly occur as acute reactions but heal within weeks of treatment. Fibrosis and telangiectasia occur at times as late complications. Local radionecrosis involving skin or deeper tissues is an occasional hazard and a painful, unhealed ulcer or osteomyelitis with sequestration is at times encountered. Pulmonary fibrosis with pronounced dyspnoea may follow excessive chest irradiation and simulate advanced malignancy. Stricture, fistula and obstruction involving bowel, ureter, bladder or vagina are serious and important sequelae. Nonetheless more accurate localisation obtained by modern investigations such as CT scanning and meticulous attention to planning details to obtain the optimum distribution of radiotherapy have all helped to decrease the incidence of severe radiation damage.

Chemotherapy

Many cytotoxic agents have some anticancer effect due to their ability to damage actively dividing cells. They are not specific for malignant tissue and their use may therefore produce toxic effects. Cytotoxic drugs are employed at various stages of the disease depending on its nature. There are some tumours such as Hodgkin's, Wilm's and teratomas in which a proportion of patients can be cured by chemotherapy. It can also be used in those with advanced disease to improve survival rate and in some instances effective palliation may be obtained. It may also be helpful as an adjuvant to surgery and radiotherapy.

There may be acute side effects such as drug leakage on injection into tissues outside a vein, or there may be nausea, vomiting or gastric mucositis. Haemopoeitic depression can occur and frequent estimation of the haemoglobin, white cell and platelet counts are necessary. Therapy should cease if the white cell count falls to 3000 per mm^3 or the platelet count below 90000 per mm^3. Later problems can include sterility, alopecia and the development of other malignancies. The general condition of the patient must be carefully assessed before any treatment is commenced and if poor, therapy should be withheld.

Four main groups of agents are in common use:

1. Alkylating agents.
2. Nutritional antagonists and antimetabolites.
3. Plant alkaloids.
4. Products from micro-organisms.

Alkylating agents

Cell death is caused by the alteration in essential cellular constituents produced by this group of drugs. The *nitrogen mustards* are perhaps the best known, and mustine or HN_2, which is used in the management of Hodgkin's disease, is given intravenously in doses totalling up to 0.4 mg per kilogram of body weight. *Chlorambucil* and *cyclophosphamide* are nitrogen mustard analogues which are useful in lymphocytic proliferations as well as in breast and ovarian malignant tumours. *Myleran*, a methane sulphonate, has produced improvement in chronic myeloid leukaemia, sometimes for many years. *Cisplatin*, whose main method of action is probably alkylation, has been recently introduced. It is successful in malignant testicular tumours, and is active against ovarian carcinoma and squamous cell carcinoma of the head and neck, and bladder.

Antagonists and antimetabolites

The action of these agents depends on the blocking of enzymatic reactions by the use of competitive substances. The two main groups are (1) folic acid antagonists, and (2) antipurine drugs. *Folic acid antagonists*, of which *amethopterine* (methotrexate) is an example, are mainly used for acute leukaemia. The *antipurine* drugs are antagonistic to the precursor of nucleic acid. 6-*mercaptopurine* and 6-*thioguanine* are agents of value in the management of leukaemia in children. They are not very effective in acute myeloid leukaemia in adults, but occasional remissions occur up to six months. 5-*flurouracil* is another antimetabolite and has had limited success in metastatic large bowel cancers.

Plant alkaloids and products of micro-organisms

The group of plant alkaloid drugs, *vinblastine*, *vincristine*, and *vindesine*, exert considerable chemotherapeutic effects. Vinblastine is mainly used in the control of Hodgkin's disease and is employed when the alkylating agents have failed. Vincristine is effective against lymphoblastic leukaemia and non-Hodgkin's lymphoma. These drugs are employed in *combination chemotherapy* in a wide range of adult and childhood neoplasms. They are given intravenously and spillage outside the vein is dangerous. The main side-effect of vincristine and vindesine is neurotoxicity, whilst vinblastine predominantly causes marrow depression. Alopecia may occur with all these drugs.

Certain antibiotics also have a very definite antitumour effect. Adriamycin has a wide range of activity and is commonly used in combination with other agents. Bleomycin is used to treat squamous cell carcinoma and teratomas. Actinomycin D is effective against Wilm's tumour and Ewing's tumour in conjunction with surgery and radiotherapy.

Special applications. The current management in chemotherapy appears to be high dosage and multiple drug therapy, where necessary taking precautions to minimise the risks of toxicity by nursing the patient in a sterile atmosphere, such as Reverse Barrier Nursing Unit or in plastic tents, thereby reducing the risk of infection. In highly selected cases regional perfusion aimed at delivering high concentrations of anti-cancer drugs to an isolated area of the body may be of some value. An alternative procedure is by means of endolymphatic perfusion which has a limited place in some instances. Immunotherapy, using B.C.G., has been attempted to encourage a host reaction, but with only a minimum of success.

FURTHER READING

Halnan, K. E. (1982). *Treatment of Cancer*. London: Chapman and Hall.

Walter, J. (1977). *Cancer and Radiotherapy*. 2nd ed. Edinburgh: Churchill Livingstone.

31

Surgical aspects of pain

The unpleasant sensation of pain serves a useful purpose in announcing physical injury and thereby permitting evasive action to be taken before severe damage results. In a similar manner it often marks the onset of a disease process and may lead the individual to seek medical assistance. An understanding of the anatomy and physiology of pain and the application of this knowledge is helpful in both diagnosis and treatment.

Anatomy and physiology

Pain is experienced as the result of the stimulation of peripheral receptors. These transmit impulses along afferent nerve fibres to the spinal cord, through which they are conveyed to the thalamus and cerebral cortex.

The **skin** contains an abundant supply of pain receptors, thereby permitting accurate localisation. Pain occurs when a stimulus is severe enough to cause tissue destruction. A chemical such as histamine or prostaglandin E is produced which stimulates the nerve fibres. The impulses are mainly carried in slow-conducting unmyelinated fibres although myelinated fibres are also involved. These fibres pass to the dorsal root of the cord, where they relay in the substantia gelatinosa before crossing to the opposite side in the lateral spinothalamic tract. There may be other ascending fibres apart from those in the spinothalamic tract. All fibres pass up the cord to the postero-lateral nucleus of the thalamus and are then relayed to the sensory cerebral cortex. In the same way pain fibres in the cranial nerves relay to form the bulbothalamic tract and hence to the thalamus and the sensory cortex.

All other pain fibres enter the cord in a similar manner and relay in the substantia gelatinosa to form the spinothalamic tract. Thus visceral pain carried by the autonomic nervous system relays in the same way as the skin efferents. The area in the substantia gelatinosa where the pain fibres relay is influenced by impulses in sensory fibres entering from the periphery or others descending from the brain. As a result of their activity the pain impulse is prevented from passing to the spinothalamic tract. This 'Gate' theory helps to explain why injuries sustained in the excitement of sport can pass unnoticed at the time and be discovered later, or how torture can be borne. It also has an application in the treatment of pain by skin stimulation and possibly acupuncture.

The body has natural opiate receptors in the periventricular area of the brain and in the spinal cord where the endogenous opiates, methionine-encephalin and β-endorphin, act to modulate pain. Acupuncture appears to release these substances.

The **peritoneum, pleura and pericardium** have both somatic and splanchnic afferent fibres. The parietal layer is supplied by somatic nerves and responds to stimuli in the same way as the overlying skin. In the case of the central part of the diaphragm, which is supplied by the phrenic nerve, pain is referred to the tip of the corresponding shoulder.

The visceral layers of intestine, heart and lung differ in being insensitive to heat or incision. Distension, ischaemia, chemical agents and stretching of ligaments all produce visceral pain, but the precise mechanism is unknown. An increase in the intraluminal pressure of the bowel by the exaggerated peristalsis of intestinal obstruction is responsible for the characteristic cramp-like pain. Ischaemia causes pain through an accumulation of metabolites, an example being angina pectoris, whilst the action of gastric hydrochloric acid on peptic ulcer is a further instance of a chemical agent producing pain.

The fibres which carry visceral pain are conveyed in the autonomic nervous system to the posterior horn. The level in the cord to which visceral afferents pass is dependent on the segments from which they have developed. Visceral pain is poorly localised and often referred to the somatic area supplied by the same segment. The appendix and small intestine originate in the tenth thoracic segment and pain is therefore referred to this distribution at the level of the umbilicus. This mechanism of referred pain is not completely understood. It may be a mistake in cortical appreciation due to the greater frequency of skin pain impulses which have established a pattern, or it may be the result of a spill-over of splanchnic impulses which affect the somatic fibres in the cord. Although visceral disease does give rise to pain which is poorly localised and often referred, once the parietal layer is involved accurate localisation occurs.

Deep somatic structures react in a similar manner to the viscera. Muscle is insensitive to pricking and cutting but pain results from increased tension such as that produced by the injection of hypertonic saline. This pain has a characteristic aching quality, is poorly localised and referred to the corresponding dermatome.

The **parenchyma of solid structures** such as the liver, lung or brain is probably insensitive to stimuli such as cutting or pricking. A secondary deposit may be present in these organs without producing discomfort, but a sudden increase in tension as a result of haemorrhage causes pain through stretching of the covering membrane.

Compact and cancellous bone react differently, the former being insensitive. Pain is a feature of bony metastases and can occur even in the absence of periosteal involvement or pathological fracture. The source of such pain may thus originate in the cancellous portion of the bone.

Arteries and veins are surrounded by a plexus of nerves, branches passing to the muscular wall and adventitia; the supply to the arteries is considerably greater than that to the veins. Afferent fibres reach the adventitia but it is uncertain whether they penetrate to the media; the intima has no afferent or efferent nerve supply. The arterial wall is sensitive to needling, pulsation and infection. The throbbing migrainous headache is believed to be due to increased pulsation in the external carotid artery, whilst temporal arteritis gives rise to pain in the region of the diseased vessel. The vein wall is not usually sensitive to needling.

Pathological change or compression of the sensory fibres of the **central nervous system** may induce pain. In tabes dorsalis, where there is destruction of such fibres in the posterior nerve root, spontaneous severe lightning pains occur which may simulate an acute abdominal emergency. In herpes zoster, viral infection of the posterior root ganglion results in paraesthesiae in the corresponding dermatome, whilst nerve root pressure due to a prolapsed intervertebral disc causes pain in a similar peripheral segment.

Pain can follow injury to the nervous system and there are essentially two main types. The first is causalgia, a rare condition characterised by burning pain often in relation to the median and sciatic nerves (p. 415). It is probable that there is initially a leak of impulses from the post-ganglionic sympathetic fibres to the afferent system, but changes in the cord may occur later and result in chain reactions which perpetuate the condition. The second is characterised by spontaneous pain and hyperaesthesia. The pain is not of a burning nature as in causalgia; a familiar example is experienced after amputation in the painful phantom limb. A glomus tumour gives rise to severe radiating pain but the mechanism involved in this instance is not clearly understood.

Hyperalgesia exists when pain is produced by stimuli which are usually innocuous. It can occur in skin as a result of bacterial infection or after a burn. Referred pain may also be associated with hyperalgesia, occurring in the shoulder from diaphragmatic stimuli and in the back due to cholecystitis.

Diagnosis

The determination of the cause of a particular pain which is merely a symptom and the diagnosis of the underlying condition can be an involved problem. There are a number of variables which may exist and accurate diagnosis is dependent on their assessment and interpretation. Differences in appreciation occur commonly and varying degrees of response to stimulation take place in those with a high or low threshold of pain. Difficulties in communication may arise, particulary in small children or in the semiconscious, and clinical acumen must be diligently applied. Interpretation of the degree of pain by the surgeon is a further variable in which experience and judgment are important. Full discussion of the pain and any associated symptoms, using as a comparison other types of pain, is of value. The following points should be considered.

1. Onset

This may be sudden as in the perforation of a viscus, or arise gradually and slowly increase in severity. The time of day or relationship to a particular stimulus should be noted. The duration may be momentary or extend over several hours or days. It is unusual for severe pain to persist without remissions, but the pain of malignant disease may be intractable.

2. Type

This is often characteristic. Inflammatory pain is throbbing in nature and often described as dull and heavy. Short, sharp bursts of colic can be associated with urinary or biliary calculi or intestinal obstruction. Cardiac ischaemia pain is characteristically likened to a vice or constriction around the chest.

3. Severity

The degree of pain threshold varies and assessment can be difficult. Evaluation is mainly dependent on clinical experience and judgment of the type of patient. Severe colic may produce uncontrollable writhing and facial contortion, whilst in a perforated ulcer reluctance to move indicates the severe nature of the pain.

4. Site

There may be localisation to the site of causation or the symptom may be referred. The reference of visceral pain has been discussed (p. 442). A further example is pain experienced in the knee due to a lesion of the hip, both joints receiving a supply from the obturator nerve.

5. Radiation

Radiation from the initial site is often characteristic. Renal pain typically commences in the loin and radiates around the abdomen to the testis or labium majus; prolapse of a cervical or lumbar disc causes initial local back pain, later extending to upper or lower limb.

6. Aggravating and relieving factors

It is important that these should be ascertained. Undue exercise adversely affects the pain of cardiac ischaemia or intermittent claudication. Prolonged fasting may exacerbate a peptic ulcer. Nocturnal pain can occur in the same disease, or the symptom in other instances is exaggerated by a loss of the distraction of outside interests. Support and rest relieve inflammation; food and alkalis are of value in peptic ulceration.

7. Psychological factors

Pain is worse in a patient who is depressed and may be tolerable if the depression is treated. Patients with intractable pain often become depressed. Anxious people are also more susceptible to pain.

Treatment

Attention should be initially directed to a removal of the causative agent. Specific therapy for the primary inflammatory, neoplastic or ischaemic lesion should be instituted, and this is considered under the appropriate section. Rest, splintage and support are simple aids which alleviate many inflammatory states. Superficial or deep heat and the use of antibiotics are valuable, whilst incision of an abscess can produce dramatic relief of pain. Physiotherapy and manipulation can benefit certain orthopaedic lesions.

Simple non-habit-forming drugs can be employed as an initial measure, asprin, 0.3 to 1 g, compound codeine, 1 to 2 tablets, or paracetamol (Panadol),

0.5 to 1 g, being widely used. Pentazocine, 30 to 60 mg, pethidine, 50 to 100 mg, or morphine, 10 to 20 mg, may be required in more severe cases, and in the presence of vomiting the intramuscular or intravenous route is preferable. These more powerful drugs should not be administered (a) for abdominal pain until a definite diagnosis has been ascertained, or the clinical picture may be obscured; (b) in cases of head injury, where the level of consciousness may be masked, or depression of the respiratory centre may take place; (c) for any condition associated with respiratory depression, which might then become aggravated. Pethidine does not increase sphincteric tone and is to be preferred to morphine in biliary colic. Antispasmodics such as hyoscine butylbromide (Buscopan), 10 to 20 mg, or propantheline (Probanthine), 15 to 30 mg, are also of help in renal and biliary colic.

In severe chest or head injuries when a mechanical ventilator is required additional stress is present. Relief may be obtained by the use of neuroleptic drugs such as butyrophenone derivatives (droperidol), which act on the central nervous system to produce a state of detachment or indifference to the pain. Their efficacy is increased by combining them with an analgesic. In some instances ventilation may be avoided by adequate pain relief.

Local anaesthetics can provide valuable analgesia either by surface use or by injection. Lignocaine (Xylocaine) jelly or ointment may be applied to endotracheal or nasogastric tubes to diminish discomfort and reduce restlessness. It is also used in the management of painful fissures. The injection of lignocaine or bupivacaine (Marcain) directly on to intercostal nerves in multiple rib fractures or into the epidural space as is performed in childbirth is often helpful.

Many minor painful investigations, or procedures such as dressings in a Burns Unit, can be performed without conventional anaesthesia. Ketamine, a derivative of phencyclidine, can be used. It produces a feeling of indifference to pain by dissociating cortical from brainstem function in association with profound analgesia. The protective reflexes are only partially diminished but hallucinations during emergence are a disadvantage. Methoxyflurane (Penthrane) or trichlorethylene in air mixtures and nitrous oxide in oxygen (Entonox) are examples of inhalation methods which can provide analgesia for minor procedures.

Post-operative pain requires a wide range of drugs for its relief, from morphine or pethidine in the immediate post-operative period to mild analgesics as the pain decreases. Care should be taken to avoid respiratory depression due to excessive doses. An anti-emetic drug such as perphenazine (Fentazin) is a valuable adjunct to relieve nausea and vomiting. The combination of analgesics with tranquillising drugs, such as amitriptyline (Tryptizol) or diazepam (Valium), is advantageous when anxiety is an aggravating factor. This may be necessary in the post-operative period or in prolonged illness, particularly from malignant disease. Local anaesthetic blocks such as epidural or intercostal or the use of epidural opiates can be helpful.

Management of prolonged pain

In most hospitals Pain Relief Clinics have been set up to aid the management of intractable pain. These are generally run by anaesthetists and treat all types of chronic pain, such as post-herpetic neuralgia, trigeminal neuralgia, causalgia, musculo-skeletal pain, ischaemic pain and malignant pain; the last may amount to 30 per cent of the cases. The pain of malignancy is often not severe throughout the illness and simple measures such as aspirin, paracetamol or codeine will often suffice. When codeine is used care should be taken to ensure regular bowel action as the drug is constipating and in a debilitated patient faecal impaction may supervene. Intractable pain does occur especially in advanced forms of malignancy necessitating more powerful agents. Sublingual preparations of the partial opiate agonists phenazocine (Narphen) and buprenorphine (Temgesic) can be effective and have prolonged action. Pethidine and morphine, now available as a long-acting preparation, can be administered orally, but should be used with care where the prognosis is good because of the addictive potential. The latter drugs are antagonists to the partial agonist. A mixture of aspirin and opiate, methadone (Physeptone) or pethidine, can be useful. Increasing dosage becomes necessary but the addition of an ataractic such as chlorpromazine (Largactil) will potentiate their action. In the terminal stage a mixture containing cocaine, morphine, honey and gin may be fully adequate.

Injection therapy should be delayed but is employed when the oral route is ineffective or unsatisfactory. Pethidine, 50 to 100 mg, or methadone (Physeptone), 5 to 10 mg, is efficient whilst phenazocine is also recommended. Papaveretum (Omnopon), 10 to 20 mg is less liable than morphine to produce vomiting. Diamorphine (heroin), 5 to 10 mg, causes early addiction and in some countries is restricted in supply. Pentazocine (Fortral) and buprenorphine have the advantage of not being addicting and may be advised. The dosage of all drugs should be small initially but can be increased gradually as required. Anxious people are more susceptible to pain than others but chronic or recurring pain can also cause an anxiety state. The use of appropriate drugs in combination with analgesics is beneficial, and chlorpromazine (Largactil) and chlordiazepoxide (Librium) have been used successfully in this way.

Although the relief of pain may be of paramount importance, except in the terminal state prolonged drowsiness or semicoma is to be avoided. Apart from the obvious dangers of hypostatic pneumonia and deep vein thrombosis, it is desirable for the patient to make reasonable contact with both relatives and visitors. Skill is required in arranging medication in order to avoid such a drowsy state, at the same time preventing acute awareness of a hopeless and worsening clinical condition. Despite the rapid addiction which exists for heroin it is at times useful in the terminal days since the analgesia it produces is associated with a powerful euphoria. The problem of nausea and vomiting may be alleviated by anti-emetic drugs such as metoclopramide (Maxolon) or perphenazine (Fentazin).

Surgical methods. These have a definite use but because many are not permanent they are particulary useful when life expectancy is short. They do have the great advantage that the patient may be able to enjoy a relatively normal time for the rest of his life, possibly free from medication. The pain of pelvic cancer can be relieved by the use of long-acting local anaesthetics, phenol or alcohol in thecal, lumbar or sacral extradural regions, although retention of urine can be a complication. Coeliac plexus block relieves the pain from intra-abdominal malignancy, particularly carcinoma of the pancreas. Peripheral nerves may be frozen with a specially modified cryoprobe which produces analgesia for 7 to 60 days. The nerve always recovers. Interruption of the spinothalamic tract has been used for many years for the relief of chronic pain. Formerly a laminectomy was necessary but it is now usually performed by a percutaneous method in the cervical region. It is particulary useful for unilateral pain but good results have also been achieved when it is bilateral. The latter patients are liable to bladder complications and difficulty with breathing. Carbamazepine (Tegretol) is often effective in the treatment of trigeminal neuralgia and surgical methods are only used when it is unsuccessful. Sensory fibres can be sectioned in the posterior fossa, at the same time preserving the corneal reflex. Some benefit has been achieved by thermocoagulation of the Gasserian ganglion using a percutaneous method. It follows from the 'Gate' theory that pain may be relieved by stimulating the large fibre afferents. This is obtained by using electrodes in the same afferent area and by electrical stimulation producing a tingling sensation. It has been tried in a wide variety of chronic pain states but with only limited success. Prefrontal leucotomy has an occasional place in treating an exaggerated psychological response to intractable pain. When the cause is localised, particularly in secondary neoplasms, radiotherapy may be of value in diminishing pain.

FURTHER READING

Hannington-Kiff, J. G. (1981) *Pain*. 2nd ed. London: Update Publications Ltd.

Ed. Harcus, A. W., Smith, R. & Whittle, B. (1977). *Pain–New Perspectives in Measurement and Management*. Edinburgh: Churchill Livingstone.

Ed. Swerdlow, M. (1981). *The Therapy of Pain*. Current Status of Modern Therapy, Vol. 6. Lancaster: MTP Press.

Index

D

G

I

M

N

Q

R

T

X

Y

Z